...book of

VETERINARY PAIN
MANAGEMENT

Handbook of

VETERINARY PAIN MANAGEMENT

SECOND EDITION

James S. Gaynor, DVM, MS
Diplomate, American College of Veterinary Anesthesiologists
Diplomate, American Academy of Pain Management
Certified Veterinary Acupuncturist, International Veterinary Acupuncture Society
Director, Animal Anesthesia & Pain Management Center
Colorado Springs, Colorado

William W. Muir III, DVM, PhD
Diplomate, American College of Veterinary Anesthesiologists
Diplomate, American College of Veterinary Emergency and Critical Care
Regional Director, American Academy of Pain Management
Veterinary Clinical Pharmacology Consulting Services
Columbus, Ohio

MOSBY

ELSEVIER

MOSBY
ELSEVIER

11830 Westline Industrial Drive
St. Louis, Missouri 63146

HANDBOOK OF VETERINARY PAIN MANAGEMENT,   ISBN: 978-0-323-04679-4
SECOND EDITION

NOTICE
Veterinary medicine is an ever-changing field. Standard safety precautions must be followed,
but as new research and clinical experience broaden our knowledge, changes in treatment
and drug therapy will become necessary. Readers are advised to check the most current
product information provided by the manufacturer of each drug in order to verify the
recommended dose, the method and duration of administration, and contraindications.
It is the responsibility of the licensed veterinarian, relying on experience and knowledge
of the patient, to determine dosages and the best treatment for each individual patient.
Neither the publisher nor the editor assumes any liability for any injury and/or damage to
persons or property arising from this publication.

ISBN: 978-0-323-04679-4

Vice President and Publisher: Linda Duncan
Senior Acquisitions Editor: Anthony Winkel
Developmental Editor: Maureen Slaten
Publishing Services Manager: Patricia Tannian
Senior Project Manager: John Casey
Designer: Andrea Lutes

Printed in China

Last digit is print number: 9 8 7 6 5 4 3 2 1

CONTRIBUTORS

Steven C. Budsberg, DVM, MS, DACVS
Professor
Department of Small Animal Medicine and Surgery
College of Veterinary Medicine
The University of Georgia
Athens, Georgia
Nonsteroidal Antiinflammatory Drugs

James S. Gaynor, DVM, MS, DACVA, DAAPM, CVA (IVAS)
Director, Animal Anesthesia & Pain Management Center
Colorado Springs, Colorado
Definitions of Terms Describing Pain
Pain Behaviors
Other Drugs Used to Treat Pain
Local and Regional Anesthetic Techniques for the Alleviation of Perioperative Pain
Acute Pain Management: A Case-Based Approach
Chronic Pain Management: A Case-Based Approach
Cancer Pain Management

Peter W. Hellyer, DVM, MS, DACVA
Assistant Dean for the Professional Veterinary Medical Program
Professor of Anesthesiology
Department of Clinical Sciences
College of Veterinary Medicine and Biomedical Sciences
Colorado State University
Fort Collins, Colorado
Objective, Categoric Methods for Assessing Pain and Analgesia

Sandra L. Hudson, BS, MBA, CCRP
Owner and Rehabilitation Practitioner
Canine Rehabilitation and Conditioning Center of Texas
Round Rock, Texas
Rehabilitation Methods and Modalities for the Cat

Matthew S. Johnston, VMD, DABVP (Avian)
Assistant Professor of Zoological Medicine
James L. Voss Veterinary Teaching Hospital
College of Veterinary Medicine and Biomedical Sciences
Colorado State University
Fort Collins, Colorado
Clinical Approach to Analgesia in Ferrets and Rabbits

Leigh A. Lamont, DVM, MS, DACVA
Assistant Professor of Anesthesiology
Department of Companion Animals
Atlantic Veterinary College

University of Prince Edward Island
Charlottetown, Prince Edward Island, Canada
α2-Agonists

Phillip Lerche, BVSc, DACVA
Assistant Professor—Clinical
Department of Veterinary Clinical Sciences
College of Veterinary Medicine
The Ohio State University
Columbus, Ohio
Pain Management in Horses and Cattle

Khursheed R. Mama, BVSc, DVM, DACVA
Associate Professor
Department of Clinical Sciences
College of Veterinary Medicine and Biomedical Sciences
Colorado State University
Fort Collins, Colorado
Local Anesthetics
Local and Regional Anesthetic Techniques for Alleviation of Perioperative Pain

Patrice M. Mich, DVM, DABVP (Canine/Feline)
Resident in Anesthesiology
Department of Clinical Sciences
College of Veterinary Medicine and Biomedical Sciences
Colorado State University
Fort Collins, Colorado
Objective, Categoric Methods for Assessing Pain and Analgesia

Darryl L. Millis, MS, DVM, DACVS, CRP
Professor of Orthopedic Surgery
Department of Small Animal Clinical Sciences
College of Veterinary Medicine
The University of Tennessee
Knoxville, Tennessee
Physical Therapy and Rehabilitation in Dogs

Craig Mosley, DVM, MSc, DACVA
Assistant Professor, Anesthesiology
College of Veterinary Medicine
Oregon State University
Corvallis, Oregon
Clinical Approaches to Analgesia in Reptiles

William W. Muir III, DVM, PhD, DACVA, DACVECC
Professor
Department of Veterinary Clinical Sciences
College of Veterinary Medicine
The Ohio State University
Columbus, Ohio
Physiology and Pathophysiology of Pain
Pain and Stress

Pain Behaviors
Pharmacologic Principles and Pain: Pharmacokinetics and Pharmacodynamics
Drugs Used to Treat Pain
Selecting Analgesic Drugs and Routes of Drug Administration
Acute Pain Management: A Case-Based Approach
Chronic Pain Management: A Case-Based Approach
Drug Antagonism and Antagonists
Pain Management in Horses and Cattle

Andrea M. Nolan, MVB, PhD, DVA, DECVA, DECVPT, MRCVS
Professor
Veterinary Cell Sciences
Institute of Comparative Medicine
Faculty of Veterinary Medicine
University of Glasgow
Glasgow, Scotland
Quality of Life Issues

Joanne Paul-Murphy, BS, DVM, DACZM
Clinical Associate Professor
School of Veterinary Medicine
University of Wisconsin–Madison
Madison, Wisconsin
Pain Management for the Pet Bird

Jacqueline A. Reid, BVMS, PhD, DVA, DECVA, MRCVS
Honorary Senior Research Fellow
Companion Animal Sciences
Institute of Comparative Medicine
Faculty of Veterinary Medicine
University of Glasgow
Glasgow, Scotland
Quality of Life Issues

Sheilah A. Robertson, BVMS, PhD, DACVA
Professor
Anesthesiology & Pain Management Section
Large Animal Clinical Sciences
College of Veterinary Medicine
University of Florida
Gainesville, Florida
Pain Management in the Cat

Narda G. Robinson, DO, DVM, MS, DABMA, FAAMA
Assistant Professor of Complementary and Alternative Medicine
Department of Clinical Sciences
College of Veterinary Medicine and Biomedical Sciences
Colorado State University
Fort Collins, Colorado
*Complementary and Alternative Medicine (CAM) for Pain Management
    in Veterinary Patients*

Bernard E. Rollin, PhD
University Distinguished Professor
Professor of Philosophy, Biomedical Sciences and Animal Sciences
Department of Philosophy
Colorado State University
Fort Collins, Colorado
The Ethics of Pain Management

Richard A. Sams, PhD
Professor
College of Veterinary Medicine
University of Florida
Gainesville, Florida
Pharmacologic Principles and Pain: Pharmacokinetics and Pharmacodynamics

E. Marian Scott, BSc, PhD, CStat
Professor
Department of Statistics
University of Glasgow
Glasgow, Scotland
Quality of Life Issues

Tami Shearer, DVM
VCA Sawmill Animal Hospital
Columbus, Ohio
Hospice and Palliative Care

Mary O. Smith, BVM&S, PhD, MRCVS, DACVIM (Neurology)
Affiliated Veterinary Specialists
Maitland, Florida
Glucocorticoids

Ann E. Wagner, DVM, MS, DACVP (Clinical Pathology), DACVA
Professor
Department of Clinical Sciences
College of Veterinary Medicine and Biomedical Sciences
Colorado State University
Fort Collins, Colorado
Opioids

M. Lesley Wiseman-Orr, BSc, PhD
Honorary Research Assistant
Companion Animal Sciences
Institute of Comparative Medicine
Faculty of Veterinary Medicine
University of Glasgow
Glasgow, Scotland
Quality of Life Issues

A COMPANION'S PAIN

Labored into the world
Vibrant life ripped from flesh
Flung towards days of wagging ease.
Comfort razed in an instant
A shrouded attack within
Writhe, recoil
Stifled whimper
Not too close! Trust growls distant
Flee, retreat, curl up close
Wrapped tight while hope tremors.
Pleading glance; lights wane and ebb
The tearless eye reveals nature's sting
On stoic souls;
Bearing it wisely
Grasping on instinct
Eased by the graciousness of man
Or Mercy.

– Kristine J. McComis

The second edition of this handbook was developed after considering the suggestions and ideas of many veterinarians and veterinary students who had used the first edition. The second edition contains updated drugs, doses, and protocols and incorporates a complete revision and expansion in a number of areas. New chapters cover pain relief, specifically targeting cats, birds, horses, cows, reptiles, ferrets, and rabbits. We have also included dedicated chapters to physical rehabilitation in dogs and cats, quality of life issues, and hospice care. This expansion has allowed us to provide more complete information for the alleviation of pain and suffering of many common species.

This edition of the handbook is designed for both busy practitioners and students who need and desire accurate and clinically useful information in a timely manner. We have worked very hard to provide the most recent information and dosing.

As stated in our previous edition, the science of pain and its therapy has garnered everyone's attention and interest during the past several decades due in no small part to the literal exponential growth of scientific information regarding pain mechanisms and management and the ever-increasing number of therapeutic modalities. Although all veterinarians take an oath to use their scientific knowledge and skills for "the relief of animal suffering," the treatment and prevention of pain has only recently become a singular objective. Excellent textbooks describing the neuroanatomy, neurophysiology, pathophysiology, and treatment of pain have been published only since the early 1980s. These textbooks, particularly *The Textbook of Pain,* edited by Patrick D. Wall and Ronald Melzack, serve as the foundation of current understanding and practice. The goal of this handbook is not to replace these textbooks but to supplement them by providing a species oriented, rapid, clinically applicable resource for use by all who witness and treat animal pain. The handbook serves as a quick reference for pertinent physiologic and pharmacologic information, including drugs and complementary therapeutic modalities used to treat pain. Uniquely, this handbook also provides an extensive array of acute and chronic case examples that can be used to provide a framework for discussion of pain therapy by practicing veterinarians, professional students, interns, residents, and veterinary technical support staff that are responsible for the day-to-day evaluation and care of patients. Significantly and somewhat unfortunately, some information has been extrapolated from the human experience. Ideally, future basic and clinical investigations conducted in animals will remedy this shortcoming, since most if not all therapies are tested in animals before they are applied to humans.

We would like to thank all of the contributors for the time and effort they have dedicated to making this handbook a reality. We also greatly appreciate the talented efforts of Tim Vojt and Dr. Michelle Murray, whose artwork has made written concepts visually understandable. Finally we would like to thank all those who have contributed their time, energy, and efforts toward improving the quality of life for all animals.

James S. Gaynor
William W. Muir III

VETERINARIAN'S OATH

Being admitted to the profession of veterinary medicine,

I solemnly swear to use my scientific knowledge and skills for the benefit of society through the protection of animal health, the relief of animal suffering, the conservation of livestock resources, the promotion of public health, and the advancement of medical knowledge.

I will practice my profession conscientiously, with dignity, and in keeping with the principles of veterinary medical ethics.

I accept as a lifelong obligation the continual improvement of my professional knowledge and competence.

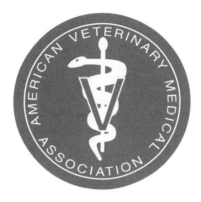

Adopted by the American Veterinary Medical Association (AVMA) House of Delegates, July, 1969.

CONTENTS

PART FOUR   ACUTE AND CHRONIC PAIN MANAGEMENT

Handbook of

VETERINARY PAIN
MANAGEMENT

ONE

PRINCIPLES OF PAIN MANAGEMENT

1

THE ETHICS OF PAIN MANAGEMENT

BERNARD E. ROLLIN

HISTORY OF ETHICS OF ANIMAL TREATMENT

For most of human history, civilized society has expressed a social ethic consensus regarding animal treatment, albeit a minimalistic one. This ethic, found even in the Bible, forbids cruelty toward animals, where *cruelty* is defined as deliberate, purposeless, willful, sadistic, deviant, unnecessary infliction of pain and suffering, such as muzzling an ox when it is being used to thresh grain. Historically, the concept of cruelty has been used in part to protect the animals but in equal measure to identify sadists and psychopaths who, common sense and recent science tell us, begin by torturing animals and graduate to harming people. In this spirit, "accepted," "necessary," and "nondeviant" infliction of pain and suffering have been invisible to the anticruelty laws and ethic they instantiate. Thus, practices such as steel-jawed trapping, hot iron branding, castration without anesthesia, training of animals with severe negative reinforcement, poisoning, fracturing, or invasive use of animals in research—in short, as one law put it, "anything done to minister to the necessities of man"—do not fall under the purview of cruelty.

During the past 30 years, however, society has considerably expanded the old ethic. For a variety of reasons, the public, at least in North America, Western Europe, and Australia and New Zealand, has grown increasingly concerned about a wide array of animal suffering, well beyond what arises out of cruelty. Most evident, perhaps, are the laws and policies that have been adopted to protect the interests of research animals in Great Britain, the United States, the Netherlands, Sweden, Australia, New Zealand, Switzerland, and Germany—all aimed at minimizing the pain and suffering of animals used in science. Laws and bills relevant to control of animal pain and suffering in all areas of human use have proliferated all over the world, ranging from the abolition or severe curtailment of confinement agriculture to protection of dolphins from tuna nets.

All of this marks a major departure from traditional social concern with cruelty alone. For example, in the 1890s, a judge refused to stop a service club–sponsored tame pigeon shooting competition under the anticruelty laws on the grounds that the persons participating were upstanding citizens who were working for charity and who were no threat to the community. In today's world, in most urban and suburban jurisdictions, such an activity, if not stopped by the judge, would be eliminated by public pressure or a city council mandate merely because of the unnecessary suffering and pain incurred by the animals.

Today's social ethic is thus concerned first of all with eliminating unnecessary pain and suffering in a much broader sense than the traditional anticruelty ethic. As society has become more urbanized, more sensitive, and less tolerant of animal suffering, the bar for what counts as cruelty has naturally been lowered. Since 1986, some 40 states have elevated animal cruelty from a misdemeanor to a felony offense, and what counts as cruelty has been significantly expanded. Consider one example. In 1997, during an attempt by the U.S. Department of Agriculture (USDA) to bolster dairy prices by buying a large number of dairy cows, the agency did not trust the farmers not to rebuy the cattle and return them to their herds. In an attempt to forestall such undercutting of the program, the USDA mandated face branding of all purchased milk cows with a USDA identification mark. Dairy farmers (who generally do not brand any part of the cow) and Humane Society members were appalled by this barbaric decree and brought the USDA to court in New York State on charges of cruelty. The judge ruled that the agency was guilty of cruelty, for it had failed to examine or use alternative, less invasive methods of identification. In earlier eras, although society always defined cruelty as inflicting "unnecessary" suffering, it defined *necessary* as that which was inconvenient, too expensive, or not customary to alleviate. Today that definition has changed radically, and increasingly, when someone says that "unnecessary suffering" is unacceptable, he or she means suffering that is possible, if inconvenient, to alleviate. Necessary suffering, then, is suffering that is impossible to alleviate. In another era, it might have been considered acceptable to train a horse by using considerable negative reinforcement. Today, because our sensitivities and expertise in training have increased, we are aware that positive reinforcement can accomplish more than negative reinforcement. Thus someone who beats a horse severely in the process of training is likely to be seen as cruel by society in general, even if some of his or her peers endorse such training methods.

Today, society is far less willing to tolerate animal pain and suffering in any area of animal use, regardless of whether such use is seen as frivolous (and hence possible to eliminate) or as essential to human well-being, as in the case of research and agriculture (and hence not seen as possible to eliminate), but traditionally exempt from the purview of anticruelty laws. These latter uses have elicited new ethical principles in the form of legislation (ethics "written large," as Plato said) aimed at minimizing animal pain and suffering attendant on these activities.

For example, consider the 1985 federal laboratory animal laws. On one hand, society realized that researchers are not cruel and yet also saw that some pain, suffering, and death must inevitably and necessarily accompany the study of disease, toxicity, new surgical procedures, and stress. On the other hand, society was unwilling to forsake the benefits of biomedicine, despite the inevitability of some animal suffering, and thus would not forbid animal experimentation. However, society also did not believe that researchers were doing the best they could for animals used in research. This belief was evident when it was discovered, for example, that analgesics were rarely used, social animals such as chimpanzees were housed in tiny individual cages, and atrocities were documented. Society acted to "write large" in law its moral commitment to the best possible treatment of animals consonant with biomedical use by mandating pain control, eliminating multiple use, preventing the administration of paralytic agents without anesthetics, and providing enriched environments.

The key moral concept encoded in the 1985 amendments to the Animal Welfare Act and in the National Institutes of Health Reauthorization Act—the latter putting the National Institutes of Health Guidelines for Laboratory Animal Care and Use into law—is the need to control laboratory animal pain not directly required by the nature of the research (for example, pain research). In some countries, such as Great Britain, the research must be terminated if the animal experiences intractable pain. In the United States, such a move depends on the discretion of the Institutional Animal Care and Use Committee, which may move to stop research under conditions of uncontrollable pain but need not do so. However the laws are written, it is manifest that society wants to see virtually all pain managed. Because this moral mandate is encoded in federal law, the highest law of the land, it therefore becomes the standard of practice for veterinary medicine. The ethic embodied in the laboratory animal laws has or will have ramifications for all veterinary practice.

The same point about minimizing pain and suffering holds true for animal agriculture in Europe. People wish to consume animal products, but as the 1965 British Brambell Commission stated, they also wish to see animals live decent lives, such as those provided by husbandry agriculture. Industrialized agriculture grew without people explicitly realizing what it entailed. As soon as people did (e.g., in Great Britain and Sweden), laws were passed that underscored public commitment to decent lives for animals; abolished sow stalls, veal crates, and battery cages; and required pain control for management procedures.

Research is seen by society as essential to human life, and animal agriculture is seen as essential to the food supply (most persons are not prepared to be vegetarians). Thus society uses the new ethic to shape these activities. Horse tripping, tame pigeon shoots, and dog fighting are not seen as essential or desirable by most citizens but are seen to cause animal suffering; therefore, society has moved to abolish them.

ROLE OF VETERINARY MEDICINE IN PAIN CONTROL

This ethic suggests that a fundamental role for veterinary medicine in society is finding modalities to control pain and suffering in the use of animals because such control seems to be the main point of the new ethic and the laws it has engendered. The track record of veterinary medicine in this area is not good, however. The reasons for this neglect are worth detailing because few veterinarians have actively thought them through.

First, in the twentieth century, human and veterinary medicine became increasingly science-based, essentially perceived as applied biologic science, with physics and chemistry serving as the exemplar of ideal science. In this light, emphasis on the individual and idiosyncratic aspects of a disease (what composed the "art of medicine") became subordinate to the universal captured in medical science. Second, in keeping with an ideologic emphasis on science dealing only with what is testable and observable, talk of subjective states, such as pain and suffering, tended to disappear as unscientific. Even psychology became the science of observable behavior. Third, physicians and veterinarians measured success by prolonging life or function, focusing on quantity of life rather than quality of life and emphasizing cure rather than care because quality is difficult to measure and impossible to quantify. Pain became more of a concern to the patient than to the clinician. Several articles by Frank McMillan[1,2] have eloquently documented the untoward effects of this attitude in veterinary medicine. Thus, in essence, control of pain became increasingly irrelevant in scientific medicine, a tendency that unfortunately continues to this day.

The most dramatic and egregious example of the supposed irrelevance of pain in the history of human medicine is the failure to control pain in 80% of human patients with cancer, even though 90% of such pain is controllable. Equally horrifying is the fact that until the late 1980s, neonatal surgeons regularly performed open heart surgery on newborns after administration of paralytic drugs and still perform a variety of procedures from colonoscopy and setting broken limbs to bone marrow aspiration with the use of nonanesthetic, nonanalgesic amnesiacs such as short-acting benzodiazepines (diazepam [Valium] and midazolam [Versed, Dormicum]).

If human medicine was cavalier in dealing with pain and suffering in its patients during most of the twentieth century (the term *suffering* does not even appear in medical dictionaries), this is even more true of veterinary medicine because for most of the twentieth century, society placed little moral value on control of animal pain.

Until the late 1960s, veterinary medicine was overwhelmingly ancillary to agriculture, and the veterinarian's task was strictly dictated by the economic value of the animal; the control of pain was not of concern to producers and thus not expected of veterinary medicine. This attitude is epitomized in Merillat's 1905 veterinary surgery textbook[3] in which he laments the almost total disregard of anesthesia in veterinary practice, with the episodic exception of the canine practitioner, whose clients presumably valued their animals enough in noneconomic terms to demand anesthesia.

These practical considerations were further compounded by the persistence of the Cartesian belief that possession of language is a precondition for the ability to feel pain, a notion that until recently (2001) existed in the definition of pain of the International Pain Society.

The denial of the experience of pain by animals in veterinary medicine was so powerful that when the first textbooks of veterinary anesthesia (by Lumb,[4] and Lumb and Jones[5]) were published in the United States in 1964 and 1972, they did not list the control of felt pain as a reason for using anesthesia and had no discussion of analgesia. When I went before Congress in 1982 to defend the laboratory animal laws we had drafted, I was asked by Congress to prove that there was a need for such legislation. I did so by doing a literature search on laboratory animal analgesia in particular and "animal analgesia" in general. I found two papers—one that said that there ought to be papers on this subject, and the other one summarizing in one page the scanty knowledge available.

Many veterinarians who are more than 40 or 50 years of age still use the phrase *chemical restraint* as synonymous with *anesthesia;* some were trained in the 1960s to castrate horses using curariform (paralytic) drugs such as succinylcholine, which not only do not mask or diminish pain but probably intensify it by the fear they create. Others erroneously speak of anesthesia as *sedation,* although most sedatives neither mask nor diminish pain. For too many years, ketamine alone was used in cat spays, despite the fact that it is not analgesic for visceral pain. And though we know anecdotally that some animals, like some persons, experience "bad trips" and flashbacks when dosed with ketamine, this is not yet a concern in veterinary circles.

Of equal concern are the ideologic rationalizations still invoked by some (particularly older) veterinarians to justify withholding postsurgical or posttraumatic analgesia from animals. These rationalizations include the belief that anesthesia is more stressful than the surgical procedure performed without anesthesia. Other beliefs are the following: Postsurgical analgesics are not needed because animals supposedly will eat immediately after surgery. Analgesics are not to be used because without the pain, the animal will inexorably reinjure the damaged body part. Post-surgical howling and whining are not signs of pain; they are aftereffects of anesthesia. Anatomic differences, such as the presence of an anatomic mesenteric sling, vitiate the need for pain control after abdominal surgery in the dog. Animals do not need postsurgical analgesia because we can watch them behave normally after surgery. Young animals feel less pain than older ones and thus do not need surgical anesthesia for procedures such as tail docking or castration, which are performed with "bruticaine." Analgesia deadens the coping ability of predators and thus is more discomfiting to an animal than the pain is. Liver biopsies do not hurt.

Although adequate, even definitive, responses to this spurious reasoning exist, they persist as barriers to pain management. One drug company executive has even told me that, by the company's reckoning, approximately one third of veterinarians do not use analgesia. This is buttressed by a statement made by the executive director of one large state veterinary association who expressed amazement that so many veterinarians fail to supply pain control, even though it is easy to achieve, lucrative, and causes remarkable changes in the animal's demeanor.

Finally, many veterinarians do not know a great deal about pain management. In a 1996 study, Dohoo and Dohoo[6] showed that veterinarians' knowledge is limited and that what practitioners do know is typically not acquired in veterinary school, although I suspect that this is rapidly changing as society increases its demand for pain control in animals. A variety of factors provide strong arguments in favor of the idea that pain control is one of the chief issues facing veterinary medicine.

THE CHANGING SOCIAL ETHICS AND SOCIAL ROLE OF ANIMALS

As previously discussed, society has become increasingly concerned about animal welfare. Central to the new ethic is the realization that uncontrolled pain and suffering probably represent the greatest harm that can be visited upon animals and thus that control of pain and suffering in all areas of animal use is a major moral imperative.

In particular, the new role that companion animals play in persons' lives militates in favor of client concern for their pain and suffering. We live, particularly in urban areas, in a society that has become more and more of what German sociologists call *Gesellschaft* (a mixture, a haphazard, unconnected assemblage of persons) rather than *Gemeinschaft* (a compound, an organic unity). One can be lonelier in New York City than in rural Wyoming; where the distance separating persons in Wyoming is merely physical, in New York it is psychological. We have lonely divorced persons, lonely elderly persons, and lonely children. In such a world, companion animals become bonded to us by love and need; an animal can literally become a *raison d'être* for an elderly person, a reason to get up in the morning and go out. More than anything else, Hurricane Katrina demonstrated this new relationship, when individuals refused to be evacuated without their animals, thereby risking their lives. In such a world, animal owners are sensitive to pain and suffering on the part of their animals to an unprecedented extent.

NEW PHILOSOPHICAL REFLECTIONS ON ANIMAL EXPERIENCE

Better philosophy than we have had in the past strongly argues in favor of the view that animals have thoughts, mental states, and feelings. The fact that some such mental states are in many ways probably not like ours, since animal thoughts and feelings are not mediated by language, does not obviate the need for serious concern about their pain, fear, and distress. Possibly, animal pain is worse than human pain because, lacking language and sophisticated reasoning skills and temporal concepts, animals cannot understand the reasons for and causes of pain and thus lack the ability to hope for and anticipate its cessation.

LAWS

New laws articulating the new ethic have specifically flagged pain control as the major moral concern about animal treatment. The essence of the 1985 U.S. laboratory animal laws, originally the first laws in America articulating the new ethic for animals, embody the control of pain and distress as their major edict. Unfortunately, before the advent of these laws, virtually no literature on animal pain control existed. Thus the goal of pain control needs to be sought not only for research animals but also for animals in all other areas of human use, including farm and companion animals. Countries such as Sweden have articulated the need for pain control in farm animals. Treatment of companion animals may be the only area in which concern for pain in animals is not trumped, diluted, or submerged by economic considerations and can be wholly realized. In the 20 years since the U.S. laboratory animal laws went into effect, the literature on animal analgesia and its use has grown exponentially. Compared with the two papers I found in 1982, we now enjoy a literature that, according to my colleagues in anesthesiology, numbers between 5000 and 10,000 papers. And the use of analgesia is axiomatic to today's young graduate.

The laws are also helping to drive another revolution. The original statutes of 1985 required control of "pain and distress." USDA initially focused on pain, wisely realizing that overcoming ideology was of necessity incremental. Now that pain control is well established, USDA has moved to monitor "distress." Distress seems to be a generic term for the variety of other noxious experiences animals can suffer: for example, fear, loneliness, boredom, stimulational deprivation, and restricted movement. Ironically but predictably, many scientists to whom pain is axiomatic express doubts about these other modalities— so much so that when I addressed a conference on animal distress in 2004, I felt compelled to remind the attendees that I encountered the same sort of agnosticism about pain 25 years earlier at a conference that I was now experiencing regarding distress, and that 25 years hence, the same degree of acceptance of these now alien concepts would be found.

PREVENTION OF SUFFERING

If we keep these animals to give and receive love, as members of our families, we have an insurmountable obligation not to let them suffer. Equally important, it is now definitively known that uncontrolled pain is not only morally problematic when allowed to persist in human beings or animals, it is biologically deleterious. Unmitigated pain is a major biologic stressor and affects numerous aspects of physical health, from wound healing to resistance to infectious disease. One remarkable study showed that when pain in rats with cancer was controlled with analgesia versus not controlled, the rats given analgesia had 80% fewer metastatic lesions. The conclusion is inescapable: uncontrolled pain damages health and well-being and can even, if pain is severe enough, engender death. Ironically, the new edition of Lumb and Jones's veterinary textbook[7] stresses this dimension of pain management, a major salubrious change since the publication of the 1970s edition.

PRESERVING THE ROLE OF VETERINARIANS AS THE RECOGNIZED HEALTH CARE PROVIDERS FOR ANIMALS

One of the unexpected consequences of ignoring pain and suffering in human and animal medicine in the twentieth century has been the fueling of the development of alternative, non–evidence-based, nonscientific "therapies." To put it crudely, patients and animal owners have reasoned that if doctors do not worry about human or animal suffering, they will find others who will. Also, many alternative practitioners approach human and animal patients with empathy and understanding of the full significance of pain and suffering. Unfortunately, however, compassion is not cure and is only part of care. Recognition that a being is suffering is not alleviation of that suffering, although it is surely a necessary condition for such alleviation. If veterinary clients are drawn to alternative unproven therapies that may be fueled by compassion but do not work to control pain, the animal may be cheated of a proven modality for pain control, creating an intolerable moral situation for the animal owner and a loss of credibility for veterinarians because clients may not be able to judge when pain is (or is not) alleviated. If veterinarians will not manage pain, they also risk a grave loss of credibility among the public, who may then seek to remove the special status of scientifically based veterinary medicine and open animal medicine to the forces of the free market, at an incalculable cost in animal suffering.

MEETING ONE'S PROFESSIONAL OBLIGATIONS

It does not appear that animals fear death, lacking after all the concepts to understand, in Heidegger's masterful phrase, "the possibility of the impossibility of their being." Yet they clearly fear pain. We urge death in veterinary medicine as a merciful tool for escape from pain. (There is reason to believe that human beings also fear pain more than death, and it is often suggested that if we truly attacked pain in terminally ill patients with all of our medical armamentarium and with no absurd fears that they will become addicted, patients would not seek euthanasia as much as they do and would die with far more dignity, as the hospice movement has shown.) It is thus reasonable to say of animals that letting them live in unalleviated pain is the worst thing we can do to them. If the veterinarian's *raison d'être* is, as is so often remarked, the health and well-being of the animals in his or her care, then the assiduous pursuit of eliminating or at least managing pain should be his or her top priority. The fact that it has not been so in the past only makes it all the more imperative to make it so in the future. Further, there is now a vast literature showing that uncontrolled pain is a major stressor, retarding healing and increasing the likelihood of infection.

> ### Sources of Information Regarding Regulations Governing Animal Welfare
>
> Animal Welfare Act and Regulations
>   Animal Welfare Information Center
>   U.S. Department of Agriculture
>   Agricultural Research Service
>   National Agricultural Library
>   *www.nal.usda.gov/awic/legislat/usdaleg1.htm*
> AVMA Guidelines on Euthanasia (American Veterinary Medical Association, June 2007)
>   *www.avma.org/issues/animal_welfare/euthanasia.pdf*
> U.S. Department of Agriculture Animal and Plant Health Inspection Animal Care Policy
>   Manual
>   *www.aphis.usda.gov/animal_welfare/policy*
> Office of Laboratory Animal Welfare
>   *http://grants.nih.gov/grants/olaw/olaw.htm*
>   *http://oacu.od.nih.gov/ARAC/tablesbyspecies.pdf*

PROLIFERATION OF TREATMENT MODALITIES

During the past 2 decades, more and more treatment modalities that were developed in human medicine have been exported to veterinary medicine. These modalities include an exponential growth in oncology, transplantation, and dialysis, with clients willing to spend essentially unlimited amounts on their animals. This is good for veterinary medicine and good for animals but raises new ethical challenges; for example, managing the animals' pain and suffering under heroic medical conditions, including pressing euthanasia on clients when the suffering cannot be alleviated. The recently developed concept of "pawspice"—hospice for animals—is a double-edged sword, promising state-of-the-art management of suffering but also presenting the real risk of affluent clients' extending treatment too long. Whereas once veterinarians were primarily advocates to forestall clients' euthanizing animals too early, they now must additionally advocate for animal euthanasia in the face of clients' wishing to continue treatment beyond a reasonable endpoint.

References

1. McMillan FD: Influence of mental states on somatic health in animals, *JAVMA* 214:1221-1223, 1999.
2. McMillan FD: Stress, distress and emotion: distinctions and implications for animal well-being. In McMillan FD, editor: *Mental health and well-being in animals,* Ames, Ia, 2005, Blackwell.
3. Merillat LA: *Principles of veterinary surgery,* Chicago, 1906, Alexander Eger.

4. Lumb WV: *Small animal anesthesia,* Philadelphia, 1963, Lea & Febiger.
5. Lumb WV, Jones EW: *Veterinary anesthesia,* Philadelphia, 1973, Lea & Febiger.
6. Dohoo SE, Dohoo IR: Factors influencing the postoperative use of analgesics in dogs and cats by Canadian veterinarians, *Can Vet J* 37(9):552-556, 1996.

SUGGESTED READINGS

Dohoo SE, Dohoo IR: Postoperative use of analgesics in dogs and cats by Canadian veterinarians, *Can Vet J* 37(9):546-551, 1996.

Ferrel BR, Rhiner M: High-tech comfort: ethical issues in cancer pain management for the 1990s, *J Clin Ethics* 2:108-115, 1991.

Humane Society of Rochester v. Ling, 633f. Supp. 480, U.S. District Court, WDNY, NY 1986.

Kitchell R, Guinan M: The nature of pain in animals. In Rollin B, Kesel M, editors: *The experimental animal in biomedical research,* vol 1, Boca Raton, Fla, 1989, CRC Press.

McMillan F: Comfort as the primary goal in veterinary medical practice, *J Am Vet Med Assoc* 212(9):1370-1374, 1998.

McMillan F: Effects of human contact on animal well-being, *J Am Vet Med Assoc* 215(11):1592-1598, 1999.

McMillan F: Influence of mental states on somatic health in animals, *J Am Vet Med Assoc* 214(8):1221-1225, 1999.

McMillan F: Quality of life in animals, *J Am Vet Med Assoc* 216(12):1904-1910, 2000.

Page GG, Ben-Eliyahu J, Yirmiyah R et al: Morphine attenuates surgery-induced enhancement of metastatic colonization in rats, *Pain* 54:21-28, 1993.

Rollin BE: *Animal rights and human morality,* ed 2, Buffalo, 1992, Prometheus Books.

Rollin BE: Pain and ideology in human and veterinary medicine, *Semin Vet Med Surg (Small Anim)* 12(2):56-60, 1997.

Rollin BE: *The unheeded cry: animal consciousness, animal pain, and science,* ed 2, Ames, 1998, Iowa State University Press.

Rollin BE.: Some conceptual and ethical concerns about current views of pain, *Pain Forum* 8(2):78-83, 1999.

Rollin BE: Equine welfare and emerging social ethics, *J Am Vet Med Assoc* 216(8): 1234-1237, 2000.

Rollin BE: The ethics of pain control in companion animals. In Hellebrekers L, editor: *Animal pain: a practice-oriented approach to an effective pain control in animals,* Utrecht, Netherlands, 2000, Van Der Wels.

Rollin BE: *Science and ethics,* New York, 2006, Cambridge University Press.

Rollin BE: *An introduction to veterinary medical ethics: theory and cases,* ed 2, Ames, Iowa, 2006, Blackwell Publishing Professional.

2

PHYSIOLOGY AND PATHOPHYSIOLOGY OF PAIN

WILLIAM W. MUIR III

Pain is a sensory experience that is frequently but not always associated with nerve or tissue damage. The study of pain encompasses all the individual biologic basic sciences, especially anatomy, physiology, pharmacology, and pathology. A functional appreciation of each of these areas as they pertain to the generation, transmission, and recognition of painful stimuli is fundamental to understanding pain and pain processes. The following discussion is meant to provide an overview of the important aspects of the nervous system, sensory pathways, and pain processing. As in all areas of biologic science, jargon is used, such as *afferent* (toward the central nervous system [CNS]) and *efferent* (away from the CNS). Terms are defined when first mentioned. Pain itself is usually described in terms of a noxious stimulus, meaning a damaging or potentially tissue-damaging stimulus. Another term frequently encountered in descriptions of pain is *neuroplasticity.* This term implies that the nervous system can be changed (shaped or molded), depending on the environment (outside) and biologic processes (inside) that are responsible for painful sensations. The neuroplasticity of the nervous system should be kept in mind during attempts to assess the severity of pain, especially severe acute or chronic pain, and in the design of treatment protocols. Another term that arises during discussions of pain management in animals is *anthropomorphize,* which means to attribute a human form or personality to an animal. Human nature is to project personal experiences and feelings onto our animal patients because they cannot verbally describe to us how they feel; however, it is inappropriate to attribute human feelings to something not human. Alternatively, it is morally and ethically appropriate to adopt and use an anthropocentric viewpoint when assessing and treating pain in animals.

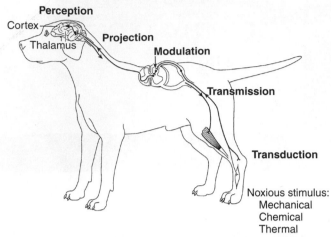

FIG. 2-1. Pathways involved in producing painful sensations. Noxious stimuli (mechanical, chemical, thermal, electrical) are transduced (transduction) into electrical signals that are transmitted (transmission) to the spinal cord, where they are modulated (modulation) before being relayed (projection) to the brain for final processing and awareness (perception). Descending pathways from the brain modulate sensory input, and outputs from the spinal cord regulate skeletal muscle contraction.

NEUROPHYSIOLOGY OF SENSATION

Peripheral nerves can be thought of as an extension of the CNS, consisting of sensory, motor, and autonomic nerve fibers. They are the electrical cables over which sensory and motor information are transmitted. The terminal ends of sensory nerve fibers recognize and transform (transduce) various environmental stimuli into electrical signals (action potentials) that are carried (transmitted) to the dorsal horn of the CNS, where they are immediately changed (modulated) and relayed (projected) to the brainstem and brain. The signal is then integrated, recognized, identified (perceived), and transformed (secondary modulation) into appropriate self-preserving experiences and motor responses that are protective and remembered (Fig. 2-1).

TRANSDUCTION

The detection of innocuous and noxious information is accomplished by specialized encapsulated and bare (free) nerve endings that transform environmental stimuli into electrical signals called *action potentials* (Table 2-1). These receptors vary in their sensitivity to mechanical, thermal,

TABLE 2-1	Important Receptors in Somatic Sensation	
Receptor	**Modality**	**Nerve Fiber Type**
CUTANEOUS AND SUBCUTANEOUS	**TOUCH**	
Pacini's	Vibration	Aα,β
Ruffini's	Skin stretch	Aα,β
Merkel's	Pressure	Aα,β
Meissner's	Stroking	Aα,β
MUSCLE AND SKELETAL MECHANORECEPTORS	**LIMB PROPRIOCEPTION**	
Muscle spindles	Muscle length and stretch	Aα,β
Golgi tendon	Muscle contraction	Aα
Joint capsule	Joint angle	Aβ
Stretch	Excessive stretch	Aδ
THERMAL	**TEMPERATURE**	
Heat nociceptors	Hot temperature	Aδ
Cold nociceptors	Cold temperature	C
NOCICEPTORS	**PAIN**	
Mechanical	Sharp, pricking	Aδ
Thermal-mechanical	Burning, freezing	Aδ, C
Polymodal	Slow burning	C

and chemical stimuli (low- and high-threshold), providing a seamless response to innocuous through noxious sensations.

The minimal stimulus required to elicit a transmittable electrical signal (action potential) from a peripheral sensory receptor is considered to be its *threshold*. The sensory receptors located on Aβ, Aδ, and C fibers demonstrate a large degree of sensory overlap, providing for a continuum of sensations. Once the threshold for a receptor is reached, stronger stimuli elicit more action potentials. The longer the duration of the suprathreshold stimulus, the longer the train of electrical signals produced (Fig. 2-2).

Specialized Nerve Endings

Specialized low-threshold (high-sensitivity) nerve endings or receptors (e.g., Meissner's, Merkel's, Pacini's, and Ruffini's) in the skin, muscles, and joints respond to innocuous mechanical stimulation. These receptors are primarily concerned with touch, vibration, pressure, movement, and proprioception. The information transduced by these nerve receptors is conveyed to the CNS by Aβ nerve fibers. The nerve terminals of Aβ fibers are normally responsible for transducing innocuous sensory information.

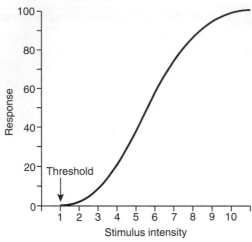

FIG. 2-2. The pain threshold is the point at which stimulus intensity is just strong enough to be perceived as painful. Stronger stimuli elicit greater and greater responses until the maximum response possible is produced.

The $A\delta$ and C nerve fibers terminate as free nerve endings in the skin, subcutaneous tissue, periosteum, joints, muscles, and viscera. Free nerve ending pain receptors (nociceptors) respond to low-intensity (nonpainful) and high-intensity (painful) mechanical, thermal, and chemical stimuli. The terminals of $A\delta$ and C nerve fibers are essential for detection of all pain sensations. Approximately 75% of the $A\delta$-fiber and 10% to 15% of the C-fiber nociceptors respond to low-intensity stimuli. The remainder respond only to high-intensity tissue-threatening or tissue-damaging stimuli. Some nociceptors respond only to intense mechanical stimulation and are referred to as *high-threshold mechanical nociceptors,* whereas others respond to noxious mechanothermal stimulation, and still others respond to noxious mechanical, thermal, and chemical stimuli (polymodal nociceptors).

Aδ Nociceptors.   The $A\delta$ nerve terminals can be nociceptive or nonnociceptive and are composed of low-threshold (<75%) and high-threshold (>25%) mechanoreceptors and mechanothermal receptors. The latter are referred to as $A\delta$ heat nociceptors. High-threshold $A\delta$ nociceptors respond only to tissue-threatening or tissue-damaging stimulation. Many of the $A\delta$ nociceptors respond only to specific stimuli, whereas others are polymodal and respond to mechanical, chemical, and thermal stimulation. The $A\delta$-fiber nociceptors discharge at higher rates than C fiber nociceptors, providing more discriminative information to the CNS, and are responsible for the pricking and sharp qualities associated with the initiation of pain ("first pain"). Activation of Aδ-fiber and C-fiber nociceptors occurs during the generation of acute pain.

C-Fiber Nociceptors. Almost all C-fiber nociceptors are high-threshold and polymodal. The C-fiber nociceptors are found in large numbers in the skin, skeletal muscle, and joints. Although they are abundant, fewer C-fiber nociceptors are found in visceral tissues. C-fiber activation is responsible for second (slow-onset) pain and occurs after the initial insult. Second pain is characterized by a burning, aching quality and signals tissue damage and inflammation. The pain produced by tissue damage and inflammation initiates self-preservation behaviors (avoidance, guarding) and disuse. Tissue damage and inflammation also intensify the sensation of pain (activate and sensitize nociceptors), producing hyperalgesia.

Silent or Sleeping Nociceptors. The Aδ fibers and C fibers contain "silent" or "sleeping" nociceptors that can be activated by tissue-damaging events.

TRANSMISSION

Sensory and motor electrical impulses (action potentials) to and from the spinal cord, respectively, are transmitted by peripheral nerves. Peripheral nerves are categorized according to their anatomy, size, and mean conduction velocity (Table 2-2). Peripheral nerves contain afferent (sensory) and efferent (motor) nerve fibers. The peripheral processes of sensory nerves diverge to form multiple branches, ending in specialized (low-threshold) or free (high-threshold) nerve endings (see "Specialized Nerve Endings"). The afferent fibers of peripheral nerves form the dorsal root near the spinal cord. The efferent fiber from the spinal cord forms the ventral root (Fig. 2-3). The area of the skin innervated by the dorsal root is called a *dermatome*. Adjacent dermatomes overlap, minimizing sensory deficits that may occur as a result of dorsal root injuries.

Once a peripheral afferent nerve is activated and the stimulus is transduced into an action potential, it is transmitted to the dorsal horn of the spinal cord. Under normal circumstances, nonnoxious sensory information is transmitted by myelinated Aβ nerve fibers, whereas nonnoxious and some noxious information is transmitted by minimally myelinated Aδ nerve fibers. Noxious information is transmitted by unmyelinated C fibers.

Receptive Fields

The receptive field defines the area innervated by a sensory nerve fiber. The receptive fields of high-threshold nociceptors consist of collections of 2 to 20 spots, each with an area of less than 1 mm². Receptive fields

TABLE 2-2	Classification of Nerve Fibers		
Group	Innervation	Myelination	Velocity (m/s)
Aα	Motor to skeletal muscle	Myelinated	70-120
Aβ	Sensory: touch, vibration, pressure, proprioception	Myelinated	30-70
Aγ	Motor to muscle spindles	Myelinated	15-30
Aδ	Mechanoreceptors, thermo-receptors, nociceptors	Thinly myelinated	12-30
B	Sympathetic Preganglionic	Unmyelinated	3-15
C	Mechanoreceptors, thermo-receptors Sympathetic postganglionic Nociceptors	Unmyelinated	0.5-3

are small on the face and head (1 to 2 mm^2), are larger on the body surface, and provide discriminatory capability. The receptive fields of C-fiber nociceptors are generally much smaller than those of Aδ-fiber nociceptors, and considerable overlap exists between Aδ-fiber and C-fiber nociceptive fields. Nociceptive afferent nerve fibers from the thoracic and abdominal viscera are sparse compared with cutaneous fibers and constitute less than 10% of the sensory nervous input to the spinal cord. Furthermore, the smaller number of visceral afferent fibers innervates a much larger area and demonstrates almost 100% overlap, which helps explain the diffuse nature of visceral pain sensations.

Dorsal Root and Cranial Nerve Ganglia

The cell bodies of sensory afferent peripheral nerve fibers are located in the dorsal root ganglia of the spinal nerves and sensory ganglia of cranial nerves (V, VII, IX, and X). The nerve branches divide as they leave the cell body, with one branch traveling centrally to the spinal cord and the other branch traveling through the formed peripheral nerve and its divisions to reach the sensory nerve endings in the skin, subcutaneous tissues, muscles, bones, and joints. These branches are called somatic sensory fibers. Some of the sensory processes of sensory afferent nerves accompany the sympathetic and parasympathetic nerves to innervate the viscera and are called visceral sensory nerve fibers (Fig. 2-3). The cell bodies of the dorsal root ganglion produce a variety of enzymes and neurotransmitters that are important in signal transmission and nerve cell viability. Among the more prevalent neurochemicals are substance P, calcitonin gene-related peptide (CGRP), cholecystokinin,

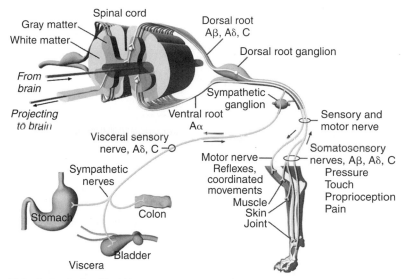

FIG. 2-3. A simplified illustration of sensory (visceral and somatic) nerve fibers (Aβ, Aδ, C) as they travel to the dorsal root ganglia and then via the dorsal root nerves to the gray matter of the spinal cord. Many of the Aδ and C sensory nerve fibers innervating the viscera travel with the sympathetic nerves, passing through the sympathetic ganglia before reaching the dorsal root ganglia.

somatostatin (SOM), vasoactive intestinal peptide, bombesin, galanin (GAL), dynorphin (DYN), endorphin (END), enkephalin (ENK), and corticotropin-releasing factor (Box 2-1).

MODULATION

Peripheral sensory nerve impulses are modulated (amplified or suppressed) in the spinal cord. The spinal cord is divided into white matter (axons of nerve fibers) and gray matter (nerve cells). The gray matter is divided into three distinct regions: the dorsal horn, the intermediate zone, and the ventral horn. The gray matter of the dorsal horn contains interneurons (interconnecting nerves) and ascending neurons that receive, transmit, and project sensory information to the brain. The ventral horn contains interneurons and motor neurons that control skeletal muscle function. The gray matter of the intermediate zone contains autonomic preganglionic neurons that mediate visceral control and transmit information to higher centers. Primary sensory afferent nerve fibers enter the spinal cord through the dorsal nerve root and synapse with neurons in the dorsal horn of the gray matter.

BOX 2-1

Prevalent Neurochemicals that are Important in Signal Transmission and Nerve Cell Viability

Bombesin
Calcitonin gene-related peptide
Cholecystokinin
Corticotropin-releasing factor
Dynorphin
Endorphin

Enkephalin
Galanin
Somatostatin
Substance P
Vasoactive intestinal peptide

Many of the sensory afferent nerve fibers bifurcate, sending branches that ascend and descend several spinal cord segments (Lissauer's tract) before entering and synapsing in the dorsal horn. Sensory nerve fibers can synapse directly with projection neurons in the gray matter, which relay incoming sensory information to the brain, or indirectly with local excitatory and inhibitory interneurons that regulate and modify sensory information before it is relayed to projection neurons and higher centers.

Gray Matter

The gray matter of the spinal cord has been subdivided into 10 laminae (Rexed's laminae) based on the presence of neuronal cells with similar function. Gray matter sensory neurons are basically of two types: (1) those that process high-threshold, nociceptive-specific information and have small receptive fields that are organized somatotopically and (2) those that process low- and high-threshold information (wide-dynamic-range neurons), are nociceptive-nonspecific, and have large receptive fields. Information from the various peripheral sensory nerve fiber types (Aβ, Aδ, C) is transmitted to the various laminae, where amino acids (e.g., glutamate) and peptides (e.g., substance P) activate a variety of postsynaptic receptors.

◆ The gray matter of the dorsal horn contains projection neurons, propriospinal neurons, and interneurons that relay sensory information to the brain and activate descending control systems, which control the sensitivity of dorsal horn neurons to excitatory and inhibitory impulses. Propriospinal neurons transfer sensory information from one segment of the spinal cord to the next and ultimately to the brain, and local interneurons modulate (excite and inhibit) and transmit sensory information for a short distance within the spinal cord.

◆ The gray matter of the ventral horn contains interneurons and motor neurons that control skeletal muscle activity.

♦ The gray matter of the intermediate zone contains preganglionic neurons of the autonomic nervous system that control visceral functions and transmit afferent information to the brain.

White Matter

The white matter contains the axons of the spinal cord and has been anatomically divided into three bilaterally paired spinal columns that relay information to and from the brain:

♦ Dorsal columns: The dorsal columns are medial to the dorsal horn and relay somatic sensory information to the medulla.

♦ Lateral columns: The lateral columns are lateral to the gray matter, relay somatic sensory information to the brain, and contain nerve fibers from sensory, motor, and autonomic control centers in the brain.

♦ Ventral columns: The ventral columns are medial to the ventral horns and are primarily composed of neurons descending from the brain that control skeletal muscle.

Spinal Cord Laminae

Laminae I to VI compose the dorsal horn, lamina VII composes the intermediate zone, and laminae VIII to IX compose the ventral horn (Fig. 2-4). These laminae extend the entire length of the spinal cord and fuse cranially in the medulla. Lamina X surrounds the central canal of the spinal cord. The laminar anatomy refers to the location of specific cell bodies:

♦ Lamina I: The most superficial lamina, or marginal layer, of the dorsal horn serves as an important sensory relay junction for pain and temperature. Lamina I contains nociceptive-specific neurons, wide-dynamic-range neurons, and projection neurons. This lamina receives the majority of its input from sympathetic Aδ and C fibers originating in the skin, skeletal muscle, joints, viscera, and trigeminal structures.

♦ Lamina II *(substantia gelatinosa):* Lamina II is divided into outer (IIo) and inner (IIi) layers, which receive afferent sensory information predominantly from small nonmyelinated C fibers and thinly myelinated Aδ fibers that project to lamina I. Lamina II contains a large number of second-order multireceptive or wide-dynamic-range neurons, almost all of which are interneurons; this suggests the importance of lamina II as a site for the modulation of synaptic transmission. Few visceral afferent nerves terminate in lamina II.

♦ Laminae III to VI *(nucleus proprius):* Lamina III integrates sensory input with information descending from the brain and contains neurons that project sensory information to the brain. Lamina IV receives sensory information from large-diameter Aβ fibers from the skin, which synapse

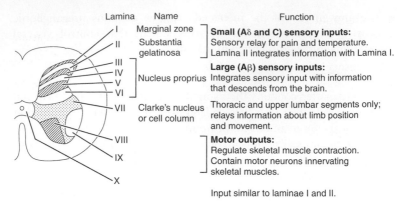

Lamina	Name	Function
I	Marginal zone	**Small (Aδ and C) sensory inputs:** Sensory relay for pain and temperature. Lamina II integrates information with Lamina I.
II	Substantia gelatinosa	
III		**Large (Aβ) sensory inputs:** Integrates sensory input with information that descends from the brain.
IV	Nucleus proprius	
V		
VI		
VII	Clarke's nucleus or cell column	Thoracic and upper lumbar segments only; relays information about limb position and movement.
VIII		**Motor outputs:** Regulate skeletal muscle contraction. Contain motor neurons innervating skeletal muscles.
IX		
X		Input similar to laminae I and II.

FIG. 2-4. The gray matter of the spinal cord is divided into functionally distinct nerve cells (Rexed's laminae). The dorsal horn of the gray matter receives sensory input from Aβ, Aδ, and C nerve fibers. The ventral horn of the spinal cord contains motor nerves that innervate and regulate skeletal muscle contraction. The white matter that surrounds the gray matter is divided into columns of myelinated nerves. The dorsal column relays somatic sensory information to the brain. The intermediate column contains sensory motor and autonomic nerve fibers descending from the brain and sensory pathways ascending to the brain. The ventral column contains nerve fibers descending from the brain that control skeletal muscle contraction.

with low-threshold mechanoreceptors responding to innocuous tactile and thermal stimuli. Lamina IV also receives some input from small-diameter Aδ and C fibers in the skin, muscle, and viscera. Lamina V predominantly contains wide-dynamic-range neurons, which receive sensory information from Aβ fibers and sympathetic Aδ and C fibers, which synapse with neurons that project to the brain.

♦ Laminae VII to IX: Laminae VII, VIII, and IX contain interneurons that are important in regulating skeletal muscle contraction and limb movement.

♦ Laminae X: Lamina X surrounds the central canal and receives sensory information similar to that received by laminae I and II.

Spinal Cord Neurotransmitters and Receptors

As stated previously, the dorsal horn of the spinal cord receives and processes sensory information and relays this information to the brain. A multitude of neurotransmitters—including peptides (substance P, CGRP, SOM, neuropeptide Y, GAL), excitatory (glutamate, aspartate) and inhibitory (γ-aminobutyric acid [GABA], glycine) amino acids, nitric oxide (NO), prostaglandins, adenosine triphosphate (ATP), endogenous opioids, and monoamines (serotonin, norepinephrine)—are responsible for transmitting peripheral information to spinal cord neurons. These neurotransmitters act on excitatory (α-amino-3-hydroxy-5-methyl-4-isoxazole propionic acid [AMPA], kainate [KAI], N-methyl-D-aspartate [NMDA]) and inhibitory (GABA, glycine) receptors on neurons that relay sensory information to the brain.

◆ AMPA, KAI, and neurokinin receptors: Most transmissions between the periphery and dorsal horn of the spinal cord occur as a result of glutamate acting on postsynaptically located AMPA and KAI ionotropic receptors. Activation of AMPA and KAI receptors is responsible for tactile sensations and, with neurokinin (NK) receptors, the acute response to brief and tonic noxious (painful) sensations. The activation of AMPA and NK receptors is believed to be responsible for signaling the location, intensity, and duration of peripheral stimuli.

◆ NMDA receptors: The activation of ionotropic glutamate NMDA receptors, caused by substantial and prolonged afferent input from Aδ and C fibers, is responsible for the development of slower-onset and longer-lasting pain states. NMDA receptors are involved in long-term potentiation and central (spinal cord) sensitization. Their activation is facilitated by the simultaneous stimulation of substance P–sensitive AMPA and NK receptors, and the removal of magnesium from the NMDA receptor channel.

◆ Metabotropic receptors: Activation of metabotropic glutamate receptors (mGluR) stimulates the production of intracellular second messengers (inositol-1,4,5-triphosphate, DAG, NO), which increase intracellular calcium levels, leading to increases in cellular metabolism, potentiation in synaptic transmission, and alterations in gene expression (central neuroplasticity). Activation of NMDA and mGluR is believed to be responsible for integrating spatial and temporal pain-related events.

◆ GABA and glycine receptors: Activation of GABA and glycine receptors modulates and reduces (inhibits) the effects of excitatory sensory input to the spinal cord.

Spinal Cord Modulation of Sensory Input

The complexity of neural inputs (peripheral, local, ascending, descending) and networks (parallel, converging, diverging) within the spinal cord suggests that sensory homeostasis is maintained by a balance of activity between peripheral nerve inputs and descending excitatory and inhibitory influences from the brain. Although this description may seem overly simplistic, the selective stimulation of peripheral afferent nerve input, the release of local endogenous modulators of synaptic transmission, and the activation of descending inhibitory pathways modify sensory input and the response to a painful stimulus (Table 2-3).

TABLE 2-3	Modulators of Excitatory and Inhibitory Synaptic Transmission
Modulator	**Effect**
EXCITATORY	
γ-Aminobutyric acid	Inhibition
Opioid	Inhibition
Serotonin:	
5-hydroxytryptamine$_1$	Inhibition
5-hydroxytryptamine$_2$	Facilitation
Norepinephrine	Inhibition
Adenosine triphosphate	Facilitation
Tachykinin:	
Substance P	Facilitation
Neurokinin A	Facilitation
Prostanoids	Facilitation
Brain-derived neurotrophic factor	Facilitation
Kainate	Inhibition
INHIBITORY	
Serotonin	Facilitation
Norepinephrine	Facilitation
Acetylcholine	Facilitation
Adenosine	Inhibition

◆ Gate control theory (Fig. 2-5): The idea of a gating mechanism for the transfer of nervous system information was first proposed by Melzack and Wall and suggested that low-threshold Aβ fibers and high-threshold C fibers modulate the activity of inhibitory interneurons located in the spine. Inhibitory interneurons normally reduce the output of spontaneously active projection neurons, which relay sensory information to the brain. Activation of the low-threshold Aβ fibers, which normally transmit nonpainful stimuli, increases inhibitory interneuron effects on projection neurons, thereby reducing the transmission of painful stimuli to the brain.

◆ Endogenous opioids: Painful stimuli can initiate the release of endogenous opioids (e.g., ENK, END, and DYN). These chemicals act at a variety of opioid receptors (μ, δ, κ) to suppress nociceptive responses in the periphery, spinal cord, and brain. One of the effects of these chemicals is to inhibit the release of local excitatory neurotransmitters, including glutamate and substance P.

◆ Modulators of excitatory and inhibitory spinal cord transmission: Excitatory and inhibitory synaptic transmission are modulated in the spinal cord by various neuromodulators. GABA, opioids, serotonin, and norepinephrine inhibit excitatory synaptic transmission, whereas

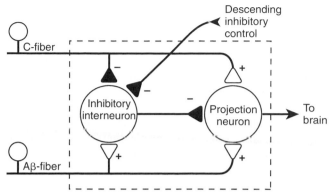

FIG. 2-5. The gate control theory is a simplified view of pain modulation in the central nervous system. Inputs from large myelinated Aβ sensory nerve fibers, which normally transmit innocuous sensory information (touch), activate (+) inhibitory interneurons in the spinal cord, inhibiting projection neurons to the brain. Note that the activation of Aδ and C sensory nerve fibers, which carry noxious inputs, inhibits (–) the inhibitory interneurons.

ATP, substance P, and prostanoids are facilitative. Conversely, serotonin, norepinephrine, and acetylcholine facilitate inhibitory synaptic transmission, and ATP is inhibitory (Table 2-3).

Supraspinal Modulation of Sensory Input

Descending axons of serotoninergic and noradrenergic neurons from the brain synapse with opioid-containing inhibitory interneurons. Once activated by a stressful event (e.g., pain, fear, or hypoxia), opioid-like analgesic effects are produced. Activation of these pathways is thought to be responsible for "stress-induced analgesia." Interestingly and somewhat paradoxically, activation of these same pathways suppresses the release of the inhibitory neurotransmitter GABA from inhibitory interneurons, leading to local disinhibitory effects and a potential increase in pain perception. This latter effect is believed to be more important in chronic pain states.

PROJECTION

Nociceptive information is conveyed to the brain by bundles of neurons (nerve tracts) that originate in the laminae of the dorsal horn. Some controversy exists regarding the relative importance of the various nerve tracts in nociceptive processing, so only the pathways of primary importance are mentioned.

- Spinothalamic tract: The spinothalamic tract is the most prominent ascending nociceptive pathway and originates from laminae I and IV to

VII of the spinal cord. This tract contains axons of nociceptive-specific and wide-dynamic-range neurons, which terminate in the thalamus.

◆ Spinoreticular tract: Spinoreticular tract axons originate at locations similar to those of the spinothalamic tract neurons but terminate in the reticular formation (RF) and the thalamus.

◆ Spinomesencephalic tract: Axons of the spinomesencephalic tract originate in laminae I and V and terminate in the midbrain (periaqueductal gray region, limbic system, hypothalamus).

◆ Spinohypothalamic tract: Axons originating from neurons in laminae III and IV project information to the hypothalamus and ventral forebrain.

PERCEPTION

The integration, processing, and recognition of sensory information (perception) occurs in multiple specific areas of the brain, which communicate via interneurons to produce an integrated response that reflects the coordinated contributions of arousal, somatosensory input, and autonomic and motor output (Fig. 2-6). Somatosensory modalities take specific routes to the brain: the dorsal column–medial lemniscal system and the anterolateral system. The use of several neural pathways (redundancy) to convey information from a specific body part is called *parallel processing* and helps to ensure adequate input to the CNS. Neurons in the dorsal column–medial lemniscal system originate from laminae III, IV, and V; ascend to synapse with neurons in the caudal medulla (brainstem); and relay information concerning tactile sensation, including touch, vibration, and limb proprioception.

◆ The reticular activating system (RAS), located in the brainstem, is a critical center for the integration of these sensory experiences and the subsequent affective and motivational aspects of pain through projections to the medial thalamus and limbic system. The RAS also mediates motor, autonomic, and endocrine responses. The anterolateral system originates from neurons in laminae I and V, which synapse in the RF of the pons and medulla, the midbrain (periaqueductal gray matter [PAG]), and the thalamus. The PAG and thalamus serve as relay points for sensory information transfer: the former transfers information to the thalamus and hypothalamus, and the latter transfers information to the cerebral cortex. The three major pathways of the anterolateral system are the spinothalamic, spinoreticular, and spinomesencephalic tracts (see "Projection"), which are primarily involved in relaying painful and temperature-related sensations.

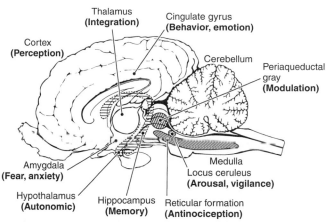

FIG. 2-6. Regions of the brain that are linked to various functions and responses. The thalamus serves as the central integrating and transmission point for pain perception and subsequent responses.

♦ The thalamus relays information to the somatosensory cortex, which in turn projects the information to adjacent cortical association areas, including the limbic system. The limbic system includes the cingulate gyrus (behavior, emotion), amygdala (conditioned fear, anxiety), hippocampus (memory), hypothalamus (sympathetic autonomic activity), and locus ceruleus (arousal, vigilance, behavior; Fig. 2-6). The caudal extension of the limbic system, the PAG, receives descending information from the cortex, amygdala, and hypothalamus and ascending projections from the medulla, RF (including the locus ceruleus), and spinal cord.

♦ The PAG is considered to be an important relay for descending facilitative and inhibitory (endogenous opioid) modulation of nociceptive input. The PAG connects with the rostral ventromedial medulla (RVM) and medullary RF, from which adrenergic and serotoninergic fibers descend to the dorsal horn of the spinal cord, inducing inhibitory or analgesic effects. Descending facilitation from the RVM is thought to be a critical component of many chronic pain states.

♦ Collectively, these centers process sensory information that elicits fear, anxiety, and aggression and activate efferent pathways that mediate autonomic, neuroendocrine, and motor (skeletal and visceral) responses. Furthermore, all of these areas can be conditioned by visual, olfactory, auditory, and somatic or visceral stimuli that prepare the CNS for fearful or stressful (painful) events. The physiologic, biochemical, cellular, and molecular changes that occur in response to stressful or noxious events emphasize the tremendous plasticity of the CNS and highlight the importance of chronic stress in the development of pathologic pain.

MEMORY

The memory of pain is shaped by several factors, including the animal's behavior pattern, the environment, the expectation of pain, and the intensity of painful events. The peak intensity of pain is the single most important factor in determining the memory of pain. *Neuroplasticity* refers to the ability of the nervous system to change or adapt its biochemical and physiologic functions in response to internal and external stimuli (including chronic drug use): the implication is that multiple minor sensory events or a single major sensory event can change the stimulus-response characteristics of the nervous system. Patients who have an inherent memory of pain or of a significant painful event are harder to treat, and those patients in whom pain has been allowed to persist for periods of more than 12 to 24 hours are less responsive to analgesic therapy.

PAIN

Pain has been and remains difficult to define, both in scope and consequence (see Chapter 4). The complexity of its ubiquity is highlighted by the myriad of neurochemical, peripheral, and central neuroanatomic and biochemical events involved in pain production (Table 2-4). Pain is not nociception (the detection of tissue damage by specialized receptors) but is the conscious experience of nociception, which is only partly determined by the stimulus-induced (mechanical, thermal, chemical, electrical) activation of afferent neural pathways. Pain encompasses nociception—the perception of pain, suffering, and pain-related behaviors—and is defined by the International Association for the Study of Pain as "an unpleasant sensory and emotional experience associated with actual or potential tissue damage, or described in terms of such damage." The inability to communicate (verbally or because of altered consciousness) does not negate the fact that pain may exist. Pain can occur in the absence of input from peripheral nociceptors (e.g., phantom limb pain and CNS-induced pain) and depends on but is not limited to somatic and visceral sensory input, conditioned environmental cues, memory, and activity. In other words, pain is a homeostatic mechanism that is not homogenous but represents a continuum of varied physiologic and behavioral responses that are unique to each animal.

TABLE 2-4	Activation and Sensitization of Nociceptors ("Sensitizing Soup")	
Substance	**Origin**	**Effect**
Hydrogen ion	Damaged cells	Activation
Potassium ion	Damaged cells	Activation
Prostaglandins (E$_2$)	Damaged cells	Sensitization
Leukotrienes	Damaged cells	Sensitization
Bradykinin	Plasma	Activation
Serotonin	Platelets, mast cells	Activation
Histamine	Mast cells	Activation
Substance P	Sensory nerve endings	Sensitization
Nerve growth factor	Sensory nerve endings	Sensitization

TAXONOMY

Pain has been categorized based on disease (arthritis, pancreatitis, cancer), anatomy (bladder, pancreatic, back, orthopedic), general location (superficial, visceral, deep), duration (transient, acute, chronic), intensity (mild, moderate, severe), and response to manipulation (palpation, response to commands, algesiometers). Each category attempts to suggest potential causes for pain, its severity, and by association, the most appropriate therapy. Although these categorizations are descriptive, none of these methods identifies the mechanism(s) responsible for pain and therefore provides minimal therapeutic insight. Ultimately, pain should be categorized based on the mechanism(s) responsible for its production. Current conceptual mechanisms include alterations in nociceptive transduction, peripheral sensitization, altered excitability, central sensitization, phenotypic modulation, synaptic reorganization, and disinhibition. As these mechanisms are studied and become better understood, rational pain therapy will follow. Until that time, the best approach to categorizing pain is to understand its evolution from purely physiologic and protective to pathologic and harmful:

◆ Physiologic pain: Pain is frequently referred to as *nociceptive pain* because it depends on the activation of high-threshold peripheral pain receptors (nociceptors) by excessive pressure, heat, cold, chemical, or electrical irritants. This is the type of pain an animal feels when it is pinched, poked, or aggressively palpated or when it briefly comes in contact with a potentially harmful entity. Physiologic or nociceptive pain is highly localized, often transient, serving to warn the body of potential danger or tissue damage. Pain intensity is highly correlated to reflex withdrawal responses. All other types of pain can be considered pathologic or clinical, arising for the most part from tissue (inflammatory) or nerve (neuropathic) damage.

◆ Pathologic pain: Pathologic pain occurs in the presence or absence of a stimulus or in response to innocuous stimuli (allodynia), often producing an exaggerated (hyperalgesia) and prolonged (hyperpathia) response. The acute form of pathologic pain, like physiologic pain, serves a protective function leading to disuse, rest and recuperation, guarding, and avoidance, thereby minimizing further injury and promoting repair processes (Fig. 2-7). Exaggerated (extensive trauma) or prolonged (chronic) pain has significant impact on an animal's quality of life far exceeding any protective role and disrupts homeostasis, initiating pathophysiologic changes and considerable suffering and producing abnormal and unexpected behaviors that may contribute to the clinical decision to euthanize an animal (Table 2-5). Abnormal (reluctance to move, lack of interaction) or unexpected behaviors (aggression) are common in spite of or because of the administration of analgesic drugs, emphasizing the need for careful evaluation before selection of the appropriate analgesic therapy.

◆ Aggression or escape behaviors are recognized as one of the most common abnormal behaviors in dogs and cats and can be induced by pain and many drugs used to produce analgesia and sedation (release of suppressed behavior). Aggression is particularly common in dogs and cats when they are frightened and experiencing pain and during the postoperative period. During this time the clinician or veterinary technician must be particularly astute in identifying abnormal behavior and determining whether it is pain-related, thereby facilitating appropriate therapy and avoiding unnecessary drug administration.

PAINFUL SENSATIONS

Although truly rational therapeutic approaches cannot be developed until most, if not all, of the specific mechanisms responsible for physiologic and pathologic pain are known, the use of simple yet detailed pain scoring systems can help categorize the intensity, duration, and topography of pain, thereby suggesting potential treatments or the benefits of treatment (see Chapter 6). Pain scoring systems, however, are of little value in suggesting therapy until the evaluator has a general understanding of the physiologic and pathophysiologic processes involved in the production of pain (Box 2-2). An understanding of these processes implies an understanding of the reasons for tissue hypersensitivity, peripheral sensitization, primary and secondary hyperalgesia, central sensitization, allodynia, spontaneous and referred pain, and the differences between somatic and visceral pain. All of these changes modify the gain of the system and can lead to CNS modification and

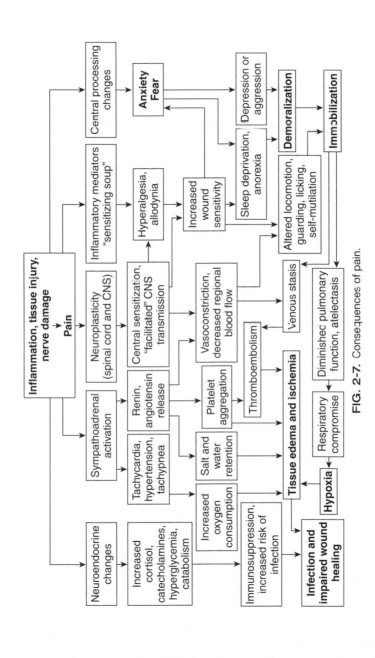

FIG. 2-7. Consequences of pain.

TABLE 2-5	Pathophysiologic Consequences of Pain
Source of Pain	**Symptoms**
Cardiovascular	Tachycardia, hypertension, vasoconstriction, increased cardiac work and oxygen consumption
Pulmonary	Hypoxia, hypercarbia, atelectasis; decreased cough; ventilation/perfusion mismatch, predisposition to pulmonary infection
Gastrointestinal	Nausea, vomiting, ileus
Renal	Oliguria, urine retention
Extremities	Skeletal muscle pain, limited mobility, thromboembolism
Endocrine	Vagal inhibition; increased adrenergic activity, increased metabolism, increased oxygen consumption
Central nervous system	Anxiety, fear, sedation, fatigue
Immunologic	Impairment

BOX 2-2

Mechanisms Responsible for Prolonged and Exaggerated Pain

- Peripheral sensitization (inflammatory soup)
- "Windup" (temporal summation of sensory inputs)
- Central sensitization
- Increased sympathetic innervation and excitation of dorsal root ganglion
- Disinhibition of inhibitory modulation of sensory inputs
- Redistribution of Aβ inputs from laminae III and IV to lamina II
- Abnormal patterns of spinal cord interneuronal communication
- Altered phenotype of damaged sensory nerve fibers
- Abnormal patterns of peripheral nerve regeneration after trauma

---

phenotypic (physical characteristics) changes. To rephrase an often-quoted saying, "No gain, no pain."

◆ Pain is produced by activation of functionally specialized Aδ and C nerve terminal nociceptors, which transduce noxious stimuli dependent on distinct thermal, mechanical, chemical, and electrical thresholds. The free nerve endings of these afferent pain-processing fibers encode noxious stimuli, depending on the modality, intensity, duration, and location of the stimulus.

◆ The intensity of the stimulus that produces pain is considerably greater than that required to elicit innocuous sensations and is the most important factor in determining the severity of pain. Intensity can be quantitatively defined by a stimulus intensity-response relationship similar to that of other somatosensations (Fig. 2-2).

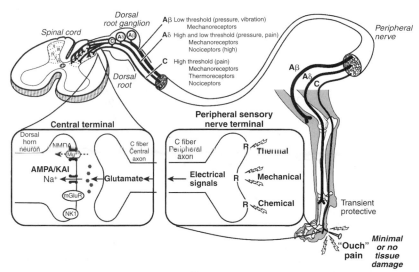

FIG. 2-8. Physiologic pain: Non–tissue-damaging stimuli activate peripheral pain receptors (nociceptors; *R*), which produce electrical signals that are transmitted by Aδ and C sensory nerve fibers to the spinal cord and brain. Glutamate is the primary neurotransmitter released at the nerve terminal in the spinal cord (central terminals). Glutamate primarily activates α-amino-3-hydroxy-5-methyl-4-isoxazole propionic acid/kainate, producing transient or temporary ("ouch") pain.

♦ In the absence of tissue damage, nociceptor-mediated pain is considered to be physiologic, warning the animal of potentially harmful stimuli (Fig. 2-8). Most pathologic pain occurs after tissue or nerve damage and, as stated previously, has been clinically categorized as inflammatory or neuropathic.

♦ Pathologic pain is caused by tissue damage or alterations in the physiology or anatomy of the sensory nervous system. The temporal aspects of pathologic pain continuously change (dynamic plasticity) and are characterized by a reduction in the intensity of the stimulus required to initiate pain (hypersensitivity) and a leftward shift in the stimulus-response curve (Fig. 2-9). The development of tissue hypersensitivity (nociceptive sensitization) is responsible for allodynia, hyperalgesia, and hyperpathia.

PERIPHERAL SENSITIZATION

Peripheral sensitization is produced by neurochemical alterations caused by tissue damage and inflammation at the site of injury and in the immediately surrounding tissues, resulting in hyperalgesia at the site of injury (primary hyperalgesia). The release and activation of intracellular components from damaged cells, inflammatory cells (lymphocytes, neutrophils, mast

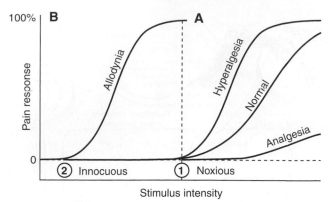

FIG. 2-9. The normal stimulus intensity-pain response curve is shown **(A)**. Increased responsiveness to a given stimulus that shifts the curve to the left is termed *hyperalgesia*. A decrease in the response to a given stimulus that shifts the curve to the right or flattens the curve is termed *analgesia* or *anesthesia*. A large left shift in the curve such that innocuous stimuli begin to elicit a painful response **(B)** is termed *allodynia*.

cells, macrophages), postganglionic sympathetic efferent nerve terminals, and the primary nerve fiber itself excite and increase the sensitivity of peripheral nociceptors (Table 2-5). Direct tissue damage results in the local release and spread of ATP, ions (H^+, K^+), prostaglandins, bradykinin, and nerve growth factors. Lymphocytes, neutrophils, and macrophages release cytokines (interleukin-1 [IL-1], IL-6, and tumor necrosis factor α). Mast cell degranulation increases the local concentration of 5-hydroxytryptamine (serotonin) and histamine. Sympathetic nerve fibers release substances (catecholamines, neuropeptide Y) that potentiate inflammatory mediators that amplify the local inflammatory response. Primary afferent sensory nerve fibers release neuropeptides (substance P, CGRP) that cause degranulation of mast cells, local vasodilation, and plasma extravasation, resulting in a further amplification of the inflammatory response and a spread of hypersensitivity to surrounding tissues (secondary hyperalgesia). Together these substances produce a "sensitizing soup," which changes high-threshold nociceptors to low-threshold nociceptors and activates the "sleeping" or silent nociceptors (10% to 40% of the total nociceptor population) found in joints and visceral and cutaneous tissues, amplifying the pain response (Fig. 2-10).

CENTRAL SENSITIZATION

Central sensitization is produced by a change in the excitability of neurons in the spinal cord and/or activation of spinal cord glial cells and contributes to primary hyperalgesia. Central sensitization is responsible for

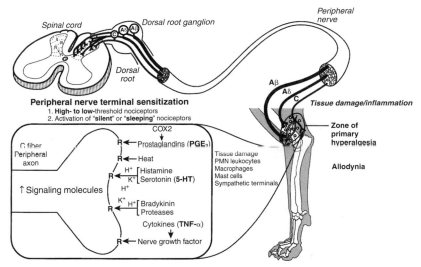

FIG. 2-10. Peripheral sensitization: Inflammation and tissue damage produce a variety of nociceptor-sensitizing substances, including prostaglandins, histamine, serotonin, bradykinin, proteases, cytokines (tumor necrosis factor α), and nerve growth factor. This "sensitizing soup" lowers the nociceptor threshold to painful stimuli and activates "silent" or "sleeping" nociceptors, resulting in hyperalgesia and allodynia.

pain hypersensitivity outside the area of primary hyperalgesia (secondary hyperalgesia, extraterritorial pain). Mild, infrequent, noxious stimuli generate fast excitatory potentials within the CNS (spinal cord, brainstem, and brain) that indicate the onset, duration, intensity, and location of the painful stimulus (Box 2-2). This fast excitatory transmission is transmitted by Aδ and C fibers and is mediated by glutamate acting on AMPA and KAI ligand-gated ion channels within the dorsal horn of the spinal cord. The sensory input is focused by descending activation of inhibitory neurons that co-release glycine and GABA, two CNS inhibitory neurotransmitters. Frequent (chronic) or severe peripheral nociceptor input initiated by inflammation or tissue damage, by contrast, results in the central release of neuroexcitatory substances (substance P, neurokinin A, CGRP) including glutamate, which activates NMDA (removes the magnesium block), neurokinin, and mGluR receptors. The temporal and spatial summation ("windup") of neuroexcitatory input from noxious stimuli produces a prolonged sensitization (long-term potentiation) of neurons in the dorsal horn of the spinal cord. Sensitization of dorsal horn neurons can last for hours and is believed to be responsible for increases in the receptive field properties (spatial, threshold, temporal, modality), secondary hyperalgesia, and allodynia (Fig. 2-11). Decreases in phasic and tonic inhibition from higher CNS centers and a loss of segmental inhibitory interneurons in the dorsal horn can also contribute to dorsal horn hyperexcitability, resulting in the perception of pain from otherwise innocuous stimuli carried by Aβ nerve fibers (receptive field plasticity). Nerve cell injury can also stimulate the growth of the central terminals of low-threshold mechanoreceptors (Aβ fibers), which normally terminate in lamina IV. Their infiltration into lamina II, the location of C-fiber terminals, produces an anatomic substrate for tactile pain hypersensitivity and spontaneous pain.

◆ Central sensitization is fundamentally different from peripheral sensitization in that it enables low-intensity stimuli and low-threshold Aβ sensory fibers to produce pain as a result of changes in sensory processing in the spinal cord.

◆ Central sensitization, phenotypic switches, and disinhibition are responsible for increases in the responsiveness of dorsal horn neurons to sensory input (allodynia), receptive field plasticity, continued pain even after amputation (phantom limb pain), and the discomfort and agony experienced by severely injured patients and patients with chronic diseases.

◆ Windup, central sensitization, and the development of a structurally reorganized hyperactive CNS represent a continuum of the pain process, which exists as a consequence of continuous, unrelenting, and untreated pain.

◆ The development of central sensitization within the CNS and, more specifically, the brain may be responsible for memory patterns, or at least the modification of memory. Continued noxious stimuli lasting longer than several hours result in the up-regulation of immediate-early genes (c-fos, c-jun), which are regulated by the cyclic adenosine monophosphate response element-binding protein and are responsible for activity-dependent plasticity and long-term structural changes (neuroplastic) within the CNS.

VISCERAL PAIN

Nociceptive-specific fibers do not appear to be present in the viscera. Visceral afferent painful stimuli originating from visceral organs (e.g., gut, liver, spleen, kidney, and bladder) are transmitted by Aδ and C fibers that travel along sympathetic and parasympathetic pathways. Parasympathetic, principally vagal, and splanchnic afferent nerve fibers are also responsible for transmitting noxious inputs from visceral organs, including the distal colon (rectum) and bladder. This difference (transmission by sympathetic and parasympathetic pathways) means that most inputs coming from

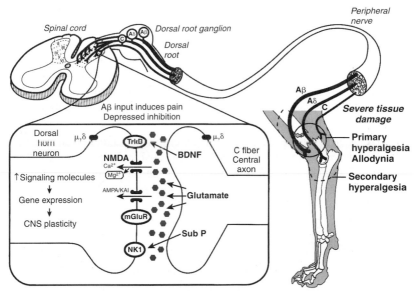

FIG. 2-11. Central sensitization: Severe (high-intensity) or chronic painful stimuli activate C fibers, causing the release of glutamate, substance P (*Sub P*), and brain-derived neurotrophic factor (*BDNF*) at central nerve terminals; this results in the activation of α-amino-3-hydroxy-5-methyl-4-isoxazole propionic acid/ kainate, N-methyl-D-aspartate, neurokinin, and Trk B receptors, producing acute and long-lasting dull, aching, burning pain sensations. Collectively, the activation of these receptors increases the activity of a host of signaling molecules that alter gene expression and change the responsiveness (sensitize) of the central nervous system to subsequent input. Chronic painful stimulation may result in neurochemical changes (neuroplasticity) in the spinal cord such that all stimuli produce pain.

viscera may not be perceived. Local clamping, burning (cautery), and cutting generally produce no pain when applied to visceral structures. Generalized or diffuse inflammation, ischemia, and mesenteric stretching or dilation (e.g., gastric dilatation-volvulus), however, produce severe unrelenting pain associated with a significant sympathetic component (tachycardia, tachypnea). Inflammation and tissue damage are also known to activate a large population of "silent" nociceptors in the gut and bladder, which produce mechanosensitivity in response to otherwise innocuous smooth muscle contractile activity.

- ◆ Visceral nociception is much more responsive to κ-opioid receptor agonists. The systemic and local administration of the κ-opioid receptor agonist butorphanol may be more effective in treating visceral (colonic, urinary bladder) pain (milligram/milligram basis) than morphine, a classic μ-opioid agonist.

- Visceral afferent nerve fibers are important in modulating the enteric nervous system, including the gastroesophageal, duodenogastric, colonogastric, rectocolonic, peritoneogastrointestinal, and voiding reflex loops.
- Reflex regulation of visceral structures also includes motor-secretory and motor-vascular reflexes triggered by extrinsic innervation and axon reflexes, extraspinal and spinal pathways, and splanchnovagal and vagovagal pathways.
- Vagal afferent fibers terminate in the brainstem. The nucleus tractus solitarius is the major projection site for vagal and splanchnic afferent inputs, and the dorsal motor nucleus of the vagus nerve also plays a role in the integration of sensory information passing to the PAG and thalamus.

REFERRED PAIN

As the name implies, referred pain is pain (tenderness, allodynia, and hyperalgesia) that is felt in uninjured, intact tissues remote from the presumed causative lesion. Referred pain develops slowly, is generally triggered by deep somatic and visceral rather than superficial injury, and conforms to the "dermatomal rule," whereby pain is often referred to regions derived from the same dermatome. The best examples of referred pain are those associated with stimulation of the visceral afferent nerve fibers and the referral of pain to muscles, tendons, and joints in the same dermatome. Potential explanations for referred pain include (1) the peripheral branching of primary sensory nerve fibers to cutaneous and deep tissues or the branching of primary sensory nerve fibers to an injured and uninjured area, (2) the activation of primary sensory nerve fibers that project to both (left and right) dorsal horns of the spinal cord, and (3) the convergence of primary sensory nerve fibers from different tissue beds on the same population of dorsal horn neurons. The latter explanations emphasize a potential central mechanism as a cause for referred pain and the potentiation of reflexes from remote tissue regions.

MEMORY OF PAIN

In human beings, the perception and memory of pain correlates strongly with the peak intensity of pain but, interestingly, not with its duration. "In primitive life forms whose genome we have inherited, memory subserves only nociception." Furthermore, pain is more likely to occur and be more severe in patients who have a history of injury, suggesting that injury produces CNS neurochemical changes that influence nociceptive behavior. The same types of biologic processes and genetic modifications are known to occur in animals in response to painful stimuli. Furthermore, if painful stimuli establish the memory of pain, then therapies that prevent central sensitization and the neuroplastic changes that occur should be beneficial in maintaining or restoring normal pain sensitivity. This argument is the basis for preventing pain from being perceived and the practice of "preemptive" analgesia, in which analgesic therapy is administered before a painful event with the goal of preventing or reducing subsequent pain and analgesic requirements. Once hyperexcitability (central sensitization) is established, large doses of analgesic agents are required to treat pain or the therapy becomes ineffective. In other words, all pain should be treated as early as possible and preemptively when possible.

CONCLUSION

The mechanisms responsible for the production and maintenance of pain continue to unravel. Sensory nerve endings and the nervous system transduce and transmit sensations to the brain. Alternative mechanisms regarding pain perception, however, are emerging and suggest that pain can be elicited by the production of inflammatory molecules that travel to the brain through the bloodstream ("humoral" signaling). These molecules increase the concentration of inflammatory signaling molecules in the brain (IL-1β), leading to the enhanced expression of cyclooxygenase-2 and prostaglandin E synthase (two prominent pain inducers) in the cerebrospinal fluid and enhanced pain response and hypersensitivity. The blood-borne inflammatory molecules remain unknown but provide fertile ground for the continued exploration of mechanisms that initiate and transmit painful events and suggest new avenues for the development of pain therapies. Understanding the mechanisms responsible for pain is the basis for rational and effective pain therapies.

REFERENCE

1. Melzack R, Wall PD: Pain mechanisms: a new theory, *Science* 150:971-979, 1965.

SUGGESTED READINGS

Byers MR, Bonica JJ: Peripheral pain mechanisms and nociceptor plasticity. In Loeser JD, Butler SH, Chapman CR et al, editors: *Bonica's management of pain*, ed 3, Philadelphia, 2001, Lippincott Williams & Wilkins.

Craig AD: Interoception: the sense of the physiological condition of the body, *Curr Opin Neurobiol* 13:500-505, 2003.

Dray A: Inflammatory mediators of pain, *Br J Anaesth* 75:125-131, 1995.

Fields HL, Basbaum AI: Central nervous system mechanisms of pain modulation. In Wall PD, Melzack R, editors: *Textbook of pain*, ed 4, Edinburgh, 1999, Churchill Livingstone.

Fields HL, Heinricher MM, Mason P: Neurotransmitters in nociceptive modulatory circuits, *Annu Rev Neurosci* 14:219-245, 1991.

Kandel ER: Nerve cells and behavior. In Kandel ER, Schwartz JH, Jessel TM, editors: *Principles of neural science*, ed 3, Norwalk, Conn, 1991, Appleton & Lange.

Koltzenburg M: The changing sensitivity in the life of the nociceptor, *Pain Suppl* 6:S93-S102, 1999.

Levine JD, Reichling DB: Peripheral mechanisms of inflammatory pain. In Wall PD, Melzack R, editors: *Textbook of pain*, ed 4, Edinburgh, 1999, Churchill Livingstone.

Maier SF, Watkins LR: Cytokines for psychologists: implications of bidirectional immune-to-brain communication for understanding behavior, mood, and cognition, *Psychol Rev* 105:83-107, 1998.

Melzack R, Wall PD: Pain mechanisms: a new theory, *Science* 150:971-979, 1965.

Milan MJ: The induction of pain: an integrative review, *Prog Neurobiol* 57:1-164, 1999.

Muir WW 3rd, Woolf CJ: Mechanisms of pain and their therapeutic implications, *J Am Vet Med Assoc* 219:1346-1356, 2001.

Raja SN, Meyer RA, Ringkamp M et al: Peripheral neural mechanisms of nociceptor. In Wall PD, Melzack R, editors: *Textbook of pain*, ed 4, Edinburgh, 1999, Churchill Livingstone.

Rexed B: The cytoarchitectonic organization of the spinal cord in the cat, *J Comp Neurol* 96:415-466, 1952.

Ru-Rong J, Woolf CJ: Neuronal plasticity and signal transduction in nociceptive neurons: implications for the initiation and maintenance of pathological pain, *Neurobiol Dis* 8:1-10, 2001.

Sandkuhler J: The organization and function of endogenous antinociceptive systems, *Prog Neurobiol* 50:49-81, 1996.

Snider WD, McMahon SB: Tackling pain at the source: new ideas about nociceptors, *Neuron* 20:629-632, 1998.

Watkins LR, Milligan ED, Maier SF: Glial activation: a driving force for pathological pain, *Trends Neurosci* 24:450-455, 2001.

Willert RP, Woolf CJ, Hobson AR et al: The development and maintenance of human visceral pain hypersensitivity is dependent on the N-methyl-D-aspartate, *Gastroenterology* 126:683-692, 2004.

Willis WD, Coggeshall RE: *Sensory mechanisms of the spinal cord*, New York, 1991, Plenum Press.

Willis AD, Westlund KN: Neuroanatomy of the pain system and of the pathways that modulate pain, *J Clin Neurophysiol* 14:2-31, 1997.

Woolf CJ: Pain: moving from symptom control towards mechanism-specific pharmacologic management, *Ann Intern Med* 140:441-451, 2004.

Woolf CJ, Chong M: Preemptive analgesia: treating postoperative pain by preventing the establishment of central sensitization, *Anesth Analg* 77: 362-379, 1993.

Woolf CJ, Costigan M: Transcriptional and posttranslational plasticity and the generation of inflammatory pain, *Proc Natl Acad Sci U S A* 96: 7723-7730, 1999.

Woolf CJ, Salter MW: Neuronal plasticity: increasing the gain in pain, *Science* 288:1765-1768, 2000.

Yaksh TL: Spinal systems and pain processing: development of novel analgesic drugs with mechanistically defined models, *Trends Pharmacol Sci* 20: 329-337, 1999.

3

PAIN AND STRESS

WILLIAM W. MUIR III

Animal well-being should include the "five freedoms": freedom from hunger and malnutrition, freedom from discomfort, freedom from disease, freedom from injury, and freedom from pain (Box 3-1). Stress is the biologic response that an animal exhibits when homeostasis is threatened. Stress occurs when animals perceive a threat. Conscious (e.g., physical restraint or pain) and unconscious (e.g., pain caused by surgery) stressors can elicit stress. Historically, most authors have concerned themselves with the response of the body to injury and surgical trauma. The role of the central nervous system (CNS) in modifying the response of the body to various stressors (e.g., pain, surgery, restraint, and confinement) varies among and within species and can be modified by domestication and training. Auditory and visual stimuli produce and potentiate somatosensory input to the CNS, eliciting systemic responses identical to those produced by tissue trauma. This input can modify the animal's memory, evoking predictable behavioral changes characterized by startle, fear, an attempt to escape, aggression (fight or flight), or submission. Dogs and cats, like all animals, respond to stressors by exhibiting one or more biologic defense mechanisms targeted toward avoiding injury and maintaining homeostasis. Stress then serves a protective role of diverting the biologic resources of the body to cope with the stressor. Normally, bodily homeostatic mechanisms function to maintain a continual internal state of well-being. Ineffective responses to stress, particularly stress caused by trauma, results in dysfunction, disability, disease (systemic inflammatory response), distress, and suffering, collectively constituting a "sickness syndrome" that hastens death (Fig. 3-1).

Whether animals perceive pain and suffer in the same way that human beings do is uncertain because of differences in their ability to comprehend pain and the potential for impending doom. Most

> ### BOX 3-1
> ### The Five Freedoms
>
> Freedom from thirst, hunger, and malnutrition
> - Access to fresh water and a healthful diet
>
> Freedom from discomfort
> - Suitable environment, shelter, and a resting place
>
> Freedom from pain, injury, and disease
> - Prevention of cruelty and illness by care and rapid treatment
>
> Freedom to express normal behavior
> - Provision of space, facilities, and company of the animal's own kind
>
> Freedom from fear and distress
> - Assurance of conditions that avoid stress and mental suffering

animals are aware of the present with little or no regard for the past or future; they live in "the now." Animals do not comprehend death. The animal's health and interaction with its environment and ongoing external events determine its well-being. These processes incorporate feeling, perceiving, and awareness and are the simplest of the cognitive processes. In other words, if an animal perceives an event as threatening, its responses will be the same, whether the event is threatening or not. Everyone at some time has probably witnessed the "fight or flight" response in a dog or cat put in a new environment, whether the environment was threatening or not. Therefore, it is ethical and humane to minimize animal stress because all animals react adversely to real or perceived threats or life-threatening events. Pain normally serves a protective function by warning the animal of real or impending tissue damage. Acute and chronic pain are capable of producing stress, and when severe, can be responsible for dramatic increases in neuroendocrine activity, temporary periods of "stress-induced analgesia," and profound behavioral changes. Even without a painful stimulus, environmental factors (e.g., environment, loud noise, restraint, and predators) can produce a state of anxiety or fear that sensitizes and amplifies the stress response to a painful stimulus. Distress, an exaggerated form of stress, is present when the biologic cost of stress negatively affects biologic functions critical to the animal's well-being. Therefore, pain should be thought of in terms of the magnitude of the stress response that it produces, its potential to produce distress, and the degree of animal suffering incurred. In practical terms, the severity and duration of pain determine the consequences of the patient's pain on the continuum of stress and suffering.

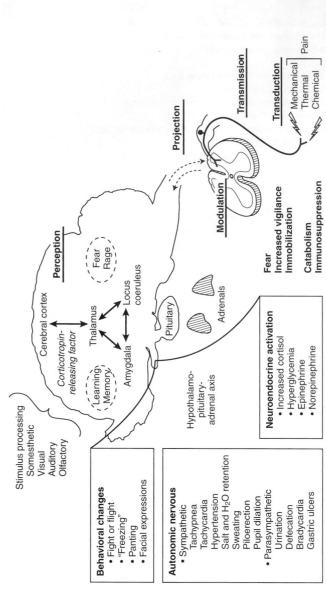

FIG. 3-1. Stress response: Activation of the neural circuits (transduction, transmission, modulation, projection, perception) responsible for producing pain stimulates the thalamus, locus ceruleus (*LC*), and amygdala, which induce fear, anxiety, and rage in animals, resulting in behavioral, autonomic, and neuroendocrine changes. Acute pain often produces fear, increased vigilance, and immobilization ("freezing" stance) in some animals, and chronic unrelenting pain can lead to loss of appetite, tissue catabolism, and immunosuppression and can alter learning patterns and memory.

DEFINING TERMS

PAIN

Pain is often defined as "an unpleasant sensory and emotional experience associated with actual or potential tissue damage or described in terms of such damage" (see Chapter 4). Pain produces physical or physiologic changes that are exhibited as mild behavioral discomfort or distress to acute, often unbearable, agony. Pain may be diffuse or localized and usually produces a desire to avoid, escape, or destroy (autonomy) the factors responsible for its production. Untreated or prolonged pain promotes an extended and destructive stress response, characterized by neuroendocrine dysregulation, fatigue, dysphoria, myalgia, abnormal behavior, and altered physical performance.

STRESS

Stress is the animal's biologic response to factors that disrupt or threaten homeostasis. A stressor is a physical, chemical, or emotional factor (e.g., trauma or fear) to which the animal fails to make a satisfactory adaptation and that causes physiologic tensions that can contribute to causes of disease.

DISTRESS

Distress is the state produced when the biologic cost of stress negatively affects biologic functions critical to the animal's well-being. Distress also means to cause pain or suffering or to make miserable.

SUFFERING

Suffering is defined as a perception or feeling of impending destruction or harm; the endurance of or submission to physical or mental stress, pain, or loss.

BIOLOGIC COMPONENTS OF THE STRESS RESPONSE

The stress response is an adaptive pattern of behavioral, neural, endocrine, immune, hematologic, and metabolic changes directed toward the restoration of homeostasis (Box 3-2).

Most stress is short-lived because of the removal of or short duration of exposure to the stressor. The nature, magnitude, and duration of the

---

BOX 3-2

Biologic Stress Response

- Behavioral
- Autonomic nervous system
- Neuroendocrine
- Immunologic
- Hematologic
- Metabolic
- Morphologic

---

specific stimulus are important factors in determining the magnitude and extent of the adaptive responses elicited in the animal. Manipulation of a dog's hip joint or physical restraint of a cat, for example, generally elicits only a brief stress response. During more threatening circumstances, the stress response prepares the animal for emergency situations and fosters survival in threatening circumstances (fight or flight). Acute pain is capable of producing a significant stress response in dogs and cats. Pain induced by surgical or accidental trauma evokes responses characterized by activation of the sympathetic nervous system, secretion of glucocorticoids (primarily cortisol), hypermetabolism, sodium and water retention, and altered carbohydrate and protein metabolism (Box 3-3). When stress is severe or allowed to continue for an extended time, it becomes maladaptive, producing distress and triggering self-sustaining neural and endocrine cascades that upset homeostasis. Severe pain produces behavioral, autonomic, neuroendocrine, and immunologic responses that are responsible for self-mutilation, immune incompetence, and a "sickness syndrome" that can culminate in death. Prior experience (memory) and current physical status (health, pain state) play an important role in determining the animal's adaptive and behavioral responses.

BEHAVIORAL INDICATORS OF STRESS AND PAIN

Pain is a stressor and is responsible for changes in brain chemistry (neural plasticity) resulting in behavioral modifications, the level of alertness, learning performance, and memory (Box 3-4). Intense stimulation of sensory (somatosensory, visual, acoustic) inputs to the brain activates the locus ceruleus (LC), limbic regions (e.g., hypothalamus, hippocampus, and amygdala), and cerebral cortex, which together are involved in

---

BOX 3-3

Systemic Effects of the Stress Response

- Activation of central nervous system
    Hypothalamus, amygdala, locus ceruleus
- Increases in central nervous system sympathetic output
    Catecholamines
- Endocrine "stress" response
    Pituitary hormone secretion
    Adrenal hormone secretion
- Glucosemia
- Insulin resistance
- Cytokine production
- Acute-phase reaction
- Neutrophil leukocytosis
- Immunologic and hematologic changes

BOX 3-4

Behavioral Indicators of Stress and Pain

- Activity
- Aggression
- Appearance
- Appetite
- Attitude
- Facial expression
- Locomotion
- Posture
- Response to handling
- Vocalization

---

adaptive responses to stress. Stress as mild as a cat being confronted by a dog, for example, can double or triple neuronal activity, leading to concurrent activation of a "stress response" and behavioral changes. Pain-induced increases in the concentration of corticotropin-releasing factor (CRF) in the hypothalamus, amygdala, and LC, for example, result in an increased startle response, anxiety, fear, and in some animals, rage. Therefore, CRF serves as an excitatory neurotransmitter in the LC, resulting in the release of adrenocorticotropic hormone (ACTH), cortical norepinephrine, dopamine, and 5-hydroxytryptamine and hyperresponsiveness, hyperarousal, vigilance, and agitation. Prolonged stress impairs the animal's ability to learn and can change the animal's behavior.

Pain in dogs and cats is frequently indicated by changes in behavior (see Chapter 5). Lameness, for example, is an obvious indicator of acute pain or chronic injury. Observation of changes in a dog's or cat's behavior may be the most noninvasive and promising method for determining the severity of an animal's pain and associated stress.

AUTONOMIC NERVOUS SYSTEM

Activation of the sympathetic nervous system is one of the principal effects initiated by stress. Sensory activation of the hypothalamus results in graded increases in CNS sympathetic output, resulting in increases in heart rate and arterial blood pressure, sweating, piloerection, and pupil dilation. The secretion of cortisol by the adrenal cortex and catecholamines from the adrenal medulla and the spillover of norepinephrine from postganglionic sympathetic nerve terminals augment central effects.

NEUROENDOCRINE AXIS

The neuroendocrine axis can be defined as the biologic interface for afferent sensory input and humoral communication between the CNS and the peripheral glands or organs that are responsible for mobilizing the stress response (Fig. 3-2). Auditory, visual, and somatosensory afferent sensory information is transmitted to the thalamus or directly to the amygdala, activating the hypothalamo-pituitary-adrenocortical (HPA) system axis (Table 3-1). This afferent information stimulates the secretion of CRF and vasoactive intestinal peptide (VIP), which in turn stimulates the pituitary gland to release ACTH, melanocortin, prolactin, vasopressin, thyroid-stimulating hormone (TSH), and growth hormone (GH). The metabolic consequences of these hormonal changes are increased catabolism, the mobilization of substrates to provide energy for tissue repair, and salt and water retention to maintain fluid volume and cardiovascular homeostasis. CRF, ACTH, and corticosterone are significant modulators of learning and memory processes.

RELEASE OF CORTICOTROPIN-RELEASING FACTOR IN THE BRAIN

The release of CRF in the brain is one of the major components of the stress response, if not the most important. CRF acts synergistically with vasopressin to stimulate the production of ACTH and β-endorphin, thereby enhancing cell survival and producing analgesic effects, respectively. CRF also stimulates the adrenomedullary release of ACTH and catecholamines. CRF is an excitatory neurotransmitter

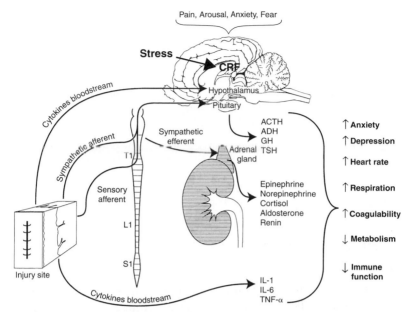

FIG. 3-2. Acute surgical stimulation initiates the release of cytokines (interleukin1, interleukin-6, tumor necrosis factor α) into the bloodstream and activation of the hypothalamo-pituitary-adrenocorticol (*HPA*) system axis and sympathetic nervous system. Activation of hypothalamus and pituitary releases adrenocorticotropic hormone (*ACTH*), vasopressin (or antidiuretic hormone [*ADH*]), growth hormone (*GH*), and thyroid-stimulating hormone (*TSH*). Sympathetic nervous system activation initiates the release of epinephrine, norepinephrine, cortisol, aldosterone, and renin. Together these changes can alter hemodynamics, which elevates heart rate; increase the coagulability of blood, predisposing to thrombosis; increase metabolism and caloric requirements; and when exaggerated, depress immune function.

in the brain, producing increased cortical norepinephrine release and excitation.

ADRENOCORTICOTROPIC HORMONE

ACTH release is stimulated by CRF, catecholamines, vasopressin, and VIP. The primary function of ACTH is to stimulate the adrenal cortex to secrete cortisol, corticosterone, aldosterone, and androgenic substances. ACTH also stimulates the adrenomedullary secretion of catecholamines. ACTH, cortisol, and epinephrine levels are increased during emergence from anesthesia without surgery, suggesting that anesthesia alone can induce a stress response in animals.

TABLE 3-1	Neurohumoral Response to Stress	
Endocrine Gland	**Hormone**	**Change**
Pituitary	Adrenocorticotropic hormone	Increase
	Growth hormone	Increase
	Vasopressin	Increase
	Thyroid-stimulating hormone	Increase or decrease
Adrenal cortex	Cortisol	Increase
	Aldosterone	Increase
	Catecholamines	Increase
Pancreas	Insulin	Often decreases
	Glucagon	Increase
Thyroid	Thyroxine	Decrease

CORTISOL

Serum cortisol concentration is an indicator of the severity of stress in most species. The mortality rate is increased in animals that are not able to increase serum cortisol concentrations. Etomidate, an injectable hypnotic recommended for anesthesia in high-risk cases, is known to increase the mortality rate in very ill human patients because it suppresses serum cortisol concentrations. Cortisol stimulates gluconeogenesis, increases proteolysis and lipolysis, facilitates catecholamine effects, and produces antiinflammatory actions.

CATECHOLAMINES

Serum concentrations of norepinephrine, epinephrine, and dopamine are increased by CRF. Epinephrine causes glycogenolysis, gluconeogenesis, inhibition of insulin release, peripheral insulin resistance, and lipolysis. The release of these catecholamines can be responsible for elevations in heart rate, respiratory rate, arterial blood pressure, and cardiac output. Increases in skeletal muscle blood flow prepare the animal for fight or flight.

GLUCAGON AND INSULIN

Endogenous endorphins, GH, epinephrine, and glucocorticoids are capable of stimulating glucagon and insulin (β-adrenergic effect) secretion by the pancreas. More typically, however, surgical procedures increase glucagon secretion and decrease (α_2 effect) insulin secretion, leading to hepatic glycogenolysis, gluconeogenesis from amino acids, glucosemia, and glucosuria.

OTHER HORMONES

A variety of other hormones, including GH, TSH, and vasopressin, act together to protect cellular function and restore homeostasis.

Growth Hormone

GH stimulates protein synthesis and inhibits protein breakdown, promotes lipolysis, and produces antiinsulin effects. GH spares glucose for use by the nervous system.

Thyroid Hormones

Thyroxine and triiodothyronine are secreted into the systemic circulation from the thyroid gland during stimulation by TSH. Thyroid hormones stimulate carbohydrate metabolism and heat production and increase and sensitize β-adrenergic receptors in the heart, thereby sensitizing it to the effects of circulating catecholamines.

Vasopressin

Vasopressin, also known as the *antidiuretic hormone,* promotes water retention. Production and release of vasopressin into the systemic circulation in conjunction with increased concentrations of renin (sympathetic effect) increase the circulating blood volume, vascular tone, and vascular responsiveness, thereby improving cardiovascular homeostasis.

METABOLISM

The net effect of the majority of the neurohumoral changes produced is an increase in the secretion of catabolic hormones, promoting the production of food substrates from the breakdown of carbohydrates, fats, and proteins.

CARBOHYDRATE METABOLISM

Hyperglycemia is produced and may persist because of the production of glucagon and relative lack of insulin, although insulin levels may periodically increase. Pain can be responsible for increases in blood glucose, which is known to be associated with an increased incidence of wound infection, morbidity, and mortality.

FAT METABOLISM

Lipolytic activity is stimulated by cortisol, catecholamines, and GH, resulting in an increase in circulating glycerol and free fatty acids. Glycerol in turn serves as a source for gluconeogenesis in the liver.

PROTEIN METABOLISM

Protein catabolism is a common occurrence and a major concern after severe trauma or extensive surgical procedures. Cortisol increases protein catabolism, resulting in the release of amino acids. These amino acids can be used to form new proteins and to produce glucose and other substrates. Protein supplementation (e.g., glutamine and arginine) during and after surgery results in fewer infections and shorter overall recovery time. Prostaglandins (PGs; e.g., PGE_2) and cytokines may promote protein catabolism indirectly by increasing the energy expenditure of the body.

IMMUNE SYSTEM

Although the immune system is primarily thought of in relation to the identification and destruction of foreign substances, it also functions as a diffusely distributed sense organ that communicates injury-related information to the brain. The immune system can be activated or depressed by stress (Box 3-5). Thus pain, whether accidental or intentional (e.g., surgery), modulates the immune response. The key elements in determining the immune response to pain are its intensity and duration (Box 3-6). Chronic pain can produce sustained increases in circulating concentrations of cortisol, epinephrine, norepinephrine, and glucagon, suppressing the humoral and cellular immune responses. The systemic release of endogenous opioids (endorphin and enkephalin) may contribute to immunosuppression. Mild to moderate pain associated with extensive tissue trauma may activate the immune response (Fig. 3-3). The messengers of the immune system are cytokines (e.g., interleukin 1 [IL-1], IL-6, and tumor necrosis factor α [TNF-α]).

CYTOKINES

A variety of low-molecular-weight proteins and cytokines are produced from activated leukocytes, fibroblasts, and endothelial cells in response to tissue injury. Their role is to protect the body by destroying and removing foreign invaders. These proteins and cytokines are responsible for the

---

BOX 3-5

Immunologic and Hematologic Response to Severe Stress

- Cytokine production
- Acute-phase response
- Neutrophil leukocytosis
- Lymphopenia
- Immune system depression

BOX 3-6

Neurotransmitters, Neuropeptides, Neurohormones, and Neuroendocrine Effector Molecules that are Affected by Stress and can Modulate Immune System Function*

- Neurotransmitters
  - Acetylcholine
  - Dopamine
  - 5-Hydroxytryptamine (serotonin)
  - Norepinephrine
  - Opiates
- Neuropeptides
  - Arginine vasopressin
  - Cholecystokinin
  - Melatonin
  - Oxytocin
  - Substance P
  - Vasoactive intestinal polypeptide
- Neurohormones
  - Corticosteroid
  - Corticotropin
  - Corticotropin-releasing factor
  - Growth hormone
  - Prolactin
- Neuroendocrine effector molecules
  - Epinephrine
  - Sex steroids
  - Thyroxine

*These categories are not mutually exclusive. For example, the neuropeptides oxytocin and arginine vasopressin are also considered to be neurohormones.

---

production of a local inflammatory response. When tissue trauma is severe, the excessive production of cytokines can lead to a systemic effect called the *systemic inflammatory response syndrome* (SIRS). Although pain has never been reported to cause SIRS, pain can contribute to the production of SIRS because it induces similar autonomic and endocrine effects. The major cytokines produced during stress are TNF-α, IL-1, and IL-6:

- IL-1 and IL-6 induce the release of acute-phase (inflammatory) reactants, cause fever, and initiate PG production (e.g., PGE_2). IL-1 and IL-6 can stimulate the secretion of ACTH from the pituitary gland and the subsequent release of cortisol.

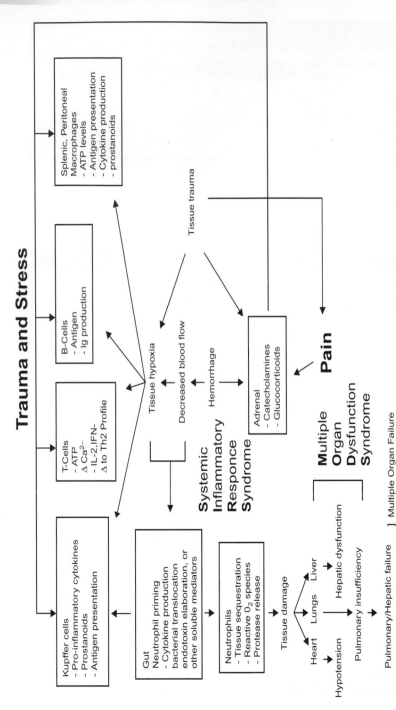

FIG. 3-3. Schematic of the immune response to trauma and stress. Trauma-pain-stress results in a multitude of hematologic and immune-mediated responses that can provoke and support the systemic inflammatory response syndrome (*SIRS*) and lead to the development of multiple organ dysfunction syndrome (*MODS*).

♦ TNF-α produces signs of shock, including hypotension, hemo-concentration, hyperglycemia, hyperkalemia, nonrespiratory acidosis, and activation of the complement cascade.

ACUTE-PHASE RESPONSE

The acute-phase response can be triggered by severe stress from any cause. The main feature of the acute-phase response is the release of proteins from the liver, which act as inflammatory mediators and scavengers in tissue repair. These proteins include C-reactive protein, fibrinogen, macroglobulin, and antiproteinases. C-reactive protein is an excellent biomarker of physiologic stress, infection, and morbidity. Excessive production of these proteins can contribute to SIRS.

HEMATOLOGY

The peripheral blood white cell count generally reflects a stress leukogram typified by an elevated number of mature and immature polymorphonuclear leukocytes (left shift) and reduced numbers of lymphocytes.

MORPHOLOGIC CHANGES

Morphologic changes associated with chronic stress or pain are typical of long-term aversive stimuli and include failure to thrive, hair loss or poor coat condition, weight loss, and acceleration of aging.

Suggested Readings

Carr DB, Goudes LC: Acute pain, *Lancet* 353:2051-2058, 1999.

Carstens E, Moberg GP: Recognizing pain and distress in laboratory animals, *ILAR J* 41(2):62-71, 2000.

Chapman CR, Garvin J: Suffering: the contributions of persistent pain, *Lancet* 353:2233-2237, 1999.

Charney DS, Grillon C, Bremner JD: The neurobiological basis of anxiety and fear: circuits, mechanisms, and neurochemical interactions (part I), *Neuroscientist* 4:35-44, 1998.

Charney DS, Grillon C, Bremner JD: The neurobiological basis of anxiety and fear: circuits, mechanisms, and neurochemical interactions (part II), *Neuroscientist* 4:122-132, 1998.

Clark JD, Rager DR, Calpin JP: Animal well-being. I. General considerations, *Lab Anim Sci* 47(6):564-570, 1997.

Clark JD, Rager DR, Calpin JP: Animal well-being. II. Stress and distress, *Lab Anim Sci* 47(6):571-585, 1997.

Curcio K, Bidwell LA, Bohart GV et al: Evaluation of signs of postoperative pain and complications after forelimb onychectomy in cats receiving buprenorphine alone or with bupivacaine administered as a four-point regional nerve block, *J Am Vet Med Assoc* 228(1):65-68, 2006.

Davis M: The role of the amygdala in fear-potentiated startle: implications for animal models of anxiety, *Trends Pharmacol Sci* 13:35-41, 1992.

Desborough JP: The stress response to trauma and surgery, *Br J Anaesth* 85(1):109-117, 2000.

Imbe H, Iwai-Liao Y, Senba E: Stress-induced hyperalgesia: animal models and putative mechanisms, *Front Biosci* 11:2179-2192, 2006.

Khuseyinova N, Koenig W: Biomarkers of outcome from cardiovascular disease, *Curr Opin Crit Care* 12(5):412-419, 2006.

Nasraway SA Jr: Hyperglycemia during critical illness, *JPEN J Parenter Enteral Nutr* 30(3):254-258, 2006.

Weissman C: The metabolic response to stress: an overview and update, *Anesthesia* 73:308-327, 1999.

Yates AR, Dyke PC 2nd, Taeed R et al: Hyperglycemia is a marker for poor outcome in the postoperative pediatric cardiac patient, *Pediatr Crit Care Med* 7(4):351-355, 2006.

4

DEFINITIONS OF TERMS DESCRIBING PAIN

JAMES S. GAYNOR

A working understanding of the terminology surrounding pain and analgesia is important to have. By knowing the terminology, practitioners can speak intelligently and accurately to one another when discussing cases. The following are definitions, arranged alphabetically, that are commonly used when discussing pain and may be used throughout this handbook.

DEFINITIONS

Acupuncture—The practice of inserting needles at certain points in the skin to achieve specific effects such as pain relief.

Acute pain—Pain that follows some bodily injury, disappears with healing, and tends to be self-limiting.

Allodynia—Pain caused by a stimulus that does not normally cause pain.

Analgesia—The loss of sensitivity to pain.

Anesthesia—Total or partial loss of sensation.

Breakthrough pain—A transient flare-up of pain in the chronic pain setting that can occur even when chronic pain is under control.

Cancer pain—Pain that can be acute, chronic, or intermittent and is related to the disease itself or to the treatment.

Chronic pain—Pain that lasts several weeks to months and persists beyond the expected healing time when nonmalignant in origin.

Epidural space—The space above the dura mater. An injection into this area is commonly referred to as an *epidural*.

Hyperalgesia—An increased response to a stimulation that is normally painful (a heightened sense of pain) at the site of injury or in surrounding undamaged tissue. Stimulated nociceptors respond to noxious stimuli more vigorously and at a lower threshold.

Hyperesthesia—Increased sensitivity to sensation.

Hyperpathia—A painful syndrome characterized by an increased reaction to a stimulus, especially if it is repetitive.

Hypoalgesia—Decreased sensitivity to pain.

Hypoesthesia—Decreased sensitivity to stimulation.

Interventional pain management—An invasive procedure to treat or manage pain through an injection of a drug or implantation of a drug-delivery device.

Local anesthesia—The temporary loss of sensation in a defined part of the body without loss of consciousness.

Multimodal analgesia—The use of multiple drugs with different actions, which may act at different levels of the nociceptive pathways, to produce optimal analgesia.

Myofascial pain—A syndrome of focal pain in a muscle or related tissues, stiffness, muscle spasm, and decreased range of motion.

Neuropathic pain—Pain that originates from injury or involvement of the peripheral or central nervous system and is described as burning or shooting, possibly associated with motor, sensory, or autonomic deficits.

Nociception—The reception, conduction, and central nervous system processing of nerve signals generated by the stimulation of nociceptors; the physiologic process that leads to the perception of pain.

Opioid—A drug that is related naturally or synthetically to morphine.

Pain—An unpleasant sensory and emotional experience associated with actual or potential tissue damage or described in terms of such damage.

Pain threshold—The least experience of pain that a patient can recognize.

Pain tolerance level—The greatest level of pain that a patient can tolerate.

Pathologic pain—Pain that has an exaggerated response much beyond its protective usefulness. This is often associated with tissue injury incurred at the time of surgery or trauma.

Physiologic pain—Pain that acts as a protective mechanism to incite individuals to move away from the cause of potential tissue damage or to avoid movement or contact with external stimuli during a reparative phase.

Preemptive analgesia—The administration of an analgesic drug before stimulation to prevent sensitization of neurons and windup, thus improving postoperative analgesia.

Regional anesthesia—The loss of sensation in part of the body by interrupting the sensory nerves conducting impulses from that region of the body.

Sedation—Central nervous system depression, mediated via the cerebral cortex, in which the patient is drowsy but arousable.

Somatic pain—Pain that originates from damage to bones, joints, muscle, or skin and is described in human beings as localized, constant, sharp, aching, and throbbing.

Subarachnoid space—The space above the pia mater and below the arachnoid mater, in which cerebrospinal fluid can be found. A subarachnoid injection is also referred to as a spinal.

Sympathetic mediated pain—A syndrome in which there is abnormal sympathetic nervous system activity causing a severe debilitation that is often associated with tenderness to a light touch.

Tolerance—A shortened duration and decreased intensity of the analgesic, euphorigenic, sedative, and other central nervous system depressant effects, as well as considerable increase in the average dose required to achieve a given effect.

Tranquilization—A state of calmness, meditated through the reticular activating system, in which the patient is relaxed, awake, unaware of its surroundings, and potentially indifferent to minor pain.

Visceral pain—Pain that arises from stretching, distention, or inflammation of the viscera, and is described as deep, cramping, aching, or gnawing, without good localization.

Windup—Sensitization of nociceptors and peripheral and central pain pathways in response to a barrage of afferent nociceptive impulses resulting in expanded receptive fields and an increased rate of discharge.

RECOGNITION AND EVALUATION OF PAIN

5 PAIN BEHAVIORS

WILLIAM W. MUIR III and JAMES S. GAYNOR

- Every animal experiences and demonstrates pain in a unique way. Just because a patient does not display a pain-related behavior, however, does not mean that the patient is not in pain. Although it may be difficult to quantify pain, there are characteristic body positions and behaviors that become recognizable in any animal that is experiencing pain (Box 5-1). Interactive and unprovoked (noninteractive) behavior assessments are useful.
- One must remember that no behavior by itself is pathognomonic for pain. Behavior at home may be considerably different from behavior in a strange environment.
- The behavior displayed by an animal depends on many factors, including species, age, breed, sex, personality, and the severity and duration of pain (Box 5-2).
- Many animals may display little outward behavior indicative of pain in the presence of human beings or other animals, especially potential predators. This behavior may be an innate protective mechanism to prevent a predator from recognizing easy prey.

PAIN BEHAVIORS

BODY POSTURE AND ACTIVITY

Dogs and cats assume characteristic postures or become reluctant to change position or move as pain intensity increases. Some animals become anxious, restless, and aggressive. These animals may begin to lick or chew at the site of pain. Most importantly, their routine pattern of behavior changes can only truly be assessed by someone who knows the animal's behavior.

BOX 5-1

Common Indicators of Pain in Dogs and Cats

Dogs
- Decreased social interaction
- Anxious expression
- Submissive behavior
- Refusal to move
- Whimpering
- Howling
- Growling
- Guarding behavior
- Aggression; biting
- Loss of appetite
- Self-mutilation

Cats
- Reduced activity
- Loss of appetite
- Quiet/loss of curiosity
- Hiding
- Hissing or spitting
- Excessive licking/grooming
- Stiff posture/gait
- Guarding behavior
- Attempts to escape
- Cessation of grooming
- Tail flicking

BOX 5-2

Behavioral and Physiologic Characteristics Associated with Pain in Dogs and Cats

Abnormal Posture
Hunched-up guarding or splinting of abdomen
"Praying" position (forequarters on the ground, hindquarters in the air)
Sitting or lying in an abnormal position
Not resting in a normal position (e.g., sternal or curled up)
Statuelike appearance
Abnormal body part position (e.g., extended head and neck)

Abnormal Gait
Stiff
Partial or no weight bearing on injured limb
Lameness, slight to obvious limp
Reluctance to move

Abnormal Movement
Thrashing
Restlessness
Circling
Continuous activity

Vocalization
Screaming, howling, barking, meowing
Whining (intermittent, constant, or when touched)
Crying (intermittent, constant, or when touched)
None

—Continued

BOX 5-2

Behavioral and Physiologic Characteristics Associated with Pain in Dogs and Cats—*cont'd*

Miscellaneous

Looking, licking, or chewing at the painful area
Hyperesthesia or hyperalgesia
Allodynia

Pain-Associated Characteristics That May Also Be Associated with Poor General Health (Medical Problems)

Restlessness or agitation
Trembling or shaking
Tachypnea or panting
Tucked tail or tail flicking (cats)
Low carriage of tail
Depressed or poor response to caregiver
Head hanging down
Not grooming
Appetite decreased, picky, or absent
Dull, depressed
Lying quietly and not moving for hours
Stuporous
Urinates or defecates and makes no attempt to move
Recumbent and unaware of surroundings
Unwilling or unable to walk
Bites or attempts to bite caregivers

Pain-Associated Characteristics That May Also Be Associated with Apprehension or Anxiety

Restlessness or agitation
Trembling or shaking
Tachypnea or panting
Weak tail wag
Low tail carriage
Slow to rise
Depressed (poor response to caregiver)
Not grooming
Bites or attempts to bite caregiver
Ears pulled back
Restless
Barking or growling (intermittent, constant, or when approached by caregiver)
Growling or hissing (intermittent, constant, or when approached by caregiver)
Sitting in the back of the cage or hiding (cat)

—Continued

BOX 5-2

Behavioral and Physiologic Characteristics Associated with Pain in Dogs and Cats—*cont'd*

Pain-Associated Characteristics That May Be Normal Behavior
Reluctant to move head (eye movement only)
Stretching all four legs when abdomen is touched
Penile prolapse
Cleaning (licking) a wound or incision

Physiologic Signs That Can Be Associated with Pain
Tachypnea or panting
Tachycardia (mild, moderate, or severe)
Dilated pupils
Hypertension
Increased serum cortisol and epinephrine

From Mathew KA: Vet Clin North Am Small Anim Pract 30(4):729-752, 2000.

Reluctance to Move

Animals that are reluctant to move usually have moderate to severe pain (Figs. 5-1 to 5-3). This behavior provides protection against movement-induced (incident) pain. Usually, slight movement results in some other behavior associated with an abnormal gait (e.g., limping or stilted gait), aggression, or vocalization.

Reluctance to Lie Down

Reluctance to lie down is often associated with acute abdominal or thoracic pain (Fig. 5-4). Dogs or cats with abdominal pain may sit for hours or assume a "praying" position (Figs. 5-4 and 5-5). Some animals frequently attempt to sit or remain standing for hours. Some animals commonly fall asleep, slump down, wake up abruptly because of the pain, and then resume their original position (Fig. 5-6).

Changing Positions

Restlessness and frequent changes in body position indicate that an animal is not comfortable. Some dogs may shift from side to side or get up and lie down multiple times (Fig. 5-7). As stated previously, some animals change positions frequently because of a full bladder and may need to have their bladders expressed. Good nursing practices should not be forgotten when caring for animals in pain:

◆ Dogs and cats experiencing severe pain are often anxious and restless (getting up and lying down) and may become unmanageable. Some become aggressive.

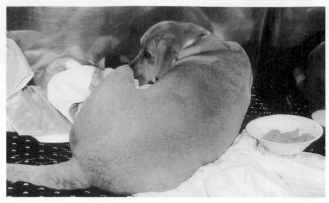

FIG. 5-1. Reluctance to move and unresponsive. Abdominal pain caused this dog to lie facing the back of the cage for hours. Note the depressed expression.

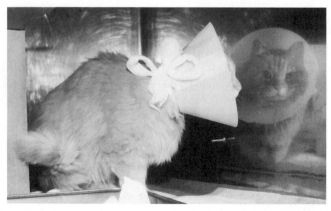

FIG. 5-2. Reluctance to move. Abdominal (bladder) pain caused this cat to sit in the litter box facing the back of the cage.

- Some animals become submissive or mentally depressed because of acute pain (Fig. 5-8). Depression can be associated with chronic pain, and the animal may be reluctant to move or engage in any activity.
- Dogs and cats may become increasingly protective and aggressive, even those that have never displayed aggression, as their pain becomes more severe (Fig. 5-9).
- Aggression is frequently observed in association with severe acute pain. Often, the slightest manipulation stimulates the patient to attempt to bite the handler.
- Some dogs may become much more vigilant, timid, and fearful.
- Cats are much more likely to hide or attempt to escape (Fig. 5-10).

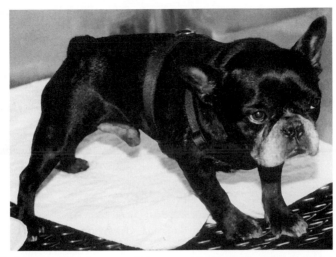

FIG. 5-3. Reluctance to move. Pain caused by trauma to a cervical disk in a dog. Note the statuelike appearance.

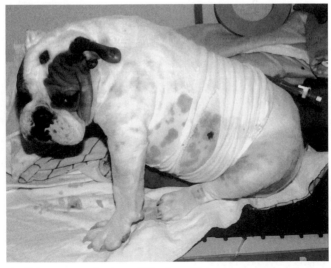

FIG. 5-4. Reluctance to lie down. This dog with traumatic peritonitis would not lie down until exhausted.

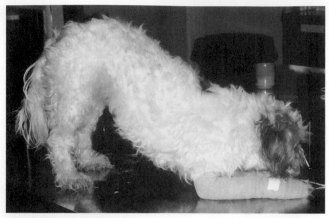

FIG. 5-5. Reluctance to lie down. The so-called praying position characteristic of dogs and cats with abdominal pain.

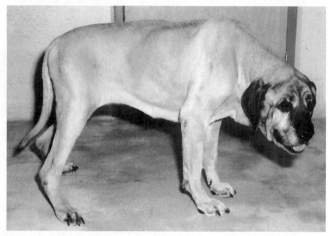

FIG. 5-6. Reluctance to lie down. This dog with chronic bloat and abdominal pain remained standing in one spot until exhausted. Note the tense abdomen, open mouth breathing, and head-down, anxious expression.

LOCOMOTOR ACTIVITY

Limping and guarding (protecting an injured area from further insult) are clearly the most obvious signs of limb pain, whether long bone, joint, or soft tissue in origin (Fig. 5-11). Limping is a protective behavior potentially to prevent further damage and to decrease pain associated with weight bearing. Stilted gaits, placing excessive weight on the front limbs (hip osteoarthritis), and reluctance to move are also signs of acute or chronic pain (Fig. 5-12).

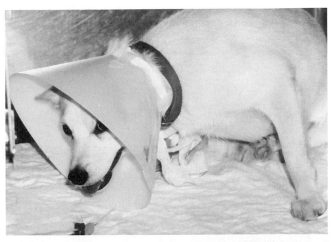

FIG. 5-7. Shifting positions. This dog with abdominal pain would frequently get up and lie down. The dog was careful not to induce more pain, taking several minutes to lie down.

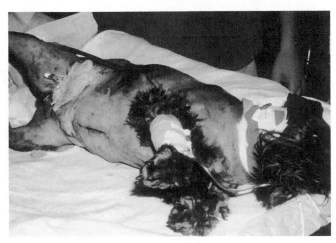

FIG. 5-8. Submissive position. This dog with abdominal trauma demonstrated a submissive posture (on back, rear legs apart, ears flat) when approached.

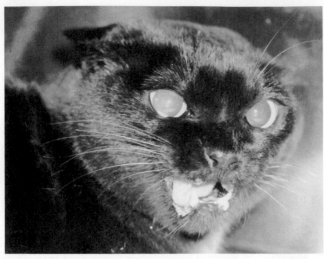

FIG. 5-9. Aggression. Expression of aggression in a cat with a femoral fracture. Note the dilated pupils, flattened ears, and open mouth.

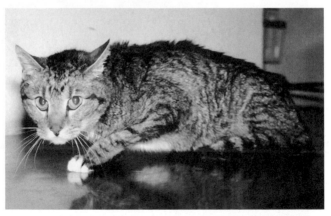

FIG. 5-10. Escape behavior. This cat with chronic pancreatitis attempted to hide or escape when approached. Note the dull, ungroomed hair coat.

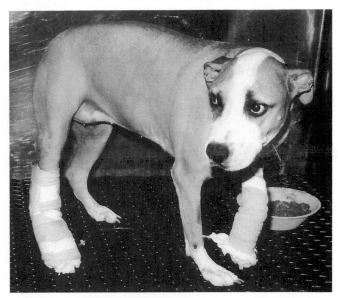

FIG. 5-11. Acute pain. Left foreleg lameness in a dog. Pain causes the dog to lift its left foreleg and walk with a limp.

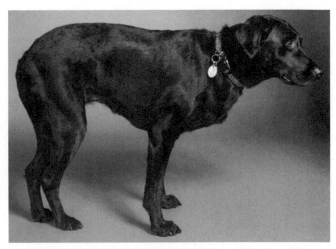

FIG. 5-12. Chronic pain. Severe hip osteoarthritis in a dog. Note that the majority of the dog's weight is being carried on the front legs.

VOCALIZATION

- ◆ Vocalization can be associated with painful situations that are mild to severe, depending on the animal's behavior pattern and the environmental circumstances.
- ◆ Vocalization is nonspecific. Most veterinarians have experienced situations in which animals are anesthetized for minor surgical procedures and wake up vocalizing. Some animals vocalize postoperatively as a result of emergence delirium associated with recovery from anesthesia. This frequently resolves in a short period.
- ◆ Some animals will not display signs of pain until the pain is severe, at which time they may begin to whimper or vocalize.
- ◆ Vocalization may also be an example of the animal's exhaustion of protective mechanisms (e.g., avoidance or escape) and increased anxiety.
- ◆ Vocalization in dogs likely manifests as groaning, whining, whimpering, or growling.
- ◆ Cats frequently groan, growl, or purr.
- ◆ Some animals whine postoperatively. Whining can also indicate a full bladder and the need to urinate. Good nursing practices should not be forgotten when caring for animals in pain.

ALTERED FACIAL EXPRESSIONS AND APPEARANCE
Dogs

See Fig. 5-13.
- ◆ Fixed glare, focused
- ◆ Glazed appearance
- ◆ Oblivious
- ◆ Depressed
- ◆ Ungroomed

Cats

See Fig. 5-14.
- ◆ Furrowed brow
- ◆ Squinted eyes (Fig. 5-15)
- ◆ Depressed
- ◆ Poor hair coat, ungroomed

APPETITE

Anorexia is common in dogs or cats with significant acute or chronic pain. These animals may be misdiagnosed as having some other systemic

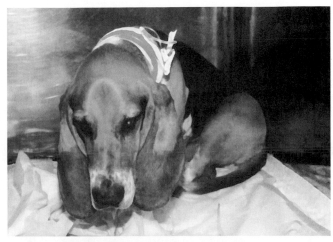

FIG. 5-13. Facial expression. Note the head-down, fixed-gaze, and depressed expression. The dog was oblivious to its environment.

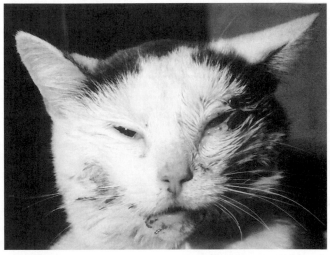

FIG. 5-14. Facial expression. Note the squinted dull eyes and abnormal facial expression.

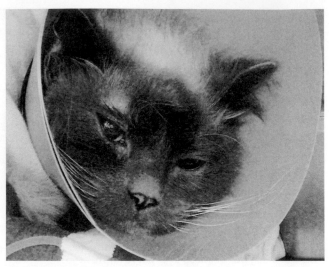

FIG. 5-15. Facial expression. Note the hanging head and squinted eyes.

problem. One must determine whether there are concurrent problems that could predispose to anorexia.

APPEARANCE

◆ Dogs and cats with chronic pain or stress often lose hair coat sheen (Fig. 5-16; see Chapter 3).
◆ Cats with chronic pain often fail to groom themselves, resulting in an unkempt appearance (Fig. 5-10).

RESPONSE TO MANIPULATION

◆ Dogs and cats frequently respond with purposeful movement and occasionally become aggressive in response to palpation of a painful area. Abdominal splinting or tenseness is often due to abdominal pain, which can be determined only by abdominal palpaton (Fig. 5-17). During palpation, animals may try to bite the handler (Fig. 5-18).
◆ Animals may also become defensive by protecting the area or by withdrawing to avoid being touched.
◆ Passive animals may freeze or look at the area in question (Figs. 5-18, 5-19, and 5-20).

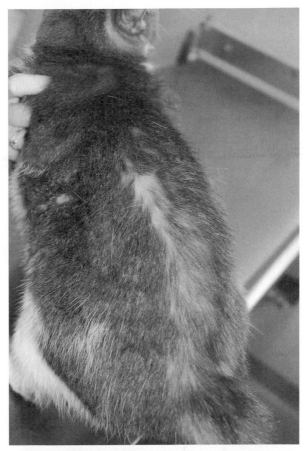

FIG. 5-16. Some cats that are chronically stressed will lose their hair coat. This is particularly noticeable along the spine.

URINARY AND BOWEL HABITS

◆ Dogs and cats experiencing pain commonly lose their house training, presumably because they are too uncomfortable to go outside.

◆ Dogs and cats may urinate frequently because of painful distention of the bladder or irritation (inflammation) of the bladder or urethra. One must remember that animals that have been administered opioids (e.g., morphine or hydromorphone) may be comfortable but still experience urinary retention as a side effect of the drugs.

◆ Cats may also lose their house training as pain increases, which manifests as failure to use the litter box.

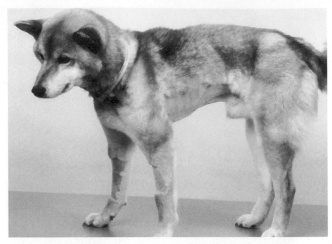

FIG. 5-17. Note the facial expression and tense abdomen in this dog with abdominal pain of unknown origin.

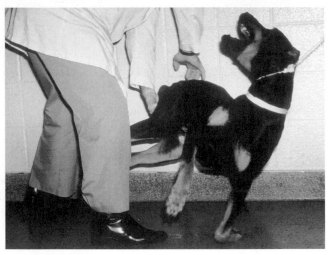

FIG. 5-18. Response to manipulation. This dog became aggressive any time its pelvis was palpated.

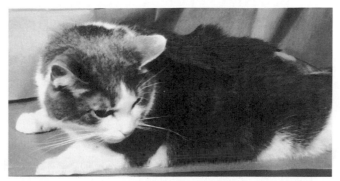

FIG. 5-19. This cat would sit and stare at its rear end. Its tail had been traumatized in an automobile accident.

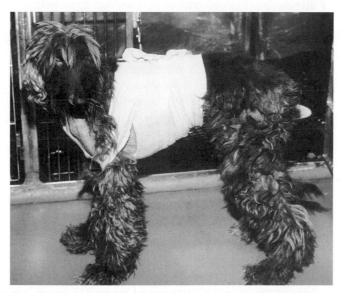

FIG. 5-20. This dog would stare at its left chest wall after a thoracotomy.

Suggested Readings

Bateson P: Assessment of pain in animals, *Anim Behav* 3:87-107, 1991.

Carstens E, Moberg GP: Recognizing pain and distress in laboratory animals, *ILAR J* 41:62-71, 2000.

Hansen B: Through a glass darkly: using behavior to assess pain, *Semin Vet Med Surg Small Anim* 12:61-74, 1997.

Mathew KA: Pain assessment and general approach to management, *Vet Clin North Am Small Anim Pract* 30(4):729-752, 2000.

6

OBJECTIVE, CATEGORIC METHODS FOR ASSESSING PAIN AND ANALGESIA

PATRICE M. MICH AND PETER W. HELLYER

Veterinarians are well trained at assessing organ system function/ dysfunction using a wide variety of measurable and quantifiable parameters. For example, changes in blood urea nitrogen, creatinine, and urine specific gravity can be used to assess the degree of renal failure and the response to treatment. Unfortunately, no similar set of objective and easily measured parameters is available to assess pain in people or animals. The treatment of acute pain in people and animals is hampered by a lack of objective criteria to measure pain intensity and a reluctance of medical personnel to thoroughly evaluate, ask questions, or rely on patients' self-reports (signs) of pain. Understanding and appropriately treating chronic pain in animals is even more complex, re-quiring an accurate assessment of the amount and type of tissue injury in addition to specific psychosocial, behavioral, and psychological factors.[1]

It can be especially difficult to assess the degree of pain experienced by animals and the ability of an animal to cope with that pain.[2] In a survey of Canadian veterinarians, Dohoo and Dohoo[3] found that one of the main factors influencing whether veterinarians routinely administered analgesic drugs postoperatively was the veterinarians' perception of the degree of pain felt by animals. The fact that 51.5% of those veterinarians surveyed were considered to be analgesic nonusers (never used analgesics) highlights the clinical importance of being able to recognize pain in the species under a veterinarian's care. In a subsequent survey, animal health technologists in Canada had higher pain perception scores than did veterinarians.[4] A majority (55%) of the animal health technologists surveyed agreed that risks of potent opioids (morphine or oxymorphone) outweighed the analgesic benefits, suggesting a lack of experience in treating and evaluating dogs and cats for pain. Even among veterinary personnel committed to treating pain, it can be difficult determining whether the benefits of the analgesic protocol selected (i.e., decreased pain intensity) outweigh the side effects (e.g., sedation and nausea). Complicating the evaluation of pain is the fact that one set of criteria to measure pain cannot be used to assess all species and all types of pain: acute, chronic, superficial, deep, or neuropathic. There is no question that as more studies focus on species-specific pain behaviors, the ability to recognize and treat pain in animals will improve. Nevertheless, the assessment of pain in animals remains a subjective and inaccurate undertaking for the foreseeable future. One truth remains certain: ignoring pain simply because one has trouble measuring it condemns patients to undue suffering. Endeavoring to assess and treat pain in animals is a worthwhile and laudable goal of veterinary professionals notwithstanding current uncertainties.

The evaluation methods described in this chapter are primarily designed to assess acute postoperative and traumatic pain in dogs. These methods can be adapted to chronic pain conditions and pain in cats and other species provided that the caregiver recognizes that pain behaviors are likely to be different between species. *Importantly, all of the methods described are categorical, subjective, and prone to the error of underestimating or overestimating the degree of pain. Even if the amount of pain is correctly estimated, how well the individual animal is coping with the pain may be difficult to ascertain. In addition, all of the current pain scales are subject to some degree of interobserver variability. Finally, it should be recognized that pain results in stress and suffering* (see Chapter 3), adversely affecting the animal's quality of life (QOL). Quality-of-life assessments should be performed by both veterinarians and owners and are essential for evaluating treatment regimens, focusing veterinarian-owner therapeutic goals, and as independent predictors of survival.

LIMITATIONS OF OBJECTIVE AND CATEGORIC ASSESSMENT OF PAIN

NO ESTABLISHED "GOLD STANDARD" TO ASSESS PAIN

- No "gold standard" exists to assess pain in people, although caregivers can ask the patient if the patient is painful, if the analgesic treatment has improved pain control, and how well the patient is coping with the pain. Self-reports of pain in people are frequently ignored. Individuals that complain of postoperative pain may be viewed as "bad patients."[5]
- Likewise, no "gold standard" exists to assess pain in animals or to compare one type of scale or measurement instrument to another. Most pain scales have been used to assess acute postoperative pain in dogs and cats. These scales are likely to be ineffective at assessing other types of pain, such as acute pain/distress caused by pancreatitis, sepsis, or vasculitis. These scales are probably not useful in the assessment of emotional or psychological pain or in the assessment of chronic pain, such as osteoarthritis or cancer pain.

1. All of the pain scales used in animals rely on the recognition and/or interpretation of some behavior. The most useful scales rely on the determination of the presence or absence of specific behaviors while minimizing the interpretation of those behaviors.
2. All pain scales have a subjective component and are vulnerable to observer error and bias.

PHYSIOLOGICAL ASSESSMENT CAN BE MISLEADING

♦ By no means is it clear that physiological data (e.g., changes in heart rate, respiratory rate, arterial blood pressure, and pupil dilation) are useful in assessing response to a noxious (harmful) stimulus. For example, physiological measurements, including heart rate, respiratory rate, rectal temperature, plasma cortisol and β-endorphin concentrations, did not differentiate between cats that underwent surgery (tenectomy, onychectomy) and control cats that were anesthetized and bandaged but had no surgery.[6]

1. Cardiopulmonary reflexes may obtund the easily recognizable changes in physiological parameters in response to pain.
2. Physiological parameters are not specific enough to differentiate pain from other stressors such as anxiety, fear, or physiological responses to metabolic conditions (e.g., anemia).[7]
3. Holton et al.[8] found that heart rate and respiratory rate were not useful indicators of pain in hospitalized dogs following surgery. Pupil dilation was significantly correlated with the pain score (numeric rating scale) in dogs following surgery. Nevertheless, the authors indicated that pupil size is unlikely to be a useful parameter to assess pain in hospitalized dogs.

♦ Note that some of the pain scales presented in this chapter use physiological data and some do not. In the authors' opinion, physiological parameters are useful in assessing responses to noxious stimuli in patients under general anesthesia or for transient periods in conscious patients. The longer a conscious patient experiences pain, the less useful are physiological parameters in assessing the degree of pain.

BEHAVIORAL ASSESSMENT IS SUBJECT TO INTERPRETATION

♦ Evaluation of pain in animals relies on behavioral assessment and interpretation by an observer. Please refer to Chapter 3 for examples of behaviors indicative of pain in dogs.

♦ Behavioral changes indicative of pain may be too subtle or take too long to be recognized under routine clinical situations. This was verified in the most extensive evaluation to date of pain behaviors in dogs following ovariohysterectomy.[9] Using two evaluation methods, a numeric scoring system and quantitative behavioral measurements, Hardie et al. evaluated dogs following anesthesia only and anesthesia plus surgery, with or without analgesia. Surgery resulted in an increase in pain score, sedation score, time spent sleeping, and a decrease in greeting behaviors during timed interactions with caregivers. Importantly, dogs that received oxymorphone (preoperatively and 6, 12, and 18 hours later) had a faster return to more normal greeting behaviors than did dogs that had surgery and placebo. Quantitative behavioral measurements were able to differentiate postoperatively the dogs that were administered oxymorphone from placebo-treated dogs, whereas the numeric scoring system was not.

♦ Sporadic observation of animal behavior may not reveal signs of pain. Except in the most severe circumstances, the signs of pain may be "masked" by behavior that is stereotypical of the species being observed. For instance, dogs may wag their tail and greet an observer at the cage door in spite of being in pain. Cats may simply hide in the back of their cage and demonstrate no behaviors that would suggest to a casual observer that they are painful. Flock animals, such as sheep, may be startled when an observer approaches and attempt to conceal any signs of pain by staying bunched up with the rest of the flock (personal observations).

♦ Behavioral changes indicating pain may not be what one expects. A cat sitting quietly in the back of the cage after surgery may be painful; however, pain would not be recognized if the caregiver expects to see more active signs of pain such as pacing, agitation, or vocalization.

1. A lack of familiarity with normal behaviors typical of a particular species or breed makes recognition of pain-induced behaviors difficult or impossible.[10] Specific pain scales have not been developed for most species, dogs being a notable exception.

2. Pain tolerance of individual animals within a species may vary greatly. A genetic predisposition to pain tolerance may explain some of the variability observed in clinical patients.[11]

GUIDELINES FOR USE OF PAIN SCALES

RECOGNIZE THE INTENDED PURPOSE OF THE ASSESSMENT METHOD

Regardless of the scale or method used to assess pain, it is critical that the caregiver recognize the limitations of the scale and the purpose for which the scale was developed. For example, if a scale uses lack of grooming and unkept appearance as a criterion for pain, it is unlikely that a caregiver could draw any reasonable conclusions about grooming in the immediate postoperative period. Thus lack of grooming would not be expected to be a helpful criterion during the first 12 to 24 hours after surgery. Likewise, inactivity is a difficult, if not impossible, parameter to assess if the animal is never let out of its cage and allowed to explore its surroundings.

♦ The evaluation of acute surgical and traumatic pain in dogs and cats has received a fair amount of attention in recent years.[9,12-15] Many of the criteria commonly used—such as vocalizing, trying to escape, and thrashing—are not applicable to chronic pain. In addition, clinical criteria used to assess chronic pain—such as lack of exercise, lack of grooming, inappetence, weight loss—are not incorporated into these scales for reasons already mentioned. In general, responses to acute surgical and traumatic pain are likely to be more marked and readily recognizable than clinical signs associated with chronic pain.

♦ The clinical signs of pain/discomfort associated with acute, nonsurgical diseases (e.g., pancreatitis, pleuritis, and vasculitis) might not be recognizable using pain scales developed for acute surgical pain. For example, how does one assess the discomfort/suffering associated with constant vomiting, fever-induced myalgia, or abdominal pain/cramping? If a dog vomits 5, 10, or 20 times an hour, are there simply concerns about stopping the vomiting and rehydrating the patient, or might there be concerns regarding abdominal pain/discomfort associated with the vomiting? How many times have veterinarians diagnosed abdominal pain in puppies with parvovirus, yet analgesics were not administered? What does a clinical sign such as head pressing or head banging on the side of the cage indicate in a dog with acute septic peritonitis? Does the clinical sign indicate the development of secondary neurologic symptoms, or does it represent the desperate attempts of the animal to cope with its pain and suffering? Assessing this type of patient with a standard pain scale developed to evaluate a dog following surgery would likely result in a score that was too low to prompt analgesic therapy. Thus, care must be taken so that overreliance on a particular pain scale does not preclude the use of good clinical judgment and assessment of the patient.

♦ Cancer pain may have components of acute pain (e.g., expansion of a tumor or side effects of surgical, radiation, or chemotherapy treatment) and components of chronic pain. Thus, assessment of cancer pain requires the caregiver to use methods that can detect behavioral changes associated with acute and chronic pain. Indeed, an increase in pain-related behaviors may indicate the progression of disease and prompt further diagnostic and therapeutic interventions, as well as changes in analgesic therapy.

> ### BOX 6-1
>
> ## Key Points Related to Pain Scales
>
> 1. Pain scales should be used to ensure that pain is assessed and treated in every patient.
> 2. Pain scales are an adjunct to good physical examinations and thorough patient evaluation.
> 3. All pain scales have their limitations.
> 4. Individual behaviors frequently prompt analgesic therapy regardless of pain score.
> 5. Effective analgesic therapy should result in a low pain score and an animal that appears comfortable.

◆ Evaluation of the degree of lameness of the affected limb(s) is often used to assess chronic orthopedic pain. In addition, observations of owners are essential to detect more subtle signs of chronic pain such as lack of activity, change in attitude or interaction with family members, and changes in appetite. Response to therapy, such as increased activity after administering a nonsteroidal antiinflammatory drug, may provide important information regarding the role that pain has played in behavioral changes that was not illuminated by the pain scale and that may even surprise owners.

USE PAIN SCALE TO GUIDE THERAPY

The purpose of any pain scale is to help guide analgesic, medical, or surgical treatment and to provide diagnostic/prognostic information regarding the onset of healing and the resolution of tissue injury (Box 6-1).

◆ Pain scales may be used to ensure that individual animals are comfortable during the recuperative phase following surgery, trauma, invasive diagnostic procedures, or medical conditions. This is particularly important in animals that are unlikely to demonstrate overtly recognizable signs of pain, such as cats or "stoic" dogs.

◆ Pain scales may encourage the frequent evaluation of patients that are likely to be in pain, ensuring that pain does not go unrecognized or undertreated.

  1. Many human hospitals in the United States are now required to monitor pain as one of the patients' vital signs. Pain, like heart rate, respiratory rate, and body temperature, is considered to be a critical clinical sign.
  2. An institutional commitment to the treatment of pain is required in order to make certain that pain is not overlooked or ignored.[16]

3. The American Animal Hospital Association has incorporated pain management standards as a component of its Standards of Accreditation.

◆ Pain scales should not be used to deny analgesic therapy to an animal that is likely to be in pain. Rather, the pain scale should be used to determine whether analgesic therapy needs to be increased or can be tapered off.
   1. Do not use rigid minimum scores to prompt therapy.
   2. Individual behaviors suggestive of animal pain/distress should overrule results of pain score.
   3. If the procedure was likely to be painful, but the pain score is too low to prompt treatment, try a test dose of analgesic and observe the patient's response.

◆ Sedated, critically ill, or compromised animals may not be able to elicit behaviors required to prompt treatment using the pain scale.
   1. Consider low-dose opioid therapy in the animal likely to be painful that is slightly obtunded. Increased awareness of surroundings, but not agitation, suggests a beneficial effect of analgesic therapy.

◆ If one is unsure that the patient is painful, but tissue trauma has occurred, treat for pain conservatively and observe results.

FREQUENTLY OBSERVE THE ANIMAL

The health status of the animal, extent of surgery/injuries, and anticipated duration of analgesic drugs determine the frequency and interval of evaluations.

◆ In general, evaluations should be made at least hourly for the first 4 to 6 hours after surgery, provided the animal has recovered from anesthesia, has stable vital signs, and is resting comfortably.

◆ Animals not recovering as anticipated from anesthesia/surgery and critically ill animals require much more frequent evaluations until they are stabilized.

◆ Patient response to analgesic therapy and expected duration of analgesic drug(s) administered help to determine frequency of evaluations. For example, if a dog is resting comfortably following the postoperative administration of morphine, it may not need to be reassessed for 2 to 4 hours. Animals should be allowed to sleep following analgesic therapy. Vital signs can often be checked without unduly disturbing a sleeping animal. In general, animals are not awakened to check their pain status.

◆ Continuous, undisturbed observations, coupled with periodic interactive observations (open the cage, palpate wound) are likely to provide more information than occasionally observing the animal through the cage door.[9] Unfortunately, continuous observations are not practical for most clinical situations.

◆ In general, the more frequent the observations, the more likely that subtle signs of pain will be detected.

SUBJECTIVE AND SEMIOBJECTIVE PAIN SCALES FOR ACUTE SURGICAL AND TRAUMATIC PAIN

PREEMPTIVE SCORING SYSTEM

The preemptive scoring system is a subjective scoring system based on the amount of pain an individual observer feels the animal will experience following a given procedure.

◆ Preemptive scoring systems assign a degree of pain (none, mild, moderate, severe) based on the procedure performed and the amount of tissue trauma involved (Box 6-2).[17] In general, the greater the amount of tissue trauma, the greater the assigned level of pain.

BOX 6-2

Preemptive Scoring System

Minor Procedures: No Pain or Temporary Pain
Grooming
Nail trim
Physical examination, restraint
Radiography
Suture removal, cast application, bandage change*

Minor Surgeries: Minor Pain
Abscess lancing
Dental cleaning
Ear examination and cleaning
Removal of cutaneous foreign bodies
Suturing, débridement
Urinary catheterization

Moderate Surgeries: Moderate Pain
Anal sacculectomy
Cutaneous mass removal
Cystotomy
Dental extraction
Feline onychectomy
Ovariohysterectomy, castration, cesarean section
Severe laceration repair

Major Surgeries: Severe Pain
Ear canal ablation
Fracture repair, cruciate ligament repair
Limb amputation
Thoracotomy, laminectomy, exploratory laparotomy

Preemptive scoring system used to anticipate the amount of pain induced by surgical procedures. Modified from *A roundtable discussion: rethinking your approach to sedation, anesthesia, and analgesia,* Lenexa, Kan, 1997, Veterinary Medicine Publishing.
The pain categories are only a "best guess" of the amount of pain a certain procedure induces. In general, the more tissue trauma, the greater the pain. Individual animals may have more or less pain than the category suggests.
*Setting of fractures and some bandage changes can be very painful.

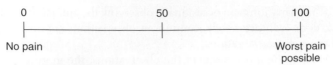

FIG. 6-1. Visual analog scale (*VAS*) used to estimate an animal's current pain status. The scale is a 100-mm line representing the entire spectrum of pain, from no pain to the worst pain possible. The observer draws a line that best represents the animal's estimated pain.

♦ The advantages of preemptive scoring systems include simplicity and their utility as an aid in planning perioperative analgesic strategies. For example, procedures inducing moderate to severe pain often require the use of multiple analgesic drugs and techniques to manage pain adequately.

♦ One of the primary disadvantages of preemptive scoring systems is they are not useful in determining the degree of pain felt by an individual patient. As a result of species, breed, temperament, and individual variability, a given patient may experience more or less pain than predicted by the preemptive pain scale. Additionally, preemptive scoring systems are not useful in assessing response to therapy.

VISUAL ANALOG SCALE

♦ The visual analog scale (VAS) is a semiobjective scoring system used to quantify pain intensity.

♦ The VAS is typically a straight, horizontal line, 100 mm in length, bracketed with descriptors of pain intensity (e.g., No Pain, [Very Extreme] Worst Pain Possible) on either end of the line (Fig. 6-1).

♦ The patient draws a vertical line across the scale that best represents the patient's degree of pain. The patient may be asked to assess pain at the current time or the worst pain that occurred since the last assessment.

♦ The VAS has been used extensively in human beings and is generally completed by the patient experiencing the pain. The scale avoids the use of imprecise descriptive terms and provides many points from which to choose. In people, bracketing the VAS with terms such as "no relief of pain" and "complete relief of pain" may provide more clinically useful information because patients do not all start with the same degree of pain.[18]

   1. The primary advantage of the VAS is its ease of use as a quantitative mechanism providing a general assessment of trends (i.e., whether pain is getting worse or improving). This scale is not species-specific.

BOX 6-3
Simple Descriptive Scale
0 = No pain 1 = Mild pain 2 = Moderate pain 3 = Severe pain

Simple descriptive scale used to estimate an animal's current pain status.

2. Disadvantages of the VAS include the concept that pain is a multidimensional experience and pain intensity as measured by the VAS is only one aspect of that experience[19]; the use of the VAS may result in greater variability of pain scores than a simple descriptive scale (see the following); and the VAS may erroneously appear as a more sensitive scale compared with other scales, resulting in overinterpretation or excessive confidence in the results.[13]

♦ The use of the VAS in veterinary medicine relies on an observer to identify and interpret pain behaviors in the patient. Advantages and disadvantages of the VAS as used in animals are similar to those noted before. Additionally, consider the following:
   1. Observer bias may play a key role in assessing pain, leading to the possibility of overdiagnosing or underdiagnosing pain.
   2. Variability of visual acuity among observers may affect the accuracy of the VAS.[13]
   3. Observer variability, when more than one observer evaluates an animal, affects the accuracy of the VAS.[13]
   4. In human beings, at least one study has shown that an individual's score must move at least 13 mm along the 100-mm scale in order for a significant change in acute, traumatic pain to be clinically significant. Even if there is a 50% change in VAS score, it is not known whether that represents an adequate degree of pain relief unless the patient is asked.[18,20] The sensitivity of the VAS has not been determined in animals; therefore, changes in VAS score should be interpreted in light of overall patient appearance.

SIMPLE DESCRIPTIVE SCALE

♦ The simple descriptive scale (SDS) is a semiobjective scoring system.
♦ The SDS usually consists of four or five categories or descriptions of pain intensity (Box 6-3). Each description is assigned a number, which becomes the patient's pain score.[13] This differs from the preemptive

scoring system in that the SDS assigns a score based on observation of the individual animal and not the nature of the procedure performed.

◆ Advantages of the SDS are that it is simple to use, it is not species-specific, and the results are not affected by visual acuity (no drawing of a line required). The SDS can be used to follow response to therapy and thereby guide therapy. Unlike the VAS, the SDS better addresses the multidimensional aspects of pain.

◆ Disadvantages of the SDS are that it is not a sensitive scale (consists of only 4 or 5 categories); therefore, it may overestimate or underestimate the degree of pain and the efficacy of analgesic therapy. In addition, observer bias may play a key role in determining pain score; and like the VAS, observer variability, when more than one observer evaluates an animal, affects accuracy.

NUMERICAL RATING SCALE

◆ The numerical rating scale (NRS) is a semiobjective scoring system.

◆ The NRS consists of multiple categories with descriptive definitions of pain for each category (Table 6-1).[21] The NRS generally uses categories that are assigned whole numbers, and the importance of each category is not weighted.[12]

◆ The NRS prompts the observer to evaluate certain aspects of the patient that might otherwise go unnoticed (e.g., appearance of the eyes, interactive behaviors, and physiological parameters).

◆ Advantages of the NRS include a more thorough patient evaluation than what is prompted by the VAS or SDS, an easy method to tabulate the score, and numerous categories on which to base an assessment of patient comfort and response to therapy.

◆ Disadvantages of the NRS include lack of accuracy and little improvement over the SDS.[12]

   1. Categories are generally scored by whole numbers, suggesting that equal differences exist between categories when in fact that may not be true.[12]

   2. In spite of numerous categories, painful animals may go undiagnosed. For example, a dog with severe abdominal pain may not receive a high enough number to be considered painful when using a scale designed to assess surgical pain.

   3. In the postsurgical patient, the NRS may be too insensitive to detect differences in some animals that receive analgesics and those that go untreated.[9] Thus the NRS may only be able to identify those animals with extreme pain that overtly demonstrate pain behaviors and would have been identified otherwise.

4. The NRS may not be useful in species other than dogs.
5. The NRS does not account for the residual or adverse effects of anesthesia in scoring. Examples include dysphoria and persistent sedation.

BEHAVIORAL PAIN SCALES FOR ACUTE SURGICAL AND TRAUMATIC PAIN

THE UNIVERSITY OF MELBOURNE PAIN SCALE: A BEHAVIORAL AND PHYSIOLOGICAL RESPONSES SCALE

◆ The University of Melbourne Pain Scale (UMPS) is a scale based on specific behavioral and physiological responses.[12]
◆ The UMPS includes multiple descriptors in six categories of parameters or behaviors related to pain (Table 6-2).
◆ Advantages of the UMPS may include increased accuracy over the preemptive scoring system, VAS, SDS, or NRS and an ability to weight the importance of certain behaviors or parameters.
   1. Multiple factors evaluated increase the sensitivity and specificity of the UMPS.
   2. The UMPS relies on behavioral observations, thereby limiting interpretation and observer bias.
   3. The UMPS evaluates changes in behavior or demeanor, adding to the sensitivity of the scale.
◆ Disadvantages of the UMPS include limited validation to date. The specific types of patients and procedures in which the UMPS would be expected to be accurate have not been elucidated.
   1. The UMPS may not be sensitive enough to detect small changes in pain behaviors, particularly if patient evaluations are performed only periodically.
   2. The UMPS was designed to evaluate dogs following surgery. The accuracy of the scale for other uses or for use in other species has not been established.
   3. The UMPS requires some knowledge of the demeanor (mental and behavioral status) of the dog before anesthesia and surgery. Although the veterinary staff usually knows this, the dog's actual temperament when truly comfortable at home will probably not be known. In other words, the demeanor of the dog after surgery will be compared with an already altered demeanor that exists simply because the dog is in a veterinary hospital and away from familiar surroundings. An important consideration is that previous experiences may play a significant role in the response of a patient and may alter the accuracy of the scale.

TABLE 6-1	Numerical Rating Scale Previously Used at the Colorado State University James L. Voss Veterinary Medical Center

Observation	Score	Patient Criteria
Comfort	0	Asleep or calm
	1	Awake; interested in surroundings
	2	Mild agitation; obtunded and uninterested in surroundings
	3	Moderate agitation; restless and uncomfortable
	4	Extremely agitated; thrashing
Movement	0	Normal amount of movement
	1	Frequent position changes or reluctance to move
	2	Thrashing
Appearance	0	Normal
	1	Mild changes: eyelids partially closed; ears flattened or carried abnormally
	2	Moderate changes: eyes sunken or glazed; unkempt appearance
	3	Severe changes: eyes pale; enlarged pupils; "grimacing" or other abnormal facial expressions; guarding; hunched-up position; legs in abnormal position; grunting before expiration; teeth grinding
Behavior (unprovoked)	0	Normal
	1	Minor changes
	2	Moderately abnormal: less mobile and less alert than normal; unaware of surroundings; very restless
	3	Markedly abnormal: very restless; vocalizing; self-mutilation; grunting; facing back of cage
Interactive behavior	0	Normal
	1	Pulls away when surgical site is touched; looks at wound; mobile
	2	Vocalizing when wound is touched; somewhat restless; reluctant to move but will if coaxed
	3	Violent reaction to stimuli; vocalizing when wound is not touched; snapping, growling, or hissing when approached; extremely restless; will not move when coaxed

Vocalization	0	Quiet; responds to calm voice and stroking
	1	Crying; responds to calm voice and stroking
	2	Intermittent crying or whimpering; no response to calm voice and stroking
	3	Continuous noise that is unusual for this animal
Heart rate	0	0%-15% above presurgical value
	1	16%-29% above presurgical value
	2	30%-45% above presurgical value
	3	>45% above presurgical value
Respiration rate	0	0%-15% above presurgical value
	1	16%-29% above presurgical value
	2	30%-45% above presurgical value
	3	>45% above presurgical value
Total score (0-24) ____		

Numeric rating scale used to assess pain in dogs and cats. Adapted from Hellyer PW, Gaynor JS: *Compend Contin Educ* 20:140-153, 1998. *It is not the intent of this form to require that animals prove they are in pain before therapy is initiated.* Instead, this form is intended to aid in the evaluation of dogs and cats that may be in pain after surgery or trauma. The exact score that will indicate that treatment for pain is appropriate and will vary from individual to individual. Animals that are expected to be in moderate to severe pain, based on the surgical procedure performed, should be treated *before* assessment indicates severe pain. Many animals will receive analgesics before pain is detected based on this scoring system. Regardless of score, if there is evidence that the animal is in pain, a test dose of analgesic should be administered and changes in behavior noted.

TABLE 6-2   University of Melbourne Pain Scale

Category	Descriptor	Score
1. Physiologic data		
a.	Physiologic data within reference range	0
b.	Dilated pupils	2
c. Choose only one	Percentage increase in heart rate relative to preprocedural rate	
	>20%	1
	>50%	2
	>100%	3
d. Choose only one	Percentage increase in respiratory rate relative to preprocedural rate	
	>20%	1
	>50%	2
	>100%	3
e.	Rectal temperature exceeds reference range	1
f.	Salivation	2
2. Response to palpation (choose only one)	No change from preprocedural behavior	0
	Guards/reacts* when touched	2
	Guards/reacts* before touched	3
3. Activity (choose only one)	At rest: sleeping	0
	At rest: semiconscious	0
	At rest: awake	1
	Eating	0
	Restless (pacing continuously, getting up and down)	2
	Rolling, thrashing	3

4. Mental status (choose only one)	Submissive	0
	Overtly friendly	1
	Wary	2
	Aggressive	3
5. Posture		
a.	Guarding or protecting affected area (includes fetal position)	2
b. Choose only one	Lateral recumbency	0
	Sternal recumbency	1
	Sitting or standing, head up	1
	Standing, head hanging down	2
	Moving	1
	Abnormal posture (e.g., prayer position or hunched back)	2
6. Vocalization[†] (choose only one)	Not vocalizing	0
	Vocalizing when touched	2
	Intermittent vocalization	2
	Continuous vocalization	3

Modified from Firth AM, Haldane SL: *J Am Vet Med Assoc* 214:651-659, 1999.

The pain scale includes six categories. Each category contains descriptors of various behaviors that are assigned numeric values. The assessor examines the descriptors in each category and decides whether a descriptor approximates the dog's behavior. If so, the value for that descriptor is added to the patient's pain score. Certain descriptors are mutually exclusive (e.g., a dog cannot be in sternal recumbency and standing at the same time). These mutually exclusive descriptors are grouped together with the notation "choose only one." For the fourth category, mental status, the assessor must have completed a preprocedural assessment of the dog's dominant/aggressive behavior to establish a baseline score. The mental status score is the absolute difference between preprocedural and postprocedural scores. The minimum possible total pain score is 0 points; the maximum possible pain score is 27 points.

*Includes turning head toward affected area; biting, licking, or scratching at the wound; snapping at the handler; or tense muscle and a protective (guarding) posture.

†Does not include alert barking.

4. The UMPS does not account for the residual or adverse effects of anesthesia in scoring. Examples include dysphoria and persistent sedation.

BEHAVIORAL RESPONSE SCALES

◆ The Glasgow Composite Measure Pain Score (GCMPS) is a scale based on specific behavioral signs believed to represent pain in the dog (Box 6-4).[22]
  1. The behaviors included in the scale were derived from a questionnaire of veterinarians.
  2. The expressions used to describe pain behaviors were reduced to specific words and validated using a variety of statistical methods.
  3. Potential advantages of this scale include the following:
     a. Limited interpretation and bias is required by the observer.
     b. Accuracy is increased over the preemptive scoring system, VAS, SDS, and NRS.
     c. Observers simply identify the presence or absence of a behavior.
     d. Terms used to describe individual behaviors are specifically defined, thereby decreasing uncertainty in using the scale.
     e. Physiological data are not included, making the scale easier to use than the UMPS and perhaps more accurate.
  4. Disadvantages of the scale are the following:
     a. Limited validation in actual animal studies
     b. Lack of a numeric scoring system that would allow for comparison of scores over time
     c. Designed for use in dogs only
     d. Does not take into account the impact of demeanor/temperament, as well as previous experience of the patient
     e. Does not account for residual effect of anesthetics
◆ Glasgow Composite Measure Pain Score Short Form (GCMPS-SF) is a modification of the Glasgow Composite Measure Pain Score and as such can be applied quickly in a clinical setting. The short form was designed as a clinical decision-making tool developed for dogs in acute pain (Box 6-5).[23]
  1. Advantages of this scale include those listed before for the original Glasgow scale as well as its use as a numeric rating scale that facilitates therapeutic decision making and comparison among observers and over time. Additionally, the shorter format allows for easier use and potentially increased use.
  2. Disadvantages include those listed before with the notable exception of *b*.

BOX 6-4

The Glasgow Composite Measure Pain Score

The questionnaire is made up of a number of sections, each of which has several possible answers. Please check the answers that you feel are appropriate to the dog you are assessing. If more than one answer is appropriate, then check all that apply. Approach the kennel and ensure you are not wearing a laboratory coat or theater "greens," because the dog may associate these with stress and/or pain. While you approach the kennel, look at the dog's behavior and reactions. From outside the dog's kennel, look at the dog's behavior and answer the following questions.

Look at the Dog's Posture; Does It Seem ...
Rigid ☐   Neither of these ☐
Hunched or tense ☐

Does the Dog Seem to be ...
Restless ☐   Comfortable ☐

If the Dog is Vocalizing, Is It ...
Crying or Whimpering ☐   Screaming ☐
Groaning ☐   Not vocalizing/none of these ☐

If the Dog Is Paying Attention to Its Wound, Is It ...
Chewing ☐   Ignoring its wound ☐
Licking, looking, or rubbing ☐

Now approach the kennel door and call the dog's name. Then open the door and encourage the dog to come to you. From the dog's reaction to you and behaviors when you were watching him/her, assess his/her character.

Does the Dog Seem to be ...
Aggressive ☐   Quiet or indifferent ☐
Depressed ☐   Happy and content ☐
Disinterested ☐   Happy and bouncy ☐
Nervous, anxious, or fearful ☐

During This Procedure, Did the Dog Seem to Be ...
Stiff ☐   None of these ☐
Slow or reluctant to rise or sit ☐ Assessment not carried out ☐
Lame ☐

The next procedure is to assess the dog's response to touch. If the animal has a wound, apply gentle pressure to the wound using two fingers in an area approximately 2 inches around it. If the position of the wound is such that it is impossible to touch, then apply the pressure to the closest point to the wound. If there is no wound, apply the same pressure to the stifle and surrounding area.

—Continued

From Holton L, Reid J, Scott EM, et al: *Vet Rec* 148(17):525-531, 2001.

BOX 6-4

The Glasgow Composite Measure Pain Score—*cont'd*

When Touched, Did the Dog...

Cry ☐

Flinch ☐

Snap ☐

Growl or guard wound ☐

None of these ☐

Definitions of expressions used in the Glasgow Composite Measure Pain Score for dogs.

Posture

Rigid: Animal lying in lateral recumbency, legs extended or partially extended in a fixed position.

Hunched: When animal is standing, its back forms a convex shape with abdomen tucked up, or, back in a concave shape with shoulders and front legs lower than hips.

Tense: Animal appears frightened or reluctant to move; overall impression is of tight muscles. Animal can be in any body position.

Normal body posture: Animal may be in any position, appears comfortable, with muscles relaxed.

Comfort

Restless: Moving bodily position, circling, pacing, shifting body parts, unsettled.

Comfortable: Animal resting and relaxed, no avoidance or abnormal body position evident or settled, remains in same body position, at ease.

Vocalization

Crying: Extension of the whimpering noise, louder and with open mouth.

Whimpering: Often quiet, short, high-pitched sound, frequently closed mouth (whining).

Groaning: Low moaning or grunting deep sound, intermittent.

Screaming: Animal making a continual high-pitched noise, inconsolable, mouth wide open.

Attention to Wound Area

Chewing: Using mouth and teeth on wound area, pulling stitches.

Licking: Using tongue to stroke area of wound.

Looking: Turning head in direction of area of wound.

Rubbing: Using paw or kennel floor to stroke wound area.

Ignoring: Paying no attention to the wound area.

Demeanor

Aggressive: Mouth open or lip curled showing teeth, snarling, growling, snapping, or barking.

Depressed: Dull demeanor, not responsive, shows reluctance to interact.

Disinterested: Cannot be stimulated to wag tail or interact with observer.

Nervous: Eyes in continual movement, often head and body movement, jumpy.

Anxious: Worried expression, eyes wide with whites showing, wrinkled forehead.

Fearful: Cowering away, guarding body and head.

Quiet: Sitting or lying still, no noise, will look when spoken to but does not respond.

Indifferent: Not responsive to surroundings or observer.

Content: Interested in surroundings, has positive interaction with observer, responsive and alert.

Bouncy: Tail wagging, jumping in kennel, often vocalizing with a happy and excited noise.

—Continued

BOX 6-4

The Glasgow Composite Measure Pain Score—*cont'd*

Mobility

Stiff: Stilted gait, also slow to rise or sit, may be reluctant to move.

Slow to rise or sit: Slow to get up or sit down but not stilted in movement.

Reluctant to rise or sit: Needs encouragement to get up or sit down.

Lame: Irregular gait, uneven weight bearing when walking.

Normal mobility: Gets up and lies down with no alteration from normal.

Response to touch

Cry: A short vocal response. Looks at area and opens mouth, emits a brief sound.

Flinch: Painful area is quickly moved away from stimulus either before or in response to touch.

Snap: Tries to bite observer before or in response to touch.

Growl: Emits a low prolonged warning sound before or in response to touch.

Guard: Pulls painful area away from stimulus or tenses local muscles in order to protect from stimulus.

None: Accepts firm pressure on wound with none of the aforementioned reactions.

BOX 6-5

Glasgow Composite Measure Pain Score—Short Form

Dog's Name: _____ Hospital Number: _____

Date: _____ Time of Assessment: _____ Assessor: _____

Surgery: Yes / No   Routine Analgesic Intervention: Yes / No

Procedure or Condition:

_____

Do you think this dog needs analgesia? Yes / No

A. Look at dog in kennel. *Is the dog?*

(i)

Quiet	0
Crying or whimpering	1
Groaning	2
Screaming	3

(ii)

Ignoring any wound or painful area	0
Looking at wound or painful area	1
Licking wound or painful area	2
Rubbing wound or painful area	3
Chewing wound or painful area	4

◆ In the case of spinal, pelvic, or multiple limb fractures, or where assistance is required to aid locomotion, do not carry out section B and proceed to C. Please mark if this is the case, and then proceed to C.

—Continued

> **BOX 6-5**
>
> ## Glasgow Composite Measure Pain Score—Short Form —cont'd
>
> **B. Put lead on dog and lead out of kennel.** *When the dog walks/rises, is it?*
> (iii)
>
> | | |
> |---|---|
> | Normal | 0 |
> | Lame | 1 |
> | Slow or reluctant | 2 |
> | Stiff | 3 |
> | It refuses to move | 4 |
>
> **C. If it has a wound or painful area, including abdomen, apply gentle pressure 2 inches around site.** *Does it?*
> (iv)
>
> | | |
> |---|---|
> | Do nothing | 0 |
> | Look around | 1 |
> | Flinch | 2 |
> | Growl or guard area | 3 |
> | Snap | 4 |
> | Cry | 5 |
>
> **D. Overall.** *Is the dog?*
> (v)
>
> | | |
> |---|---|
> | Happy and content or happy and bouncy | 0 |
> | Quiet | 1 |
> | Indifferent or nonresponsive to surroundings | 2 |
> | Nervous or anxious or fearful | 3 |
> | Depressed or nonresponsive to stimulation | 4 |
>
> (vi)
>
> | | |
> |---|---|
> | Comfortable | 0 |
> | Unsettled | 1 |
> | Restless | 2 |
> | Hunched or tense | 3 |
> | Rigid | 4 |
>
> **TOTAL SCORE** (i + ii + iii + iv + v + vi) = _____

From Reid J, Scott M, Nolan A: *Vet Anaesth Analg* 32(6):7, 2005.

RECOMMENDED PAIN SCALE: COLORADO STATE UNIVERSITY VETERINARY MEDICAL CENTER ACUTE PAIN SCALES (CANINE AND FELINE)

A modified pain scale is presented in Figs. 6-2 to 6-4. This scale is a composite scale derived from the UMPS, GCMPS, GCMPS-SF, and the SDS. The format is intended to incorporate the most practical features of the other scales in a single-page, user-friendly design. The scale uses an observational period and a hands-on evaluation of the patient. In general, the assessment begins with quiet observation of the patient in its cage at a relatively unobtrusive distance. Afterward, the patient as a whole (wound and the entire body) is approached to assess reaction to gentle palpation, indicators of muscle tension and heat, and response to interaction.

- The scale uses a generic 0-to-4 scale with quarter marks as its base (Fig. 6-5) along with a color scale as a visual cue for progression along the 5-point scale.

- Realistic artist's renderings of animals at various levels of pain add further visual cues. Additional drawings provide space for recording pain, warmth, and muscle tension; this allows documentation of specific areas of concern in the medical record. A further advantage of these drawings is that the observer is encouraged to assess the overall pain of the patient in addition to focusing on the primary lesion.

- The scale includes psychological and behavioral signs of pain and palpation responses. Further, the scale uses body tension as an evaluation tool, a parameter not addressed in other scales.

- There is a provision for nonassessment in the resting patient. To the authors' knowledge, this is the only scale that emphasizes the importance of delaying assessment in a sleeping patient while prompting the observer to recognize patients that may be inappropriately obtunded by medication or a more serious health concern.

- Advantages of this scale include ease of use with minimal interpretation required. Specific descriptors for individual behaviors are provided, which decreases interobserver variability. Additionally, a scale is provided for the dog and the cat. This is the first comprehensive feline pain scale as of this date.

- A disadvantage of this scale is a lack of validation by clinical studies comparing it with other scales. Further, its use is largely limited to and is intended for use in acute pain. As of this writing, scales have not been developed for other species.

THE OHIO STATE UNIVERSITY VETERINARY TEACHING HOSPITAL

PAIN MANAGEMENT PLAN

"Pain assessment is considered part of every patient evaluation, regardless of presenting complaint."

PATIENT ID CARD

Date: _____   Department: _____

Pulse rate:	Temperature:	°C / °F	
Respiratory rate:	Weight:	lbs / kg	Attitude:

Is pain present upon admission? Y ☐ N ☐   Pain on palpation only? Y ☐ N ☐   Cause of pain: _____

Signs of pain (Check all that apply):

Descriptors (Circle):

Behavior:	Normal ☐	Depressed ☐	Excited ☐	Agitated ☐	Guarding ☐	Aggressive ☐	Restless	Not grooming
Vocalization:	None ☐	Occasional ☐	Continuous ☐	Other ☐			Agitated	Obtund
Posture:	Normal ☐	Frozen ☐	Rigid ☐	Hunched ☐	Recumbent ☐	Reluctant to move ☐	Trembling	Inappetent
Gait:	Sound ☐	Lame weight bearing ☐		Lame non-weight bearing ☐	Non-ambulatory ☐		Nervous	Biting or Licking area

Other signs of pain: _____

Previous Analgesic History: _____

Classification of pain (Check):

Anatomical location of pain (Circle):

Ventral   Dorsal

Left

Right

Comments: _____

Diagnosis: _____

Acute ☐
Acute recurrent ☐
Chronic (>weeks) ☐
Chronic progressive ☐

Superficial ☐
Deep ☐
Visceral ☐

Inflammatory ☐
Neuropathic ☐
Both (Infl/Neuro) ☐
Cancer ☐

Primary hyperalgesia ☐
Secondary hyperalgesia ☐
Central analgesia ☐

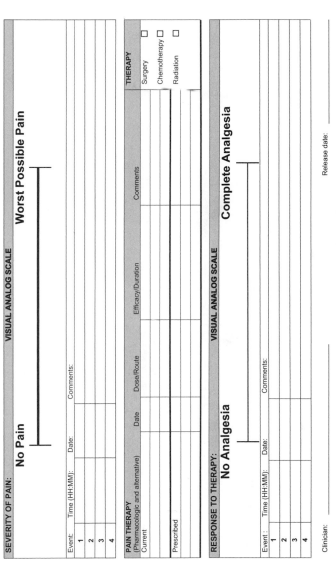

FIG. 6-2. Generic vertical pain scale used as a more versatile adaptation of the simple descriptive scale in the Colorado State University Veterinary Medical Center Acute Pain Scale.

Date _____

Time _____

Colorado State University
Veterinary Medical Center
Canine Acute Pain Scale

Rescore when awake | ☐ Animal is sleeping, but can be aroused - Not evaluated for pain
☐ Animal can't be aroused, check vital signs, assess therapy

Pain Score	Example	Psychological & Behavioral	Response to Palpation	Body Tension
0		☐ **Comfortable** when resting ☐ **Happy, content** ☐ Not bothering wound or surgery site ☐ Interested in or curious about surroundings	☐ **Nontender** to palpation of wound or surgery site, or to palpation elsewhere	Minimal
1		☐ Content to **slightly unsettled** or restless ☐ **Distracted easily** by surroundings	☐ **Reacts to palpation** of wound, surgery site, or other body part by **looking around, flinching,** or **whimpering**	Mild

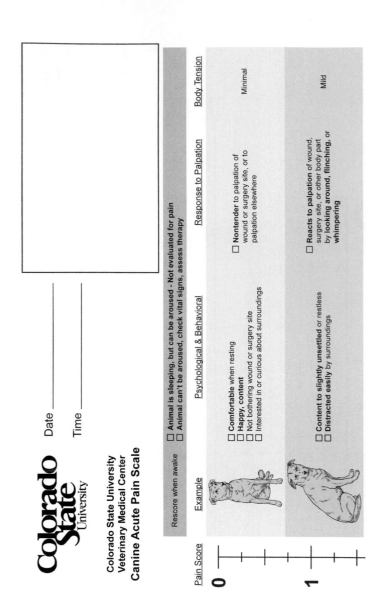

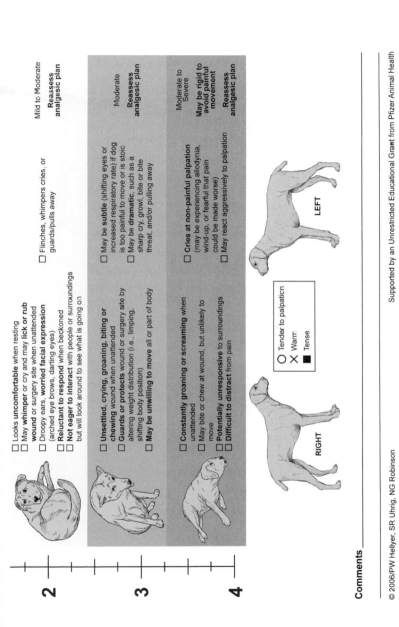

Mild to Moderate

Reassess analgesic plan

☐ Looks **uncomfortable** when resting
☐ May **whimper** or cry and may **lick or rub wound** or surgery site when unattended
☐ Droopy ears, **worried facial expression** (arched eye brows, darting eyes)
☐ **Reluctant to respond** when beckoned
☐ **Not eager to interact** with people or surroundings but will look around to see what is going on

☐ Flinches, whimpers cries, or guards/pulls away

Moderate

Reassess analgesic plan

☐ **Unsettled, crying, groaning, biting or chewing** wound when unattended
☐ **Guards or protects** wound or surgery site by altering weight distribution (i.e., limping, shifting body position)
☐ **May be unwilling to move** all or part of body

☐ May be **subtle** (shifting eyes or increased respiratory rate) if dog is too painful to move or is stoic
☐ May be **dramatic**, such as a sharp cry, growl, bite or bite threat, and/or pulling away

Moderate to Severe

May be rigid to avoid painful movement

Reassess analgesic plan

☐ **Constantly groaning or screaming** when unattended
☐ May bite or chew at wound, but unlikely to move
☐ **Potentially unresponsive** to surroundings
☐ **Difficult to distract** from pain

☐ **Cries at non-painful palpation** (may be experiencing allodynia, wind-up, or fearful that pain could be made worse)
☐ May react aggressively to palpation

○ Tender to palpation
✕ Warm
■ Tense

RIGHT

LEFT

2

3

4

Comments _____

© 2006/PW Hellyer, SR Uhrig, NG Robinson

Supported by an Unrestricted Educational Grant from Pfizer Animal Health

FIG. 6-3. Colorado State University Veterinary Medical Center Canine Acute Pain Scale. (Courtesy Peter Hellyer, Samantha Uhrig, Narda Robinson.)

Colorado State University
Veterinary Medical Center
Feline Acute Pain Scale

Date _____

Time _____

Pain Score		Example	Psychological & Behavioral	Response to Palpation	Body Tension
0	Rescore when awake		☐ Animal is sleeping, but can be aroused - Not evaluated for pain ☐ Animal can't be aroused, check vital signs, assess therapy		
			☐ **Content and quiet** when unattended ☐ **Comfortable** when resting ☐ Interested in or **curious** about surroundings	☐ **Not bothered** by palpation of wound or surgery site, or to palpation elsewhere	Minimal
1			☐ **Signs are often subtle and not easily detected in the hospital setting**; more likely to be detected by the owner(s) at home ☐ Earliest signs at home may be **withdrawal from surroundings or change in normal routine** ☐ In the hospital, may be content or slightly unsettled ☐ **Less interested** in surroundings but will look around to see what is going on	☐ May or may not react to palpation of wound or surgery site	Mild

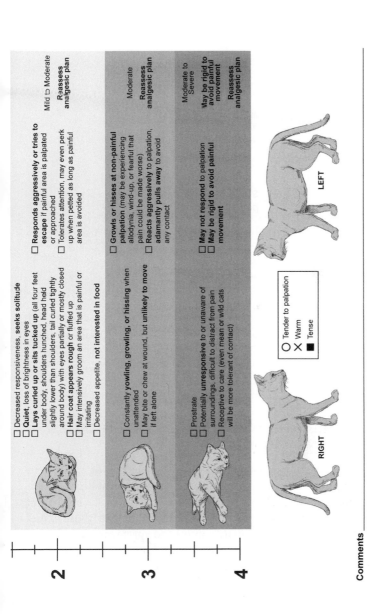

2

- ☐ Decreased responsiveness, **seeks solitude**
- ☐ **Quiet**, loss of brightness in eyes
- ☐ **Lays curled up or sits tucked up** (all four feet under body, shoulders hunched, head held slightly lower than shoulders, tail curled tightly around body) with eyes partially or mostly closed
- ☐ **Hair coat appears rough or fluffed up**
- ☐ May intensively groom an area that is painful or irritating
- ☐ Decreased appetite, **not interested in food**

- ☐ **Responds aggressively or tries to escape** if painful area is palpated or approached
- ☐ Tolerates attention, may even perk up when petted as long as painful area is avoided

Mild to Moderate

Reassess analgesic plan

3

- ☐ **Constantly yowling, growling, or hissing** when unattended
- ☐ May bite or chew at wound, but **unlikely to move if left alone**

- ☐ **Growls or hisses at non-painful palpation** (may be experiencing allodynia, wind-up, or fearful that pain could be made worse)
- ☐ Reacts aggressively to palpation, adamantly pulls away to avoid any contact

Moderate

Reassess analgesic plan

4

- ☐ Prostrate
- ☐ Potentially **unresponsive** to or unaware of surroundings, difficult to distract from pain
- ☐ Receptive to care (even mean or wild cats will be more tolerant of contact)

- ☐ **May not respond to palpation**
- ☐ **May be rigid to avoid painful movement**

Moderate to Severe

May be rigid to avoid painful movement

Reassess analgesic plan

RIGHT   LEFT

○ Tender to palpation
✕ Warm
■ Tense

Comments _____

© 2006/PW Hellyer, SR Uhrig, NG Robinson   Supported by an Unrestricted Educational Grant from Pfizer Animal Health

FIG. 6-4. Colorado State University Veterinary Medical Center Feline Acute Pain Scale. (Courtesy Peter Hellyer, Samantha Uhrig, Narda Robinson.)

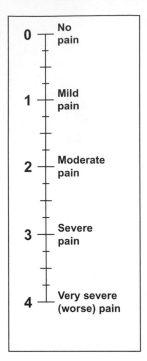

FIG. 6-5. The Ohio State University Veterinary Teaching Hospital Pain Scale and Pain Management Form. (Courtesy W.W. Muir.)

HEALTH RELATED QUALITY OF LIFE SCALES (CANINE AND FELINE)

Quality of life in animals can be assessed by the use of multi-item questionnaires that incorporate general yes or no or multiple option responses that address three primary factors: physical, behavioral (psychological), and social.[24-26] Physical factors include those issues that are associated with animals' ability to perform daily living activities including but not limited to locomotion, appetite, and sleep. Behavioral factors include level of consciousness, sense of well-being, and cognitive functioning. Social factors include both quantitative and qualitative consideration of owner-animal, social relationships, and societal integration. All pain assessment tools should *(must)* be used in conjunction with QOL assessment to maximize animal well-being (Fig. 6-6).

Date: _____   Animal name: _____

Case#: _____   Type of disease: _____

Domain	Classification of QOL		
	Regularly	**Sometimes**	**Rarely**
Physical			
Is your pet's energy level normal?			
Is your pet capable of completing normal everyday tasks (playing, working, going up stairs, etc.)?			
Is your pet eating normal amounts of food?			
Does your pet get up to greet you?			
Does your pet run around the house?			
Can your pet get up easily?			
Is your pet breathing normally?			
Does your pet let you touch the painful area?			
Behavioral			
Is your pet behaving normally?			
Does your pet groom itself?			
Does your pet sleep comfortably?			
Is your pet urinating and defecating normally?			
Does your pet ever seem depressed?			
Is your pet ever anxious or nervous?			
Does your pet cry out unexpectedly?			
Is your pet ever aggressive?			
Is your pet reacting adversely to any medications?			
Do you think your pet is happy?			
Social			
Is your pet happy to see you when you get home?			
Does your pet interact normally with you and other people?			
Does your pet interact normally with other animals?			

Clinician: _____

What is your pet's quality of life?

Quality of life could not be worse   Quality of life could not be better

0_____10

FIG. 6-6. Quality-of-life questionnaire.

REFERENCES

1. Turk CD, Okifuji A: Pain: assessment of patients' reporting of pain—an integrated perspective, *Lancet* 353:1784-1788, 1999.
2. Mathews KA: Pain assessment and general approach to management, *Vet Clin North Am Small Anim Pract* 30:729-755, 2000.
3. Dohoo SE, Dohoo IR: Factors influencing the postoperative use of analgesics in dogs and cats by Canadian veterinarians, *Can Vet J* 37:552-556, 1996.
4. Dohoo SE, Dohoo IA: Attitudes and concerns of Canadian animal health technologists toward postoperative pain management in dogs and cats, *Can Vet J* 39:491-496, 1998.
5. Salmon P, Manyande A: Good patients cope with their pain: postoperative analgesia and nurses' perceptions of their patients' pain, *Pain* 68:63-68, 1996.
6. Cambridge AJ, Tobias KM, Newberry RC, Sarkar DK: Subjective and objective measurements of postoperative pain in cats, *J Am Vet Med Assoc* 217:685-689, 2000.
7. Carroll GL: *Small animal pain management,* Lakewood, Colo, 1998, AAHA Press.
8. Holton LL, Scott EM, Nolan AM et al: Relationship between physiological factors and clinical pain in dogs scored using a numerical rating scale, *J Small Anim Pract* 39:469-474, 1998.
9. Hardie EM, Hansen BD, Carroll GS: Behavior after ovariohysterectomy in the dog: what's normal? *Applied Animal Behaviour Science* 51:111-128, 1997.
10. Dobromylskyj P et al: Pain assessment. In Flecknell P, Waterman-Pearson A, editors: *Pain management in animal,* London, 2000, WB Saunders.
11. Mogil JS: The genetic mediation of individual differences in sensitivity to pain and its inhibition, *Proc Natl Acad Sci U S A* 96:7744-7751, 1999.
12. Firth AM, Haldane SL: Development of a scale to evaluate postoperative pain in dogs, *J Am Vet Med Assoc* 214:651-659, 1999.
13. Holton LL, Scott EM, Nolan AM et al: Comparison of three methods used for assessment of pain in dogs, *J Am Vet Med Assoc* 212:61-66, 1998.
14. Hansen BD, Hardie EM, Carroll GS: Physiological measurements after ovariohysterectomy in dogs: what's normal? *Applied Animal Behaviour Science* 51:101-109, 1997.
15. Smith JD, Allen SW, Quandt JE: Changes in cortisol concentration in response to stress and postoperative pain in client-owned cats and correlation with objective clinical variables, *Am J Vet Res* 60:432-436, 1999.
16. Ferrell BR, Dean GE, Grant M, Coluzzi P: An institutional commitment to pain management, *J Clin Oncol* 13:2158-2165, 1995.
17. *A roundtable discussion: Rethinking your approach to sedation, anesthesia, and analgesia,* Lenexa, Kan, 1997, Veterinary Medicine Publishing.
18. McQuay HJ, Moore RA: Methods of therapeutic trials. In Wall PD, Melzack R, editors: *Textbook of pain,* ed 4, Edinburgh, 1999, Churchill Livingstone.
19. Melzack R, Katz J: Pain measurement in persons in pain. In Wall PD, Melzack R, editors: *Textbook of pain,* ed 4, Edinburgh, 1999, Churchill Livingstone.

20. Todd KH, Funk KG, Funk JP, Bonacci R: Clinical significance of reported changes in pain severity, *Ann Emerg Med* 27:485-489, 1996.
21. Hellyer PW, Gaynor JS: How I treat: acute postsurgical pain in dogs and cats, *Compend Contin Educ* 20:140-153, 1998.
22. Holton L, Reid J, Scott EM et al: Development of a behaviour-based scale to measure acute pain in dogs, *Vet Rec* 148(17):525-531, 2001.
23. Reid J, Scott M, Nolan A: Development of a short form of the Glasgow Composite Measure Pain Scale (CMPS) as a measure of acute pain in the dog, *Vet Anaesth Analg* 32(6):7, 2005.
24. McMillan FD: Quality of life in animals, *J Am Vet Met Assoc* 216:1904-1910, 2000.
25. McMillan FD: Maximizing quality of life in ill animals, *J Am Animal Hosp Assoc* 39:227-235, 2003.
26. Wiseman ML, Nolan AM, Reid J et al: Preliminary study on owner-reported behavior changes associated with chronic pain in dogs, *Vet Rec* 148:423-424, 2001.

7

PHARMACOLOGIC PRINCIPLES AND PAIN: PHARMACOKINETICS AND PHARMACODYNAMICS

WILLIAM W. MUIR III AND RICHARD A. SAMS

The administration of drugs to painful animals is an everyday occurrence. Knowledge of the general principles that define drug doses and dosage regimens, however, is often incomplete or absent. Veterinary clinical pharmacology is the study of drug administration and drug effects in animals, many of which are sick or injured. For example, if it is known that drug elimination is decreased by renal failure, then the dose of that drug must be reduced for an animal with renal failure. Familiarity with the pharmacokinetics and pharmacodynamics of a drug is a prerequisite to understanding clinical pharmacology. At first glance, pharmacokinetic-pharmacodynamic relationships may seem undecipherable, for they are based on a quagmire of confusing terms, mathematical formulas, and complex computer-based models—each claiming to more accurately represent the drug disposition in living animals. Regardless, a knowledge of pharmacokinetic and pharmacodynamic principles is essential to a rational understanding of drug therapy and the selection of therapeutic regimens that are safe and efficacious. This last statement is important for drugs that are used to treat pain because of the potential for analgesic drugs to produce side effects and toxicity.

1. Fundamental principles described by clinical pharmacology
   a. Factors affecting drug absorption, metabolism, distribution, and elimination
   b. Relationships between drug concentration and effect
   c. Calculation of drug dose and dosage regimens
   d. Effect of route of administration on drug concentration and effect

PHARMACOKINETICS

Pharmacokinetics is a quantitative approach to the determination of drug or drug metabolite disposition in the body. The time course of drug elimination is determined from blood or plasma, although other fluids such

113

as cerebrospinal fluid (CSF), tears, and saliva have been used to determine whether therapeutically relevant drug concentrations have been achieved. Once administered, drugs distribute into theoretic compartments (central, peripheral) that do not necessarily correspond to any physiologically relevant space (e.g., extracellular water; Fig. 7-1). Once in the body, all drugs are subjected to a multitude of metabolic and excretory processes that result in their inactivation and elimination. Drug concentration versus time profiles a graphic representation of the disposition of a drug in the body.

◆ Plasma is the most commonly assayed fluid for the detection of drug. Most of the time, the rate of drug elimination from the plasma depends on the concentration of drug in the plasma, so-called first-order elimination (one exponential term [Fig. 7-2]). In other words, the rate of drug elimination from the plasma decreases as the concentration of drug in the plasma decreases. A plot of the log concentration of the drug versus time produces a straight line. More complex multiple compartment models are used when the plot of the drug log concentration versus time curve is not linear (Fig. 7-3). Nonlinear drug log concentration-time profiles suggest complex drug metabolism or elimination processes.

◆ The rates of drug absorption, distribution, metabolism, and elimination are used to derive mathematically the pharmacokinetic variables (volume of distribution [V_d], clearance, half-life) that are used to describe the disposition of a drug in the plasma, standard doses, and dosage regimens.

◆ Physiologically based pharmacokinetic modeling is a quantitative attempt to model exactly the drug disposition in the body in terms of physiologically identifiable compartments and thereby to predict tissue concentrations within specific organs (liver, kidney), tissues (skin, muscle), and fluids (blood, CSF, urine). This latter approach provides minimal additional clinically relevant information regarding drug-dosing regimens and therefore is not discussed further.

FACTORS AFFECTING DRUG ABSORPTION AND DISTRIBUTION

Drugs administered by routes other than the intravenous route (e.g., transcutaneous, subcutaneous, intramuscular, or oral) must be absorbed into the body so that they can be distributed to the target site. Drugs that are administered intravenously depend on the injection technique used (bolus, incremental injection, infusion) and factors that promote (increased tissue blood flow) or limit (high protein binding) drug access to the target site.

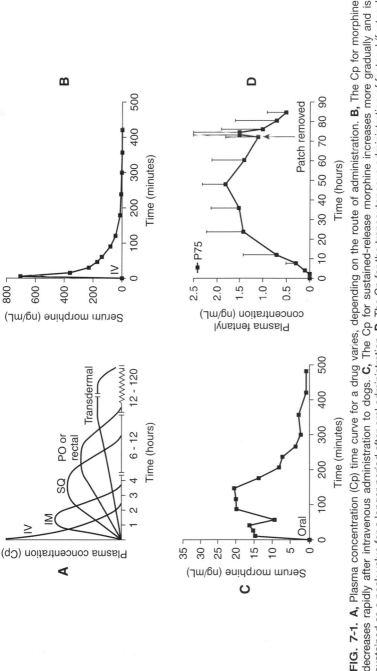

FIG. 7-1. A, Plasma concentration (Cp) time curve for a drug varies, depending on the route of administration. **B,** The Cp for morphine decreases rapidly after intravenous administration to dogs. **C,** The Cp for sustained-release morphine increases more gradually and is sustained as a peak value for a longer period after oral administration. **D,** The Cp for the transcutaneous administration of fentanyl (fentanyl patch; 75 μg/h) in dogs increases slowly before it reaches steady-state concentrations (up to 24 hours). The effects of the drug are expected to parallel the Cp. (From Dohoo SE, Tasker RAR: *Can J Vet Res* 61:251-255, 1997; Egger CM, Duke T, Archer J, Cribb PH: *Vet Surg* 27:159-166, 1998.)

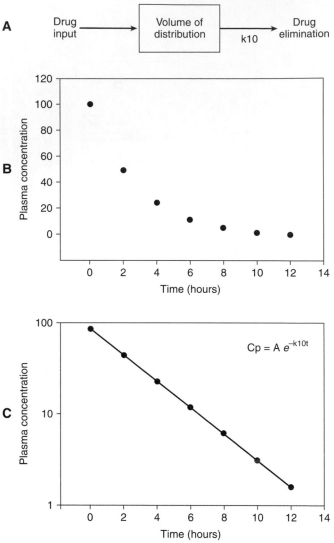

FIG. **7-2.** One-compartment model of intravenous drug disposition. **A,** Pharmacokinetic models are used to describe drug disposition (drug concentration versus time profiles). **B,** The disposition of many drugs can be described by a first-order or one-compartment mode (e.g., ketoprofen), in which the rate of drug elimination depends on the drug plasma concentration (Cp; i.e., the rate of decrease in Cp decreases as Cp decreases). **C,** A plot of the log concentration of Cp is a straight line.

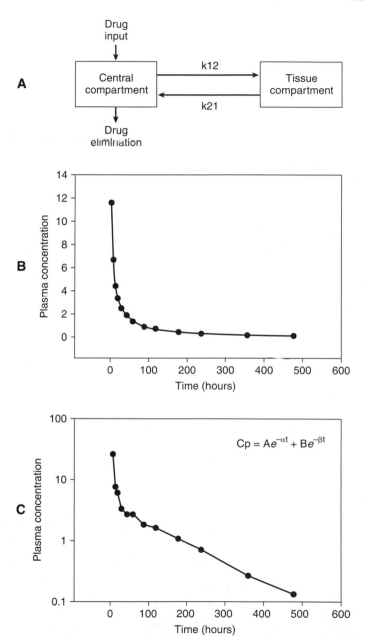

FIG. 7-3. Two-compartment model of intravenous drug disposition. **A,** Multiple compartment models are used when **B,** a plot of the Cp versus time, and **C,** log of Cp versus time, curves show curvature. Two-compartment models are common for many drugs (opioids, α_2-agonists).

ABSORPTION

A drug must pass through several different membranes to reach its site of action. The nature of the membranes determines the rate of passage of the drug through them (diffusion) and, consequently, the rate at which the drug response occurs. The rate of passage of a drug through a membrane can range from zero (i.e., no movement of drug across the membrane) to the rate of blood flow to the membrane (i.e., the drug moves across the membrane as fast as it is delivered). Biologic membranes are composed of a bimolecular layer of lipid molecules coated on either side by a protein layer. Hydrophilic drugs have a difficult time crossing lipid (hydrophobic) membranes. Many biologic membranes appear to contain pores that permit passage of small molecules. Some biologic membranes have mechanisms that transport specific molecules across the membrane. Examples of various transport mechanisms include diffusion, ultrafiltration, and carrier-mediated transport.

Diffusion

The following are determinants of rates of diffusion across biologic membranes:

◆ Concentration gradient: The concentration difference across a biologic membrane determines the direction of diffusion (high concentration to low concentration) and its rate (i.e., the rate of diffusion is directly proportional to the concentration difference).

◆ Lipid solubility: *Lipophilicity* is a term used to describe the solubility of the drug in fatty or oily solutions and is measured by determining the oil/water partition coefficient *(P=lipophilicity)*. The lipophilicity is determined by the number and type of chemical constituents that are attached to the primary chemical molecule (Table 7-1). The oil/water partition coefficient of a drug is a major determinant of the rate of drug diffusion across biologic (lipid/hydrophobic) membranes. The rate of diffusion across a membrane increases linearly with log P up to a maximum value. The optimal value is log P = 0.5 to 2.0.

$$[Drug]_{oil} : [Drug]_{water}$$

$$P = \frac{[Drug]_{oil}}{[Drug]_{water}}$$

◆ Membrane characteristics (anatomic and structural characteristics) and the permeability of different membranes may vary considerably. For example, most capillary membranes are highly permeable, but capillary

TABLE 7-1	Relative Lipophilicity of Drugs	
Drug	**Key Chemical Substituents**	**Relative P**
Most NSAIDs	COO–, COOH	Poor
Procaine, xylazine	NH_2	
Morphine	OH	Intermediate
Lidocaine, bupivacaine	$NHCH_2\,H_5$	
Oxymorphone	=O	Good
Butorphanol	CH_2-cyclobutyl	
Fentanyl	$CH_3, N(CH_3)_2$	
Naloxone	$CH_2CH=CH_2$	Excellent
Barbiturates	C_6H_5	

P, Lipophilicity; *NSAIDs,* nonsteroidal antiinflammatory drugs.

membranes of the brain contain glial cells that are much less permeable to the diffusion of less lipophilic molecules. (The blood-brain barrier is not a barrier to the diffusion of lipophilic molecules because they readily diffuse through the membrane.) Drugs that have a low molecular weight, are not electrically charged, or are highly lipophilic readily diffuse into the various tissue compartments (e.g., extracellular space, intracellular space, and CSF). The epidural or intrathecal administration of analgesic drugs provides a good example of the practical importance of lipophilicity. Highly lipid-soluble drugs (e.g., fentanyl and oxymorphone) rapidly diffuse out of the epidural space or CSF into surrounding tissues, producing a relatively short duration of analgesic effect. Morphine is less lipid soluble than fentanyl or oxymorphone and therefore produces a much longer duration of analgesia when administered by the epidural route.

◆ Small molecules (e.g., electrolytes, water, and ethanol) appear to diffuse through membranes via aqueous pores. Very large molecules do not readily diffuse through membranes.

Ultrafiltration

Water and relatively small molecules (molecular weight <30,000 D) are forced through certain membranes (e.g., glomerular filtration) by the hydrostatic pressure of the blood. Drug molecules bound to plasma proteins are not filtered because the proteins are generally too large to pass through the membrane.

Carrier-Mediated Transport

Many membranes possess specialized transport mechanisms that regulate the movement of drugs and other molecules across cell membranes. These transport mechanisms generally use a carrier molecule that may or may not require energy. Carrier-mediated transport is particularly important for the transfer of drugs across the renal tubules, biliary tract, gastrointestinal tract, and the blood-brain barrier.

◆ Carrier-mediated transport may or may not limit diffusion but often has a maximum value (becomes saturated). Competitive inhibition of transport may occur if a second molecule binds to the carrier, thereby interfering with the transport of the first molecule.

◆ Active transport is usually coupled to an energy source such as adenosine triphosphate and can transport molecules against an electrochemical gradient (e.g., transport of essential nutrients from the gastrointestinal tract against a concentration gradient). Active transport is usually specific and competitive.

  1. Specificity: The transport mechanism is usually specific for a single substance or a group of closely related substances (e.g., transport of anions from the blood into the renal tubule in the nephron).

  2. Competitive: The transport process is competitively inhibited by other molecules also transported by the system (e.g., probenecid competitively inhibits transport of various penicillins in the renal tubules).

◆ Facilitated transport promotes the equilibration of the transported substance. For example, the transport of a molecule in the same direction as its electrochemical gradient (Na^+ flux into renal tubules).

DISTRIBUTION

The distribution of a drug to the active site is governed by four factors: *drug binding, ionization, perfusion,* and *diffusion* (discussed previously). Once a drug enters the blood, it is distributed throughout all the tissues of the body based on their total blood flow. The tissues can be categorized based on the percentage of cardiac output they receive into vessel-rich group (e.g., heart, lung, brain, liver, and kidney), muscle group, fat group, and vessel-poor group (e.g., tendons, ligaments, and joint spaces). Skin can be a vessel-rich or vessel-poor group tissue, depending on temperature. Vessel-rich group tissues receive the majority (greatest percentage) of the cardiac output and are expected to receive the greatest amount of drug in the shortest time. A decrease in cardiac output prolongs the time necessary for drug distribution and, as a result of compensatory homeostatic responses, alters drug distribution. Animals in shock, for example, have a greater percentage of their cardiac output (and therefore any intravenously administered drug) delivered to vessel-rich group (heart, lungs, and brain) tissues.

Blood Flow Rate

Drugs are delivered rapidly to highly perfused tissues and slowly to poorly perfused tissues. The rate of diffusion of a drug across a membrane depends on its rate of delivery to the tissue if the drug rapidly passes through the membrane; this is known as *blood-flow rate-limited diffusion.*

The rate of diffusion of a drug across a membrane depends on the membrane permeability characteristics if the membrane is a barrier to drug passage; this is known as *membrane-limited diffusion.*

Protein Binding

Many drugs bind reversibly to macromolecules such as plasma proteins (e.g., albumen, α_1-acid glycoprotein) and tissue proteins (Drug + Protein = Drug-protein complex). A bound drug is not free to diffuse or interact with receptors; some active transport processes strip bound drugs from binding sites.

◆ Drug protein binding in the blood reduces the concentration of *free drug* available for diffusion across membranes; therefore the rate of diffusion across the membrane is decreased when a drug is extensively protein bound.

◆ At equilibrium, the concentration of free drug is the same on both sides of the membrane; the concentration of the total drug (bound and unbound) may be different on the two sides of the membrane, depending on how much of it is bound to proteins.

Differential Ionization

Ionized substances do not *diffuse* across biologic membranes. Differences in pH exist across many biologic membranes (e.g., the pH of gastric contents ranges from about 2 to 3 and that of plasma is 7.4). These differences lead to accumulation of more total drug (i.e., ionized plus nonionized) on that side of the membrane where the drug is more ionized.

The partitioning (tissue-to-plasma ratio [$R_{T/P}$] of a drug between two regions of differing pH) is described by the Henderson-Hasselbalch equation:

$$R_{T/P} = \frac{\left(1 + antilog\left[pKa - pH_T\right]\right)}{\left(1 + antilog\left[pKa - pH_P\right]\right)}$$

where pH_T and pH_P are the pH values of a tissue and plasma, respectively, and pKa is the dissociation constant of the drug. Although the pH of the plasma is maintained within narrow limits, the pH of injured or infected tissues can vary considerably.

DRUG ELIMINATION

Two principal mechanisms, metabolism and excretion, determine drug elimination from the body. The liver and kidneys are the two major organs of elimination for most drugs, although the plasma (Hoffman elimination) and lungs are potential sites for the metabolism and elimination of some drugs (nitrous oxide [N_2O]) and vapors (inhalant anesthetics). The metabolism of drugs and other foreign substances is a protective mechanism that usually results in a decrease in the lipophilicity of a drug, protein binding, or its ionization. Occasionally, drug metabolism results in the activation of drug effects (e.g., prodrugs such as parecoxib) or toxicity (drug metabolites; lidocaine).

METABOLISM IN THE LIVER

Liver metabolism depends highly on the cytochrome P_{450} enzyme system, a heterogeneous group of highly active and efficient enzymes. Synthesis of some of these enzymes is induced by exposure to drugs such as phenobarbital and rifampin, and some of these enzymes are inhibited by exposure to drugs (chloramphenicol). The capacity of the cytochrome P_{450} enzyme to metabolize drugs is very high; therefore, most drugs administered at therapeutic concentrations rarely saturate the system. Consequently, the rate of drug metabolism is generally proportional to drug concentration (first order); however, in cases of poisoning, the enzyme system may saturate, and the rate of metabolism is slowed.

◆ The anatomic position of the liver requires that drugs absorbed from the gastrointestinal tract pass through the liver before reaching the systemic circulation; if the drug is rapidly and extensively metabolized by the liver, the substance undergoes extensive *first-pass metabolism* (Fig. 7-4) with only a small fraction of the dose reaching the systemic circulation (e.g., isoxsuprine, propranolol, morphine, and lidocaine). First-pass metabolism is the reason many drugs (opioids) are ineffective when administered orally to dogs and cats.

◆ Major metabolic pathways in mammals include the following:
  1. Phase I pathways: Oxidation, reduction, hydrolysis (Esterases are also found in plasma.)
  2. Phase II pathways: Conjugation (e.g., reaction of a drug or phase I metabolite with glucuronic acid). Note that glucuronic acid conjugation is deficient in cats. Differences between species are frequently due to the absence of a particular enzyme system in one species versus another; for example, in cats the ability to conjugate most substances with glucuronic acid is deficient.

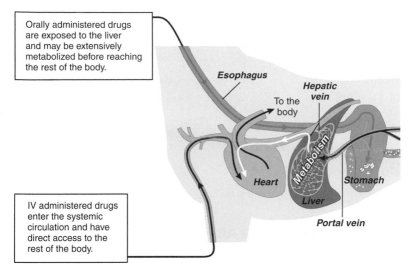

Orally administered drugs are exposed to the liver and may be extensively metabolized before reaching the rest of the body.

IV administered drugs enter the systemic circulation and have direct access to the rest of the body.

FIG. 7-4. First-pass elimination. The effects of many drugs are greatly reduced (e.g., oral opioids) or rendered biologically inactive by metabolism in the liver or by biliary excretion during first passage through the liver.

3. Spontaneous decomposition occurs in the plasma at physiologic pH and near-normal temperature by means of a base-catalyzed reaction (Hoffman elimination). In this reaction, protons (H^+) are cleaved from the α-carbon atom of the molecule, resulting in subsequent metabolism and inactive by-products (e.g., etomidate and atracurium).

EXCRETION OF DRUGS AND DRUG METABOLITES

Excretion of drugs and drug metabolites involves the kidneys, biliary mechanisms, and other routes (sweat, saliva, feces).

Renal Excretion

Renal excretion is the most important route of *excretion;* it involves three mechanisms: glomerular filtration, tubular secretion, and passive reabsorption.

- *Glomerular filtration* of unbound drug (Highly bound drugs such as the nonsteroidal antiinflammatory drugs [NSAIDs] are not excreted by glomerular filtration.)
- *Tubular secretion* of anions (e.g., NSAIDs, penicillins, cephalosporins, glucuronic acid conjugates) and cations (e.g., cimetidine) occurs with many drugs.

◆ *Passive reabsorption* of lipophilic drugs (The pH of urine can have profound effects on the extent of tubular reabsorption.)

Biliary Excretion

Biliary excretion is an active process usually restricted to drugs or metabolites above a species-specific molecular size; drug conjugates are frequently secreted in the bile.

Enterohepatic cycling involves the intestinal reabsorption of a drug excreted by the liver into the bile and the intestine.

Other Routes of Excretion

Excretion of drugs occurs in sweat, saliva, and feces.

ROUTES OF DRUG ADMINISTRATION

The advantages and disadvantages of various routes of drug administration are described in more detail elsewhere in this text (see Chapter 8). From a pharmacokinetic viewpoint, a drug can be administered by intravenous and extravascular routes with conventional or modified (prolonged release) delivery systems.

INTRAVENOUS BOLUS DOSE

An intravenous bolus dose refers to the rapid injection of a drug directly into a vein; the dose is usually expressed in terms of mass (e.g., milligrams or grams) or mass per unit of body weight (bw; e.g., milligrams/kilogram bw), not in milliliters/kilogram.

INTRAVENOUS INFUSION

Intravenous infusion is slow, continuous injection of the drug directly into a vein; the dose is usually expressed in terms of mass and time (e.g., milligrams/minute or grams/hour) or mass per unit of bw per unit of time (e.g., micrograms/kilogram per minute). A variety of commercially available infusion pumps are available for the infusion of drugs.

EXTRAVASCULAR ADMINISTRATION

Extravascular administration is administration of a drug by a route other than the vascular system (e.g., oral, rectal, intramuscular, subcutaneous, intraarticular, or transcutaneous).

PROLONGED-RELEASE DOSAGE FORMS

Drug formulations designed to release the drug at a slow rate (e.g., slow-release tablets, liposome-encapsulated) are available. Prolonged-release dosage forms designed for use in human beings may not work in animals.

PHARMACOKINETIC CONCEPTS

Pharmacokinetic variables help to understand drug disposition and the duration of drug action in the body. The basic variables include V_d, clearance, and half-life. These data are used to determine loading dose, maintenance dose, and dosing interval. Additional variables such as mean resonance time and bioavailability are used to adjust and refine initial calculations.

VOLUME OF DISTRIBUTION

The V_d is the apparent volume within which the drug is distributed. The word *apparent* is used because some drugs are bound to tissues, resulting in V_d much larger than the total volume of body water they truly occupy. Simply explained, if 10 mg of drug were injected into the body and the plasma concentration (Cp) was 0.002 mg/ml, then the V_d would be 5000 ml (5 L). The V_d of morphine is 6.1 L/kg in the dog and 1.35 L/kg in the cat. The V_d of lidocaine is 4.9 L/kg in the dog and 3.6 L/kg in the cat. These examples emphasize species differences and the much smaller V_d of morphine in the cat compared with that in the dog. The V_d calculated during the elimination phase is described by the relationship between the amount of drug injected into the body and the Cp of the drug before elimination begins or at time 0 (Cp_0):

$$V_d = \frac{Amount\ injected\ into\ body}{Cp_0}$$

The V_d calculated at steady-state equilibrium (V_{dss}) defines the extent of drug dilution at the peak of drug distribution and is a more accurate assessment of drug dilution in the body. The V_{dss} is calculated as follows:

$$V_{dss} = \frac{Dose}{AUC?}$$

where *AUC* is area under the curve.

- Units of V_d are volume (e.g., milliliter or liter) or volume per unit of bw (e.g., milliliter/kilogram bw).

♦ A large V_d implies extensive distribution of the drug to tissues, whereas a small V_d implies more limited distribution.

♦ The lower limit for V_d is the plasma volume; there is no upper limit, but values of 5 to 10 L/kg bw for lipophilic (e.g., propranolol) or highly tissue-bound (e.g., digoxin) drugs are not uncommon.

♦ The *mean resonance time (MRT)* is a term used to describe the average time that the drug stays in the body or the time it takes for 63.2% of a drug injected into the body to be eliminated. The MRT can be used to calculate V_{dss}:

$$V_{dss} = \frac{Dose}{AUC \times MRT}$$

CLEARANCE

Plasma clearance (CL) is the volume of biologic fluid (blood, plasma) that is completely freed (cleared) of drug by all routes of elimination. Units for clearance are flow (e.g., milliliters/minute) or flow per unit of bw (e.g., milliliters/minute per kilogram bw). These units (milliliters/minute per kilogram) emphasize that clearance is not the amount of drug being removed from the body but the amount of biologic fluid "cleared" of drug. Clearance can be calculated as the rate of elimination of the drug by all routes divided by the Cp of the drug:

$$CL = \frac{Rate\ of\ elimination}{Cp}$$

♦ The lower limit for clearance by an organ of elimination is zero. The upper limit is the plasma flow to the organ. Individual organ clearances can be added together for the total body clearance:

$$CL_T = CL_H + CL_R + CL_{other}$$

where CL_T is the total clearance, CL_H is the hepatic clearance, CL_R is the renal clearance, and CL_{other} represents the sum of all other clearance processes.

♦ The total clearance is considered the most useful pharmacokinetic parameter because it is a direct indicator of organ function and can be used to predict the average concentration or steady-state concentration of drug in the blood or plasma. For example, if the CL is 0.1 ml/min per kilogram and the rate of drug administration is 0.1 µg/kg per minute, then the average drug concentration of the plasma is 1.0 µg/ml (0.1 µg/min per kilogram divided by 0.1 ml/min per kilogram). Knowing the total clearance provides the ability to adjust the drug dose rate during administration.

◆ The total clearance of all of the elimination processes in the body is calculated by dividing the dose administered by the total area under the Cp time curve (AUC) from the time of dosing until drug concentrations can no longer be measured (CL = Dose/AUC). In other words, if the target steady-state Cp and clearance for a drug are known, then the dose rate can be calculated by the equation Dose rate = Cp × CL. For example, if the target Cp is 80 µg/ml and the clearance is 0.125 ml/min per kilogram, then the dose rate will be 10 µg/min per kilogram (80 µg/ml × 0.125 ml/min per kilogram) or 3.6 mg every 6 hours.

HALF-LIFE

The elimination half-life ($t_{1/2}$) is the time required for the Cp of the drug to decrease to 50% of an earlier value (Box 7-1). The units for half-life are expressed as time (minutes, hours).
◆ The half-life of a drug can also be used to determine the time required for an infused drug to reach steady state (Box 7-2).
◆ The $t_{1/2}$, total clearance, and V_d are related by the following equation:

$$t_{1/2} = \frac{0.693 \times V_d}{CL}$$

◆ Changes in total clearance or V_d alter the $t_{1/2}$. For example, reduced renal clearance resulting from renal disease or toxicity decreases total clearance and increases $t_{1/2}$.

BOX 7-1

Estimated Time for Drug Removal

1 half-life—50% eliminated
2 half-lives—75% eliminated
3 half-lives—87.5% eliminated
3.3 half-lives—90% eliminated
4 half-lives—93.75% eliminated
5 half-lives—97% eliminated

BOX 7-2

Estimated Time Required to Reach Steady State

1 half-life—50% of steady state
2 half-lives—75% of steady state
3 half-lives—87.5% of steady state
3.3 half-lives—90% of steady state

BIOAVAILABILITY

The term *bioavailability* is the amount of drug that reaches the systemic circulation after being administered by a nonintravenous route. For example, the bioavailability of many opioids is relatively low in dogs after oral administration because of erratic absorption and metabolism by the liver (first-pass effect) before the drug reaches the systemic circulation.

BIOEQUIVALENCE

Bioequivalence is a term that is used when two drugs are compared. Two drugs are considered to be bioequivalent when the Cp versus time profiles and pharmacologic, therapeutic, and toxic effects are the same after administration of equal doses by the same route. Although the peak and trough Cps of two drugs may not necessarily be exactly the same, they are considered to be bioequivalent when the maximum and minimum Cps and the time required to produce a predetermined response are the same.

CALCULATION OF DOSAGE REGIMENS

The ability to estimate and calculate drug dosage regimens is critical to producing an appropriate therapeutic effect and avoiding adverse drug effects.

Maintenance Dose

The maintenance dose is the dose administered throughout a dosage regimen to maintain effective drug concentrations (Fig. 7-5). The maintenance dose (MD) is equal to the desired Cp times the total body clearance.

$$MD = Cp \times CL$$

◆ For example, calculate the maintenance dose for a drug with a V_d of 2000 ml/kg bw and clearance of 20 ml/min per kilogram bw to be administered to a 10-kg dog to achieve a steady-state plasma drug concentration of 2 µg/ml:

$$MD = 2 \, \mu g/ml \times 20 \, ml/min \, per \, kilogram \, bw$$
$$MD = 40 \, \mu g/min \, per \, kilogram \, bw$$
$$MD = 40 \, \mu g/min \times 10 \, kg = 400 \, \mu g/min$$
$$or \, (60 \, minutes \times 6 \, hours \times 40 \, \mu g/min \, per \, kilogram) \, 14.4 \, mg \, every \, 6 \, hours$$

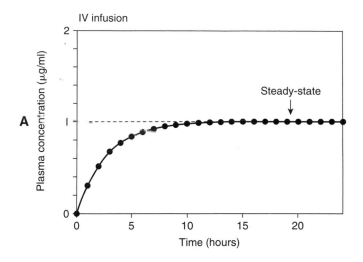

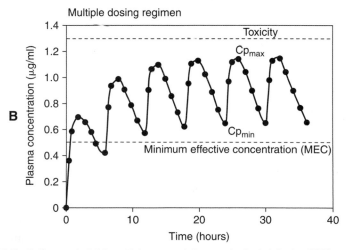

FIG. 7-5. A, Drugs administered intravenously by constant rate infusion (CRI) reach a steady-state value that can be predicted by their half-lives (i.e., 90% of steady state in 3.3 half-lives). **B,** The plasma concentration (Cp) varies between a Cp_{max} and Cp_{min} when drugs are administered at regular intervals (hours). Fluctuations between Cp_{max} and Cp_{min} at steady state increase as the dosing interval increases and can be predicted by the half-life of the drug. The Cp_{max} is equal to 2 times the Cp_{min} when the dosing interval is equal to the half-life of the drug.

♦ The time required to reach steady-state drug concentrations is determined by the terminal half-life of the drug (50% of final value in one half-life; 75% in two half-lives; 87.5% in three half-lives; 90% in 3.3 half-lives; Box 7-2). Delay in achieving desired plasma drug concentrations may be critical for certain drugs (e.g., transcutaneous fentanyl patch).

Loading Dose

The loading dose (LD) is administered at the start of a dosage regimen to achieve effective Cp rapidly. The LD is equal to the desired or target Cp multiplied by the V_d:

$$LD = Cp \times V_d$$

For example, calculate the LD required to achieve a Cp of 2 μg/ml for a drug with a V_d of 2000 ml/kg bw and clearance of 20 ml/min per kilogram bw to be administered to a 10-kg dog:

$$LD = 2 \ \mu g/ml \times 2000 \ ml/kg \ bw$$
$$LD = 4000 \ \mu g/kg \ bw \times 10 \ kg \ bw$$
$$LD = 40,000 \ \mu g/1000 \ \mu g = 40 \ mg$$

Note: The value of the clearance term was provided but was not needed for this calculation.

Dosing Interval

The dosing interval is the period between doses. An infinitely small dosing interval is a constant rate infusion (CRI). The time taken to achieve 90% of the final steady-state Cp during CRI is 3.3 half-lives. A drug with a 2½-hour half-life would take approximately 8¼ hours to reach 90% of its final steady-state Cp if administered by CRI (Fig. 7-5). Fluctuations between the maximum plasma concentration (Cp_{max}) and minimum plasma concentration (Cp_{min}) at steady state increase as the dosing interval increases. $Cp_{max} = 2 \times Cp_{min}$ when the dosing interval equals the half-life.

For example, calculate the maximum dosing interval for a drug with a V_d of 2000 ml/kg bw and a clearance of 20 ml/min per kilogram bw to achieve a Cp_{max} no more than twice Cp_{min}.

$$Dosing \ interval \ = \ t_{1/2} = 0.693 \times V_d / CL$$
$$Dosing \ interval \ = \ 0.693 \times (2000 \ ml/kg \ bw)/(20 \ ml/min \ per \ kilogram \ bw)$$
$$Dosing \ interval \ = \ 69.3 \ minutes$$

PHARMACODYNAMICS

Pharmacodynamics is a quantitative approach for describing the relationship between drug Cp and drug effect. Pharmacologic effects require that drug molecules be bound to constituents of cells or tissues to produce an effect. Most drugs exert their effects by combining with various regulatory proteins, including enzymes (NSAIDs), carrier molecules, ion channels (local anesthetics), and receptors (opioids, α_2-agonists). The term *receptor* is commonly used to mean any macromolecule (generally a protein) with which the drug combines to produce its effects. Drug concentration at the receptor site is not commonly measured but is assumed to be related to the concentration of drug in blood or plasma. The drug concentration at the receptor site, however, may not be identical to its concentration in blood because of a number of factors, including drug binding to plasma and tissue proteins, ion trapping of the drug, and slow passage of the drug through membranes. Equilibration of drug between the plasma and the receptor site generally produces a predictable relationship between Cp and effect (dose-effect relationship). The clinical goal is to develop and administer a therapeutic regimen that establishes and maintains an effective drug Cp for as long as required.

RECEPTOR PHARMACOLOGY

Many different types of drug receptors exist in the body that when occupied by drugs are capable of producing a myriad of cellular effects, including analgesia (Table 7-2). The pharmacologic response that follows drug (ligand) occupation of receptors is proportional to the number or fraction of receptors occupied.

Agonist

An agonist is a drug that binds to and activates a receptor and produces a biologic effect (Fig. 7-6). Drugs that produce the maximal response possible are called *full agonists* (i.e., the intrinsic activity is 1).

Antagonist

An antagonist is a drug that binds to a receptor and produces no biologic effect. Drug antagonists block, interfere with, or reverse the effects of agonists. A pure antagonist is assumed to produce no agonistic effects and has an intrinsic activity of zero.

♦ Competitive receptor antagonists compete for the receptor site. Their effects are said to be surmountable or reversible because they can be

TABLE 7-2	Receptor Agonists and Antagonists Known to Produce Analgesia
Receptor Agonists/Antagonists	**Receptor Subtypes**
RECEPTOR AGONISTS	
Opioid	μ, κ, δ
α_2	α_{2A}, α_{2B}, α_{2D}
Cannabinoid	$CB_{1,2}$
RECEPTOR ANTAGONISTS	
Prostaglandin	EP_{1-4}
Histamine	H_1
Calcium	N and L type
Tachykinin	NK_1
NMDA	NR_1
AMPA	iGluR1-3

NMDA, N-methyl-D-aspartate; *AMPA,* α-amino-3-hydroxy-5-methyl-4-isoxazole propionic acid.

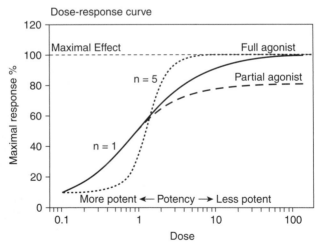

FIG. 7-6. The dose-response curve can be thought of in terms of the plasma concentration (Cp)–effect relationship and relates the drug concentration to the effect produced. Drugs that act at receptor sites (e.g., opioids, α_2-agonists) are called *full agonists* when they produce the maximal response possible (e.g., morphine, hydromorphone, and fentanyl) and *partial agonists* when they produce less than the maximal effect (e.g., buprenorphine). Drugs that produce a maximal effect at lower Cp or doses are more potent than drugs that require higher Cp. The shape (slope) of the Cp-effect curve (N) is important for estimating the therapeutic range of the drug and is important in the development of pharmacokinetic-pharmacodynamic models.

overcome by a higher dose of the agonist. Competitive antagonists shift the dose-effect curve to the right (e.g., atropine and most opioid and α_2-antagonists [opioid—nalorphine, naloxone, nalmefene; α_2—tolazoline, yohimbine, atipamezole]).

◆ Noncompetitive receptor antagonists produce an effect that cannot be overcome by increasing concentrations of the agonist (e.g., phenoxybenzamine, an α_1-antagonist]). Effects of noncompetitive receptor antagonists are irreversible until the drug is completely eliminated.

◆ Physiologic antagonism is not receptor mediated but is a term used to describe the production of an effect that is opposite to that which is not wanted (e.g., dopamine administration to raise blood pressure during hypotension).

Partial Agonist

A partial agonist is a drug that interacts with a receptor but produces less than the maximal effect (Fig. 7-6). A partial agonist produces less than full agonist effects (i.e., intrinsic activity is between 0.0 and 1.0) and is by definition less efficacious than a full agonist. Partial agonists may also act as partial antagonists (e.g., buprenorphine).

Intrinsic Activity

The term *intrinsic activity* refers to the maximal possible effect that can be produced by a drug. Intrinsic activity is determined by the drug-receptor relationship for a drug that acts on receptors. Receptor pharmacology assumes that the effect of a drug is proportional to the number of receptors occupied, implying that a greater effect is produced by occupation of more receptors and that a maximal effect can be produced without occupation of all the receptors of the drug. Low-efficacy opioids (e.g., butorphanol) or partial agonists (e.g., buprenorphine) must by definition occupy more receptors to produce a given effect than higher-efficacy opioids (e.g., fentanyl) and demonstrate a ceiling effect in which larger doses of the drug do not produce a greater degree of analgesia because all the receptors are occupied. Intrinsic efficacy for opioids is as follows: fentanyl > hydromorphone > morphine > buprenorphine > butorphanol > nalbuphine.

Potency

Drug potency depends on the affinity of a drug for the receptor (i.e., tendency for the drug to bind to the receptor) and efficacy (i.e., ability to produce an effect). Potency is the intensity of effect produced for a given drug dose. Two drugs can be equiefficacious (i.e., produce the same maximal response) but vary in potency (dose required to produce the response). The drug that requires the larger dose to produce the desired effect is said to be less potent.

Spare Receptors

The term *spare receptors* or *receptor reserve* is used to describe situations in which a drug produces a maximal effect by occupying only a small fraction of the total number of receptors, leaving the remaining receptors as spares or in reserve. More potent drugs (high intrinsic activity) occupy a smaller number of receptors than less potent drugs to produce a given effect and therefore have a larger receptor reserve.

Racemic Mixtures

Some drug molecules have two or more three-dimensional structures. Drugs that have the same chemical formula but two different structures are termed *isomers* of one another. Isomers that have different structures as a result of the interchange of any two groups around a central carbon atom are termed *enantiomorphs*. A drug that has an asymmetric carbon atom (an asymmetric center is termed a *center of chirality*) and exists as an equimolar mixture of optical (mirror image) isomers is called a *racemic mixture*. The two components of racemic mixtures may have similar or different receptor effects. Medetomidine is a racemic mixture of dexmedetomidine and levomedetomidine. Levomedetomidine is believed to be pharmacologically inactive.

PHARMACODYNAMIC MODELS

As stated previously, pharmacodynamics is the study of the relationship between drug concentration and effect. Pharmacokinetics and pharmacodynamics share drug concentration as a common feature, allowing them to be combined to describe the dose-effect relationship. The most commonly used and simplest model for describing the dose-effect relationship over a range of drug concentrations is derived from the Hill equation, which relates the drug effect to the maximum drug effect (E_{max}), Cp, and the drug concentration required to produce 50% of the maximum effect (EC_{50}):

$$E = \frac{E_{max} \times Cp}{EC_{50} + Cp}$$

This equation usually produces a hyperbolic or sigmoid drug Cp-effect curve, which permits the estimation of drug effects at differing drug doses and provides insight into the pharmacodynamics of the drug (Fig. 7-6).

PHARMACOKINETIC-PHARMACODYNAMIC MODELS

Pharmacokinetic-pharmacodynamic models are valuable in designing drug dosage regimens, particularly when the desired effect is known. In addition, information obtained from these models is valuable in defining the therapeutic index and lethal dose of a drug (Fig. 7-7).

Median Effective Dose

The median effective dose (ED_{50}) is the dose of drug required to produce a predetermined specified effect in 50% of treated animals.

Median Lethal Dose

The median lethal dose (LD_{50}) is the dose of drug required to cause death in 50% of treated animals.

Therapeutic Index

The therapeutic index (TI) is a measure of the margin of safety of a drug and is determined by dividing the LD_{50} by the ED_{50}:

$$TI = \frac{LD_{50}}{ED_{50}}$$

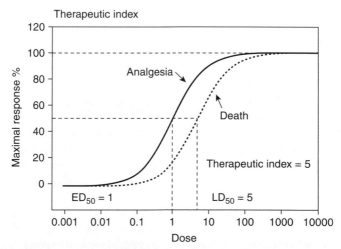

FIG. 7-7. The therapeutic index of a drug is determined by dividing the median lethal dose by the median effective dose and provides a measure of the margin of safety for that drug.

The TI may vary depending on the predetermined pharmacologic endpoint desired (e.g., analgesia versus sedation). In many instances, the ED_{50} increases while the LD_{50} stays the same, resulting in a decrease in the TI.

DRUG INTERACTIONS

The ability of one drug to alter the effects of another, thereby producing a different drug effect, is frequently encountered and often expected during drug therapy. Drug interactions can be pharmacokinetic or pharmacodynamic in origin and may produce beneficial, untoward, or toxic effects. Pharmacokinetic drug interactions occur when one drug alters the Cp and therefore the effects of another drug. Infusions of lidocaine, for example, are known to slow the metabolism and elimination of drugs that depend on liver metabolism (opioids, α_2-agonists), thereby intensifying and prolonging their effects. Pharmacodynamic drug interactions occur when one drug alters the effects of a second drug without changing the Cp or elimination (pharmacokinetics) of the second drug. The opioid antagonist naloxone, for example, can reverse unwanted or toxic effects (urine retention) produced by prior opioid (morphine, hydromorphone) administration.

PHARMACOKINETIC DRUG INTERACTIONS

Pharmacokinetic drug interactions occur when one drug alters the concentration and therefore the effects of another. Most pharmacokinetic drug interactions occur when one drug changes the absorption, distribution, metabolism, elimination, or protein binding of another drug. (Protein-bound drugs are inactive.)

PHARMACODYNAMIC DRUG INTERACTIONS

Pharmacodynamic drug interactions occur when one drug alters the effects of another drug without altering its Cp. The most common causes of pharmacodynamic drug interactions include the various types of drug antagonism (competitive, noncompetitive) or agonism (*potentiation, additivity,* and *supraadditivity*). Elaborate mathematical and statistical methods have been developed to determine whether various drug mixtures produce additive or supraadditive (synergistic) effects. The *isobologram* is derived by comparing the effects of two drugs alone and in combination at several fixed dosages or ratios and, in its simplest form, illustrates when a drug combination is additive, antagonistic, or synergistic (Fig. 7-8).

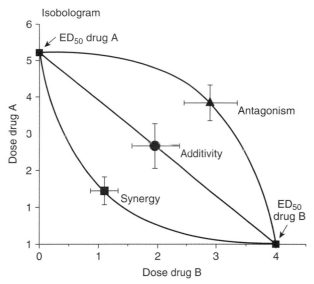

FIG. 7-8. Isobolograms are one method used to determine whether combinations of drugs are additive, synergistic, or antagonistic. The median effective dose values for two drugs are plotted on the x- and y-axes. The line that connects them is the line of additivity: a dose of drug A that produces a 25% effect and a dose of drug B that produces a 25% effect should produce a 50% effect. If lower doses than anticipated produce a 50% effect, the drug combination is said to be synergistic (concave curve), and if higher doses are required to produce the 50% effect, then the drugs are antagonistic (convex curve).

Additivity

Additivity or summation of drug effects occurs when the effects of one drug are simply additive to those of another drug. For example, if two drugs that produce analgesia are mixed together and administered, the analgesia produced is the sum of the individual analgesic activity of each drug. This is generally the case when two full opioid agonists (e.g., morphine and fentanyl) are mixed together and administered. The drug dosages need not be the same because of differences in drug potency.

Potentiation

Potentiation or synergism occurs when a mixture of two or more drugs produces a greater response than expected (i.e., greater than the sum of their individual effects; Fig. 7-8). The ability of acepromazine, a drug with little or no analgesic effects, to increase the analgesic effects of opioids (e.g., morphine and oxymorphone) is an excellent example of drug-induced potentiation or synergism. Clinically, drug synergism can be expected when drugs that act by different mechanisms of action are mixed together. Various drug combinations (e.g., NSAIDs and opioids; opioids and α_2-agonists; opioids and local anesthetics; opioid and dissociative anesthetics) frequently demonstrate synergistic effects. Synergistic drug combinations must be administered carefully, however, because unwanted and potentially toxic effects may also be potentiated (e.g., respiratory depression and bradyarrhythmias).

CLINICAL ISSUES

Therapeutic regimens, although dependent on and guided by the pharmacokinetic and pharmacodynamic principles discussed previously, must be designed and adjusted to treat disease effectively based on the severity or intensity of the disease. Patients should be treated individually after considering all of the drug-related issues. Furthermore, chronic drug use can produce a variety of altered physiological states that may be responsible for changes in the pharmacokinetic and pharmacodynamic behavior of a drug.

CLINICAL EFFICACY

Clinical efficacy refers to the ability of a drug to produce a clinically beneficial therapeutic effect, regardless of the intrinsic activity (maximal effect) of that drug and the dose required to produce that effect (potency). *Analgesic drugs are only as good as the pain being treated.* Fentanyl, for example, may be totally ineffective in the treatment of severe pain produced by a herniated disk. This last example has important clinical implications for the administration of analgesic drugs because it implies that the severity of the disease, or in this case the intensity of pain, determines the clinical efficacy of the drug. When the intensity of pain increases, the effectiveness of any drug decreases, and in the case of opioids, more receptors need to be occupied to produce a therapeutic effect. Eventually, a point is reached at which no matter how many receptors are occupied, analgesia may be difficult to produce. In other words, the intensity of the pain dictates which analgesic drugs should be used first. Low-efficacy opioids (e.g., codeine, butorphanol, and pentazocine) may be adequate for the treatment of most causes of mild to moderate pain and can be used in combination with higher-efficacy opioids (e.g., morphine and oxymorphone) to enhance analgesic effects when used to treat severe pain. The degree of analgesia produced by an opioid is therefore determined by the intensity of pain and the intrinsic activity of the opioid. If an opioid produces analgesic effects when administered alone, an additive drug interaction takes place when it is administered with another opioid.

TOLERANCE

Tolerance is said to occur when the patient requires increasing drug doses over time to maintain a desired effect. Drug tolerance can develop acutely (within hours) or chronically (over days, weeks, months) and may be attributed to pharmacokinetic (e.g., liver enzyme induction and increased clearance) or pharmacodynamic (altered cellular metabolism reducing the effects of the drug) changes. One potential mechanism for opioid tolerance is *receptor desensitization* caused by a decrease in functional opioid receptors following chronic opioid administration. Regardless of cause, the development of drug tolerance presents a significant problem in the treatment of pain, generally requiring that drug therapy be discontinued and that alternative analgesic therapy be implemented.

Drugs that require occupancy of a smaller number of receptors to produce an effect (e.g., fentanyl) are less likely to produce tolerance than less potent drugs (e.g., codeine, butorphanol, and meperidine).

PHYSICAL DEPENDENCE

Physical dependence is characterized by the development of untoward effects when a drug is acutely withheld or withdrawn. The occurrence of physical dependence in animals is unknown.

Suggested Readings

Abram SE, Mampilly GA, Milosavljevic D: Assessment of potency and intrinsic activity of systemic versus intrathecal opioids in rats, *Anesthesiology* 87: 127-134, 1997.

Dohoo S, Tasker RAR, Donald A: Pharmacokinetics of parenteral and oral sustained-release morphine sulphate in dogs, *J Vet Pharmacol Ther* 17: 426-433, 1994.

Egger CM, Duke T, Archer J, Cribb PH: Comparison of plasma fentanyl concentrations by using three transdermal fentanyl patch sizes in dogs, *Vet Surg* 27:159-166, 1998.

Holford NHG, Sheiner LB: Understanding the dose-effect relationship: clinical application of pharmacokinetic-pharmacodynamic models, *Clin Pharmacokinet* 6:429-453, 1981.

Morgan D, Cook CD, Smith MA et al: An examination of the interactions between the antinociceptive effects of morphine and various μ-opioids: the role of intrinsic efficacy and stimulus intensity, *Anesth Analg* 88:407-413, 1999.

Solomon RE, Gebhart GF: Synergistic antinociceptive interactions among drugs administered to the spinal cord, *Anesth Analg* 78:1164-1172, 1994.

Tallarida RJ: Statistical analysis of drug combination for synergism, *Pain* 49: 93-97, 1992.

Woolf CJ, Chong N: Preemptive analgesia: treating postoperative pain by preventing the establishment of central sensitization, *Anesth Analg* 77: 362-379, 1993.

8

DRUGS USED
TO TREAT PAIN

WILLIAM W. MUIR III

T he pharmacologic approach to the treatment of pain has evolved from a long history of folk remedies, herbal medicine, and more recently, the deliberate synthesis of chemical compounds specifically designed to activate or depress a wide variety of receptors or ion channels that are known or believed to be responsible for producing pain. Regardless of the significant scientific and technologic advances that have been made during the last decade, few if any drugs can be considered to produce excellent or even good analgesia for prolonged periods in dogs and cats without the risk of significant side effects or toxicity. Inadequate or unavailable scientific data, limited formulations, and an astonishing absence of controlled clinical trials further limit the chronic use of many drugs in dogs and cats. In general, currently popular drugs that have demonstrated some efficacy in the treatment of pain fall into one of five broad categories: opioids, nonsteroidal antiinflammatory drugs (NSAIDs), α_2-agonists, local anesthetics, and others. Behavior modifiers (e.g., acepromazine) and antidepressants (e.g., amitriptyline) have also been used to augment the effects of classical analgesics or to produce central analgesic effects, respectively. Each group of drugs is more or less efficacious, depending on the type and severity of the pain being treated. Many so-called adjunctive medications are known to alter central or peripheral neuronal activity (e.g., neuroleptics [tranquilizers], anticonvulsants, antidepressants, and topical preparations) or produce antiinflammatory effects (e.g., glucocorticosteroids). This chapter provides a general overview of the drugs available for the treatment of pain, emphasizing the most clinically relevant aspects of each drug group. Other chapters in this text describe and discuss the pharmacology of specific representatives of each drug group, emphasizing the drug mechanism of action, relevant pharmacology and pharmacokinetics, toxicity, and potential drug interactions (Table 8-1).

TABLE 8-1	Principal Analgesic Drugs		
	Relative Efficacy		
Drug	**Chronic Use**	**Acute Use**	**Practical Issues**
Opioids	+/−	++	Tolerance
NSAIDs	++	+/−	Efficacy, toxicity
α₂-Agonists	−	+	Sedation
Local anesthetics	−	+++	Loss of motor control, toxicity

+, Efficacious; −, minimal efficacy; *NSAIDs*, nonsteroidal antiinflammatory drugs.

OPIOIDS

The term *opioid* is preferred to the older name *narcotic* because by definition narcotics include drugs that induce sleep, but most opioid analgesics do not induce sleep, at least not in animals. Simply stated, opioids are any one of a growing number of natural or synthetic compounds that produce morphinelike effects by acting on opioid receptors (e.g., OP3 [μ], OP2 [κ], and OP1 [δ]) with the principal desired effect being the production of analgesia. From a pharmacologic perspective, opioids are of three different types: opioid agonists; opioid antagonists that are in general devoid of agonist activity and are used clinically to antagonize or reverse opioid effects; and opioid agonist-antagonists and partial agonists that produce morphinelike effects but are generally less toxic (although often less effective) than opioid agonists.

Opioids vary in their receptor specificity, potency, and efficacy at the different opioid receptors (μ, κ, δ), resulting in a wide variety of clinical effects depending on the opioid administered, the dose, and the species to which the drug is administered (e.g., dog, cat, or horse; Box 8-1). Most opioid agonists have a relatively high affinity for μ-receptors and are noted for their ability to produce analgesia and sedation (e.g., morphine, meperidine, and oxymorphone). Opioid antagonists (e.g., naloxone and naltrexone) block or reverse the effects of opioid agonists by combining with opioid receptors and producing minimal or no effects. Opioid agonists-antagonists and partial agonists act by combining with opioid receptors and producing partial or incomplete activation of the receptor, depending on the receptor (μ, κ, δ) being activated. Larger doses of opioid agonists-antagonists and partial agonists may act as antagonists for opioid agonists because of their relatively high affinity for opioid receptors and comparatively low potential for toxicity.

BOX 8-1	
Opioid Receptor Subtypes	
Receptor	**Subtype**
μ	Supraspinal, spinal, and peripheral analgesia; minimal to mild sedation; respiratory depression; bradycardia; ileus; urine retention; temperature reduction
κ	Supraspinal, spinal (?), and peripheral analgesia; minimal sedation, respiratory depression, and bradycardia
δ	Supraspinal, spinal, and peripheral analgesia; minimal sedation, respiratory depression, and bradycardia; ileus, urine retention; temperature reduction
σ	Excitement-delirium, tachycardia, hypertension

PHARMACOLOGIC CONSIDERATIONS

As suggested in Table 8-2, different opioids produce varied pharmacologic effects based on their ability to combine with and activate the various opioid receptors and receptor subtypes located in the central nervous system and periphery. The prevalence and location (central or peripheral) of the various receptors in the different species, opioid receptor selectivity, molecular size and shape, and the influence of various disease processes ultimately determine the pharmacologic effects of the opioid in any given animal. Methadone, for example, is known to act primarily at μ-opioid receptors but is also known partially to inhibit N-methyl-D-aspartate (NMDA) receptors in the spinal cord. Although the central nervous system–associated analgesic effects of opioids have been emphasized, their effects on peripheral opioid receptors should not be underestimated and is the basis for their administration intraarticularly.

CENTRAL NERVOUS SYSTEM

Opioids relieve or reduce pain by combining with opioid receptors in the central nervous system (CNS) and periphery. Opioids are generally considered to be the most effective of all analgesic medications but vary widely in their analgesic potency and clinical efficacy when used to treat pain (e.g., superficial, visceral, or deep). Fentanyl, for example, is at least 100 times more potent than morphine and produces excellent clinical analgesia when administered at what would be considered extremely small (micrograms/kilogram) doses compared with most opioid analgesics (e.g., morphine, oxymorphone, and butorphanol [milligrams/kilogram]).

Most opioid agonists produce minimal to moderate sedation when administered at recommended dosages as single-drug therapy.

TABLE 8-2	Selectivity for Opioid Receptor Subtypes			
Drug	μ	κ	δ	σ
AGONISTS				
Codeine	+	+	+	−
Fentanyl	++++	−	+	−
Hydromorphone and oxymorphone	+++	+	+	−
Meperidine	++	+	++	−
Methadone	+++	+	++	−
Morphine	+++	++	++	−
PARTIAL/MIXED AGONISTS				
Buprenorphine	(+++)	−	−	−
Butorphanol	++	(++)	−	++
Nalbuphine	+	(+++)	(++)	+
Pentazocine	+	(++)	+	++
ANTAGONISTS				
Naloxone	+++	++	+++	−
Naltrexone	+++	++	++	−
ATYPICAL OPIOID				
Tramadol	+	?	?	−

+, Mild effect; ++, moderate effect; +++, pronounced effect; ++++, very pronounced effect; (), partial agonist effects; ?, unknown; −, little or no effect.

However, opioid agonists are capable of producing profound CNS and respiratory depression or arrest when administered with tranquilizers (neuroleptanalgesia) or with injectable or inhalant anesthetics to patients that are depressed from head trauma or seizures or are clinically debilitated. Some dogs administered opioids react wildly and aggressively to loud or high-pitched noises. Increased dosages of opioids can produce nervousness, agitation, increased locomotor activity, dysphoria, and occasionally hyperthermia (cats). Cats are particularly susceptible to the neuroexcitatory effects of opioids. Early experience with morphine suggested that opioids, at least morphine, could produce excitement and mania in cats (morphine mania). This response is now known to be due to species differences and a relative drug overdose. Seizures can be triggered on rare occasions and have been attributed to drug metabolites, solution preservatives, or preexisting CNS disorders. Aged pets may be particularly susceptible to the CNS and behavioral effects of opioids, with some animals demonstrating indifference, malaise, disorientation, and agitated behavior. Other pets may become timid or aggressive when approached. The development of "release of suppressed behavior," manifesting as aggression, must be considered when any drug that alters CNS activity is administered. Changes in behavior and the development of aggression have been attributed to central neurochemical mechanisms involving opioid and dopamine receptors.

Nausea and vomiting (in dogs and cats) and panting (in dogs) are acute phenomena that are frequently observed after intramuscular opioid administration. Opioids are known to stimulate the chemoreceptor trigger zone (CTZ) and reset thermoregulatory centers in the hypothalamus, resulting in a slight fall in body temperature. Vomiting (rare in cats) may be considered an advantage in dogs that have recently eaten and are being considered as surgical candidates. Vomiting and retching, however, are problematic if the patient is believed to have a pharyngeal, esophageal, or gastric foreign body. Panting is a common clinical sign after the administration of most opioid agonists to dogs but does not provide adequate ventilation because only dead-space gas is moved in and out of the upper airways. Dogs and cats that have received opioids as preanesthetic medication may require manual or mechanical ventilation to achieve adequate ventilation and avoid respiratory acidosis during anesthesia. Shivering is common after anesthesia because body temperature may be decreased. Shivering increases postoperative oxygen and caloric requirements, which could become important in older, very young, and small patients. Shivering may also be a sign of inadequate analgesia. Some opioids (e.g., meperidine) decrease the incidence of shivering by a mechanism independent of the analgesic effects of the drug.

Most opioids depress the cough reflex by a central mechanism. Cough suppression is produced at subanalgesic doses and is prominent with less effective opioids (e.g., codeine) and opioid agonists-antagonists (e.g., butorphanol). Cough suppression may lead to the accumulation of mucous secretions in the airways of patients recovering from anesthesia, predisposing them to upper airway obstruction.

Opioids generally produce pinpoint pupils (miosis) in dogs as a result of CNS stimulation of parasympathetic segments of the oculomotor nerve. This response can be inhibited by prior administration of anticholinergic drugs (e.g., atropine and glycopyrrolate). The pupil dilates (mydriasis) in cats and horses as a result of stimulation of CNS sympathetic pathways.

RESPIRATORY SYSTEM

Opioids are notorious for their respiratory depressant effects in depressed or anesthetized animals. Opioids increase the concentration of carbon dioxide necessary to stimulate the rate and depth of breathing (increase respiratory threshold) and depress the ventilatory response to increases in inspired concentrations of carbon dioxide (decrease respiratory sensitivity). Clinically, both effects predispose patients to hypoventilation and the development of respiratory acidosis. Although of significant clinical relevance, respiratory depression is not frequently reported in dogs and cats administered opioids compared with human beings. The best explanation for this difference is that most opioids do not produce the same degree of euphoria and CNS depression in dogs or cats as they do in human beings. In other words, the severity of opioid-induced respiratory depression in dogs and cats is directly related to the amount of preexisting CNS depression. As long as the patient remains conscious, it is unlikely that respiratory depression will become problematic. Respiratory depression in patients administered tranquilizers or sedatives in conjunction with opioids before anesthesia is of greater concern, and in these patients, ventilation should be closely monitored.

Chest wall rigidity, or "woody chest syndrome," can occur in dogs or cats administered large or repeated doses of opioids (e.g., fentanyl). Increased thoracic and abdominal efforts and muscle rigidity may be related to the CNS excitation caused by larger doses of opioids. Increased respiratory effort and centrally mediated mechanisms may produce increases in body temperature resulting in hyperthermia in cats.

CARDIOVASCULAR SYSTEM

Other than bradycardia and occasional bradyarrhythmias, opioids produce relatively few if any clinically significant cardiovascular side effects in dogs and cats when administered at recommended doses. First-degree (prolonged PR interval), second-degree (P wave not followed by a QRS interval), and rarely, third-degree (no relationship between P wave and QRS complexes) atrioventricular block can occur, which is attributed to a vagally mediated increase in parasympathetic tone and is therefore responsive to anticholinergic (atropine, glycopyrrolate) therapy.

Opioids produce clinically insignificant effects on the force of cardiac contraction (inotropy), arterial blood pressure, and cardiac output unless administered as a rapid intravenous bolus. Some opioids (e.g., morphine and meperidine) are noted for producing histamine release or splanchnic sequestration of blood (dogs), which could exacerbate hypotension. The clinical impact of these effects, however, remains to be demonstrated. Histamine release in cats is signaled by increased redness of the ears and paws.

OTHER ORGAN SYSTEMS
Gastrointestinal System

Opioids, particularly µ-receptor agonists, delay gastric emptying and prolong intestinal transit time. Gastric and intestinal smooth muscle tone are increased, producing "ropy guts" that are particularly evident after the administration of an opioid to puppies or kittens. Increases in intestinal smooth muscle tone are caused by centrally mediated increases in vagal tone and activation of opioid receptors throughout the gastrointestinal tract. The onset of opioid-induced gastrointestinal effects may result in defecation and a period of diarrhea in dogs. This is followed by a decrease in propulsive peristaltic activity and absorption of water from the intestinal tract, predisposing the patient to constipation, a condition that becomes more prominent when opioids are administered for several days. Opioids increase esophageal, biliary, duodenal, and anal sphincter tone, making it difficult to perform endoscopic examinations, particularly of the duodenum. Opioids should be avoided in patients believed to have an obstructed biliary tract or biliary neoplasm. Butorphanol or butorphanol drug combinations are generally preferred for endoscopic procedures involving the gastrointestinal system because of lesser effects on gastrointestinal motility and sphincter activity.

Genitourinary System

Opioids inhibit the voiding reflex and increase external urethral sphincter tone, resulting in urine retention. Urine retention can be an important postsurgical consideration in dogs and cats that have undergone prolonged orthopedic surgical procedures or abdominal surgery or in those with preexisting bladder dysfunction. Although popular because of their analgesic and sedative effects, most opioids decrease uterine contractions, thereby prolonging labor. This issue may be of little consequence if a cesarean section is performed. Respiratory depression of the fetus is of potential concern, however, and can be treated with opioid antagonists or doxapram.

CLINICAL ISSUES

Opioids are controlled substances, making their clinical use potentially problematic because of strict ordering, storage, and record-keeping requirements. These bureaucratic issues aside, opioids are the most effective therapy for pain from all causes and are critical components of so-called multimodal therapeutic pain regimens. Opioids are less effective, however, in the treatment of pain caused by nerve injury and other forms of neuropathic pain (e.g., spinal cord compression). The routine clinical use of opioids for analgesia or as preanesthetic medication must be considered within the framework of the patient's medical problems, the severity of the patient's pain, and the potential for anesthesia. Low doses of opioid agonists-antagonists (e.g., butorphanol), for example, can be additive with opioid agonists (e.g., hydromorphone and oxymorphone). Opioid antagonist effects, however, are to be expected when large or repeated doses of an opioid agonist-antagonist (e.g., butorphanol or pentazocine) or partial agonist (e.g., buprenorphine) are administered to a patient that has received an opioid agonist (e.g., morphine or hydromorphone). Furthermore, not all opioid effects can be antagonized. The administration of the partial agonist buprenorphine, for example, after administration of an opioid agonist (e.g., morphine or hydromorphone) may lead to increased respiratory depression in some patients. As noted, low doses of opioids may produce excitatory effects in some species, especially cats and horses. It has been suggested that the administration of low doses of an opioid antagonist (naltrexone) before administration of an opioid agonist (morphine, hydromorphone) may help to prevent opioid-related excitatory effects, enhance opioid-related analgesia, and attenuate the development of tolerance associated with chronic opioid use. The clinical utility and relevance of this suggestion remains to be validated in clinical veterinary practice. Finally, diseases (liver, renal, CNS) and drugs (anesthetics) that prolong opioid metabolism and elimination may be responsible for prolonged drug effects, resulting in extended periods of depression and unconsciousness.

NONSTEROIDAL ANTIINFLAMMATORY DRUGS

NSAIDs represent a diverse group of chemical compounds that are currently the most popular analgesic drugs used in small animal veterinary practice for acute or chronic pain (Box 8-2). In addition to *analgesia,* NSAIDs are noted for their *antiinflammatory* and *antipyretic* effects. NSAIDs act by nonspecifically inhibiting the various isoforms of cyclooxygenase synthase (COX) or, in the case of the dual inhibitor tepoxalin, COX and 5-lipoxygenase (LOX), which are responsible for prostaglandin (e.g., COX: prostaglandin E_2) and leukotriene (e.g., LOX: LTB_4) production from arachidonic acid. Prostaglandins produce their algesic, proinflammatory, and pyretic effects by activating prostaglandin (EP) receptors throughout the body. Leukotrienes stimulate chemotaxis and are associated with increased neutrophil activation and their subsequent adhesion and degranulation. Leukotrienes play an important role in mediating inflammation, promoting tissue and in particular gastrointestinal mucosal damage and pain. At least two types of COX exist: COX-1 and COX-2. Although COX-1 is considered to be

---

BOX 8-2

Nonsteroidal Antiinflammatory Drugs

Salicylic Acid
Aspirin

Para-Aminophenol
Acetaminophen

Fenamic Acids
Flunixin meglumine

Pyrazolones
Dipyrone
Phenylbutazone

Propionic Acids
Carprofen
Ketoprofen
Naproxen
Ibuprofen

Oxicams
Piroxicam
Meloxicam

Acetic Acids
Ketorolac
Etodolac

Coxibs
Deracoxib
Firocoxib

Lipoxygenase/Cyclooxygenase Inhibitor
Tepoxalin

"housekeeping" COX and to be involved in cell signaling and maintaining tissue homeostasis, COX-1 and COX-2 have housekeeping roles in select tissues. COX-1 inhibition is believed to be responsible for the majority of acute and chronic toxicities of NSAIDs, especially gastrointestinal ulceration, although one theory contends that inhibition of COX-1 or both of the COX enzymes shunts substrate toward the production of leukotrienes, increasing the production of LTB_4 and thereby exacerbating mucosal damage. COX-2, often but inappropriately referred to as *inducible COX,* is the principal enzyme responsible for the overproduction of prostaglandins following acute injury or infection. Most NSAIDS that are currently available inhibit COX-1 and COX-2 isoenzymes, although several are relatively COX-2 selective (deracoxib), if not specific (firocoxib). The recent availability of a highly COX-2–selective NSAID (firocoxib) offers the potential to provide improved analgesic and antiinflammatory effects with minimal interference of gastrointestinal physiology, although this has not been borne out by clinical data. The nonsedating, analgesic, and low-toxicity profile of newer NSAIDs (e.g., carprofen, etodolac, deracoxib, and firocoxib) and the COX/LOX inhibitors (e.g., tepoxalin) has helped allay traditional concerns regarding gastrointestinal toxicity, although the potential for renal toxicity, blood clotting abnormalities, and efficacy remain controversial. Currently available NSAIDs offer reduced side effects and toxicity, improved convenience (oral and parenteral preparations), and a long duration of action (administration once a day) compared with the many nonapproved formulations.

PHARMACOLOGIC CONSIDERATIONS

Regardless of their diverse chemical structure and selectivity for COX-1 or COX-2 or LOX, most NSAIDs produce subtle and individual animal-dependent analgesic effects. Noteworthy is that NSAIDs that are COX-1 selective (e.g., aspirin and ibuprofen) inhibit platelet aggregation. Because it is not easy to determine the extent to which pain and inflammation depend on COX-1–mediated or COX-2–mediated effects, it is difficult to select the one best NSAID for the treatment of pain in every animal. Because the majority of proinflammatory prostaglandins induced by acute tissue damage or trauma are believed to be produced by the induction (up-regulation) of COX-2, it is reasonable to conclude that drugs producing more specific COX-2 effects should be more effective in producing analgesic, antiinflammatory, and antipyretic effects, but this conclusion remains unproven. Similarly, NSAIDs that interfere with normal homeostatic activity (COX-1 effects) should be more likely to produce toxicity. Clinically, these conclusions turn out to be generally true because drugs that produce COX-2 inhibitory effects exhibit good efficacy and less gastrointestinal toxicity than COX-1 inhibitors. Nevertheless, given the potential for serious toxic side effects, veterinarians should consider analgesic adjuncts (tramadol, gabapentin, amantadine) if the NSAID currently selected does not prove to be of therapeutic benefit before switching to an alternative NSAID. Also important to remember is that all current NSAIDs can produce renal toxicity.

CENTRAL NERVOUS SYSTEM

NSAIDs do not produce important CNS effects that alter the animal's level of consciousness or behavior. Peripheral analgesia, although primarily resulting from the local inhibition of prostaglandins, may also be due to the inhibition of prostaglandin generation in the CNS. The activation of glial cells and microglia within the CNS are suspected to be responsible for the production of prostaglandins that contribute to central sensitization and amplification of pain associated with chronic pain states. The use of NSAIDS that target CNS sites may have special advantage in providing analgesia for chronic pain. NSAIDs are synergistic with opioids, which are noted for their CNS analgesic effects, and reduce the amount of opioid required to produce effective analgesia.

Neurons within the hypothalamus that are responsible for regulating body temperature are affected by prostaglandins, resulting in an increase in the thermoregulatory set-point and fever. NSAIDs return the set-point to normal by inhibiting prostaglandin production.

RESPIRATORY SYSTEM

NSAIDs do not produce clinically relevant effects on the respiratory system. NSAIDs may, however, improve respiratory function in animals with respiratory- and inflammatory-mediated bronchoconstrictive diseases. On rare occasions, NSAIDs have been incriminated in the production of acute asthmalike signs. The mechanism for this is unclear, but it has been suggested that leukotriene (e.g., LTC-4 and LTD-4) production may increase when arachidonate metabolism is diverted from the COX pathway. Increased production of LTC-4 and LTD-4 causes airway hyperreactivity and bronchial contractions.

CARDIOVASCULAR SYSTEM

NSAIDs do not produce significant cardiovascular effects.

Inhibition of prostaglandin production following infection, trauma, or a generalized systemic inflammatory response can help prevent vasodilation, edema, and platelet aggregation.

Some NSAIDs, particularly those that are more COX-1 selective (e.g., aspirin), are noted for their inhibitory effect on platelet aggregation, resulting in the potential for prolonged bleeding times and the development of edema at sites of tissue injury.

NSAIDs occasionally cause fluid retention in patients with heart failure.

OTHER ORGAN SYSTEMS
Gastrointestinal System

Prostaglandins play an important role in the development of a protective gastric barrier to intraluminal acidity by stimulating mucous production and bicarbonate secretion and promoting blood flow. Prostaglandins also sustain cell turnover and repair and maintain normal gut motility. The use of NSAIDs predisposes animals to gastric erosions and ulceration, particularly in animals with gastrointestinal disease (Box 8-3).

Genitourinary System

Prostaglandins play an important role in maintaining normal renal tubular function. The use of NSAIDs may promote renal blood flow and produce diuretic effects in some animals.

> ### BOX 8-3
>
> **Treatment of Gastrointestinal Side Effects of Nonsteroidal Antiinflammatory Drugs**
>
> - Discontinue nonsteroidal antiinflammatory drug
> - Initiate antibiotic therapy
> - Sucralfate, 0.5 to 1.0 g PO
> - Ranitidine, 2.5 mg/kg IV q12h
> - Famotidine, 0.5 to 1 mg/kg IV q12h
> - Misoprostol, 0.7 to 5 µg/kg PO q8h

CLINICAL ISSUES

NSAIDs are, in general, effective for the treatment of mild to moderate pain. Although most effective for treating pain caused by tissue damage (e.g., inflammation and trauma), NSAIDs rarely eliminate all pain and are relatively ineffective for treating severe pain. Gastrointestinal, renal, or hepatic toxicity and excessive bleeding are potential problems associated with the clinical use of NSAIDs. These issues are particularly important in very young or old animals and in animals that are immunocompromised or have preexisting cardiovascular, renal, or liver disease. The potential for altered platelet function and blood dyscrasias should be considered if NSAIDs are to be administered chronically. Significant differences between drugs and their metabolism by different species (dogs versus cats) emphasize the importance of strictly adhering to dose recommendations and dosing schedules if toxicity is to be prevented.

α_2-AGONISTS

α_2-Agonists were initially developed for use as antihypertensive agents (e.g., clonidine) in human beings and for their sedative, muscle relaxant, and analgesic effects in animals (Box 8-4). Moderate to excellent analgesia can be produced, but only with moderate to profound degrees of sedation. α_2-Agonists produce their clinically relevant pharmacologic effects by activating a variety of α_2-receptor subtypes (e.g., α_{2A}, α_{2B}, α_{2C}, and α_{2D}) in the CNS and periphery. The discovery of a receptor-based mechanism has led to the identification and synthesis of α_2-receptor antagonists (e.g., yohimbine, tolazoline, and atipamezole). Based on differences in chemical structure, some α_2-agonists are capable of activating imidazoline receptors (I_1, I_2) and producing direct effects (e.g., xylazine). The diversity in chemical structure, receptor specificity, and receptor density and location among α_2-agonists is responsible for considerable differences in drug dosages and effects of α_2-agonists among and within species. Notorious

---

BOX 8-4

α_2-Agonists

- Clonidine
- Detomidine
- Dexmedetomidine
- Medetomidine
- Romifidine
- Xylazine

---

for the frequency, scope, and severity of their cardiovascular side effects, particularly bradycardia and bradyarrhythmias, α_2-receptor antagonists must be administered with caution to very young, aged, or debilitated patients and are contraindicated in most patients with cardiovascular diseases. Future α_2-agonists will be designed to activate specific receptor subtypes, ideally limiting their CNS depressant actions and decreasing the frequency of side effects.

PHARMACOLOGIC CONSIDERATIONS

More than any other group of drugs that produce analgesic effects, the clinical use of α_2-agonists centers on their associated CNS (sedative), cardiovascular, and respiratory effects. Consideration must be given to the potential for the development of profound sedation with unexpected or aggressive behavioral changes, significant bradycardia, and respiratory depression. The potential for drug interactions (particularly with anesthetics) and amplification of toxic side effects is high.

CENTRAL NERVOUS SYSTEM

α_2-Agonists activate presynaptic and postsynaptic α_2-receptors in the CNS, producing sedation and analgesia. Sedation in dogs and cats is attributed to activation of CNS α_{2A}-receptors in areas of the brain that are responsible for awareness, arousal, and vigilance. Activation of α_1 and imidizoline receptors may play some part in the pharmacology of most α_2-receptor agonists because most currently available α_2-receptors can activate both types of receptors. Large and potentially toxic doses of currently available α_2-agonists can produce an initial period of reduced or poor sedation attributed to activation of CNS α_1-receptors. Like other calming drugs (e.g., acepromazine), α_2-agonists are capable of eliciting a release of "suppressed behavior." Dogs or cats that appear sedated may become suddenly aroused and aggressive if disturbed. Many dogs, cats, and especially horses seem to demonstrate increased sensitivity to sound and initial tactile contact.

Activation of α_2-receptors in the brain and spinal cord decreases pain-related neurotransmitters and interferes with sensory transmission. α_2-Agonists also act peripherally at α_2-receptors to produce analgesia, and some α_2-agonists (e.g., xylazine) produce local anesthetic effects.

Vomiting is a common side effect in dogs and cats after the intravenous administration of an α_2-agonist. Activation of α_2-receptors within the CTZ is responsible for nausea and retching.

All α_2-agonists impair the control of body temperature through CNS-mediated dose-dependent effects on temperature thresholds for sweating, vasoconstriction, and shivering. These effects predispose dogs and cats to hypothermia, particularly during the postoperative period. However, α_2-agonists are also an effective treatment for shivering. Occasionally, the administration of α_2-agonists is responsible for triggering hyperthermia resulting from intense peripheral vasoconstriction and an inability to dissipate heat. Hyperthermia is more likely to occur in hot, humid environments.

RESPIRATORY SYSTEM

α_2-agonists agonists produce a dose-dependent rate and volume that parallels the degree of CNS depression. Pronounced CNS depression is associated with a decrease in respiratory center response (increased threshold to Pco_2) and sensitivity (decreased response to Pco_2) to carbon dioxide. Both effects combine to produce significant respiratory acidosis and hypoxemia in older or sick animals. Clinical doses generally produce mild respiratory acidosis of little consequence unless the patient becomes unconscious or anesthetized.

α_2-Agonists cause considerable relaxation of upper airway muscles in the pharynx and larynx, which can result in irregular breathing patterns, inspiratory dyspnea, and upper airway obstruction, particularly in brachycephalic breeds.

CARDIOVASCULAR SYSTEM

The α_2-agonists are capable of producing multiple and at times profound cardiovascular effects. Chief among these effects are decreases in heart rate. Sinus bradycardia and bradyarrhythmias are common following the administration of α_2-agonists. First- and second-degree atrioventricular block are the most common bradyarrhythmias to occur, although third-degree atrioventricular block and sinus arrest with ventricular escape beats are occasionally observed. Atrioventricular block and decreases in heart rate are caused by the combined effects of decreases in CNS sympathetic output and increases in vagally mediated parasympathetic tone, indicating that the administration of an anticholinergic (e.g., atropine or glycopyrrolate) may be effective in preventing or inhibiting bradycardia and atrioventricular block. One must remember, however, that the administration of an anticholinergic to dogs or cats that have been given an α_2-agonist may predispose them to the development of cardiac arrhythmias, including ventricular tachycardia and rarely ventricular fibrillation. Therefore, anticholinergics and α_2-agonists should not be administered to animals with preexisting ventricular arrhythmias, myocardial contusion, heart failure, or any other cause of ventricular electrical instability. Some α_2-agonists (e.g., xylazine) transiently sensitize the heart to catecholamine-induced arrhythmias. The clinical relevance of this effect, however, has not been established.

Arterial blood pressure usually increases transiently and then decreases from baseline values after the administration of an α_2-agonist. The early period of vasoconstriction and hypertension is initiated by stimulation of peripheral vascular α_1- and α_2-receptors and is partly responsible for the development of bradyarrhythmias because of increases in baroreceptor reflex activity and vagal tone. The long-term decrease in arterial blood pressure parallels decreases in CNS sympathetic output and heart rate.

Cardiac output decreases almost immediately after the administration of an α_2-agonist, primarily because of a decrease in heart rate ($CO = HR \times$ Stroke volume, where CO is cardiac output and HR is heart rate). The short-term and long-term decreases in cardiac output also can be attributed to vasoconstriction (increased afterload) and decreases in CNS sympathetic output, resulting in a decrease in cardiac contractile force and stroke volume.

OTHER ORGAN SYSTEMS
Gastrointestinal System

Vomiting and retching are common consequences of α_2-agonist administration to dogs and cats. Lower doses and subcutaneous administration help decrease this side effect, which is mediated by α_2-receptor effects in the CTZ in the CNS. α_2-Agonists produce immediate and pronounced decreases in gastrointestinal motility in dogs and cats, which can last for several hours. Gastrointestinal stasis is caused by stimulation of α_2-receptors in the gut and increases in serum gastrin concentration. This effect is dose-dependent but is believed to be responsible for postoperative ileus, gas accumulation, and potentially, the development of "bloat" in dogs.

Endocrine System

α_2-Receptors modulate the release of insulin by the pancreas, causing a transient decrease in serum insulin concentration and an increase in serum glucose, resulting in glycosuria. This effect is mediated by α_2-receptor modulation of insulin secretion by beta cells in the pancreas.

Genitourinary System

α_2-Agonists promote diuresis by their glucosuric effects and direct actions on the renal tubules to decrease renal tubular salt and water absorption. Labor can be delayed and prolonged as a result of sedative and muscle relaxant effects.

CLINICAL ISSUES

Although potentially useful as analgesics for minor medical or surgical procedures or as preanesthetic medication for general anesthesia, the routine use of α_2-agonists as analgesics has been hampered by side effects, especially bradyarrhythmias. The administration of an anticholinergic for the treatment of bradycardia, although indicated, may precipitate ventricular arrhythmias. The best approach to the treatment of severe bradycardia with hypotension may be the administration of an α_2-antagonist (atipamezole). α_2-Agonists are excellent anxiolytics, however, and the administration of low doses (≤ 2 µg/kg) or infusions (0.2 to 1.0 µg/kg per hour) with opioids or NSAIDs as part of a multimodal approach for the treatment of postoperative pain should be explored. α-Agonists may have considerable benefit as analgesics when administered into the epidural or subarachnoid space, but these routes of administration and others await detailed clinical evaluation on dogs and cats.

LOCAL ANESTHETICS

All local anesthetics block the initiation and conduction of electrical impulses (action potentials) in nerves (Table 8-3). Small-diameter (C, Aδ) nerve fibers are blocked first in preference to large myelinated fibers (Aβ), thereby producing a loss of sensation (analgesia) and varying degrees of paralysis (i.e., loss of motor function). More specifically, local anesthetics block sodium ion channels in neuronal cells and other tissues, thereby preventing an influx of sodium ions, membrane depolarization, and a decrease in propagated action potentials. Nonspecific membrane effects similar to those produced by inhalant anesthetics may be partially responsible for CNS-mediated analgesic activity. Analgesia is a direct

TABLE 8-3	Local Anesthetic Drugs
Drug	**Route of Administration**
Bupivacaine	I, NB, E, S
Cetacaine (benzocaine, butamben, and tetracaine hydrochloride)	T
Lidocaine	IV, T, I, NB, E, S
Mepivacaine	I, NB, E, S
Mexiletine	PO
Ropivacaine	I, NB, E, S

E, Epidural; *I,* infiltration; *IV,* intravenous (systemic or regional); *NB,* nerve block; *PO,* oral; *S,* spinal; *T,* topical.

result of sodium ion channel blockade and membrane stabilization. Local anesthetics are most frequently administered at specific sites (topical, local) or on nerves (regional) to produce analgesia.

PHARMACOLOGIC CONSIDERATIONS

Although noted for their local analgesic effects after topical or local infiltration, most local anesthetic drugs produce mild CNS depressant (anesthetic-sparing), antiarrhythmic, mild antiinflammatory, antishock, and gastrointestinal promotility effects. Significant differences exist among local anesthetics regarding their metabolism, elimination, and potential to produce toxicity in dogs, cats, and horses. Cats and horses (Chapter 22), for example, are much more susceptible to the neurotoxic side effects of local anesthetics than dogs.

CENTRAL NERVOUS SYSTEM

Local anesthetics, as their name implies, produce analgesia by suppressing or blocking electrical activity in sensory and motor nerves. The preferential blocking of small unmyelinated nerves suggests that smaller doses should limit motor dysfunction, but this is difficult, if not impossible, to take advantage of clinically.

Low doses of local anesthetics produce negligible effects on the CNS. Mild sedation may occur as a result of membrane-stabilizing effects, a generalized decrease in neuronal activity, and a centrally mediated decrease in sympathetic activity. Most local anesthetics potentiate the effects of injectable (e.g., thiopental and propofol) and inhalant anesthetics (e.g., isoflurane and sevoflurane), resulting in a decrease in the amount of anesthetic required (anesthetic sparing) to produce unconsciousness and surgical anesthesia.

Large doses of local anesthetics are capable of producing CNS stimulation typified by nervousness, disorientation, nystagmus, nausea, excitement, agitation, and convulsions. These effects are believed to be caused by the inhibition of inhibitory neurons within the CNS, and when severe, can result in death from respiratory paralysis.

RESPIRATORY SYSTEM

Recommended doses of local anesthetics produce minimal if any significant effects on the respiratory system other than those associated with their effects on the CNS.

Solutions containing local anesthetic drugs have the potential to produce respiratory paralysis when administered by epidural or spinal (subarachnoidal) routes. The migration of the local anesthetic cranially to the C5-C6 nerve roots can paralyze the diaphragm, resulting in hypoventilation and apnea.

CARDIOVASCULAR SYSTEM

Therapeutic doses of local anesthetics produce minimal cardiovascular effects in otherwise healthy dogs and cats. Heart rate may increase as a result of sympathetic suppression, arteriolar dilation, and decreases in arterial blood pressure.

A large dose or rapid intravenous administration of a local anesthetic drug decreases cardiac output, arterial blood pressure, and heart rate. The decrease in cardiac output is caused by decreases in CNS sympathetic output, myocardial contractile force, and venous return. These effects are more prominent in stressed or sick animals that depend on high sympathetic tone for maintaining homeostasis.

All local anesthetics produce antiarrhythmic effects but have the potential to produce sinus bradycardia and bradyarrhythmias and hypotension when administered too rapidly by the intravenous route. Local anesthetics should not be administered to dogs or cats with high-grade (two or more blocked P waves) second-degree or third-degree atrioventricular block because they can cause further depression of conduction and suppress ventricular escape beats, leading to cardiac arrest.

OTHER ORGAN SYSTEMS
Gastrointestinal System

High sympathetic tone can cause complete gut stasis and may be responsible for the development of ileus in the postsurgical patient. Local anesthetics promote gastrointestinal motility by suppressing sympathetic tone.

Hematopoietic System

Some local anesthetics (e.g., Cetacaine [benzocaine, butamben, and tetracaine hydrochloride], benzocaine, and dibucaine) can produce methemoglobinemia. This is particularly important in puppies and cats of all ages.

CLINICAL ISSUES

The most clinically relevant issues associated with the administration of currently available local anesthetic drugs are their lack of selectivity for sensory nerve fibers, their potential to cause motor paralysis, and the unavailability of effective oral preparations. Local anesthetics produce good to excellent analgesia when administered topically or injected locally but at the expense of motor impairment (temporary paralysis when administered epidurally), which can become problematic in some surgical patients (cesarean section, fracture repair) and induce untoward behavioral responses in others. The systemic infusion of lidocaine produces clinically relevant analgesia and anesthetic-sparing effects when administered as adjunctive therapy with inhalant (e.g., isoflurane or sevoflurane) or injectable (e.g., ketamine or propofol) anesthetics, opioids, or α_2-agonists. Mexiletine ("oral lidocaine") can be used as an alternative to injectable lidocaine for this purpose. Toxicity (CNS and cardiovascular) is most likely to occur after accidental intraarterial injection, overdose, during high infusion rates, or when multiple bolus injections of smaller doses are administered over a short period. Cats and horses are particularly more susceptible to the CNS side effects of local anesthetics than are dogs, mandating a reduction in intravenous drug dosage (>0.5 mg/kg IV). Cimetidine and other drugs that impair liver metabolism can prolong the elimination of local anesthetics and increase the potential for toxicity.

NONTRADITIONAL ANALGESICS FOR THE TREATMENT OF PAIN

A growing number of chemicals representing widely diverse drug families are being increasingly prescribed as adjunctive and adjuvant therapy for the treatment of acute and, more commonly, chronic pain (Tables 8-4 and 8-5). Corticosteroids, local anesthetics, anticonvulsants, antidepressants, antiviral and anticancer agents, herbal remedies, and a variety of nutritional supplements are capable of producing analgesic or adjuvant analgesic activity. Anticonvulsants (gabapentin, pregabalin) and

TABLE 8-4	Adjuvant Analgesic Drugs	
Drug Category	**Possible Side Effects**	
CORTICOSTEROIDS		
Prednisone	Tissue edema, immune suppression	
Prednisolone		
Dexamethasone		
LOCAL ANESTHETICS		
Lidocaine	Central nervous system toxicity,	
Mexiletine	cardiovascular depression	
TRANQUILIZERS/MUSCLE RELAXANTS		
Acepromazine	Central nervous system	
Chlorpromazine	depression, hypotension	
Diazepam		
Midazolam		
ANTICONVULSANTS		
Carbamazepine	Disorientation, depression	
Gabapentin		
Phenytoin		
ANTIDEPRESSANTS		
Amitriptyline	Behavioral changes,	
Clomipramine	anticholinergic effects	
CALCIUM ANTAGONISTS		
Diltiazem	Bradycardia, hypotension	
SYMPATHOLYTICS		
Atenolol	Bradycardia, hypotension	
Prazosin		
Propranolol		
MISCELLANEOUS DRUGS		
Alendronate	Disorientation, depression	
Amantadine		
Clonidine		
Codeine		
Dextromethorphan		
Ketamine		
Magnesium salts ($Mg^{-2}SO_4^{-2}$)		
Tramadol		

behavior-modifying drugs (e.g., amitriptyline and clomipramine) may be efficacious for treating chronic pain syndromes, particularly neuropathic pain. Several drugs have weak but potentially relevant NMDA receptor blocking activity (amantadine, dextromethorphan) and have been used in conjunction with NSAIDs and opioids to control chronic pain.

TABLE 8-5	Adjuvant Analgesic Drug Dosages	
Drug	**Dosage in Dogs**	**Dosage in Cats**
CORTICOSTEROIDS		
Dexamethasone	0.10-0.15 mg/kg SC, PO	0.10-0.15 mg/kg SC, PO
Prednisolone	1.0-2.2 mg/kg PO	1-2 mg/kg PO
Prednisone	1.0-2.2 mg/kg PO	1-2 mg/kg PO
LOCAL ANESTHETICS		
Lidocaine	2-4 mg/kg IV bolus and then 25-75 μg/kg IV infusion	0.25-1.0 mg/kg IV bolus and then 10-40 μg/kg IV infusion
Mexiletine	4-10 mg/kg PO	—
TRANQUILIZERS/MUSCLE RELAXANTS		
Acepromazine	0.025-1.13 mg/kg IV, SC, IM	0.05-2.25 mg/kg IM, SC, IV, PO
Chlorpromazine	0.05-0.50 mg/kg SC, IM; 0.8-4.4 mg/kg PO	0.5 mg/kg IM, IV; 2-4 mg/kg PO
Diazepam	2-5 mg/kg IV; 0.5-2.2 mg/kg PO	2-5 mg/kg IV; 0.5-2.2 mg/kg PO
Midazolam	0.066-0.22 mg/kg IV, IM	0.066-0.22 mg/kg IV, IM
ANTICONVULSANTS		
Carbamazepine	Not recommended	—
Gabapentin	1-3 mg/kg PO, initial dose	—
Phenytoin	20-35 mg/kg PO	2-3 mg/kg PO
ANTIDEPRESSANTS		
Amitriptyline	1-2 mg/kg PO	1-2 mg/kg PO
Clomipramine	1-3 mg/kg PO	1-5 mg/kg PO
CALCIUM ANTAGONISTS		
Diltiazem	0.5-1.5 mg/kg PO	1.75-2.5 mg/kg PO
SYMPATHOLYTICS		
Atenolol	0.25-1.0 mg/kg PO	2-3 mg/kg
Prazosin	1 mg/15 kg PO	—
Propranolol	0.125-1.10 mg/kg PO	0.4-1.2 mg/kg PO
MISCELLANEOUS DRUGS		
Alendronate	10-20 mg/kg PO	
Amantadine	3-5 mg/kg PO	3-5 mg/kg PO
Clonidine	10 μg/kg IV	10 μg/kg IV
Codeine	1-2 mg/kg PO	—
Dextromethorphan	0.5-2 mg/kg PO, SC, IV	—
Ketamine	0.5 mg/kg SC 20 μg/kg per minute IV	0.5 mg/kg SC 5-10 μg/kg per minute IV
Magnesium salts ($Mg^{-2}SO_4^{-2}$)	5-15 mg/kg IV	5-15 mg/kg IV
Tramadol	2-5 mg/kg PO, bid-tid	1-3 mg/kg PO, sid-bid

Tramadol acts at both opioid receptors, inhibits the reuptake of serotonin and norepinephrine, and has been administered alone or as adjunctive therapy with NSAIDs to control chronic pain. Tramadol should not be administered in conjunction with tricyclic antidepressants (amitriptyline) because of the potential for behavioral abnormalities. Many drugs used to produce anxiolysis and produce muscle relaxation before surgery (e.g., acepromazine and diazepam) produce adjunctive analgesic effects when combined with inhalant (e.g., isoflurane and sevoflurane) or injectable (e.g., ketamine and propofol) anesthetics, opioids, or α_2-agonists. The potential to produce significant drug interactions and side effects and to enhance the toxicity of the primary analgesic drug presents a risk. The coadministration of acepromazine and opioids, for example, may improve overall analgesic efficacy by 2 to 3 times but also increases the potential for increased respiratory depression and the development of respiratory acidosis. To date, there are no controlled clinical trials demonstrating the efficacy or safety of most if not all of the drugs considered to be useful for producing adjuvant analgesia. Ideally, future studies will fill this void.

Suggested Readings

Boothe DM: *Small animal clinical pharmacology and therapeutics,* Philadelphia, 2001, WB Saunders.

Carroll GL, Simonson SM: Recent developments in nonsteroidal antiinflammatory drugs in cats, *JAAMHA* 41:347-354, 2005.

Dahl JB, Moiniche S: Pre-emptive analgesia, *Br Med Bull* 71:13-27 2004.

Hobbs WR, Rall RW, Verdoorn TA: Hypnotics and sedatives: ethanol. In *Hardman JG et al,* editors: *Goodman & Gillman's the pharmacological basis of therapeutics,* ed 9, New York, 1996, McGraw-Hill.

Muir WW: Pain. In Muir WW, Hubbell JAE, Skarda RT et al: *Handbook of veterinary anesthesia,* ed 3, St Louis, 2000, Mosby.

Reisine T, Pasternak G: Opioid analgesics and antagonists. In *Hardman JG et al,* editors: *Goodman & Gillman's the pharmacological basis of therapeutics,* ed 9, New York, 1996, McGraw-Hill.

Wieseler-Frank J, Maier SF, Watkins LR: Central proinflammatory cytokines and pain enhancement, *Neurosignals* 14:166-174, 2005.

9

OPIOIDS

ANN E. WAGNER

DEFINITION

An *opioid* can be defined as any natural or synthetic drug that has opiate-like activities, exerting its effects by interacting with opiate receptors of cell membranes (Box 9-1).

ANALGESIC EFFICACY

Opioids, which characteristically *produce analgesia without loss of proprioception or consciousness,* are currently the most efficacious systemic means of controlling acute or postoperative pain.

OTHER EFFECTS

In addition to their analgesic effects, opioids may cause side effects (see Side Effects/Toxicity).

OPIATE RECEPTORS

- *Function:* Opiate receptors mediate the various effects of opioids (Table 9-1).
- *Classification:* The location, identification, and actions of various opiate receptors are subject to ongoing investigation, and consequently, the classification of opioid drugs and receptors presented may not reflect the latest findings. (For instance, there may actually be seven subtypes of the μ-receptor; see also Relevant Pharmacology.)
- *Locations*
  1. Central nervous system: Traditionally, it was believed that opiate receptors were located only in the central nervous system, particularly in the brain and in the dorsal horn of the spinal cord,

---

BOX 9-1
Definitions

- A pure opioid *agonist* binds to one or more types of receptor and causes certain effects, such as analgesia or respiratory depression (e.g., morphine).
- An opioid is considered a *partial agonist* if its binding at a given receptor causes an effect that is less pronounced than that of a pure agonist (e.g., buprenorphine).
- An opioid *antagonist* binds to one or more types of receptor but causes no effect at those receptors. By competitively displacing an agonist from a receptor, the antagonist effectively "reverses" the effect of the agonist (e.g., naloxone).
- An opioid *agonist-antagonist* binds to more than one type of receptor, causing an effect at one but no effect or a less pronounced effect at another (e.g., butorphanol).

TABLE 9-1 — Classification of Opiate Receptors and Their Effects

Class	Effects
μ-1	Supraspinal analgesia
μ-2	Respiratory depression
	Bradycardia
	Physical dependence
	Euphoria
μ-3	Hyperpolarization of peripheral nerves induced by inflammation/ immune response
κ	Analgesia
	Sedation
	Miosis
δ	Modulation of μ-receptor activity

where impulses from peripheral nerves are modulated before being transmitted to higher centers.

2. Peripheral tissues: Although recent studies suggest that opioid receptors and activities also occur in some peripheral tissues, the clinical applications of these findings have yet to be fully evaluated.

PROTOTYPE AND MEMBERS

AGONISTS

*Morphine**

DESCRIPTION: *Morphine is the principal alkaloid derived from opium and the prototype opioid agonist to which all others are compared (Table 9-2).*

---

*Morphine, Morphine Sulfate Injection; Elkins-Sinn, Cherry Hill, N.J.

For many reasons, morphine is generally considered a primary analgesic in small animal practice.

ANALGESIC EFFICACY: *Although other opioids may be more potent, to date, none is more effective than morphine at relieving pain. Cats do not produce the active metabolite of morphine after intramuscular administration, and only 50% of cats produce it after intravenous morphine administration. Therefore, morphine is less efficacious in most cats than in dogs.*

MAIN EFFECT: *Analgesia without loss of sensation or proprioception*

POSSIBLE SIDE EFFECTS

1. Depression of the respiratory center, resulting in decreased minute volume and increased arterial carbon dioxide tension
2. Depression of the cough center
3. Stimulation of the chemoreceptor trigger zone and increased intestinal peristalsis, which may cause defecation shortly after administration, along with stimulation of gastrointestinal sphincters, which can lead to eventual constipation
4. Increased antidiuretic hormone, with urine production decreased by up to 90%
5. Histamine release: Morphine should be administered slowly and in conservative doses if given intravenously because of the potential for endogenous histamine release, which may occur within 1 minute and persist for at least 60 minutes.
6. Cardiovascular effects: Morphine generally causes minimal depression of cardiac contractility but can cause bradycardia, which is generally responsive to anticholinergic agents. Histamine release, if it occurs, may result in hypotension.
7. Excitement/dysphoria: Morphine may cause excitement or dysphoria in some animals, with dogs generally being less affected than cats and horses.

DURATION: *Analgesic effects of systemically administered morphine may last up to 4 hours, an advantage in the management of acute pain associated with trauma or surgery.*

COST: *Morphine is inexpensive enough that cost should not be an excuse for inadequate treatment of pain.*

Oxymorphone*

DESCRIPTION: *A semisynthetic opioid*

ANALGESIC EFFICACY AND DURATION: *Similar to morphine*

---

*Oxymorphone, P/M Oxymorphone HCl Injection; Mallinckrodt, St. Louis, Mo.

TABLE 9-2	Comparative Potencies, Suggested Dosages, and Dosing Frequencies of Common Opioid Analgesics			
Opioid Analgesic	**Relative Potency**	**Dog Dose (mg/kg)**	**Cat Dose (mg/kg)**	**Comments**
Morphine	1	0.5-2 q2-4h	0.2-0.5 q3-4h	Oral tablets and suspension also available Use caution when given intravenously (histamine release)
Morphine, sustained release (oral)		2-5 q12h		Bioavailability is poor when morphine is given orally
Oxymorphone	10	0.05-0.4 q2-4h	0.02-0.1 q3-4h	Minimal to no histamine release
Hydromorphone	10-15	0.05-0.2 q2-6h	0.05-0.1 q2-6h	Minimal to no histamine release
Methadone	1-1.5	0.5-1	0.1-0.5	
Meperidine	0.1	3-5 q1-2h	3-5 q1-2h	Not recommended for intravenous use (histamine release)
Fentanyl	100	*Loading:* 2-5 µg/kg	*Loading:* 1-3 µg/kg	Constant rate infusion (CRI) required for sustained effect
		CRI: 2-5 µg/kg per hour (pain management); 10-45 µg/kg per hour (surgical analgesia and minimum alveolar concentration reduction)	*CRI:* 1-4 µg/kg per hour (pain management); 10-30 µg/kg per hour (surgical analgesia)	
Sufentanil	1000	5 µg/kg loading; 0.1 µg/kg per minute	?	Unpredictable sedation; may require tranquilizer

Drug	Dose		Notes
Alfentanil	10	?	Rapid onset, short duration (10 minutes?)
Remifentanil	50	?	Extremely rapid elimination
	Loading: 4-10 µg/kg		
	CRI: 4-10 µg/kg per hour (pain management); 20-60 µg/kg per hour (surgical analgesia)		
Butorphanol	3-5		
	0.1-0.4 q1-4h	0.1-0.4 q2-6h	
Butorphanol, oral	0.5-2 q6-8h	0.5-1 q6-8h	
Buprenorphine	25		May be difficult to antagonize
	0.005-0.02 q8-12h	0.005-0.02 q8-12h;	Cats: Instill in cheek pouch for transmucosal absorption.
		0.01-0.02 PO, tid, qid	
Nalbuphine	1		
	0.5-1 q1-4h	0.2-0.4 q1-44h	
Pentazocine	0.25-0.5		
	1-3 q2-4h	1-3 q2-4h	

Drugs may be administered intravenously, intramuscularly, and subcutaneously unless otherwise stated. Dosages are milligrams/kilogram unless otherwise stated. Required dosages and duration of analgesia vary from individual to individual; these are guidelines only.

OTHER EFFECTS

1. Oxymorphone does not cause histamine release; therefore, it is safer for intravenous (IV) administration than morphine.
2. Clinical impression suggests that oxymorphone may be less likely to produce excitement than morphine.
3. Oxymorphone is more likely to induce panting than morphine. Panting results from a resetting of the thermoregulatory center, so the animal "thinks" it needs to cool off despite a normal or low body temperature.

COST: *Oxymorphone is approved for use in dogs and cats but is considerably more expensive than morphine.*

Hydromorphone*

DESCRIPTION: *A semisynthetic opioid*
ANALGESIC EFFICACY: *Hydromorphone has nearly the same efficacy and potency as oxymorphone. Hydromorphone may actually produce better analgesia in cats than does morphine.*
DURATION: *Similar to morphine and oxymorphone*
COST: *Currently, hydromorphone is considerably less expensive than oxymorphone, so it has been recommended as a lower-cost alternative to oxymorphone.*
OTHER COMMENTS: *Although hydromorphone can induce some histamine release, the effect is apparently mild and unlikely to cause vasodilation and hypotension, so IV administration is considered relatively safe. Hydromorphone produces less sedation than morphine or oxymorphone in dogs and cats. Cats may become hyperthermic after hydromorphone administration.*

Methadone†

DESCRIPTION: *A synthetic opioid*
ANALGESIC EFFICACY: *Similar to morphine*
DURATION: *2 to 6 hours*
OTHER COMMENTS: *Methadone is the least likely of the µ-agonist opioids to cause vomiting. Methadone may have N-methyl-D-aspartate receptor antagonist activity, which may add another dimension to its analgesia and may help prevent development of opioid tolerance.*

Meperidine‡

DESCRIPTION: *Meperidine is a synthetic opioid about one tenth as potent as morphine. Because of its short duration and possible*

*Hydromorphone, Hydromorphone HCl; Wyeth-Ayerst, Philadelphia.
†Methadone (Dolophine); Eli Lilly, Indianapolis, Ind.
‡Meperidine, Meperidine HCl; Astra, Westborough, Mass.

cardiovascular effects, meperidine is less satisfactory for long-term analgesia than morphine.

ANALGESIC EFFICACY: *Similar to morphine*

DURATION: *Appears to be of much shorter duration in animals, with analgesia lasting generally less than 1 hour*

OTHER COMMENTS

1. Negative inotropy: Unlike other opioids, meperidine reportedly may have significant negative inotropic effects.

2. Histamine release: Like morphine, meperidine can induce histamine release. For this reason, IV administration is not recommended

Fentanyl*

DESCRIPTION: *A short-acting synthetic opioid*

ANALGESIC EFFICACY: *Similar to morphine. Fentanyl can decrease the minimum alveolar concentration (MAC) requirement for inhaled anesthetics by up to 63%.*

DURATION: *The effects of fentanyl last only about 30 minutes after a single injection. For clinical application, the duration of fentanyl is commonly extended by administering it as a constant rate infusion—intraoperatively to augment surgical analgesia and to reduce the requirement for inhalation anesthetics (10 to 45 µg/kg per hour) and postoperatively for pain management (2 to 5 µg/kg per hour). Despite the supposed short duration of fentanyl, there is a great deal of individual variation in recovery time from infusions.*

OTHER COMMENTS

1. The use of fentanyl intraoperatively may be especially advantageous in patients with compromised cardiac function because (unlike inhaled anesthetics) it causes minimal cardiovascular depression or hypotension while contributing to significant reduction in the MAC requirement.

2. Experimental findings and clinical impression suggest that tolerance to fentanyl can occur, perhaps as soon as 3 hours after administration is begun.

Sufentanil†

DESCRIPTION: *A synthetic opioid about 1000 times as potent as morphine*

DURATION: *About half as long as that of fentanyl*

OTHER COMMENTS: *Currently, sufentanil is not commonly used for pain management in animals.*

---

*Fentanyl, Fentanyl Citrate Injection; Abbott Laboratories, North Chicago.
†Sufentanil (Sufenta); Taylor Pharmaceuticals, San Clemente, Calif.

Alfentanil*

DESCRIPTION: *A synthetic opioid about 25 times as potent as morphine*
DURATION: *Shorter in duration than fentanyl*
OTHER COMMENTS: *Currently, alfentanil is not commonly used for pain management in animals.*

Remifentanil†

DESCRIPTION: *Remifentanil is another synthetic opioid that is about half as potent as fentanyl and is unique among opioids in that it is metabolized by nonspecific esterases that occur in blood and tissues throughout the body (mainly in skeletal muscle). This gives remifentanil the clinical advantage of extremely rapid clearance that does not depend on liver or kidney function.*
DURATION: *Because of this rapid clearance, constant rate infusion is required for sustained analgesia. Recovery is generally expected to occur within 3 to 7 minutes after termination of an infusion.*
OTHER COMMENTS: *Remifentanil may be useful in situations in which intense analgesia is needed for a short or variable period.*

Carfentanil‡

DESCRIPTION: *Synthetic opioid approximately 10,000 times more potent than morphine*
OTHER COMMENTS: *Used mainly for capture of wild and feral animals; not normally used in pain management*

AGONIST-ANTAGONISTS
Butorphanol §

DESCRIPTION: *Butorphanol is a synthetic opioid believed to exert its effects mainly at κ-receptors, producing varying degrees of analgesia and sedation with minimal cardiopulmonary depression. Butorphanol binds to, but has minimal effect at, μ-receptors and, consequently, is labeled a μ-receptor antagonist.*
ANALGESIC EFFICACY: *Butorphanol appears to be a less effective analgesic than morphine and other pure μ-agonist opioids.*

---

*Alfentanil (Alfenta); Taylor Pharmaceuticals.
†Remifentanil (Ultiva); GlaxoWellcome, Research Triangle Park, N.C.
‡Carfentanil (Wildnil); Wildlife Pharmaceuticals, Fort Collins, Colo.
§Butorphanol (Torbugesic); Fort Dodge Animal Health, Fort Dodge, Iowa.

1. Plateau or ceiling effect: Although at low doses, the analgesic potency of butorphanol is about 3 times that of morphine, doses greater than about 0.8 to 1 mg/kg are associated with a plateau or ceiling effect, such that no further enhancement of analgesia occurs.
2. Butorphanol appears to be more effective for mild to moderate pain and for visceral pain than for severe or somatic pain.

DURATION: *The duration of analgesia from butorphanol is debatable and probably varies depending on the species, degree of pain, and route of administration. Some studies suggest a duration of less than an hour in dogs, whereas others indicate a longer duration of up to 6 hours, particularly in cats.*

OTHER COMMENTS

1. Interaction of butorphanol with pure agonists: Traditionally, it was thought that simultaneous or sequential administration of an agonist-antagonist such as butorphanol and a pure agonist such as oxymorphone or morphine would be counterproductive in that the agonist-antagonist might inhibit or even reverse the analgesic effects of the agonist. However, a recent study in cats, in which the colonic balloon model for visceral pain was used, suggests that combining butorphanol with oxymorphone (0.05 to 0.1 mg/kg of each) results in synergistic analgesia, minimal cardiopulmonary effects, and decreased excitement or dysphoria compared with oxymorphone alone.[1] This result suggested that a combination of an agonist-antagonist and a pure agonist may have advantages, particularly in species or individuals prone to opioid-induced dysphoria. However, another study, in which butorphanol was combined with hydromorphone in cats, found that although duration of analgesia was enhanced, the intensity of analgesia was reduced.[2]
2. Partial antagonism of pure agonists: Another use for butorphanol and other agonist-antagonists is to partially antagonize the sedative or respiratory depressant effects of a pure μ-agonist such as morphine or oxymorphone, without completely removing analgesia. This technique is particularly useful for reversal of excessive sedation and restoration of laryngeal reflexes so that a postoperative patient can be extubated in recovery. For this purpose, butorphanol, 0.1 mg/kg, administered IV, is generally effective.

*Nalbuphine**

DESCRIPTION: *A κ-agonist and partial μ-antagonist, nalbuphine produces mild analgesia with little sedation, respiratory depression, or cardiovascular effect with a duration of action of about 1 hour.*

---

*Nalbuphine, Nalbuphine HCl Injection; Astra.

OTHER COMMENTS

1. Cost: One of the main advantages of nalbuphine is that it is inexpensive.
2. Nalbuphine is not on the Drug Enforcement Administration (DEA) scheduled substance list because of its low abuse potential.
3. Partial antagonism of pure agonists: Nalbuphine, like butorphanol, may also be effective in partially antagonizing the sedative effects of a μ-agonist, at a dosage of 0.1 to 0.5 mg/kg administered IV.

Pentazocine*

DESCRIPTION: *Pentazocine is another κ-agonist and μ-antagonist similar to butorphanol and nalbuphine, producing mild analgesia of uncertain duration.*

OTHER COMMENTS: *Pentazocine appears to be less reliable than butorphanol or nalbuphine as a partial antagonist for other opioids.*

Buprenorphine†

DESCRIPTION: *Buprenorphine is different from other agonist-antagonists in that it is considered a partial agonist at μ-receptors and an antagonist at κ-receptors.*

ANALGESIC EFFICACY: *Because it is only a partial agonist, buprenorphine may not provide adequate analgesia for moderate to severe pain, such as that following orthopedic or thoracotomy procedures, and increasing dosages above those clinically recommended may actually result in reduced analgesia.*

ONSET OF ACTION: *Buprenorphine has a slower onset of action than many other opioids, with its peak effect delayed up to an hour after IV administration.*

DURATION: *Although a purported advantage of buprenorphine is its long duration of analgesia (up to 12 hours), its clinical analgesic effect in animals often seems to wane by 6 hours.*

OTHER COMMENTS:

1. Once bound to μ-receptors, buprenorphine is reportedly difficult to displace, meaning that its effects may be difficult to antagonize.
2. Buprenorphine is well absorbed when administered transmucosally (placed in the cheek pouch) in cats, with a duration of 6 to 8 hours, making this a practical analgesic for cats.

COST: *Buprenorphine is considerably more expensive than morphine.*

MECHANISM OF ACTION

◆ Inhibit pain transmission in the dorsal horn of the spinal cord
◆ Inhibit somatosensory afferent nerves at supraspinal levels
◆ Activate descending inhibitory pathways

---

*Pentazocine (Talwin); Sanofi Winthrop, New York.
†Buprenorphine (Buprenex Injectable); Reckitt & Colman Products, Richmond, Va.

◆ Bind to receptors on the terminal axons of primary afferent nerves within the substantia gelatinosa of the spinal cord, causing a decrease in the release of neurotransmitters such as substance P

EFFICACY/USE

REGIONAL OR LOCAL ADMINISTRATION

Epidural

◆ Epidural administration of morphine is widely practiced in a variety of species, including dogs, cats, and horses.
◆ Morphine, 0.1 mg/kg, administered epidurally provides analgesia with fewer side effects than systemically administered morphine.
  1. Onset: Approximately 30 to 60 minutes in small animals; longer in horses
  2. Duration: Approximately 18 hours
◆ Preservative-free morphine is recommended because preservatives may be neurotoxic. However, in horses and other large animals, preservative-containing morphine is typically used but is diluted with sterile physiologic saline.

Intraarticular

◆ Trauma or inflammation may activate opioid receptors on nociceptive nerve terminals and/or inflammatory cells (possibly μ-3 receptors).
◆ Morphine instilled into joints at the end of surgery reportedly provides up to 18 hours of analgesia.
◆ Based on human studies, application of a tourniquet proximal to the joint is recommended for 10 minutes after injection but is rarely practiced in veterinary patients.
◆ Intraarticular morphine administration may be combined with a local anesthetic such as bupivacaine for enhanced analgesia.

Topical Application on Cornea

◆ Specially prepared, pH-controlled 1% morphine sulfate solution has been applied to experimentally induced corneal ulcers in dogs.[3]
◆ Topical use of morphine on the cornea was associated with decreased pain behaviors (reduced blepharospasm and lower esthesiometer readings).[3]
◆ Healing of corneal ulcers was not affected by topical morphine.[3]

TRANSDERMAL ADMINISTRATION

Fentanyl is available in a transdermal delivery system.*
    DOSAGE: *2 to 4 µg/kg per hour*
    1. Patch sizes: 25, 50, 75, or 100 µg/h.
    2. For very small animals, remove the backing from only a portion of
        the patch that represents an appropriate dose (i.e., for a 4-kg cat,
        use a 25 µg/h patch with only half the backing removed: →12.5
        µg/h, or 3.125 µg/kg per hour).
    APPLICATION
    1. Site is the back of the neck or shoulders, lateral thorax, or metatarsus.
    2. Clip hair; clean skin with water only.
    3. Apply patch and hold firmly in place for at least 2 minutes.
    4. Apply a bandage over the patch.
    ONSET: *6 to 24 hours*
    DURATION: *72 to 104 hours*

RELEVANT PHARMACOLOGY

HISTORICAL CLASSIFICATION

Opiate receptors were originally classified as σ, κ, μ, and δ.

RESULTS OF OPIOID AGONIST OCCUPYING OPIATE RECEPTOR

Events that may occur when an opioid agonist occupies a particular
opiate receptor, which result in inhibition of activation of neurons, are
the following:
- Depression of cyclic adenosine monophosphate formation
- Activation of potassium channels, resulting in membrane
  hyperpolarization
- Activation of G proteins
- Inhibition of opening of voltage-sensitive calcium channels
- Decreased release of neurotransmitters such as substance P

LOCATION OF OPIATE RECEPTORS

Traditionally, it was thought that opiate receptors were confined to the
central nervous system. However, more recently a peripheral, local action
of opioids has also been demonstrated.

---

*Fentanyl (Duragesic); Janssen Pharmaceutical, Titusville, N.J.

Brain (Predominantly μ-Receptors)

- Mesencephalic periaqueductal gray
- Mesencephalic reticular formation
- Medulla
- Substantia nigra
- Ventral forebrain
- Amygdala

Spinal Cord (μ-, κ-, and δ-Receptors)

- Dorsal horn laminae I to V
- Substantia gelatinosa

Peripheral Receptors

Opioids may have local actions under certain conditions of inflammation with hyperalgesia, suggesting that inflammatory cells that release cytokines and other nerve-sensitizing products may contain opiate receptors that can suppress these events.

SIDE EFFECTS/TOXICITY

Possible side effects of opioid administration are many and varied, although rarely problematic enough to prevent the use of opioids in pain management. One of the major advantages of opioids in pain management is their safety.

SEDATION OR CENTRAL NERVOUS SYSTEM DEPRESSION

- Sedation commonly occurs after opioid administration in small animals, more so in dogs than in cats.
- Sedation is generally considered an advantage when an opioid is used as a preanesthetic or in the immediate postoperative period when rest is desirable.
- Sedation may be undesirable if it interferes with return to normal behaviors such as eating and drinking.
- Options for preventing excessive sedation are as follows:
  1. Reduce the dosage of opioid.
  2. Administer a low dose of an agonist-antagonist such as nalbuphine or butorphanol in conjunction with a pure agonist such as morphine.
  3. Administer a low dose of a pure antagonist such as nalmefene in conjunction with a pure agonist such as morphine.

EXCITEMENT OR DYSPHORIA

◆ Excitement occurs in some, but not all, animals after opioid administration. A great deal of species and individual variation exists, with cats, horses, and northern breeds of dogs (e.g., malamutes and huskies) apparently more susceptible to dysphoria.

◆ The recommended dosages (milligrams/kilogram) for most opioids in cats are about half those recommended for dogs to minimize the incidence of excitement. Use of lower opioid dosages may minimize dysphoria in susceptible animals.

◆ If dysphoria or agitation occurs, administration of a tranquilizer such as acepromazine (0.01 to 0.03 mg/kg) or a sedative such as xylazine (0.1 to 0.3 mg/kg) or medetomidine (0.5 to 5 µg/kg) should help to calm the animal.

◆ Another option is to use an agonist-antagonist such as nalbuphine or butorphanol to antagonize the excitatory effects of a pure agonist such as morphine, without antagonizing analgesia. A study in cats demonstrated that 0.1 mg/kg each of oxymorphone and butorphanol provided synergistic analgesia without excitement.[1]

◆ Determination of whether an agitated animal is dysphoric or in pain is important because the treatment for each situation may be different. (See Chapters 3 and 4 for more information on assessing pain and analgesia.)

BRADYCARDIA

◆ Bradycardia occurs as a result of opioid-induced medullary vagal stimulation.

◆ Bradycardia is more likely to occur in an animal not in pain (e.g., when an opioid is given as a preanesthetic).

◆ Some animals may develop second-degree atrioventricular block.

◆ Prevention and treatment: Atropine (0.02 to 0.04 mg/kg) or glycopyrrolate (0.01 to 0.02 mg/kg), administered subcutaneously, intramuscularly, or IV, is generally effective at restoring heart rate to an acceptable level.

OTHER CARDIOVASCULAR EFFECTS

◆ With the exception of meperidine, opioids generally cause little to no depression of myocardial contractility.

◆ Therefore as long as bradycardia is prevented, cardiac output and blood pressure should be minimally affected by opioid administration.

RESPIRATORY DEPRESSION

◆ Respiratory depression results from an opioid-induced decrease in responsiveness of the brainstem respiratory center to $Paco_2$.

◆ In human beings, opioid-induced respiratory depression can be profound, but in animals, clinically useful analgesic dosages of opioids *alone* are unlikely to produce clinically significant respiratory depression.

◆ However, when opioids are used in high dosages to provide surgical analgesia (such as fentanyl infusions at 20 µg/kg per hour or higher) or when they are used in conjunction with other respiratory depressant drugs (such as thiopental, propofol, or the inhaled anesthetics), assisted or controlled ventilation may be required.

PANTING

◆ Panting may occur in some dogs after opioid administration, particularly after oxymorphone administration.

◆ Panting animals do not necessarily hyperventilate; in fact, they may hypoventilate and become hypercapnic.

◆ The cause of panting is resetting of the thermoregulatory center in the thalamus, which makes a normothermic dog "think" it is hot, causing it to pant to cool off.

◆ Panting can be annoying or inconvenient, for instance, during radiography when excessive motion is problematic.

◆ Panting can also interfere with rewarming a hypothermic animal, for instance, in the postoperative recovery period. However, hypothermia should not be a reason to withhold opioid analgesics from a patient during the postoperative period; rather, external warming devices such as circulating warm water blankets or forced warm air heating blankets should be used to restore and maintain body temperature while analgesia is provided.

COUGH SUPPRESSION OR DEPRESSION OF LARYNGEAL REFLEXES

◆ Opioid-induced cough suppression can be desirable or undesirable, depending on circumstances.

◆ Many dogs can be intubated after receiving IV administration of an opioid and benzodiazepine, even though they remain conscious. This technique can be used to induce profound neuroleptanalgesia in critical patients, thus avoiding the use of more depressant anesthesia induction drugs.

- Depression of laryngeal reflexes might be desirable when a brachycephalic (or other airway-challenged) dog is recovering from anesthesia because it will allow the animal to tolerate the endotracheal tube for a longer time, during which inhaled anesthetic can be eliminated.
- Some opioid-treated dogs have excessively prolonged recoveries from anesthesia, in part because of insensitivity to the endotracheal tube. In those cases, a small dose of an agonist-antagonist such as nalbuphine or butorphanol (0.1 mg/kg IV) or a very small dose of an antagonist such as naloxone (1 to 10 μg/kg IV) may restore laryngeal reflexes to the point that the dog can be extubated safely.

HISTAMINE RELEASE

- Histamine release can occur with administration of certain opioids, such as morphine and meperidine, particularly with IV administration.
- Sequelae of histamine release include vasodilation and hypotension.
- Morphine should be given by the IV route only if given cautiously and slowly and in low dosages. Morphine should generally not be given by the IV route to an animal during general anesthesia.
- It is best to avoid IV administration of meperidine.
- No significant histamine release occurs after administration of oxymorphone, hydromorphone, or fentanyl, so these opioids are considered safe for IV use. Methadone is also commonly administered IV without apparent complication.

VOMITING AND DEFECATION

- Vomiting and defecation commonly follow administration of opioids, particularly when administered as preanesthetics to animals not in pain; these effects are less common when administered to animals in pain or those that have had surgery.
- Nausea and vomiting are caused by stimulation of the chemoreceptor trigger zone in the medulla.
- Defecation may result from an initial increase in gastrointestinal tone.

CONSTIPATION

- With long-term opioid use, increased gastrointestinal sphincter tone and reduced peristalsis may lead to constipation.

◆ Constipation is not usually a clinical problem in short-term pain management.

URINARY RETENTION

◆ Urinary retention is caused by increased detrusor muscle tone and increased vesical sphincter tone.
◆ Urinary retention is especially common after epidural morphine administration.
◆ The bladder may need to be manually expressed or catheterized.

EFFECT ON BILIARY SMOOTH MUSCLE

◆ In human beings, morphine has been shown to cause constriction of the sphincter of Oddi, causing pain from increased pressure within the common bile duct.
◆ Other opioids such as meperidine, fentanyl, and pentazocine may similarly affect this sphincter, but nalbuphine and buprenorphine appear to have minimal effect. Thus certain opioids may be contraindicated in patients with pancreatitis or biliary disease.
◆ Dogs often have separate bile and pancreatic ducts, so use of opioids in dogs with pancreatitis may not be problematic.
◆ Most cats do have a common pancreatic and bile duct, so nalbuphine or buprenorphine may be the best choice for pain management in cats with pancreatitis.

SPECIAL ISSUES

COMPREHENSIVE DRUG ABUSE PREVENTION AND CONTROL ACT (UNITED STATES)

◆ Drugs are classified according to potential for abuse.
  1. Most opioid agonists have a high potential for abuse and are listed in schedule II: morphine, hydromorphone, methadone, meperidine, and others.
  2. Butorphanol, an opioid agonist-antagonist with moderate abuse potential, is listed in schedule IV.
◆ Prescribing of controlled substances is regulated in the United States.
  1. Veterinarian must register with DEA (registration to be renewed every 2 years).
  2. Veterinarian must keep inventory of controlled substances.
  3. Controlled substances must be ordered by using special forms.

TOLERANCE AND PHYSICAL DEPENDENCE

- ◆ It has been shown that tolerance to the effects of opioids can develop rapidly.
- ◆ Nociceptive stimulation reportedly antagonizes or prevents development of tolerance to fentanyl; therefore, tolerance is less likely to occur during pain management.
- ◆ Clinically, occurrence of tolerance or physical dependence in animals is anecdotal and apparently rare.

HYPERTHERMIA

Cats may develop hyperthermia (103° to 105° F) several hours after the administration of μ-opioid agonists (morphine, oxymorphone, hydromorphone). Cats should be treated with antipyretics if necessary. Hyperthermia is not generally seen in cats given buprenorphine.

ANTAGONISTS

General comments: Opioid antagonists are often used to arouse animals that are excessively sedated or obtunded from opioid administration, for instance, when recovery from anesthesia is prolonged and the patient has not regained laryngeal/cough reflexes. One should remember that reversal of opioid effects, particularly in an animal that is potentially in pain, may result in intense acute pain with accompanying sympathetic stimulation that may be detrimental. Therefore, opioid antagonists should be used conservatively and only with good reason in animals experiencing pain. If bradycardia is the main cause for concern, an anticholinergic such as atropine or glycopyrrolate should be used instead of an opioid antagonist to restore a normal heart rate without affecting patient comfort.

Naloxone*

DESCRIPTION: *Naloxone does not induce any effects when administered alone, but when administered to an animal that has previously been given an opioid agonist such as morphine, it effectively reverses the effects of the agonist, causing increased alertness, responsiveness, and coordination, as well as increased awareness of pain.*
DURATION: *The duration of naloxone is shorter than that of many opioid agonists; an IV injection of naloxone, 0.01 mg/kg, lasts 20 to 40 minutes, whereas 0.04 mg/kg, administered intramuscularly, lasts 40 to 70 minutes.*

---

*Naloxone, P/M Naloxone HCl Injection; Mallinckrodt.

Therefore, animals should be watched for renarcotization or resedation after a dose of naloxone.

OTHER COMMENTS

1. Excitement or anxiety may accompany naloxone reversal of the effects of an opioid agonist.
2. Although not common, cardiac dysrhythmias such as ventricular premature contractions can occur after naloxone reversal of the effects of an opioid, particularly if conditions favor high levels of circulating catecholamines.
3. In potentially painful situations (such as after surgery), the dose of naloxone should be greatly reduced and given in small increments, just to the point of arousal, to avoid precipitating a painful recovery. For this purpose, a total dosage of 0.001 to 0.01 mg/kg IV may be sufficient.

Nalmefene*

DESCRIPTION: *An opioid antagonist approximately 4 times as potent as naloxone*

DURATION: *Nalmefene works as quickly as naloxone, but its duration of action is approximately 1 to 2 hours, about twice that of naloxone. Therefore, nalmefene may be advantageous in preventing renarcotization when it is used to antagonize a long-acting opioid.*

OTHER COMMENTS: *Dosages for animals have not been well-established, but in human beings, dosages may vary from 0.25 μg/kg to 30 μg/kg.*

Naltrexone†

DESCRIPTION: *Another pure opioid antagonist, about 4 times more potent than naloxone*

DURATION: *Duration is about twice that of naloxone (in human beings), but in dogs, pharmacokinetic studies suggest that naltrexone is not much longer-acting than naloxone.*

OTHER COMMENTS: *Based on these findings, a dose of 0.0025 mg/kg IV should effectively antagonize a pure agonist for approximately 2 hours.*

REFERENCES

1. Briggs SL, Sneed K, Sawyer DC: Antinociceptive effects of oxymorphone-butorphanol-acepromazine combination in cats, *Vet Surg* 27:466-472, 1998.

---

*Nalmefene (Revex); Ohmeda (Baxter), Deerfield, Ill.
†Naltrexone (Trexonil); Wildlife Pharmaceuticals.

2. Lascelles BDX, Robertson SA: Antinociceptive effects of hydromorphone, butorphanol, or the combination in cats, *J Vet Intern Med* 18:190-195, 2004.

3. Stiles J, Honda CN, Krohne SG, Kazacos EA: Effect of topical administration of 1% morphine sulfate solution on signs of pain and corneal wound healing in dogs, *Am J Vet Res* 64:813-818, 2003.

Suggested Readings

Hansen B: Pain, *Semin Vet Med Surg (Small Anim)* 12(2):55-142, 1997.

Mathews KA: Management of pain, *Vet Clin North Am Small Anim Pract* 30(4):703-970, 2000.

Tranquilli WJ, Thurman JC, Grimm KA, editors: *Lumb & Jones' veterinary anesthesia and analgesia*, ed 4, 2007, Blackwell.

10 NONSTEROIDAL ANTIINFLAMMATORY DRUGS

STEVEN BUDSBERG

Nonsteroidal antiinflammatory drugs (NSAIDs) share therapeutic actions including analgesic, antiinflammatory, and antipyretic capabilities despite differences in chemical structure. Although chemically related, these compounds vary widely in their structure, and their classification based on chemical structure still engenders some controversy.[1,2] NSAIDs have a unifying action biochemically in the inhibition of the cyclooxygenase enzymes. Historically, NSAIDs are one of the most commonly used classes of drugs in human beings.[3] The same statement is now made about NSAIDs in small animal clinical practice. Several reasons exist for the dramatic increase in NSAID use in companion animals. Veterinarians now have a better understanding of the need to manage acute and chronic pain in small animal medicine. Pain control is an important mission for the practicing veterinarian. NSAIDs provide an effective means to accomplish this goal. Furthermore, there is now the availability of NSAIDs with improved safety and efficacy targeted for small animals (primarily the dog). For the most part, currently prescribed NSAIDs are safe drugs; with only a small percentage of patients experiencing serious complications. However, these problems have achieved significant proportions based on the fact that so many patients are taking them each year; thus a small percentage becomes a large number. Because these drugs are remarkably effective, yet carry a significant risk potential, one must closely evaluate and monitor their usage in each patient.

MECHANISM OF ACTION
PROSTAGLANDIN INHIBITION

- The mechanism of actions of NSAIDs is a continually evolving story that started in the early 1970s with the publication of two manuscripts that examined the ability of aspirin to inhibit prostaglandin production.[4,5] Eicosanoids, which include the compounds known as prostaglandins, are derived from arachidonic acid. The ability of NSAIDs to interfere with eicosanoid synthesis and the subsequent alteration of different physiological systems is what explains the numerous effects seen in the body with NSAID administration.[6] A significant portion of the analgesic and antiinflammatory clinical effects seen with NSAID administration are related to the inhibition of the cyclooxygenase (COX) enzyme isoforms.

◆ The last 15 years have seen the discovery, identification, and considerable elucidation of a group of COX enzymes. Two isoforms, COX-1 and COX-2, are well established, with the presence of a third isoform, COX-3 (which is an alternative splice variant of COX-1), currently being hotly debated. Discovery of the first two isoforms generated a hypothesis that their functions were mutually exclusive, with COX-1 involved with normal physiologic functions of various systems and COX-2 involved in pathologic processes. Current data about these enzymes have shown that this initial paradigm was an oversimplification.[7] COX-1 is now primarily considered the constitutive isoform of COX, and it is responsible for basal prostaglandin production for normal homeostasis in many tissues. COX-1 normally exists in many tissues of the body, including the stomach, kidney, platelets, and reproductive tract, where it catalyzes the synthesis of prostaglandins involved in the daily "housekeeping" functions.[8] COX-1 is expressed at sites of inflammation, but this is likely a function of basal rather than induced expression.[9] COX-2 is usually thought of as the induced isoform and is found in sites of inflammation, yet it is expressed constitutively in several tissues, including the brain, kidney, reproductive system, and eye.[8] Cells that express COX-2 include endothelial cells, smooth muscle cells, chondrocytes, fibroblasts, monocytes, macrophages, and synovial cells.[9-11] Various cytokines and growth factors rapidly induce the formation of COX-2.[10]

◆ The COX enzymes initiate a complex cascade that results in the conversion of polyunsaturated acids to prostaglandins and thromboxane (Fig. 10-1).[12] Briefly, arachidonic acid is transformed into prostaglandin G_2 (PGG_2) and then PGH_2 by COX. Further enzymatic conversion of PGH_2 leads to the functionally important prostaglandins (types D, E, F, and I) and thromboxane. Regarding pain, prostaglandins, primarily PGE_2, contribute to the inflammatory response by causing vasodilation and enhancing the effects of other cytokines and inflammatory mediators. The production of PGE_2 at various sites of inflammation appears to be mediated primarily by COX-2. Thus when an inflammatory event occurs within the tissue, COX-2 enzyme production is induced followed by an increase in prostaglandin concentrations. The selective inhibition of certain prostaglandins primarily produced by COX-2 should allow for the therapeutic analgesic and antiinflammatory effects while greatly diminishing the unwanted side effects caused with COX-1 inhibition. However, complete COX-2 inhibition is detrimental to many normal physiologic functions, including the healing of gastric ulcers. Thus, it is important to assess COX-2 selectivity accurately, and current methods to make these assessments are not clear-cut. COX selectivity is a measure of the relative concentrations of a drug required to inhibit each COX isoenzyme and usually is obtained in in vitro studies. Current ex vivo and limited in vivo data have confirmed COX-2 selectivity or COX-1 sparing effects of certain compounds.[13-16] Additionally, recent studies have provided a model to show the physiologic effects of COX selectivity in target tissues in dogs with osteoarthritis.[13,17,18] Recently, a dual COX and 5-lipoxygenase (LOX) inhibitor (tepoxalin) became available on the veterinary market. These drugs are able to block the COX and the 5-LOX metabolic pathways (Fig. 10-1). Although these drugs are nonspecific inhibitors of the COX enzymes, they appear to have the same gastrointestinal toxicity as the COX-1–selective agents and less than the nonselective COX inhibitors. The exact mechanism of why this dual inhibition limits the gastrointestinal toxicity is not well described.

SITE OF ACTION

Data now support the concept that NSAIDs act on the peripheral tissue injury site and at the level of the central nervous system. NSAIDs inhibit the peripheral COX-2 enzyme to block the formation of prostaglandins such as PGE_2 and PGI_2, which function to dilate arterioles and sensitize peripheral nociceptor terminals to the actions of mediators (e.g., histamine and bradykinin) that produce localized pain and hypersensitivity.[19,20] PGE_2, produced by COX-2, plays a pivotal role in sustaining acute pain sensation by increasing nociceptor cyclic adenosine monophosphate, which decreases the nociceptor threshold of activation.[21] Centrally, COX-2–mediated prostaglandins such as PGE_2 are involved in spinal nociception[22] and central sensitization (Fig. 10-2).[23] COX-2 is expressed in the brain and spinal cord and is up-regulated in response to traumatic injury[24] and peripheral inflammation.[24-26] COX-2–activated PGE_2 lowers the threshold for neuronal depolarization, increasing the number of action potentials and repetitive spiking. The actions of COX-2 are thought to contribute to neuronal plasticity and central sensitization.[27,28]

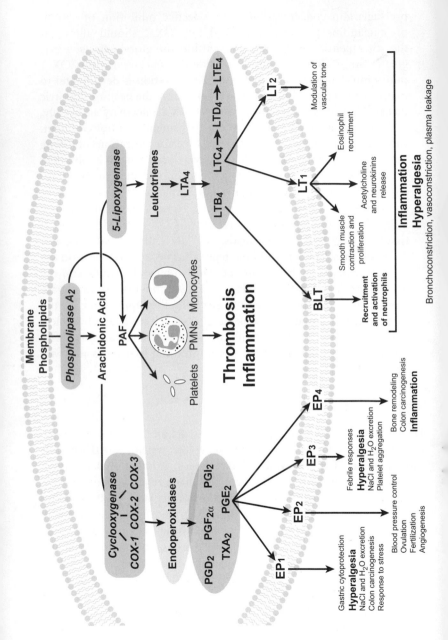

FIG. 10-1. The breakdown of membrane phospholipids and arachidonic acid cascade as influenced by cyclooxygenase and lipoxygenase leads to the production of prostaglandins and leukotrienes, which activate membrane receptors to produce a myriad of effects including pain and inflammation. See text for details.

These insights provide information into the potential value of developing centrally acting agents that alter receptor-mediated actions of prostanoids or enzyme inhibitors that can target specific sites in the prostaglandin cascade. However, this data should not lead directly to the conclusion that spinal delivery of NSAIDs is more effective over systemic delivery.[29]

CLINICAL APPLICATIONS

INDICATIONS

NSAIDs can be used to relieve pain in a variety of clinical settings. Efficacy of NSAIDs is comparable to opioids in many instances of musculoskeletal and visceral pain. However, for major pain such as fractures, data are not available to substantiate the same claim. NSAIDs can be used for cases of acute pain, traumatic or surgically induced, and for chronic pain such as osteoarthritis. Efficacy and toxicity is often individualistic, and individual monitoring is mandatory. Remember, numerous initiating pathways exist that produce pain and that are not fully understood, and it is naive to think that all pathways react the same to different drugs. Second, which in part may be intertwined with the first, heterogeneity of the patient response to a given NSAID occurs in terms of efficacy and toxicity. This individual variation may also be accounted for by slight variations in genetic expression or gene polymorphism of the COX enzymes known as the "COX continuum" hypothesis put forward recently.[30] One must also remember that in human beings, NSAID therapy has a modest effect (20% to 30%) in pain reduction, and thus to optimize treatment programs, nonpharmacologic modalities are needed and have been emphasized previously.[31]

CHOOSING AND MONITORING NSAID USAGE

◆ Use products with a history of clinical experience and good safety profiles.
◆ Use only one NSAID at a time and ensure adequate dosing.
◆ Adapt therapy to suit patient requirements. Begin with the recommended dose for an extended period (at least 10 to 14 days) in

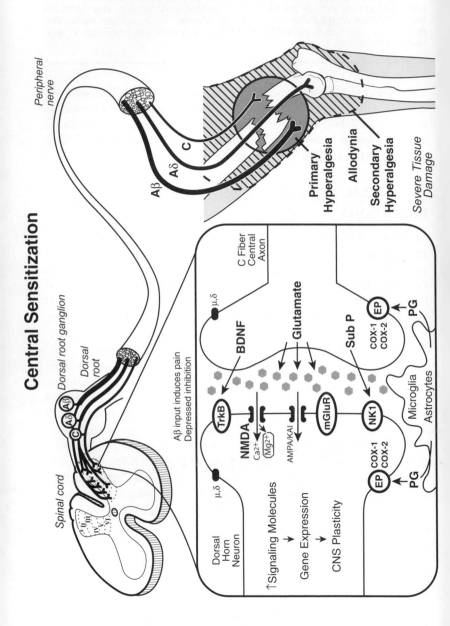

FIG. 10-2. The release of prostaglandins (PGs) from activated microglia and astrocytes within the central nervous system and spinal cord results in the exaggerated release of substance P and other excitatory amino acids from presynaptic terminals, promoting the development of central sensitization, pain facilitation, and hyperalgesia.

---

animals with chronic pain, and if efficacious, attempt to reduce the administered dose at regular intervals (e.g., weekly) until achieving the lowest dose providing the maximum benefit.

◆ Review therapy frequently, and change to alternative NSAIDs if there is a poor response to therapy.

◆ Avoid NSAIDs in patients with known contraindications to their use.

◆ Observe for potential toxicity. Increased vigilance and monitoring are required for at-risk patients. If indicated, establish renal and hepatic status of the patient before NSAID administration.

CONTRAINDICATIONS

The following recommendations are general guidelines, and the type of NSAID (e.g., COX-2 specific) may alter these recommendations as more data become available.[29]

◆ Patients receiving any type of systemic corticosteroids

◆ Patients receiving NSAIDs concurrently

◆ Patients with documented renal or hepatic insufficiency or dysfunction

◆ Patients with any clinical syndrome that creates a decrease in the circulating blood volume (e.g., shock, dehydration, hypotension, or ascites)

◆ Patients with active gastrointestinal (GI) disease.

◆ Trauma patients with known or suspected of having significant active hemorrhage or blood loss

◆ Pregnant patients or females attempting to become pregnant

◆ Patients with significant pulmonary disease (This may be less important with COX-2–specific drugs.)

◆ Patients with any type of confirmed or suspected coagulopathies (This may be less important with COX-2–specific drugs.)

SPECIFIC COMPOUNDS
Approved Compounds

Approved NSAIDs vary considerably around the world. Practitioners must remember that the clinical response to a particular drug is individualistic. Dogs may respond favorably to one product and not another, so if an NSAID is indicated in a case and the first product used does not achieve a positive clinical response, do not forsake NSAIDs, but try a different product (Table 10-1).

Carprofen. Carprofen is a member of the arylpropionic acid class of NSAIDs. Carprofen has been shown to be COX-1 sparing (COX-2 selective) in vitro and in vivo.[14,16,17,32-35] Carprofen is approved in oral and injectable formulations to treat pain and inflammation associated with osteoarthritis (OA) and postoperative pain associated with surgery in dogs. Carprofen has been shown to improve limb function in clinical trials of dogs with naturally occurring OA.[36-39] Carprofen is also effective in providing postoperative analgesia in orthopedic and soft tissue procedures.[40-46] Carprofen does not appear to affect platelet function or cause excessive bleeding in surgical procedures.[40,47,48] Adverse effects associated with carprofen are limited, with the majority related to the GI tract.[36,37,49,50] Furthermore, administration of carprofen to healthy dogs undergoing anesthesia has not been shown to cause alterations in renal function or hemostasis.[48,51-53] The association between carprofen and idiosyncratic hepatotoxicity deserves special attention (see Potential Side Effects), but the reported incidence of hepatic adverse events in dogs treated with carprofen is less than 0.06%.[50,54] In certain countries a single injectable dose in cats is approved for pain. Although ample data support single-dose use for perioperative pain in feline patients,[55-59] repetitive dosing is not recommended until additional safety and efficacy data are produced with multiple-dose protocols.[60]

Deracoxib. Deracoxib is a member of the coxib class of NSAIDs. Deracoxib has been shown to be COX-1 sparing (COX-2 selective) in vitro and in vivo.[17,61] Deracoxib is approved in an oral formulation in dogs for treatment of pain and inflammation associated with OA and postoperative pain associated with orthopedic surgery. Deracoxib has been demonstrated to provide effective analgesia for acute postoperative pain involving cruciate ligament stabilization.[62,63] Deracoxib has also been demonstrated to provide effective relief of pain in clinical OA trials in dogs.[64] Although reported adverse effects are few, a recent case series report documents serious GI complications.[65] In this report, adverse events seemed to be related to higher (3 to 4 mg/kg) dosages or concurrent use of corticosteroids or other NSAIDS. Although limited data on pharmacokinetics are available in cats, safety and efficacy have not been studied, and use in cats is not advised.[66]

Etodolac. Etodolac is a member of the pyranocarboxylic acid class of NSAIDs. In vitro data suggest that etodolac is not COX-2 selective in dogs.[14,34,35] However in vivo data are conflicting with evidence suggesting that platelet thromboxane and gastric prostaglandin PGE_1 were not inhibited by etodolac in dogs at recommended therapeutic

TABLE 10-1	Doses of Nonsteroidal Antiinflammatory Drugs in Dogs and Cats		
Drug	**Dose in Dogs**	**Dose in Cats**	**Recommendations**
NONSELECTIVE			
Acetaminophen	*10 mg/kg q12h PO*	*Not for use in cats*	NR in dogs or cats
Aspirin	10-25 mg/kg q12h PO with food	10 mg/kg q48-72h PO with food	Use carefully
Etodolac	10-15 mg/kg q24h PO	Not established	
Ketoprofen	*2 mg/kg once PO followed by 1 mg/kg q24h PO*	*2 mg/kg once PO followed by 1 mg/kg q24h PO*	NR
Naproxen	*2 mg/kg q48h PO*	*Not for use in cats*	NR
SELECTIVE			
Carprofen	2.2 mg/kg q12h PO; preoperative: 4.4 mg/kg SC	2-4 mg/kg SC once	Dosage in cats remains highly variable
Deracoxib	1-2 mg/kg q24h PO; postoperative: 3-4 mg/kg q24h PO	Not established	
Firocoxib	5 mg/kg q24h PO		
Flunixin meglumine	*1 mg/kg q24h IV, IM, SC, or PO*	*0.25 mg/kg q12-24h SC*	NR
Meloxicam	0.2 mg/kg once PO, IV, or SQ, followed by 0.1 mg/kg q24h PO, IV, or SQ	0.1-0.2 mg/kg once SC or PO, followed by 0.05-0.1 mg/kg q24h SC or PO for 1-3 days, followed by 0.1 mg per cat 2-3 times per week PO	Use lower dosages chronically
Piroxicam	0.3 mg/kg q48h PO	Not established	
COX/LOX INHIBITORS			
Tepoxalin	10 or 20 mg/kg once PO, followed by 10 mg/kg q24h PO	Not established	

NR, Not recommended; *italics*, use cautiously if at all; *COX/LOX*, cyclooxygenase /lipoxygenase.

doses.[17] Thus, it is difficult to state definitively whether etodolac is COX-1 sparing in vivo. Etodolac is approved as an oral formulation for use in managing pain and inflammation associated with canine OA. Clinically, etodolac has been shown to improve rear limb function in dogs with chronic OA.[67-69] Adverse events are primarily seen in the GI tract; however, keratoconjunctivitis sicca has also been associated with etodolac administration.[70-72]

Firocoxib. Firocoxib is a member of the coxib class of NSAIDs. In vitro data support firocoxib as a COX-1–sparing (COX-2–selective) drug; however, in vivo conformation is not yet available.[73] Firocoxib is approved, as an oral formulation, with an indication for the management of pain and inflammation associated with OA in dogs. Clinically, firocoxib has been shown to improve limb function in dogs with OA.[39,68,69] Clinical trials suggest that firocoxib may have some superiority in owner and veterinarian subjective evaluations regarding lameness resolution compared with carprofen and etodolac in dogs with lameness associated with OA.[68,69] Clinical data suggest a low rate of adverse events, limited primarily to the GI tract.[39,68,69,74]

Ketoprofen. Ketoprofen is a member of the arylpropionic acid class of NSAIDs.[75] Ketoprofen inhibits both COX isoenzymes without selectivity in dogs. Because of this inhibition of both COX enzymes, ketoprofen is expected to have significant antithromboxane activity.[14,29] Indeed, data show that although ketoprofen effectively manages postoperative pain, there is a propensity for hemorrhage perioperatively following the administration of ketoprofen.[40] Ketoprofen is approved for use in dogs and cats in Europe and Canada in oral and parenteral formulations. The only data available to the clinician regarding clinical use of this product are in an acute pain model and perioperative pain management.[29,40,76,77] Adverse events are the aforementioned excessive bleeding and GI effects (primarily vomiting).

Meloxicam. Meloxicam is a member of the oxicam family of NSAIDs. Recent in vivo and in vitro data have shown meloxicam to be COX-1 sparing (COX-2 selective).[13,14,29,34,78-80] Meloxicam is approved for use in dogs for the control of pain and inflammation associated with OA and is available in oral and parenteral formulations. Published efficacy data are available for chronic and perioperative pain management.[29,38,80-88] Meloxicam administration to dogs undergoing anesthesia has not been shown to cause alterations in renal function or hemostasis.[52,89,90] Adverse events with meloxicam are low and are primarily limited to the GI tract.[80-82,91,92]

Meloxicam is approved for use in cats, but that approval is limited to a single dose to control pain inflammation associated with orthopedic surgery, ovariohysterectomy, and castration. Several studies support the use of meloxicam for postoperative pain.[57,58,93,94] There are reports of multiple dosing regimens in cats. However, until efficacy and safety studies with specific dosing programs are performed, chronic use cannot be recommended.

Tepoxalin. Tepoxalin is a dual COX/LOX inhibitor, which means that it inhibits both COX isoenzymes and 5-LOX. These dual inhibitor drugs offer an alternative method of blocking the metabolic pathways in the management of pain and inflammation. Tepoxalin has been approved for use in dogs to control pain and inflammation associated with OA and is available in an oral formulation. In vitro and in vivo data support the ability of tepoxalin for dual COX/LOX inhibition.[79,95] Unfortunately, no published reports are available to support clinical efficacy and safety beyond data submitted for government approval. Data are available suggesting that tepoxalin does not alter hemostasis or hepatic or renal function after a single-dose surgical model.[96] Tepoxalin has also been shown not to alter renal function in healthy dogs receiving an angiotensin-converting enzyme inhibitor.[97] Adverse events with tepoxalin are low, primarily GI.

Tolfenamic Acid. Tolfenamic acid is an anthranilic acid derivative and a member of the fenamates class of NSAIDs. Tolfenamic acid is approved in Canada and Europe in an oral and parenteral formulation for dogs and cats. In vitro data support COX-1–sparing (COX-2–selective) activity.[98] However, in vivo data to confirm these actions are not available. Little clinical data are available to support the use of tolfenamic acid.[57,81,98] Strict recommendations on limiting the use of this product are apparently related to its relatively narrow therapeutic range. Most common adverse events are GI (diarrhea and vomiting) and perioperative bleeding.[29]

Compounds Used Off-Label

Nonapproved NSAIDs that have been recommended for use off-label include aspirin, piroxicam, and a plethora of human products. Be aware the vast majority of the human products have limited to no data for dogs or cats for a correct efficacy or safety dosage range.

Aspirin. Aspirin is historically the most commonly used NSAID in dogs and cats. Aspirin is relatively effective, inexpensive, and readily available. Aspirin is not COX-1 sparing (COX-2 selective). However, with the introduction of more effective and safer products, aspirin usage has declined. Adverse events are primarily GI and are common. The frequency of GI toxicity increases as the dose increases. Buffered aspirin has been demonstrated to cause less GI irritation than plain aspirin when administered to dogs.[99] Aspirin also has antithromboxane effects and is used as an anticoagulant. A final possible area of concern is the use of one of the COX-1–sparing NSAIDs concurrently or immediately after administration of aspirin. Recently, lipoxin A_4 and its

---

BOX 10-1

Nonsteroidal Antiinflammatory Drug Selectivity

Nonselective
Acetaminophen
Aspirin
Etodolac (?)
Ketoprofen
Ketorolac
Naproxen

COX-2 Selective (COX-1 Sparing)
Carprofen
Deracoxib
Etodolac (?)
Firocoxib
Flunixin meglumine
Meloxicam
Piroxicam
Tolfenamic acid

Cyclooxygenase/Lipoxygenase Inhibitor
Tepoxalin

---

epimeric counterpart, aspirin-triggered lipoxin (ATL), have been shown to exert protective effects in the stomach. Lipoxins are potent antiinflammatory lipid mediators, and there are multiple synthesis pathways of these lipoxins. ATLs diminish gastric injury most likely via release of nitric oxide from the vascular endothelium. However, concurrent administration of COX-1–sparing (COX-2–selective; Box 10-1) drugs results in the complete inhibition of ATLs and causes significant exacerbation of gastric mucosal injuries. Therefore, dogs should not receive aspirin concurrently with COX-1–sparing NSAIDs, and owners must be informed of the potential risks of such concurrent therapy. One must remember that the formation of ATLs has yet to be proved in the dog. However, it is surprising to think that ATLs are not formed because they have been found in other species.[100-103]

Piroxicam.   Piroxicam is a member of the oxicam family of NSAIDs. In vitro data suggest that piroxicam is COX-2 selective in dogs.[14,104] However, in vivo data are not available to confirm these results. Piroxicam has an elimination half-life of approximately 40 hours in the dog.[105] Piroxicam has been used as an antineoplastic agent to treat transitional cell neoplasia in dogs. Although antineoplastic activity has been linked to COX-2 inhibitory activity, other factors may also play a role in the antineoplastic activity of piroxicam. Based on clinical response and this long elimination half-life, once daily or once every other day dosing has been successfully used in the dog. Piroxicam has been administered at a dose of 0.3 mg/kg orally once daily for many

---

BOX 10-2
Key Points to Minimize Adverse Reactions
Every effort should be made to prevent rather than treat the adverse reactions associated with use of nonsteroidal antiinflammatory drugs. Chronic use is often necessary; the goal should be to decrease the dose after 10-14 days to the minimum amount of drug necessary to maintain the now improved patient function. Concurrent use of other nonsteroidal antiinflammatory drugs or corticosteriods provides no additional therapeutic benefit but does increase the potential for adverse reactions. As the patient ages or the addition of medications for nonrelated problems increases, so the monitoring for potential problems should increase.

months for the treatment of canine transitional cell neoplasia. At this dose, approximately 18% of patients demonstrated adverse GI signs.[106] Gastroendoscopic evaluation of healthy dogs given piroxicam at a dose of 0.3 mg/kg orally once daily for 28 days failed to demonstrate a difference in gastroduodenal lesion development between treated and control dogs.[107] Additional data are needed before sweeping recommendations on use in pain management can be made. Pharmacokinetic data are available in cats given single and multiple doses of piroxicam. However, until efficacy and long-term safety studies are completed in cats, piroxicam cannot be recommended.[108,109]

POTENTIAL SIDE EFFECTS

See Box 10-2.

Gastrointestinal

See Boxes 10-3 and 10-4.

The most common problems associated with NSAID administration in dogs and cats involves the GI tract. Some of the GI toxicities associated with NSAID use are believed to be due to inhibition of endogenous prostaglandins. Signs may range from vomiting and diarrhea, including hematemesis and melena, to a silent ulcer that results in perforation. Realistically, the true overall incidence of GI toxicity in dogs or cats treated with NSAIDS is unknown. Concurrent administration of other medications (especially other NSAIDs or corticosteriods), previous GI bleeding, or the presence of other systemic diseases may contribute to adverse reactions.* The effect aging has on an individual patient's ability to metabolize NSAIDs is likely to be variable. However, given the potential

---

*References 19, 29, 50, 60, 65, 110, 111.

BOX 10-3

Toxicity of Nonsteroidal Antiinflammatory Drugs

Gastrointestinal Toxicity

Clinical Signs
Abdominal tensing
Darkened stools (melena)
Depression
Diarrhea
Hematochezia
Inappetence or anorexia
Lethargy
Nausea
Vomiting

Laboratory Findings
Decreased hematocrit and total protein
Elevated leukocyte count
Increased blood urea nitrogen (BUN)
    caused by gastrointestinal
    hemorrhage

Nephrotoxicity

Clinical Signs
Oliguria or anuria
Polyuria and polydipsia
Vomiting and anorexia (as a result of
    uremic toxin production)
Other signs of chronic or acute renal
    failure

Laboratory Findings
Cast formation
Decreased urine specific gravity
Increased BUN and creatinine
Proteinuria

Hepatotoxicity

Clinical Signs
Hepatic encephalopathy
Icterus
Lethargy
Anorexia
Vomiting
Weight loss

Laboratory Findings
Increased bile acids
Increased alanine aminotransferase
Increased alkaline phosphatase
Increased aspartate aminotransferase
Possible hyperbilirubinemia
Possible hypoalbuminemia

Gastrointestinal Bleeding

Consequences of Bleeding
Dyspnea
Excessive bleeding during minor surgical
    procedures
Lethargy
Pale mucous membranes
Prolonged bleeding at venipuncture sites

---

toxicity of NSAIDs, for these patients it is appropriate initially to dose at the low end of the recommended range and to assess the response critically.[111] Various gastroprotectant strategies should be considered when NSAIDS are prescribed for chronic use (Table 10-2).

Hepatic

See Box 10-3.

Hepatotoxicosis caused by NSAIDs is generally considered to be idiosyncratic. Administration of carprofen has been associated with an idiosyncratic cytotoxic hepatocellular reaction.[54] Anorexia, vomiting, and icterus along with increased hepatic enzyme levels have been seen. The onset of signs was seen by 21 days in the vast majority of dogs but ranged from 3 to 180 days of carprofen administration. Most dogs recovered

BOX 10-4

Gastrointestinal Effects of Nonsteroidal Antiinflammatory Drugs

PGD_2, PGE_2, PGF_{2a}
↓↓
↓Mucin
↓Neutral mucosal pH
↓Bicarbonate
↓Blood flow
↑Leukocyte adherence
↑Intestinal permeability
Gastric hypermotility
Uncoupling of enterocyte
Mitochondrial oxidative phosphorylation
↓↓
Gastrointestinal erosions and ulcers
Bleeding and perforation

*PG, Prostaglandin.

with cessation of treatment and supportive care. However, other NSAIDs can induce the same problems, and liver function must be monitored with the use of all NSAIDs. Because NSAIDS are metabolized by the liver, they should not be used in animals with liver failure.

Renal

See Box 10-3.

Renal dysfunction may occur with NSAID administration as a consequence of prostaglandin inhibition (Fig. 10-3). Renal prostaglandin synthesis is very low under normovolemic conditions. When normovolemia is challenged, prostaglandin synthesis is increased and functions to maintain renal perfusion.[19,111] NSAID use must be considered carefully in hypovolemic animals. This is especially important to remember with the increasing use of NSAIDs perioperatively for pain management. It must be noted that the COX-1–sparing NSAIDs do not infer greater safety in the kidney.

Cartilage

NSAIDs are used frequently and often chronically in osteoarthritic patients. Studies have demonstrated a variety of effects on proteoglycan synthesis when chondrocytes or cartilage explants are incubated with an NSAID in vitro. The most pronounced effects have been seen in chondrocytes from OA joints, although a lesser effect has been demonstrated on normal cartilage. Aspirin is uniformly reported to cause

TABLE 10-2	Doses of Drugs Used for Treatment of NSAID Toxicity in Dogs and Cats	
Drug	**Dose**	**Recommendations**
H₂ RECEPTOR BLOCKER		
Famotidine	0.5 mg/kg q12-24h PO, SC, IM, or IV	Decrease dose in renal failure
Nizatidine	2.5-5.0 mg/kg q24h PO	
MUCOSAL PROTECTANT		
Sucralfate	Dogs: 0.5-1.0 g per dog q8-12h PO Cats: 0.25 g per cat q8-12h PO	If coadministering antibiotics, separate administration by at least 2 hours. If coadministering antacids, administer antacid at least 30 minutes after sucralfate administration. Use cautiously in renal failure. Side effect: constipation
Omeprazole	Dogs: 0.5-1.0 mg/kg q24h PO Cats: 0.7 mg/kg q24h PO	Do not administer partial tablet or capsule unless dissolved in HCO₃.*
Pantoprazole	0.7-1.0 mg/kg q24h PO or IV	
PROSTAGLANDIN ANALOG		
Misoprostol	Dogs: 3-5 µg/kg q6h PO Cats: Not established	Side effects: diarrhea, abortion
PROMOTILITY AGENT		
Metoclopramide	0.2-0.4 mg/kg q8h 30 minutes before eating, PO, IM, or SC; or 1-2 mg/kg every 24 hours given in fluids CRI	Not for use in patients with mechanical gastrointestinal obstruction, GI hemorrhage, or epilepsy. Should not be used in combination with phenothiazines, butyrophenones, or narcotics. Decrease dose in renal failure. Physically incompatible when mixed with cephalothin sodium, sodium bicarbonate, chloramphenicol sodium succinate, or tetracycline. Side effects: anxiety, agitation, tremors, twitching, and constipation
FLUID THERAPY		
Administer fluids intravenously at a diuretic rate for at least 48 hours if potential renal toxicity dose has been ingested.		
HEPATOTHERAPY		
Discontinue NSAID and begin intravenous fluid administration; administer vitamin K₁ (1-2 mg/kg PO), and control vomiting with metoclopramide (see dose above); administer S-adenosyl-L-methionine 18 mg/kg q24h PO for 1-3 months.		

*To prepare an oral suspension, dissolve 20-mg capsule or tablet in 10 ml 8.4% HCO₃ to make a 2 mg/ml solution; good for 7 days.

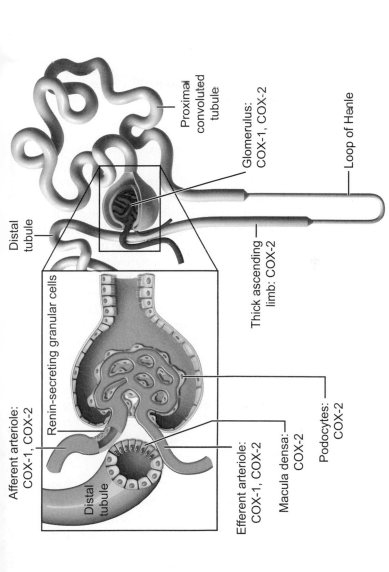

FIG. 10-3. Cyclooxygenase enzymes (COX-1, COX-2) are important regulators of renal blood flow and renal tubular function. Their inhibition by all currently available nonsteroidal antiinflammatory drugs can result in vasoconstriction of afferent and efferent blood vessels, glomerular dysfunction, and abnormal tubuloglomerular feedback, resulting in renal failure.

inhibition of proteoglycan synthesis, whereas conflicting data exist for other NSAIDs, such as etodolac, showing potential negative and positive effects; and there is a final group including meloxicam, piroxicam, and carprofen in which no effect or even some increased synthesis of proteoglycan has been noted.[112-119] The significance of these in vitro findings remains unclear, and there is now experimental data suggesting that NSAIDs and dual inhibitors can slow the progression of OA in vivo; however, the clinical significance of this data in the clinical setting with naturally occurring disease is unknown.[120-123]

Bone Healing

Pain management is an important component of the care of fracture patients. Interestingly and importantly, prostaglandins also play an important role in bone repair and normal bone homeostasis. Experimental studies support the hypothesis that nonspecific and specific COX inhibitors (COX-1 sparing) do impair bone healing. With the nonspecific NSAIDs the effects appear to be time and dose dependent. Whether COX-1–sparing drugs have the same effects on fracture healing, spinal fusions, and bone ingrowth remains controversial, but recent data support the effects of COX-1–sparing drugs also as dose and time dependent and as reversible. These statements are based on rabbit, rat, and mouse induced fracture models that show that COX-1–sparing agents alter bone healing. However, the most recent data confirm that following cessation of NSAIDs, fracture healing returns to its normal rate, and thus judicious use of postoperative NSAIDs can be recommended. Said another way, any potential adverse effects must be weighed against potential benefits that include improved analgesia and earlier return to function (mobilization of the limb/patient and weight bearing), and data support use of NSAIDs in the immediate postoperative period as long as it is not administered continuous for several weeks.[124-133]

Cardiovascular

Nonselective NSAIDs inhibit the platelet COX-1 enzyme and cause a significant decrease in the amount of thromboxane A_2 produced by clotting platelets. Thromboxane is an important activator of platelet aggregation[134] and is released by activated platelets to encourage further platelet recruitment to the site of vessel injury. Thromboxane is also a potent vasoconstrictor. A decrease in thromboxane release can result in prolongations of primary hemostasis. COX-1–sparing (COX-2 selective inhibitor) drugs do not have this effect on thromboxane production or primary hemostasis.[135] The actions of thromboxane are balanced at the vessel level by the presence of prostacyclin (PGI_2), which is produced by

COX enzymes in the vascular endothelial cells. PGI_2 is a strong inhibitor of platelet aggregation and also results in vasodilation. In the presence of endothelial inflammation (such as that caused by atherosclerotic plaques), the expression of COX-2 in the endothelial cells increases and may produce the majority of PGI_2 in that area.[136] When COX-nonselective NSAIDs are administered, the expression of thromboxane from platelets and PGI_2 from endothelial cells is decreased, preserving the balance. In certain circumstances of endothelial inflammation (e.g., with atherosclerosis), specific COX-2 inhibitors may decrease the endothelial production of PGI_2 (mainly from COX-2) without a concomitant decrease in platelet thromboxane (produced only by COX-1) and consequently may result in the development of a hypercoagulable state.[136]

REFERENCES

1. Scarpinganto C: Nonsteroidal anti-inflammatory drugs: how do they damage gastroduodenal mucosa, *Dig Dis* 13:9S-39S, 1995.
2. Humber LG: On the classification of NSAIDs, *Drug News & Perspectives* pp102-103, 1992.
3. Wolfe MM, Lichtenstein DR, Singh G: Gastrointestinal toxicity of nonsteroidal antiinflammatory drugs, *N Engl J Med* 340:1888-1898, 1999.
4. Vane JR: Inhibition of prostaglandin synthesis as a possible mechanism of action of aspirin like drugs, *Nature* 231:232-235, 1971.
5. Smith JB, Willis AL: Aspirin selectively inhibits prostaglandin production in human platelets, *Nature* 231:235-237, 1971.
6. Livingston A: Mechanism of action of nonsteroidal antiinflammatory drugs, *Vet Clin North Am Small Anim Pract* 30:773-781, 2000.
7. Patrignani P: Nonsteroidal antiinflammatory drugs, COX-2 and colorectal cancer, *Toxicol Lett* 112-113:493-498, 2000.
8. Jones CJ, Budsberg SC: Physiologic characteristics and clinical importance of the cyclooxygenase isoforms in dogs and cats, *J Am Vet Med Assoc* 217:721-729, 2000.
9. Crofford LJ, Wilder RL, Ristimaki AP et al: Cyclooxygenase-1 and -2 expression in rheumatoid synovial tissues: effects of interleukin-1β, phorbol ester, and corticosteroids, *J Clin Invest* 93:1095-1101, 1994.
10. Smith TJ: Cyclooxygenases as the principal targets for the action of NSAIDs, *Rheum Dis Clin North Am* 24:501-521, 1998.
11. Masferrer JL, Isakson PC, Seibert K: Cyclooxygenase-2 inhibitors: a new class of anti-inflammatory agents that spare the gastrointestinal tract, *Gastroenterol Clin North Am* 25:363-372, 1996.
12. Vane JR, Bakhle YS, Botting RM: Cyclooxygenases 1 and 2, *Annu Rev Pharmacol Toxicol* 38:97-120, 1998.
13. Jones CJ, Streppa HK, Budsberg SC: In vivo effect of a COX-2 selective and nonselective nonsteroidal anti-inflammatory drug (NSAID) on gastric mucosal and synovial fluid prostaglandin synthesis in dogs, *J Vet Intern Med* 15:273, 2001.

14. Streppa HK, Jones CJ, Budsberg SC: Differential biochemical inhibition of specific cyclooxygenases by various non-steroidal anti-inflammatory agents in canine whole blood, *Am J Vet Res* 63:91-94, 2002.

15. Cryer B, Feldman M: Cyclooxygenase-1 and cyclooxygenase-2 selectivity of widely used nonsteroidal anti-inflammatory drugs, *Am J Med* 104: 413-421, 1998.

16. Brideau C, Kargaman S, Liu S et al: A human whole blood assay for clinical evaluation of biochemical efficacy of cyclooxygenase inhibitors, *Inflamm Res* 45:68-74, 1996.

17. Sessions JK, Agnello KA, Reynolds LR, Budsberg SC: In vivo effects of carprofen, deracoxib, and etodolac on whole blood, gastric mucosal and synovial fluid prostaglandin synthesis in dogs with osteoarthritis, *Am J Vet Res* 66:812-817, 2005.

18. Agnello KA, Reynolds LR, Budsberg SC: In vivo effects of tepoxalin, a dual COX/LOX inhibitor, on prostanoid and leukotriene production in dogs with osteoarthritis, *Am J Vet Res* 66:966-972, 2005.

19. Bergh MS, Budsberg SC: The coxib NSAIDs: potential clinical and pharmacological importance in veterinary medicine, *J Vet Intern Med* 19:633-643, 2005.

20. Stock JL, Shinjo K, Burkhardt J et al: The prostaglandin E2 EP1 receptor mediates pain perception and regulates blood pressure, *J Clin Invest* 107:325-331, 2001.

21. Zhang Y, Shaffer A, Portanova J et al: Inhibition of cyclooxygenase-2 rapidly reverses inflammatory hyperalgesia and prostaglandin E2 production, *J Pharmacol Exp Ther* 283:1069-1075, 1997.

22. Vanegas H, Schaible HG: Prostaglandins and cyclooxygenases [correction of cycloxygenases] in the spinal cord, *Prog Neurobiol* 64:327-363, 2001.

23. Watkins LR, Hutchinson MR, Ledeboer A et al: Glia as the "bad guys": implications for improving clinical pain control and the clinical utility of opioids, *Brain Behav Immun* 21:131-146, 2007.

24. Beiche F, Scheuerer S, Brune K et al: Up-regulation of cyclooxygenase-2 mRNA in the rat spinal cord following peripheral inflammation, *FEBS Lett* 390:165-169, 1996.

25. Goppelt-Struebe M, Beiche F: Cyclooxygenase-2 in the spinal cord: localization and regulation after a peripheral inflammatory stimulus, *Adv Exp Med Biol* 433:213-216, 1997.

26. Willingale HL, Gardiner NJ, McLymont N et al: Prostanoids synthesized by cyclo-oxygenase isoforms in rat spinal cord and their contribution to the development of neuronal hyperexcitability, *Br J Pharmacol* 122:1593-1604, 1997.

27. Yamagata K, Andreasson KI, Kaufmann WE et al: Expression of a mitogen-inducible cyclooxygenase in brain neurons: regulation by synaptic activity and glucocorticoids, *Neuron* 11:371-386, 1993.

28. Kaufmann WE, Worley PF, Taylor CV et al: Cyclooxygenase-2 expression during rat neocortical development and in Rett syndrome, *Brain Dev* 19:25-34, 1997.

29. Mathews KA: Nonsteroidal antiinflammatory analgesics, *Vet Clin North Am Small Anim Pract* 30:783-804, 2000.

30. Warner TD, Mitchell JA: Cyclooxygenase-3 (COX-3): filling in the gaps toward a COX continuum? *Proc Natl Acad Sci U S A* 99:13371-13373, 2002.

31. Brandt KD, Bradley JD: Should the initial drug used to treat osteoarthritis pain be a nonsteroidal anti-inflammatory drug? *J Rheumatol* 28:467-473, 2001.

32. Fox SM, Johnston SA: Use of carprofen for the treatment of pain and inflammation in dogs, *J Am Vet Med Assoc* 210:1493-1498, 1997.

33. McKellar QA, Pearson T, Gogan JA et al: Pharmacokinetics, tolerance and serum thromboxane inhibition of carprofen in the dog, *J Small Anim Pract* 31:443-448, 1999.

34. Kay-Mugford P, Benn SJ, Lamarre J et al: In vitro effects of nonsteroidal antiinflammatory drugs on cyclooxygenases activity in dogs, *Am J Vet Res* 61:802-810, 2000.

35. Ricketts AP, Lundy KM, Seibel SB: Evaluation of selective inhibition of canine cyclooxygenases 1 and 2 by carprofen and other nonsteroidal anti-inflammatory drugs, *Am J Vet Res* 59:1441-1446, 1998.

36. Vasseur PB, Johnson AL, Budsberg SC et al: Randomized, controlled trial of the efficacy of carprofen, a nonsteroidal antiinflammatory drug, in the treatment of osteoarthritis in dogs, *J Am Vet Med Assoc* 206:807-811, 1995.

37. Holtsinger RH, Parker RB, Beale BS et al: The therapeutic efficacy of carprofen in 209 clinical cases of canine degenerative joint disease, *Vet Comp Orthop Traumatol* 5:140-144, 1992.

38. Moreau M, Dubuis J, Bonneau NH et al: Clinical evaluation of a nutraceutical, carprofen and meloxicam for the treatment of dogs with osteoarthritis, *Vet Rec* 152:323-329, 2003.

39. Pollmeier M, Toulemonde C, Fleishman C et al: Clinical evaluation of firocoxib and carprofen for the treatment of dogs with osteoarthritis, *Vet Rec* 159:547-551, 2006.

40. Grisneaux E, Pibarot P, Dupuis J et al: Comparison of ketoprofen and carprofen administered prior to orthopedic surgery for control of postoperative pain in dogs, *J Am Vet Med Assoc* 215:1105-1110, 1999.

41. Balmer TV, Irvine D, Jones RS et al: Comparison of carprofen and pethidine as postoperative analgesics in the cat, *J Small Anim Pract* 39:158-164, 1998.

42. Lascelles BDX, Cripps PJ, Jones A et al: Efficacy and kinetics of carprofen, administered preoperatively or postoperatively, for the prevention of pain in dogs undergoing ovariohysterectomy, *Vet Surg* 27:568-582, 1998.

43. Nolan R, Reid J: Comparison of the postoperative analgesic and sedative effects of carprofen and papaveretum in the dog, *Vet Rec* 133:240-242, 1993.

44. Lascelles BDX, Butterworth SJ, Waterman AE: Postoperative analgesic and sedative effects of carprofen and pethidine in dogs, *Vet Rec* 134:187-191, 1994.

45. Leece EA, Brearley LC, Harding EF: Comparison of carprofen and meloxicam for 72 hours following ovariohysterectomy in dogs, *Vet Anaesth Analg* 32:184-192, 2005.

46. Horstman CL, Conzemius MG, Evans R et al: Assessing the efficacy of perioperative oral carprofen after cranial cruciate surgery using noninvasive, objective pressure platform gait analysis, *Vet Surg* 33:286-292, 2004.

47. Hickford FH, Barr SC, Erb HN: Effect of carprofen on hemostatic variables in dogs, *Am J Vet Res* 62:1642-1645, 2001.

48. Bergmann HML, Nolte IJA, Kramer S: Effects of preoperative administration of carprofen on renal function and hemostasis in dogs undergoing surgery for fracture repair, *Am J Vet Res* 66:1356-1363, 2005.

49. Raekallio MR, Hielm-Bjorkman AK, Kejonen J et al: Evaluation of adverse effects of long-term orally administered carprofen in dogs, *J Am Vet Med Assoc* 228:876-880, 2006.

50. Hodge TM, Wahlstrom T: Three years (1997-1999) of US clinical experience with Rimadyl® (carprofen), *Technical Bulletin Dec* 2000.

51. Forsyth SF, Guilford WG, Pfeiffer DU: Effect of NSAID administration on creatinine clearance in healthy dogs undergoing surgery for fracture repair, *J Small Anim Pract* 41:547-550, 2000.

52. Crandel DE, Mathews KA, Dyson DH: Effect of meloxicam and carprofen on renal function when administered to healthy dogs prior to anesthesia and painful stimulation, *Am J Vet Res* 65:1384-1390, 2004.

53. Lobetti RG, Joubert KE: Effect of administration of nonsteroidal anti-inflammatory drugs before surgery on renal function in clinically normal dogs, *Am J Vet Res* 61:1501-1507, 2000.

54. MacPhail CM, Lappin MR, Meyer DJ et al: Hepatocellular toxicosis associated with administration of carprofen in 21 dogs, *J Am Vet Med Assoc* 212:1895-1901, 1998.

55. Lascelles BDX, Cripps P, Mirchandani S et al: Carprofen as an analgesic for postoperative pain in cats: dose titration and assessment of efficacy in comparison to pethidine hydrochloride, *J Small Anim Pract* 36:535-541, 1995.

56. Balmer TV, Irvine D, Jones RS et al: Comparison of carprofen and pethidine as postoperative analgesics in the cat, *J Small Anim Pract* 39:158-164, 1998.

57. Slingsby LS, Waterman-Pearson AE: Postoperative analgesia in the cat after ovariohysterectomy by use of carprofen, ketoprofen, meloxicam or tolfenamic acid, *J Small Anim Pract* 41:447-450, 2000.

58. Slingsby LS, Waterman-Pearson AE: Comparison between meloxicam and carprofen for postoperative analgesia after feline ovariohysterectomy, *J Small Anim Pract* 43:286-289, 2002.

59. Al-Gizawiy MM, Rude PE: Comparison of preoperative carprofen and postoperative butorphanol as postsurgical analgesics in cats undergoing ovariohysterectomy, *Vet Anaesth Analg* 31:164-174, 2004.

60. Runk A, Kyles AE, Downs MO: Duodenal perforation in a cat following the administration of nonsteroidal anti-inflammatory medication, *J Am Anim Hosp Assoc* 35:52-55, 1999.

61. McCann ME, Anderson DR, Zhang D et al: In vitro effects and in vivo efficacy of a novel cyclooxygenase-2 inhibitor in dogs with experimentally induced synovitis, *Am J Vet Res* 65:503-512, 2004.

62. Millis DL, Buonomo FC: Effect of deracoxib, a new COX-2 inhibitor, on perioperative analgesia in a stifle arthrotomy cranial cruciate ligament stabilization model in dogs, *Vet Surg* 30:502, 2001.

63. Millis DL, Conzemius MG, Wells KL et al: A multi-center clinical study on the effects of deracoxib, a COX-2 selective drug, on post-operative analgesia associated with cranial cruciate ligament stabilization in dogs, *Vet Surg* 30:502, 2001.

64. Johnston SA, Conzemius MG, Cross AR et al: A multi-center clinical study of the effects of deracoxib, a COX-2 selective drug, on chronic pain in dogs with osteoarthritis, *Vet Surg* 30:497, 2001.

65. Lascelles BD, Blikslager AT, Fox SM et al: Gastrointestinal tract perforation in dogs treated with a selective cyclooxygenase-2 inhibitor: 29 cases (2002-2003), *J Am Vet Med Assoc* 227:1112-1117, 2005.

66. Gassel AD, Tobias KM, Cox SK: Disposition of deracoxib in cats after oral administration, *J Am Anim Hosp Assoc* 42(3):212-217, 2006.

67. Budsberg SC, Johnston SA, Schwarz PD et al: Evaluation of etodolac for the treatment of osteoarthritis of the hips in dogs: a prospective multicenter study, *J Am Vet Med Assoc* 214:1-5, 1999.

68. Hanson PD, Brooks KC, Case J et al: Efficacy and safety of firocoxib in the management of canine osteoarthritis under field conditions, *Vet Ther* 7:127-140, 2006.

69. Gordon WJ, Conzemius MG, Drag M et al: Assessment of the efficacy of firocoxib and etodolac for the treatment of osteoarthritis in dogs, *Vet Surg* 33:E9, 2004.

70. Sumi N, Uchimoto H, Fujimoto S et al: Three-month oral toxicity of etodolac in dogs followed by one-month recovery test, *Oyo Yakuri/Pharmacometrics* 40:515-560, 1990.

71. Wrenn JM, Inhelder JL, Hemm RD et al: One year chronic toxicity study of etodolac, a nonsteroidal anti-inflammatory agent, in the beagle dog, *Oyo Yakuri/Pharmacometrics* 40:599-646, 1990.

72. Hampshire VA, Doddy FM, Post LO et al: Adverse drug event reports at the United States FDA Center for Veterinary Medicine, *J Am Vet Med Assoc* 225:533-536, 2004.

73. McCann ME, Andersen DR, Zhang D et al: In vitro effects and in vivo efficacy of a novel cyclooxygenase-2 inhibitor in dogs with experimentally induced synovitis, *Am J Vet Res* 65:503-512, 2004.

74. Ryan WG, Moldave K, Carithers D: Clinical effectiveness and safety of a new NSAID, firocoxib: a 1000 dog study, *Vet Ther* 7:119-126, 2006.

75. Sigurdsson GH, Youssef H: Amelioration of respiratory and circulatory changes in established endotoxic shock by ketoprofen, *Acta Anesthesiol Scand* 38:33-39, 1994.

76. Pibarot P, Dupuis J, Grisneaux E et al: Comparison of ketoprofen, oxymorphone hydrochloride, and butorphanol in the treatment of postoperative pain in dogs, *J Am Vet Med Assoc* 211:438-444, 1997.

77. Hazewinkel HA, van den Brom WE, Pollmeier M et al: Reduced dosage of ketoprofen for the short-term and long-term treatment of joint pain in dogs, *Vet Rec* 152:11-14, 2003.

78. Brideau C, Van Staden C, Chan CC: In vitro effects of cyclooxygenase inhibitors in whole blood of horses, dogs, and cats, *Am J Vet Res* 62:1755-1760, 2001.

79. Agnello KA, Reynolds LR, Budsberg SC: In vivo effects of tepoxalin, an inhibitor of cyclooxygenase and lipoxygenase, on prostanoid and leukotriene production in dogs with chronic osteoarthritis, *Am J Vet Res* 66:966-972, 2005.

80. Doig PA, Purbrick KA, Hare JE et al: Clinical efficacy and tolerance of meloxicam in dogs with chronic osteoarthritis, *Can Vet J* 41:296-300, 2000.

81. Nell T, Bergman J, Hoeijmakers M et al: Comparison of vedaprofen and meloxicam in dogs with musculoskeletal pain and inflammation, *J Small Anim Pract* 43:208-212, 2002.

82. Peterson KD, Keefe TJ: Effects of meloxicam on severity of lameness and other clinical signs of osteoarthritis in dogs, *J Am Vet Med Assoc* 225:1056-1060, 2004.

83. Budsberg SC, Cross AR, Quandt JE et al: Evaluation of intravenous administration of meloxicam for perioperative pain management following stifle joint surgery in dogs, *Am J Vet Res* 63:1557-1563, 2002.

84. Fowler D, Isakow K, Caulkett N et al: An evaluation of the analgesic effects of meloxicam in addition to epidural morphine/mepivacaine in dogs undergoing cranial cruciate ligament repair, *Can Vet J* 44:643-648, 2003.

85. Lafuente MP, Franch J, Durall I et al: Comparison between meloxicam and transdermally administered fentanyl for treatment of postoperative pain in dogs undergoing osteotomy of the tibia and fibula and placement of a uniplanar external distraction device, *J Am Vet Med Assoc* 227:1768-1774, 2005.

86. Caulkett N, Read M, Fowler D et al: A comparison of the analgesic effects of butorphanol with those of meloxicam after elective ovariohysterectomy in dogs, *Can Vet J* 44:565-570, 2003.

87. Mathews KA, Pettifer G, Foster R et al: Safety and efficacy of preoperative administration of meloxicam, compared with that of ketoprofen and butorphanol in dogs undergoing abdominal surgery, *Am J Vet Res* 62:882-888, 2001.

88. Laredo FG, Belda E, Murciano J et al: Comparison of the analgesic effects of meloxicam and carprofen administered preoperatively to dogs undergoing orthopaedic surgery, *Vet Rec* 155:667-671, 2004.

89. Kazakos GM, Papazoglou LG, Rallis T et al: Effects of meloxicam on the haemostatic profile of dogs undergoing orthopaedic surgery, *Vet Rec* 157:444-446, 2005.

90. Fresno L, Moll J, Penalba B et al: Effects of preoperative administration of meloxicam on whole blood platelet aggregation, buccal mucosal bleeding time, and haematological indices in dogs undergoing elective ovariohysterectomy, *Vet J* 170:138-140, 2005.

91. Duerr FM, Carr AP, Bebchuk TN et al: Challenging diagnosis—icterus associated with a single perforating duodenal ulcer after long-term nonsteroidal antiinflammatory drug administration in a dog, *Can Vet J* 45:507-510, 2004.

92. Reed S: Nonsteroidal anti-inflammatory drug-induced duodenal ulceration and perforation in a mature rottweiler, *Can Vet J* 43:971-972, 2002.

93. Carroll GL, Howe LB, Peterson KD: Analgesic efficacy of preoperative administration of meloxicam or butorphanol in onychectomized cats, *J Am Vet Med Assoc* 226:913-919, 2005.

94. Gassel AD, Tobias KM, Egger CM et al: Comparison of oral and subcutaneous administration of buprenorphine and meloxicam for preemptive analgesia in cats undergoing ovariohysterectomy, *J Am Vet Med Assoc* 227:1937-1944, 2005.

95. Argentieri DC, Ritchie DM, Ferro MP et al: Tepoxalin: a dual cyclooxygenase/5-lipoxygenase inhibitor of arachidonic acid metabolism with potent anti-inflammatory activity and a favorable gastrointestinal profile, *J Pharmacol Exp Ther* 271:1399-1408, 1994.

96. Kay-Mugford PA, Grimm KA, Weingarten AJ et al: Effect of preoperative administration of tepoxalin on hemostasis and hepatic and renal function in dogs, *Vet Ther* 5:120-127, 2004.

97. Fusellier M, Desfontis JC, Madec S et al: Effect of tepoxalin on renal function in healthy dogs receiving an angiotensin-converting enzyme inhibitor, *J Vet Pharmacol Ther* 28:581-586, 2005.

98. Charette B, Dupuis J, Moreau M et al: Assessing the efficacy of long-term administration of tolfenamic acid in dogs undergoing femoral head and neck excision, *Vet Comp Orthop Traumatol* 16:232-237, 2003.

99. Lipowitz A, Boulay J, Klausner J: Serum salicylate concentrations and endoscopic evaluation of the gastric mucosa in dogs after oral administration of aspirin-containing products, *Am J Vet Res* 47:1586-1589, 1986.

100. Wallace JL, de Lima OM Jr, Fiorucci S: Lipoxins in gastric mucosal health and disease, *Prostaglandins Leukot Essent Fatty Acids* 73:251-255, 2005.

101. Wallace JL, Zamuner SR, McKnight W et al: Aspirin, but not NO-releasing aspirin (NCX-4016), interacts with selective COX-2 inhibitors to aggravate gastric damage and inflammation, *Am J Physiol Gastrointest Liver Physiol* 286:G76-G81, 2004.

102. Souza MH, de Lima OM Jr, Zamuner SR et al: Gastritis increases resistance to aspirin-induced mucosal injury via COX-2-mediated lipoxin synthesis, *Am J Physiol Gastrointest Liver Physiol* 285:G54-G61, 2003 (Epub 2003 Mar 13).

103. Fiorucci S, de Lima OM Jr, Mencarelli A et al: Cyclooxygenase-2-derived lipoxin A4 increases gastric resistance to aspirin-induced damage, *Gastroenterology* 123:1598-1606, 2002.

104. Wilson JE, Chandrasekharan NV, Westover KD et al: Determination of expression of cyclooxygenase-1 and -2 isozymes in canine tissues and their differential sensitivity to nonsteroidal anti-inflammatory drugs, *Am J Vet Res* 65:810-818, 2004.

105. Galbraith EA, McKellar QA: Pharmacokinetics and pharmacodynamics of piroxicam in dogs, *Vet Rec* 128:561-565, 1991.

106. Knapp DW, Richardson RC, Chan TC et al: Piroxicam therapy in 34 dogs with transitional cell carcinoma of the urinary bladder, *J Vet Intern Med* 8:273-276, 1994.

107. Johnston SA: Personal communication, 1998.

108. Heeb HL, Chun R, Koch DE et al: Multiple dose pharmacokinetics and acute safety of piroxicam and cimetidine in the cat, *J Vet Pharmacol Ther* 28:447-452, 2005.

109. Heeb HL, Chun R, Koch DE et al: Single dose pharmacokinetics of piroxicam in cats, *J Vet Pharmacol Ther* 26:259-263, 2003.
110. Boston SE, Moens NM, Kruth SA et al: Endoscopic evaluation of the gastroduodenal mucosa to determine the safety of short-term concurrent administration of meloxicam and dexamethasone in healthy dogs, *Am J Vet Res* 64:1369-1375, 2003.
111. Johnston SA, Budsberg SC: Nonsteroidal antiinflammatory drugs and corticosteriods for the management of canine osteoarthritis, *Vet Clin North Am Small Anim Pract* 27:841-862, 1997.
112. Rainsford KD, Ying C, Smith FC: Effects of meloxicam, compared with other NSAIDs, on cartilage proteoglycan metabolism, synovial prostaglandin E2, and production of interleukins 1, 6 and 8, in human and porcine explants in organ culture, *J Pharm Pharmacol* 49:991-998, 1997.
113. Henrotin Y, Bassleer C, Reginster JY, Franchimont P: Effects of etodolac on human chondrocytes cultivated in three dimensional culture, *Clin Rheumatol* 8:36-42, 1989.
114. Redini F, Mauviel A, Loyau G et al: Modulation of extracellular matrix metabolism in rabbit articular chondrocytes and human rheumatoid synovial cell by the non-steroidal antiinflammatory drug etodolac. II. Glycosaminoglycan synthesis, *Agents Actions* 31:358-367, 1990.
115. Benton HP, Vasseur PB, Broderick-Villa GA et al: Effect of carprofen on sulfated glycosaminoglycan metabolism, protein synthesis, and prostaglandin release by cultured osteoarthritic canine chondrocytes, *Am J Vet Res* 58:286-292, 1997.
116. Ghosh P: Nonsteroidal anti-inflammatory drugs and chondroprotection, *Drugs* 46:834-846, 1993.
117. Wilbrink B, Van derVeen MJ, Huber J et al: In vitro influence of ketoprofen on the proteoglycan metabolism of human normal and osteoarthritis cartilage, *Agents Actions* 32:154-159, 1991.
118. Collier S, Ghosh P: Comparison of the effects of non-steroidal anti-inflammatory drugs (NSAIDs) on proteoglycan synthesis by articular cartilage explant and chondrocyte monolayer cultures, *Biochem Pharmacol* 41:1375-1385, 1991.
119. Dvorak LD, Cook JL, Kreeger JM et al: Effects of carprofen and dexamethasone on canine chondrocytes in a three-dimensional culture model of osteoarthritis, *Am J Vet Res* 63:1363-1369, 2002.
120. Mastbergen SC, Marijnissen AC, Vianen ME et al: Inhibition of COX-2 by celecoxib in the canine groove model of osteoarthritis, *Rheumatology* 45:405-413, 2006.
121. Pelletier JP, Boileau C, Boily M et al: The protective effect of licofelone on experimental osteoarthritis is correlated with the downregulation of gene expression and protein synthesis of several major cartilage catabolic factors: MMP-13, cathepsin K and aggrecanases, *Arthritis Res Ther* 7:R1091-R1102, 2005 (Epub 2005 Jul 19).
122. Jovanovic DV, Fernandes JC, Martel-Pelletier J et al: In vivo dual inhibition of cyclooxygenase and lipoxygenase by ML-3000 reduces the progression of experimental osteoarthritis: suppression of collagenase 1 and interleukin-1beta synthesis, *Arthritis Rheum* 44:2320-2330, 2001.

123. Pelletier JP, Lajeunesse D, Jovanovic DV et al: Carprofen simultaneously reduces progression of morphological changes in cartilage and subchondral bone in experimental dog osteoarthritis, *J Rheumatol* 27:2893-2902, 2000.

124. Goodman SB, Ma T, Genovese M et al: COX-2 selective inhibitors and bone, *Int J Immunopathol Pharmacol* 16:201-205, 2003.

125. Harder AT, Yuehuei HA: The mechanisms of the inhibitory effects of nonsteroidal anti-inflammatory drugs on bone healing: a concise review, *J Clin Pharmacol* 43:807-815, 2003.

126. Seidenberg AB, Yuehuei HA: Is there an inhibitory effect of COX-2 inhibitors on bone healing? *Pharm Res* 50:151-156, 2004.

127. Goodman SB, Ma T, Mitsunaga I, et al: Temporal effects of a COX-2 selective NSAID on bone ingrowth, *J Biomed Mater Res* 72A:279-287, 2005.

128. Bergenstock M, Min W, Simon AM et al: A comparison between the effects of acetaminophen and celecoxib on bone fracture healing in rats, *J Orthop Trauma* 19:717-723, 2005.

129. Virdi AS, De Ranieri A, Sumner DR: Bone regeneration and implant fixation strength are not adversely influenced by COX-2 inhibition, *Trans 50th Ortho Society* p 455, 2004.

130. Gerstenfeld LC, Al-Ghawas M, Alkhiary YM, et al: Selective and non-selective cyclooxygenase-2 inhibitors and experimental fracture healing: reversibility of effects after short-term treatment, *J Bone Joint Surg* 89(1):114-125, 2007.

131. Gajraj NM: The effects of cyclooxygenase-2 inhibitors on bone healing, *Reg Anesth Pain Med* 28:456-465, 2005.

132. Macalena JA, Knight RQ, Mollner TJ et al: Selective COX-2 inhibition delays remodeling of primary bone, *Trans 50th Ortho Society* p 399, 2004.

133. Einhorn TA: The science of fracture healing, *J Orthop Trauma* 19:S4-S6, 2005.

134. Johnson GJ, Leis LA, Dunlop PC: Thromboxane-insensitive dog platelets have impaired activation of phospholipase C due to receptor-linked G protein dysfunction, *J Clin Invest* 92:2469-2479, 2003.

135. Brainard BM, Meredith CP, Callan MB et al: Changes in platelet function, hemostasis and prostaglandin expression after treatment with nonsteroidal anti-inflammatory drugs with various cyclooxygenase selectivities in dogs, *Am J Vet Res* 68(3):251-257, 2007.

136. Grosser T, Fries S, FitzGerald GA: Biological basis for the cardiovascular consequences of COX-2 inhibition: therapeutic challenges and opportunities, *J Clin Invest* 116:4-15, 2006.

11 α_2-AGONISTS

LEIGH LAMONT

The α_2-agonists are a group of sedative-analgesic drugs that exert their clinical effects by interacting with α_2-adrenergic receptors in the central nervous system. Although not considered first-line analgesics like opioids or nonsteroidal antiinflammatory drugs, α_2-agonists are commonly used as analgesic adjuvants. In contrast to other classes of drugs used to manage pain, α_2-agonists are distinguished by their significant cardiovascular side effects (Box 11-1).

HISTORICAL BACKGROUND

- ◆ 1962: Xylazine was synthesized in Germany for use as an antihypertensive agent in human beings; its sedative properties in animals were recognized soon afterward.
- ◆ Early 1970s: Xylazine and xylazine/ketamine combinations became popular for inducing sedation and general anesthesia in large animals; use in small animals soon followed.
- ◆ 1981: The sedative, analgesic, and muscle relaxant properties of xylazine were linked to stimulation of central α_2-adrenoceptors.[1]
- ◆ Late 1980s: New, more specific α_2-agonists (medetomidine, detomidine, and romifidine) were introduced; drug distribution and labeling vary widely from country to country.
- ◆ 1996: Medetomidine and its specific reversal agent, atipamezole, became available in the United States (labeled for use in dogs only); veterinarians began using α_2-agonists in lower doses, often in combination with opioids, as anesthetic and analgesic adjuvants.
- ◆ Currently, medetomidine is the most commonly used α_2-agonist for analgesia in small animal practice in North America; dexmedetomidine is used occasionally, whereas romifidine and xylazine are rarely used as analgesic adjuvants .

BOX 11-1

α_2-Agonists

Clonidine
Detomidine
Dexmedetomidine
Medetomidine
Romifidine
Xylazine

MOLECULAR PHARMACOLOGY OF α_2-ADRENOCEPTORS

α_2-ADRENOCEPTOR STRUCTURE

- All α_2-adrenoceptor proteins contain 415 to 480 amino acids.[2]
- Each protein contains seven transmembrane domains with segments of lipophilic amino acids separated by segments of hydrophilic amino acids; these form an extracellular amino terminus and an intracellular carboxyl terminus with three small extracellular loops and three intracellular loops

α_2-ADRENOCEPTOR SUBTYPES

- Three distinct α_2-adrenoceptor subtypes have been recognized: α_{2A}, α_{2B}, and α_{2C}.[3]
- A fourth subtype (α_{2D}) has been identified and represents the rodent homologue of the human α_{2A}-adrenoceptor.[4]
- The genes for the three human subtypes have been cloned and are designated α_2-C10, α_2-C2, and α_2-C4 for the α_{2A}, α_{2B}, and α_{2C} subtypes, respectively.[3]
- Related subtypes have been cloned in other species including rat, mouse, pig, opossum, and fish; partial complementary DNA sequences from bovine and avian α_{2A}-receptors have also been identified.
- All three α_2 subtype genes share a common evolutionary origin; several key structural and functional domains are well conserved despite only 50% protein homology at the amino acid level.
- Most currently available α_2-agonists bind with similar affinity to all three receptor subtypes.

TABLE 11-1	Expression and Distribution of α_2-Adrenoceptor Subtypes in Different Species	
	Brainstem	**Spinal Cord**
Rodents[6]	α_2A	α_2A, α_2C
Human beings[6]	α_2A	α_2A, α_2B
Dogs[7]	α_2A	Unknown

α_2-ADRENOCEPTOR EXPRESSION

◆ Expression is somewhat species-specific, resulting in varied physiological effects and pharmacologic activity profiles and making extrapolation of data among species difficult.[5]
◆ Distribution of α_2-adrenoceptor subtypes in several species is given in Table 11-1.

α_2-ADRENOCEPTOR SUBTYPE FUNCTIONAL SIGNIFICANCE

◆ All clinically relevant analgesic, sedative-hypnotic, and anesthetic-sparing responses appear to be mediated by the α_{2A} subtype.[6-9]
◆ Hypotensive and bradycardic actions are also mediated by the α_{2A} subtype.[10]
◆ Initial increase in systemic vascular resistance appears to be mediated by the α_{2B} subtype, with lesser contribution of the α_{2A} subtype in certain vascular compartments.[10]
◆ Hypothermic effects and modulation of dopaminergic activity are mediated by the α_{2C} subtype.[6]

IMIDAZOLINE RECEPTORS

◆ Clonidine and romifidine contain an imidazole moiety that binds to and activates a second class of non-noradrenergic receptors called imidazoline receptors.[11]
◆ Imidazoline receptors are involved in central control of vasomotor tone and are located in the nucleus reticularis lateralis of the ventrolateral region of the medulla.[11]
◆ Central hypotensive effects observed after administration of clonidine or romifidine result from activation of α_{2A}-adrenoceptors and imidazoline receptors.

SIGNAL TRANSDUCTION MECHANISMS OF α_2-ADRENOCEPTORS

♦ The process by which any transmembrane receptor notifies the cell of receptor occupancy by a ligand is called *signal transduction*.

♦ α_2-Adrenoceptors are part of a larger receptor superfamily including dopaminergic, cholinergic, and serotonergic receptor systems that are coupled to guanine nucleotide binding proteins (G proteins) that function in signal transduction.

♦ G proteins link cell membrane receptors to intracellular effector mechanisms, amplify the signal, and transduce external chemical stimuli into cellular responses.

♦ Binding of a specific ligand (neurotransmitter, endogenous hormone, or exogenous drug) induces a conformational change in the α_2-adrenoreceptor, which leads to activation of specific G proteins.[3]

♦ Activated G proteins then modulate the synthesis or availability of intracellular second messenger molecules or directly alter the activity of transmembrane ion channels.[3]

♦ Relevant α_2-adrenoceptor effector mechanisms include the following:
1. Increased potassium conductance leading to hyperpolarization of membrane ion channels and a decreased firing rate of excitable cells in the central nervous system (CNS)[3]
2. Inhibition of calcium influx through N-type voltage-gated calcium channels resulting in reduced fusion of synaptic vesicles with postsynaptic membranes and reduced neurotransmitter release[2]
3. Inhibition of the enzyme adenylate cyclase, resulting in decreased intracellular cyclic adenosine monophosphate accumulation and decreased phosphorylation of target regulatory proteins[12]

MECHANISM OF ANALGESIC ACTION

♦ α_2-Adrenoceptors within the CNS are found on noradrenergic and non-noradrenergic neurons.

♦ Noradrenergic α_2-adrenoceptors are called *autoreceptors* and are located at supraspinal sites.

♦ Non-noradrenergic α_2-adrenoceptors are called *heteroceptors* and are located in the dorsal horn of the spinal cord.[13,14]

♦ Both populations of receptors appear to be involved in α_2-agonist analgesia.

ANALGESIA MEDIATED AT THE LEVEL OF THE DORSAL HORN

- α_2-Heteroceptors are located presynaptically and postsynaptically on nociceptive neurons in the dorsal horn.
- Activation by norepinephrine or an exogenous α_2-agonist produces analgesia by one of two potential mechanisms:
  1. Presynaptic α_2-heteroceptors found on primary afferent C fibers bind the agonist. This causes a G protein–mediated decrease in calcium influx (see previous section), which results in decreased release of neurotransmitters/neuropeptides such as glutamate, vasoactive intestinal peptide, calcitonin gene-related peptide, substance P, and neurotensin.[15]
  2. Postsynaptic α_2-heteroceptors found on wide-dynamic-range projection neurons also bind the agonist. This produces neuronal hyperpolarization via G protein–coupled potassium channels (see previous section) and inhibits ascending nociceptive transmission.[15]

ANALGESIA MEDIATED AT THE LEVEL OF THE BRAINSTEM

- Traditionally, it has been accepted that α_2-agonist-induced analgesia results from activation of dorsal horn α_2-heteroceptors, whereas sedative-hypnotic effects are mediated by activation of supraspinal (brainstem) α_2-autoreceptors.
- It now appears that brainstem α_2-autoreceptors also contribute indirectly to analgesia.
- α_2-Autoreceptors are concentrated in three catecholaminergic nuclei in the pons: *A5*, *A6*, (also called the *locus ceruleus*), and *A7*.[16,17]
- The locus ceruleus (LC) is the most important of these, extending noradrenergic neurons to all segments of the spinal cord and modulating noradrenergic input from higher structures such as the periaqueductal gray matter (PAG) of the midbrain.
- Activation of α_2-autoreceptors in the LC by norepinephrine or an exogenous α_2-agonist results in neuronal inhibition and a decreased release of norepinephrine.
- Dampening of LC activity *disinhibits* activity in the adjacent cell bodies of A5 and A7 nuclei, resulting in increased release of norepinephrine from their terminals in the dorsal horn, which in turn activates spinal presynaptic and postsynaptic α_2-heteroceptors to produce analgesia.[16]
- Higher supraspinal structures may also play a role: the PAG of the midbrain extends noradrenergic innervation to the LC and

may lead to α_2-mediated decreases in LC norepinephrine release, which indirectly feeds back on spinal α_2-adrenoceptors to produce analgesia.[13]

CLINICAL PHARMACOLOGY OF α_2-AGONISTS

XYLAZINE

+ Xylazine is the prototype α_2-agonist.
+ Xylazine is the least selective α_2-agonist used clinically with an α_2:α_1 binding ratio of only 160:1.[18]
+ A variety of α_2-antagonists have been used to reverse the effects of xylazine, including yohimbine, tolazoline, idazoxan, and more recently, atipamezole.
+ Although still used extensively in large animal practice as a sedative-analgesic agent, xylazine is rarely used as an analgesic adjuvant in dogs and cats.

CLONIDINE

+ An α_2-agonist approved in the United States in 1997 for use in human beings as an antihypertensive agent
+ Possesses some α_1 effects, with an α_2:α_1 binding ratio of 220:1[18]
+ Has gained popularity as an analgesic adjuvant for certain types of pain syndromes in human beings
+ Not currently used clinically in dogs and cats

DEXMEDETOMIDINE

+ Dexmedetomidine is the pure S-enantiomer of the racemic α_2-agonist medetomidine; it is considered to be twice as potent as medetomidine.[19]
+ Dexmedetomidine was approved in the United States in 1999 for use in human beings as a continuous infusion to provide sedation in intensive care unit (ICU) settings; since that time its use has expanded into anesthesia and pain management practice.
+ Although not approved for use in dogs or cats, evidence suggests that equipotent doses of dexmedetomidine and medetomidine induce similar sedative, analgesic, and cardiovascular effects in these species.[19,20]

MEDETOMIDINE

+ Medetomidine is an equal mixture of two optical enantiomers: dexmedetomidine (see previous discussion) and levomedetomidine.

- Dexmedetomidine is the active component, whereas levomedetomidine is considered pharmacologically inactive (though it may play a role in drug interactions).[19]
- Racemic medetomidine is lipophilic, facilitating rapid absorption after intramuscular administration; peak plasma concentrations are reached in approximately $\frac{1}{2}$ hour.[21]
- Elimination of medetomidine from plasma is also rapid, with reported half-lives varying between 0.96[19] hour and 1.28 hours.[21]
- Medetomidine/dexmedetomidine are the most specific α_2-agonists available clinically with an α_2:α_1 binding ratio of 1620:1.[18]
- A specific α_2-antagonist, atipamezole, was marketed alongside medetomidine and rapidly reverses all sedative, analgesic, and cardiovascular effects associated with medetomidine administration, if desired.
- Medetomidine is presently the only α_2-agonist used routinely as an analgesic adjuvant in dogs and cats, so further clinical discussions will focus on this agent.

ROMIFIDINE

- Romifidine is an imino-imidazolidine derivative of clonidine.
- Romifidine is a potent and reasonably selective α_2-agonist, producing sedative and analgesic effects comparable to those achieved with medetomidine.[22,23]
- Romifidine has a α_2:α_1 binding ratio of 340:1.
- Romifidine is not currently approved for use in dogs or cats in the United States and is not used commonly as an analgesic adjuvant at this time.

DETOMIDINE

- A weakly basic, lipophilic imidazole derivative
- Also possesses greater α_1 binding compared with medetomidine, with an α_2:α_1 binding ratio of 260:1[18]
- Not commonly used as an analgesic adjuvant in dogs and cats (Box 11-2)

BOX 11-2

Pharmacokinetic Properties of α_2-Agonists

Rapid absorption (intramuscular, subcutaneous, oral)
Rapid hepatic metabolism/renal excretion
Active metabolites possible

> **BOX 11-3**
>
> ### Clinical Use of α_2-Agonists
>
> 1. Sedative-analgesic agent for short, noninvasive procedures
> 2. Adjunct to general anesthesia
>   a. Component of total injectable anesthesia protocols
>   b. Preanesthetic sedative-analgesic agent
>   c. Supplemental continuous infusion during inhalant anesthesia
> 3. Sedative-analgesic agent in postoperative or intensive care unit patients
> 4. Epidural or intrathecal administration
> 5. Intraarticular administration
> 6. Perineural administration

CONSIDERATIONS FOR PATIENT SELECTION

- Even at the low doses advocated for analgesic supplementation, α_2-agonists may induce significant alterations in cardiopulmonary function (see Cardiovascular Effects).
- In most cases, use of α_2-agonists should be reserved for young to middle-aged animals without significant systemic disease.
- As a rule, α_2-agonists *should be avoided* in the following:
  1. Patients adversely affected by an increase in cardiac afterload or a decrease in cardiac output (e.g., mitral or tricuspid regurgitation or dilated cardiomyopathy)
  2. Patients with cardiac arrhythmias or conduction disturbances (e.g., premature ventricular contractions, atrioventricular block, or other bradyarrhythmias)
  3. Patients with preexisting hypertension
  4. Patients with an increased potential for arterial hemorrhage (e.g., traumatic arterial laceration)
  5. Patients for whom vomiting could have serious detrimental effects (e.g., upper gastrointestinal obstruction or corneal descemetocele)

CLINICAL USE AS ANALGESIC ADJUVANTS

See Box 11-3.

SEDATION AND ANALGESIA FOR SHORT, NONINVASIVE PROCEDURES

- Medetomidine is used extensively for short, noninvasive procedures in dogs and cats, whereas romifidine is used less frequently.
- Medetomidine can be used alone but is often combined with an opioid (e.g., hydromorphone, morphine, buprenorphine, or butorphanol)

TABLE 11-2	Recommended Doses of Selected α_2-Agonists for Routine Sedation/Analgesia
Drug	**Dosage**
Medetomidine*†	Dog: 0.01-0.02 mg/kg IM 0.005-0.01 mg/kg IV Cat: 0.015-0.03 mg/kg IM 0.01-0.015 mg/kg IV
Romifidine*†	Dog: 0.02-0.04 mg/kg IM 0.01-0.02 mg/kg IV Cat: 0.03-0.06 mg/kg IM 0.015-0.03 mg/kg IV

*Often combined with an opioid to enhance sedation/analgesia.
†May be reversed with atipamezole at end of procedure.

to enhance sedation and provide more intense analgesia; dosing guidelines are presented in Table 11-2.

♦ Examples of short, noninvasive procedures include radiographs, ultrasound examinations, minor laceration repair, wound débridement, bandage placement, ear canal examination and cleaning, skin biopsy, and oral examination.

♦ Despite the fact that many animals appear profoundly sedated with medetomidine/opioid combinations, it is crucial to recognize that they are *not* anesthetized and may be acutely aroused by any type of stimulation.

♦ If general anesthesia is required, an anesthetic agent must be titrated to effect (see next section).

♦ For intramuscular (IM) administration, medetomidine and opioid are mixed together in one syringe and injected 20 minutes before initiation of the procedure.

♦ For intravenous (IV) administration, lower doses of medetomidine and opioid can be mixed together in one syringe; onset time is within minutes of injection.

♦ Duration of effect is relatively short, ranging from 30 to 90 minutes; the addition of an opioid prolongs analgesia for anywhere from 1 to 4 hours depending on the opioid chosen, the dose, and the route of administration.

♦ Although concurrent use of anticholinergics remains controversial, this practice is not routinely recommended when administering medetomidine/opioid combinations.

♦ Basic hemodynamic parameters should be monitored closely when using medetomidine/opioid combinations (see Cardiovascular Effects).

♦ Reversal of all α_2-mediated effects can be accomplished by IM atipamezole administration if desired.

TABLE 11-3	Recommended Doses of Selected α_2-Agonists as Adjuncts to General Anesthesia	
	Preanesthetic Agent*	**Supplemental CRI During Inhalant Anesthesia**
Medetomidine	Dog: 0.005-0.01 mg/kg IM 0.003-0.005 mg/kg IV Cat: 0.01-0.02 mg/kg IM 0.005-0.01 mg/kg IV	Dog: 0.001 mg/kg per hour IV†
Romifidine	Dog: 0.01-0.02 mg/kg IM 0.005-0.01 mg/kg IV Cat: 0.02-0.03 mg/kg IM 0.01-0.02 mg/kg IV	
Dexmedetomidine	Dog: 0.005-0.01 mg/kg IV 0.01-0.015 mg/kg IM Cat: 0.01-0.015 mg/kg IV 0.01-0.02 mg/kg IM	Dog: 0.0005 mg/kg per hour IV[25]

*Often combined with an opioid to enhance sedation/analgesia.
†Anecdotal reports only.
CRI, Constant rate infusion.

ADJUNCT TO GENERAL ANESTHESIA

Component of Total Injectable Anesthesia Protocols

◆ Medetomidine is often used in combination with injectable anesthetic agents such as ketamine, tiletamine/zolazepam, and propofol to produce short-term general anesthesia; opioids and benzodiazepines are also commonly included in such protocols.

◆ The addition of medetomidine means that lower doses of anesthetic agents are required, analgesia is supplemented, and muscle relaxation is optimized.

◆ Numerous IM and IV drug combinations involving medetomidine have been used clinically in dogs and cats, and the reader is referred elsewhere for a review of these techniques.

Preanesthetic Sedative-Analgesic Agent

◆ Medetomidine/opioid combinations are commonly administered in the preanesthetic period before induction and transfer to an inhalant anesthetic agent.

◆ Addition of medetomidine in the preanesthetic period greatly reduces the required dose of induction agent (injectable or inhalant) and decreases the minimum alveolar concentration (MAC) needed for anesthetic maintenance.[24]

◆ Medetomidine/opioid combinations can be administered IM or IV; dosing guidelines are given in Table 11-3.

◆ Routine coadministration of an anticholinergic remains controversial but is usually not necessary in most cases; if heart rate remains low after induction of general anesthesia and the patient is hypotensive, anticholinergic administration at this time is appropriate.

◆ As with any general anesthesia protocol, hemodynamic monitoring (including heart rate, rhythm, and blood pressure) is essential (see Cardiovascular Effects).

◆ In animals undergoing surgery, routine postoperative reversal of medetomidine is not recommended because this also reverses any remaining analgesic effects.

◆ Reversal with atipamezole may be considered case by case when higher doses of medetomidine have been used and/or when excessive sedation persists in the recovery period.

Supplemental Continuous Infusion During Inhalant Anesthesia

◆ Microdose medetomidine or dexmedetomidine continuous infusions have generated interest recently for use during inhalant anesthesia maintenance.

◆ It has been proposed that the use of very low doses administered as a continuous infusion concurrently with an inhalant anesthetic may attenuate the adverse cardiovascular effects seen when larger doses are administered as boluses.

◆ To date, there is only one report in the literature evaluating this approach in the dog: dexmedetomidine was infused in isoflurane-anesthetized dogs at 0.1, 0.5, and 3 µg/kg per hour IV; MAC reductions of 18% and 59% were noted with the 0.5 and 3 µg/kg per hour infusion rates; heart rate decreased while arterial blood pressure increased at these rates, but the clinical significance of these changes at the 0.5 µg/kg per hour infusion rate was considered minimal.[25]

◆ Additional studies are warranted to explore the potential use of medetomidine and dexmedetomidine as continuous infusions in inhalant-anesthetized patients, alone or in combination with other adjunctive agents such as opioids, ketamine, and lidocaine.

SEDATIVE-ANALGESIC AGENT IN POSTOPERATIVE OR INTENSIVE CARE UNIT PATIENTS

◆ Low-dose IV bolus injections of medetomidine are useful for short-term postoperative sedation, and analgesic supplementation in selected canine and feline patients (Table 11-4)

◆ Based on experience with dexmedetomidine in human ICU patients, there is increasing interest in the use of medetomidine and

TABLE 11-4	Recommended Doses of Selected α_2-Agonists for Sedation/Analgesia in Postoperative and Intensive Care Unit Patients	
	Short-Term Sedation/ Analgesia	**Extended Sedation/ Analgesia as a CRI**
Medetomidine	Dog: 0.001-0.003 mg/kg IV bolus Cat: 0.003-0.005 mg/kg IV bolus	Dog: 0.001-0.002 mg/kg per hour IV*
Dexmedetomidine	Dog: 0.0005-0.002 mg/kg IV bolus*	Dog: 0.0005-0.001 mg/kg per hour IV*

*Anecdotal reports only.
CRI, Constant rate infusion.

dexmedetomidine administered as microdose continuous infusions in dogs and cats to provide extended periods of sedation, analgesia, and anxiolysis.

◆ Studies with dexmedetomidine infusions in human beings show significant reductions in benzodiazepine and opioid requirements in intubated, mechanically ventilated patients without inducing serious impairment of cardiopulmonary parameters.[26,27]

◆ Also, a significantly improved cumulative nitrogen balance has been documented in patients receiving α_2-agonist infusions after surgery, probably as a result of stimulation of growth hormone release.[28]

◆ To date, only one study has evaluated medetomidine (in combination with fentanyl) as a continuous infusion without the influence of concurrent inhalant anesthesia; a dose of 1.5 µg/kg per hour IV was infused with 15 µg/kg boluses of fentanyl; reductions in heart rate and cardiac index and increases in pulmonary arterial pressure were noted in this study.[29]

◆ Additional studies are needed to characterize further the cardiovascular and sedative/analgesic effects of medetomidine and dexmedetomidine infusions before their routine use can be recommended in ICU patients.

EPIDURAL/INTRATHECAL ADMINISTRATION

◆ The spinal site of action appears to be important in mediating α_2-agonist–induced analgesia.

◆ This is confirmed by the following observations:
   1. Lumbar epidural injection of α_2-agonists in human beings and animals causes more intense analgesia in the skin dermatomes innervated by the cord segments near the site of spinal administration.[30]

2. Correlation between blood α_2-agonist concentration and analgesia is poor, whereas correlation between cerebrospinal fluid (CSF) concentration and analgesia is excellent, implicating a spinal site of action.[31]

♦ Stimulation of spinal cord cholinergic interneurons also may contribute to analgesia after neuraxial α_2-agonist administration.[31-33]

♦ Although intrathecal administration is not routinely used in veterinary medicine, epidural administration is common.

♦ Incorporation of a low dose of medetomidine into an epidural protocol produces additive or synergistic analgesic effects when combined with opioids and/or local anesthetics.[34]

♦ Medetomidine may be combined with standard epidural doses of morphine, oxymorphone, buprenorphine, fentanyl, lidocaine, or bupivacaine and injected into the epidural space at the lumbosacral junction.

♦ The lipophilicity of medetomidine means that it is rapidly cleared from the CSF in the vicinity of the spinal injection site; this anatomically restricts the action of the drug, resulting in significant systemic absorption.

♦ When the total dose administered approaches that which would otherwise be given systemically, the specificity of the regional analgesic effect may be lost.

♦ The regional spinal analgesic effects of medetomidine can be optimized by administering a continuous infusion through an indwelling epidural catheter using microdoses delivered directly to the desired segment of spinal cord while minimizing medetomidine plasma levels.

♦ Clinical use of epidural medetomidine via continuous infusion remains anecdotal at this time.

INTRAARTICULAR ADMINISTRATION

♦ α_2-Adrenoceptors are located in the peripheral nervous system on terminals of primary afferent nociceptive fibers; they appear to contribute to analgesia by inhibition of norepinephrine release at nerve terminals.[31]

♦ Studies in human beings have demonstrated a peripheral analgesic effect after intraarticular administration of α_2-agonists to patients undergoing arthroscopic knee surgery that is unrelated to vascular uptake of the drug and redistribution to central sites.[35]

♦ Additive and synergistic analgesic effects have also been documented for intraarticular combinations of α_2-agonists with local anesthetics and opioids.[36]

♦ Though there are currently no studies evaluating medetomidine administered intraarticularly, extrapolation from human patients

TABLE 11-5	Recommended Doses of Medetomidine as an Adjunct to Regional Anesthesia/Analgesia Techniques		
	Epidural*	Intraarticular†	Perineural†
Medetomidine	Dog/cat: 0.001-0.005 mg/kg	Dog/cat: 0.002-0.005 mg/kg	Dog/cat: 0.002-0.005 mg/kg

*May be combined with opioids, local anesthetics, or ketamine.
†For combination with a local anesthetic.

suggests that animals undergoing routine arthrotomy may benefit from low doses of medetomidine combined with morphine, bupivacaine, or both injected into the joint at the end of surgery.

PERINEURAL ADMINISTRATION

◆ In human patients, clinical evidence suggests that α_2-agonists enhance peripheral nerve block intensity and duration when added to local anesthetics administered perineurally.

◆ Enhanced perineural blockade with α_2-agonists may be a result of the following:

1. Hyperpolarization of C fibers through blockade of a specific type of potassium channel[31]
2. Local vasoconstriction that decreases vascular removal of local anesthetic surrounding neural structures and prolongs duration of action

◆ Currently, there are no published studies evaluating the efficacy of medetomidine as an adjunct for peripheral nerve blockade in dogs and cats (Table 11-5).

CLINICAL SIDE EFFECTS OF α_2-AGONISTS

See Box 11-4.

◆ A comprehensive review of the physiological side effects of α_2-agonists used in veterinary medicine is available elsewhere[37]; the following is a brief summary of relevant points.

SEDATION, MUSCLE RELAXATION, ANXIOLYSIS

◆ α_2-Agonists consistently produce significant sedative effects in dogs and cats when administered at clinically relevant dosages.

BOX 11-4

Central Nervous System Effects of α_2-Agonists

Analgesia
Anxiolysis
Muscle relaxation
Sedation

BOX 11-5

Cardiovascular Effects of α_2-Agonists

Immediate (Peripheral) Effects
↑ Systemic vascular resistance
↑ Arterial blood pressure
↑ Heart rate (baroreceptor reflex)
↑ Cardiac output

Delayed (Central) Effects
↓ Sympathetic activity
↓ Arterial blood pressure
↓ Cardiac output

◆ The LC is a major center for control of vigilance and arousal; activation of α_2-autoreceptors produces tonic inhibition of LC adrenergic neurons and decreased release of norepinephrine, which results in sedation.

◆ Sedative-hypnotic effects are largely dose dependent; however, at higher dosages a ceiling effect is attained and further increases in dose simply prolong the duration of sedation.[38]

◆ Preexisting stress, fear, or excitement can increase circulating endogenous catecholamines and prevent the onset of α_2-agonist-induced sedation.

◆ Muscle-relaxant properties of α_2-agonists are also well recognized; this is mediated through inhibition of neuronal transmission at the level of the spinal cord.

◆ Anxiolysis is another important property; in animals and human beings, α_2-agonists are able to reduce stress and anxiety independent of their sedative effects.[39]

CARDIOVASCULAR EFFECTS

See Box 11-5.

◆ Immediately after administration, α_2-agonists bind vascular postsynaptic α_2-adrenoceptors, resulting in smooth muscle contraction and vasoconstriction.[40]

BOX 11-6

Respiratory Effects of α_2-Agonists

Low Doses (for Adjunctive Analgesia)
↓ Respiratory rate
↑ Tidal volume
Normal minute ventilation
Normal $Paco_2$, Po_2, and pH

High Doses (in Combination)
↓ Respiratory rate
↓ Tidal volume
↓ Minute ventilation
↑ CO_2, ↓ pH, ↓ PVo_2,* possible ↓ Pao_2

---

*Partial oxygen pressure in mixed venous blood.

- The increase in systemic vascular resistance produces a short-lived hypertensive phase accompanied by a compensatory baroreceptor-mediated reflex bradycardia.[39,40]
- The magnitude of initial hypertension may be less after IM administration, likely because of reduced peak plasma levels of the drug.
- Bradyarrhythmias as a result of increased vagal tone are not uncommon, with heart rates decreasing by as much as 50%.[39]
- Sinus arrhythmia, sinoatrial block, and first-degree and second-degree atrioventricular block are frequently seen; third-degree atrioventricular block and sinoatrial arrest occur rarely.
- After the transient vascular effects diminish, central α_2-adrenoceptor effects predominate; decreased sympathetic tone results in reduced blood pressure and diminished cardiac output.
- Blood pressure commonly falls by one quarter to one third of baseline values, and cardiac output decreases by one third to one half of baseline values.[39]
- Decreases in heart rate and/or cardiac output may be attenuated to some degree by coadministration with ketamine or tiletamine/zolazepam because of their sympathomimetic actions.

RESPIRATORY EFFECTS

See Box 11-6.
- Although respiratory rate decreases with administration of α_2-agonists, arterial pH, Pao_2, and $Paco_2$ are not significantly altered when using doses appropriate for adjunctive analgesia.
- The decreased respiration rate is accompanied by an increased tidal volume, which effectively maintains alveolar ventilation.[39]

BOX 11-7

Gastrointestinal Effects of α_2-Agonists

↓ Salivation
↓ Gastric secretions
↓ Gastrointestinal motility
↑ Vomiting
↓ Swallowing reflex
Predisposition to gastric dilation (large-breed dogs)?

BOX 11-8

Renal and Endocrine Effects of α_2-Agonists

Diuresis (↑ water and sodium excretion)
↓ Insulin release (hyperglycemia, glucosuria)

◆ At higher dosages, especially in combination with other CNS depressants, minute ventilation may be compromised and decreases in venous PO_2 and oxygen content have been noted; venous desaturation is presumably related to increased tissue oxygen extraction associated with decreased cardiac output.

GASTROINTESTINAL EFFECTS

See Box 11-7.

◆ Up to 20% of dogs and up to 90% of cats vomit after medetomidine administration.[41]

◆ Emesis is seen most often after subcutaneous and, less frequently, IM administration.

◆ Medetomidine also inhibits small intestinal and colonic motility in dogs.[42]

◆ Xylazine decreases esophageal sphincter pressure in dogs and may increase the likelihood of gastric reflux; acute abdominal distention has been reported in large-breed dogs after xylazine administration.[39]

RENAL EFFECTS

See Box 11-8.

◆ Significant increases in urine output are seen transiently after administration of xylazine or medetomidine to dogs and cats.[43,44]

◆ Increased urinary output may be due to one or more of the following:

1. Increased renal blood flow and glomerular filtration rate[43,44]
2. Suppression of antidiuretic hormone (ADH) release centrally[43]
3. Antagonism of ADH at the level of the renal tubule[45]

ENDOCRINE EFFECTS

♦ Xylazine and perhaps medetomidine may cause hyperglycemia because of suppression of insulin secretion.[46]
♦ Cortisol and glucagon levels do not appear to change significantly,[46] but medetomidine has been shown to attenuate the stress response induced by other anesthetic agents (opioids and ketamine).[47]
♦ Other hormonal changes include transient alterations in growth hormone, testosterone, prolactin, ADH, and follicle-stimulating hormone levels.

MISCELLANEOUS EFFECTS

♦ Increased myometrial tone and intrauterine pressure have been noted in several species after xylazine administration[48-50]; medetomidine and detomidine appear less likely to have this effect.
♦ Mydriasis has been reported after administration of xylazine and medetomidine because of central inhibition of parasympathetic innervation to the iris or direct sympathetic stimulation of α_2-receptors located in the iris and CNS.[51,52]
♦ Decreased intraocular pressure has been reported in some species after systemic administration of xylazine and medetomidine because of dampened sympathetic activity and decreased aqueous flow.

REFERENCES

1. Hsu WH: Xylazine induced depression and its antagonism by alpha-adrenergic blocking agents, *J Pharmacol Exp Ther* 218:188-192, 1981.
2. Daunt DA, Maze M: α_2-Adrenergic agonist receptors, sites and mechanisms of action. In Short CE, Van Poznak A, editors: *Animal pain*, New York, 1992, Churchill Livingstone.
3. Aanta R, Marjamaki A, Scheinin M: Molecular pharmacology of α_2-adrenoceptor subtypes, *Ann Med* 27:439-449, 1995.
4. Blaxall HS, Heck DA, Bylund DB: Molecular determinants of the alpha-2D adrenergic receptor subtype, *Life Sci* 53(17):255-259, 1993.
5. Ongioco RRS, Richardson CD, Rudner XL et al: α_2-Adrenergic receptors in human dorsal root ganglia, *Anesthesiology* 92:968-976, 2000.
6. Maze M, Fujinaga M: α_2-Adrenoceptors in pain modulation: which subtype should be targeted to produce analgesia? *Anesthesiology* 92:934-936, 2000.

7. Schwartz DD, Jones WG, Hedden TP et al: Molecular and pharmacological characterization of the canine brainstem alpha-2A adrenergic receptor, *J Vet Pharmacol Ther* 22:380-386, 1999.

8. Lakhlani PP, MacMillan LB, Guo TZ et al: Substitution of a mutant α_2A-adrenergic receptor via "hit and run" gene targeting reveals the role of this subtype in sedative, analgesic, and anesthetic-sparing responses in vivo, *Proc Natl Acad Sci U S A* 94:9950-9955, 1997.

9. MacMillan LB, Lakhlani PP, Hein L et al: In vivo mutation of the α_2A-adrenergic receptor by homologous recombination reveals the role of this subtype in multiple physiologic processes, *Adv Pharmacol* 42:493-496, 1998.

10. MacMillan LB, Hein L, Smith MS et al: Central hypotensive effects of the α_2A-adrenergic receptor subtype, *Science* 273(5276):801-803, 1996.

11. Bousquet P: Imidazoline receptors: from basic concepts to recent developments, *J Cardiovasc Pharmacol* 26(suppl 2):S1-S6, 1995.

12. Schwinn DA: Adrenoceptors as models for G protein-coupled receptors: structure, function and regulation, *Br J Anaesth* 71:77-85, 1993.

13. Budai D, Harasawa I, Fields HL: Midbrain periaqueductal gray (PAG) inhibits nociceptive inputs to sacral dorsal horn nociceptive neurons through α_2-adrenergic receptors, *J Neurophysiol* 80(5):2244-2254, 1998.

14. Millan MJ, Bervoets K, Rivet JM et al: Multiple alpha$_2$-adrenergic receptor subtypes. II. Evidence for a role of rat alpha$_{2A}$-adrenergic receptors in control of nociception, motor behavior and hippocampal synthesis of noradrenaline, *J Pharmacol Exp Ther* 270(3):958-972, 1994.

15. Buerkle H, Yaksh TL: Pharmacologic evidence for different alpha$_2$-adrenergic receptor sites mediating analgesia and sedation in the rat, *Br J Anaesth* 81:208-215, 1998.

16. Guo T, Jiang J, Butterman AE et al: Dexmedetomidine injection into the locus ceruleus produces antinociception, *Anesthesiology* 84(4):873-881, 1996.

17. Peng YB, Lin Q, Willis WD: Involvement of alpha$_2$-adrenoceptors in the periaqueductal gray-induced inhibition of dorsal horn cell activity in rats, *J Pharmacol Exp Ther* 278(1):125-135, 1996.

18. Virtanen R: Pharmacologic profiles of medetomidine and its antagonist, atipamezole, *Acta Vet Scand Suppl* 85:29-37, 1989.

19. Kuusela E, Raekallio M, Anttila M et al: Clinical effects and pharmacokinetics of medetomidine and its enantiomers in dogs, *J Vet Pharmacol Ther* 23(1): 15-20, 2000.

20. Savola JM, Virtanen R: Central α2-adrenoceptors are highly stereoselective for dexmedetomidine, the dextro enantiomer of medetomidine, *Eur J Pharmacol* 195:193-199, 1991.

21. Salonen JS: Pharmacokinetics of medetomidine, *Acta Vet Scand Suppl* 85: 49-54, 1989.

22. England GCW, Flack TE, Hollingworth E et al: Sedative effects of romifidine in the dog, *J Small Anim Pract* 37:19-25, 1996.

23. Lemke KA: Sedative effects in intramuscular administration of a low dose of romifidine in dogs, *Am J Vet Res* 60(2):162-168, 1999.

24. Tranquilli WJ, Benson GJ: Advantages and guidelines for using alpha$_2$ agonists as anesthetic adjuncts, *Vet Clin North Am Small Anim Pract* 22(2):289-292, 1992.

25. Pascoe PJ, Raekallio M, Kuusela E et al: Changes in the minimum alveolar concentration of isoflurane and some cardiopulmonary measurements during three continuous infusion rates of dexmedetomidine in dogs, *Vet Anaesth Analg* 33:97-103, 2003.

26. Venn RM, Bradshaw CJ, Spencer R et al: Preliminary UK experience of dexmedetomidine, a novel agent for postoperative sedation in the intensive care unit, *Anaesthesia* 54(12):1136-1142, 1999.

27. Hall JE, Uhrich TD, Barney JA et al: Sedative, amnestic and analgesic properties of small-dose dexmedetomidine infusions, *Anesth Analg* 90(3):699-705, 2000.

28. Mertes N, Goeters C, Kuhmann M et al: Postoperative alpha$_2$-adrenergic stimulation attenuates protein catabolism, *Anesth Analg* 82(2):258-263, 1996.

29. Grimm KA, Tranquilli WJ, Gross DR et al: Cardiopulmonary effects of fentanyl in conscious dogs and dogs sedated with a continuous rate infusion of medetomidine, *Am J Vet Res* 66(7):1222-1226, 2005.

30. Sabbe MB, Penning JP, Ozaki GT et al: Spinal and systemic action of the α_2-receptor agonist dexmedetomidine in dogs: antinociception and carbon dioxide response, *Anesthesiology* 80(5):1057-1061, 1994.

31. Eisenach J, De Kock M, Klimscha W: α2-Adrenergic agonists for regional anesthesia: a clinical review of clonidine (1984-1995), *Anesthesiology* 85: 655-674, 1996.

32. De Kock M, Eisenach J: Analgesic doses of intrathecal but not intravenous clonidine increase acetylcholine in cerebrospinal fluid in humans, *Anesth Analg* 84:800-803, 1997.

33. Eisenach JC, Hood DD, Curry R: Intrathecal, but not intravenous, clonidine reduces experimental thermal or capsaicin-induced pain and hyperalgesia in normal volunteers, *Anesth Analg* 87(3):591-596, 1998.

34. Branson KR, Ko J, Tranquilli WJ et al: Duration of analgesia induced by epidurally administered morphine and medetomidine in the dog, *J Vet Pharmacol Ther* 16:369-372, 1993.

35. Gentili M, Juhel A, Bonnet F: Peripheral analgesic effect of intra-articular clonidine, *Pain* 64(3):593-596, 1996.

36. Joshi W, Reuben SS, Kilaru PR et al: Postoperative analgesia for outpatient arthroscopic knee surgery with intraarticular clonidine and/or morphine, *Anesth Analg* 90(5):1102-1106, 2000.

37. Sinclair MD: A review of the physiological effects of α_2-agonists related to the clinical use of medetomidine in small animal practice, *Can Vet J* 44: 885-897, 2003.

38. Tranquilli WJ, Maze M: Clinical pharmacology and use of α_2-agonists in veterinary anesthesia, *Anaesthetic Pharmacology Review* 1(3):297-309, 1993.

39. Thurman JC, Tranquilli WJ, Benson GJ: Preanesthetics and anesthetic adjuncts. In Thurman JC, Tranquilli WJ, Benson GJ, editors: *Lumb & Jones' veterinary anesthesia,* ed 3, Baltimore, 1996, Williams & Wilkins.

40. Pypendop B, Verstegen JP: Hemodynamic effects of medetomidine in the dog: a dose titration study, *Vet Surg* 27:612-622, 1998.

41. Vainio O: Introduction to the clinical pharmacology of medetomidine, *Acta Vet Scand Suppl* 85:85-88, 1989.

42. Maugeri S, Ferre JP, Intorre L et al: Effects of medetomidine on intestinal and colonic motility in the dog, *J Vet Pharmacol Ther* 17(2):148-154, 1994.

43. Saleh N, Aoki M, Shimada T et al: Renal effects of medetomidine in isoflurane-anesthetized dogs with special reference to its diuretic action, *J Vet Med Sci* 67(5):461-465, 2005.

44. Grimm JB, Grimm KA, Kneller SK et al: The effect of a combination of medetomidine-butorphanol and medetomidine, butorphanol, atropine on glomerular filtration rate in dogs, *Vet Radiol Ultrasound* 42(5):458-462, 2001.

45. Gellai M, Edwards RM: Mechanism of α_2-adrenoceptor agonist-induced diuresis, *Am J Physiol* 255:317-323, 1988.

46. Ambrisko TD, Hikasa Y: Neurohormonal and metabolic effects of medetomidine compared with xylazine in beagle dogs, *Can J Vet Res* 66:42-49, 2002.

47. Ambrisko TD, Hikasa Y, Sato K: Influence of medetomidine on stress-related neurohormonal and metabolic effects caused by butorphanol, fentanyl, and ketamine administration in dogs, *Am J Vet Res* 66(3):406-412, 2005.

48. Wheaton LG, Benson GJ, Tranquilli WJ et al: The oxytocic effect of xylazine on the canine uterus, *Theriogenology* 31(4):911-915, 1989.

49. Hodgson DS, Dunlop CI, Chapman PL et al: Cardiopulmonary effects of xylazine and acepromazine in pregnant cows in late gestation, *Am J Vet Res* 63(12):1695-1699, 2002.

50. Schatzmann U, Jossfck H, Stauffer JL et al: Effects of alpha 2-agonists on intrauterine pressure and sedation in horses: comparison between detomidine, romifidine and xylazine, *Zentralbl Veterinarmed A* 41(7):523-529, 1994.

51. Hsu WH, Lee P, Betts DM: Xylazine-induced mydriasis in rats and its antagonism by alpha-adrenergic blocking agents, *J Vet Pharmacol Ther* 4(2):97-101, 1981.

52. Hsu WH, Betts DM, Lee P: Xylazine-induced mydriasis: possible involvement of a central postsynaptic regulation of parasympathetic tone, *J Vet Pharmacol Ther* 4(3):209-214, 1981.

LOCAL ANESTHETICS

KHURSHEED R. MAMA

- Local anesthetics reversibly block transmission of nerve endings or fibers.
- Autonomic nervous system blockade, anesthesia (analgesia), and/or muscle paralysis may result.
- A basic understanding of nerve physiology and drug pharmacology facilitates the appropriate clinical use of local anesthetics.

PERIPHERAL NERVE ANATOMY

NERVE FIBER CLASSIFICATION

- Size and myelination
- Specific associated functions

PERIPHERAL NERVES

- Peripheral nerves are individual nerve fibers or axons grouped together as fascicles within an outer sheath.
- Peripheral nerves may be myelinated or nonmyelinated.
- Schwann cells form multiple myelin layers around each axon of myelinated nerves and only a single membrane layer around nonmyelinated axonal fibers.
- In nonmyelinated nerves, ion channels supporting propagation of the action potential are distributed all along the axon. In myelinated nerves, these ion channels are concentrated at the nodes of Ranvier, which are periodic interruptions in the myelin sheath.

PHYSIOLOGY OF NERVE CONDUCTION

ACTION POTENTIALS

Nerve signals are conducted by action potentials, which are rapid changes in the electrical gradients across the nerve membrane.[1]

◆ Depolarization is due to the rapid inward passage of sodium ions from the extracellular to the intracellular space via sodium channels in the nerve membrane.

◆ Repolarization results from the outward flow of potassium ions and resets the nerve membrane potential to resting conditions.

◆ The action potential moves along the unmyelinated nerve fiber (conduction of the impulse) until it reaches the end of the fiber. In myelinated nerves, the impulse jumps from one node of Ranvier to the next (saltatory conduction).

SITE OF LOCAL ANESTHETIC ACTION

◆ Local anesthetics inhibit the generation and propagation (conduction) of nerve impulses by blockage of sodium channels in the nerve membrane.

◆ The most prominent hypothesis is that the anesthetic enters the lipoprotein membrane and binds to a receptor site in the sodium channel to impede or prevent sodium ion movement. Sodium-generated currents are reduced because the drug inhibits channel conformational changes, and thus drug-bound channels fail to open. This slows the rate of depolarization of the membrane, preventing attainment of the threshold potential of the membrane.

◆ To a lesser extent, movement through the channel is prevented because of the physical blockade of the ion-conducting pore by the bound drug. A sodium channel that is inhibited by a local anesthetic is functionally similar to an inactivated channel. If the sodium movement is blocked over a critical length of the nerve, propagation across the blocked area is not possible.[2,3]

DIFFERENTIAL NERVE BLOCK

◆ Because of size and presence or absence of myelination, nerve fibers differ substantially in their susceptibility to local anesthetic blockade. Myelinated fibers are blocked before unmyelinated fibers of the same diameter. Smaller fibers with higher firing rates and less distance over which such fibers can passively propagate an impulse (type B and C fibers) are blocked before larger (type A) fibers.

> **BOX 12-1**
> **Priority of Local Anesthetic Blockade**
>
> 1. Pain
> 2. Warmth
> 3. Touch
> 4. Deep pressure
> 5. Motor function

◆ Although individual variation occurs, the disappearance of nervous function in response to local anesthetic blockade, in order of first to last, is generally pain, warmth, touch, deep pressure, and finally motor function. Such variation in neural sensitivity to local anesthetics has made it possible clinically to block sensory transmission in patients without accompanying motor paralysis (differential nerve block; Box 12-1).

◆ Exceptions to this general rule include large peripheral nerve trunks where motor nerves are more circumferentially located and hence exposed to the local anesthetic agent first, allowing for motor blockade to occur before sensory blockade. Also important to remember is that in general, the mantle of the peripheral nerve trunk contains sensory innervation to the proximal aspect of an extremity, whereas the core contains distal sensory innervation. Thus, anesthesia develops proximally before distal areas become desensitized.

PHARMACOLOGY

CHEMICAL STRUCTURE

◆ The typical local anesthetic molecule consists of an unsaturated aromatic group linked by an intermediate chain to a tertiary amine end.

◆ The clinically important local anesthetics are divided into two distinct chemical groups based on their intermediate chain.

◆ Aminoamides (e.g., lidocaine and bupivacaine) have an amide link between the aromatic and amine ends, and aminoesters (e.g., procaine and benzocaine) have an ester link.

◆ These linkages, in large part, determine drug disposition within the body. Drug actions are also influenced by chemical substitutions at the aromatic or amine end of the basic molecule and are discussed in the following section (Table 12-1).

TABLE 12-1	Physicochemical Properties of Selected Local Anesthetic Agents		
Drug	**pK$_a$**	**Protein Binding (%)**	**Lipid Solubility**
ESTERS			
Procaine	8.9	6	0.6
Tetracaine	8.5	76	80
AMIDES			
Lidocaine	7.8	70	2.9
Mepivacaine	7.6	77	1
Bupivacaine	8.1	95	28
Rupivacaine	8.1	94	Less than bupivacaine

pK_a, Negative logarithm of the acid ionization constant.

STRUCTURE-ACTIVITY RELATIONSHIPS
Lipophilic-Hydrophilic Balance

The aromatic portion of a local anesthetic is considered relatively lipophilic. Alkyl substitution at the aromatic region or amine end of the basic local anesthetic molecule also imparts lipophilic characteristics to the molecule that in turn affect the tendency of a compound to associate with membrane lipids. A longer duration of action and increased anesthetic potency are correlated with increased lipid solubility.

Hydrogen Ion Concentration

Local anesthetics are weak bases with negative logarithm of the acid ionization constant (pKa) values in the range of 8 to 9. Thus the predominant form of the compound in solution at physiologic pH is the ionized or cationic form. Although this form is important for local anesthetic activity at the receptor site, it is the uncharged base that is important for rapid penetration and diffusion through biologic membranes. Thus the amount of drug in the base form at physiologic pH strongly influences the onset of drug action and the potency of the drug.

Protein Binding

The tertiary amine is considered relatively hydrophilic and bears some positive charge in the physiologic pH range. The degree of ionization has been positively correlated to protein binding, and in general, the greater the protein binding, the longer the duration of action.

Chirality

Many newer local anesthetics are asymmetric compounds that exhibit two distinct spatial arrangements (mirror images), despite having the same physicochemical properties. Pharmacodynamic and pharmacokinetic actions vary as a result of these differences in structure.

DRUG DISPOSITION

Local anesthetic agents are usually injected into a localized area of the body to block specific nerves or areas. The absorption of drug from the injection site, distribution within the body, and excretion from the body are of primary importance in determining the systemic disposition of the drug and potential for side effects.

Absorption

The rate of systemic absorption of local anesthetic agents is inversely related to the duration of effect at the site of action. In addition to drug physicochemical and pharmacologic properties, drug dose, site of injection, and use of a vasoconstrictor influence drug absorption.

◆ The effect on systemic absorption of a change in volume or concentration (at a constant dose) of local anesthetic is variable and generally not significant, but if the overall dose is increased, a higher systemic peak drug concentration is likely.

◆ The site of injection also significantly influences the peak drug concentrations in the blood. Local anesthetic deposited in a highly vascular area is absorbed more rapidly and results in higher blood levels of drug than if injected into tissue with less blood flow. Epinephrine (a vasoconstrictor) tends to reduce systemic absorption by reducing local blood flow. This effect may vary depending on the nature of the local anesthetic (i.e., concurrent use of a vasoconstrictor such as epinephrine reduces the peak blood levels of the shorter-acting drugs but has a less pronounced effect on the more lipophilic and longer-acting agents).

Distribution

◆ Because of rapid breakdown by plasma pseudocholinesterase and the resulting short plasma half-life, distribution of ester anesthetics in body tissue is limited.

◆ Conversely, amide local anesthetic agents are widely distributed in the body after an intravenous bolus injection; a two- or three-compartment model usually describes their pharmacokinetic properties.

◆ Distribution of an amide-type local anesthetic, in particular, may be further influenced by anatomic and pathophysiologic factors.

1. Hypercapnia and resulting acidosis in the central nervous system (CNS) likely increase regional blood flow and as a result increase local anesthetic concentrations in the brain and increase the risk of toxicity.

2. Conversely, drug reaching the systemic circulation may be reduced in some circumstances because the lungs are capable of extracting at least some amide local anesthetics.[4] Protein binding may influence the free drug available for activity and clearance by the liver and is inversely related to toxic plasma concentrations.

Biotransformation and Excretion

A major difference between the aminoamides and aminoesters is the pattern of metabolism. This has implications for clinical usefulness and observed toxicity for the two classes of compounds.

◆ The principal metabolic pathway of local anesthetics with ester linkages is enzymatic hydrolysis in the plasma by nonspecific pseudo-cholinesterases. The rate of plasma hydrolysis varies (chloroprocaine > procaine > tetracaine) and is inversely related to toxicity.

1. Pregnancy reduces plasma cholinesterase activity and might prolong the clearance of the ester anesthetics and increase the potential for toxicity.

2. Because of the lack of significant pseudocholinesterase activity in the cerebrospinal fluid, subarachnoid administration of ester anesthetics results in a clinical effect until the drug is systemically absorbed.

3. Products of hydrolysis can be directly excreted by the kidneys, but more commonly, they undergo metabolic transformation.

4. Para-aminobenzoic acid (PABA) is a breakdown product of the esters responsible for allergic reactions in some human patients.

5. Cocaine is an atypical ester in that it undergoes significant hepatic metabolism and urinary excretion.

◆ Amide local anesthetics are metabolized primarily in the liver. The order of clearance of amides is as follows: prilocaine (most rapid) > etidocaine > lidocaine > mepivacaine/ropivacaine > bupivacaine (least rapid).

1. A common pathway in biotransformation of amide local anesthetics is dealkylation of the parent compound to an intermediate compound. This occurs primarily in the hepatic microsomes.

2. Generally, this intermediate compound is hydrolyzed and excreted in the urine, but further conjugation (e.g., with glucuronide) before

excretion is sometimes necessary. Toxicity could occur in species (e.g., cat) that have a limited ability to perform this step.

3. Metabolism of certain compounds may also directly result in toxicity, as in the case of prilocaine, which is metabolized to o-toluidine, a compound capable of oxidizing hemoglobin to methemoglobin.

4. Changes in hepatic or renal function or blood flow (as may be induced with hypotension during regional or general anesthesia and in certain disease states) prolong the clearance of the local anesthetic drugs from the body and may increase the potential for side effects.

FACTORS INFLUENCING ANESTHETIC ACTIVITY

In addition to the chemical structure and physicochemical properties of local anesthetics that influence anesthetic potency, differential sensitivity, and onset and duration of anesthetic action, a number of other drug and patient factors are worthy of consideration. These factors include dose, site of injection, addition of hyaluronidase or vasoconstrictors to the injectate, carbonation and pH adjustment, influence of varying baricity, mixture of local anesthetics, and the influence of physiologic states such as pregnancy.

DOSE OF ANESTHETIC AGENT

A more rapid anesthetic onset is facilitated by use of a greater volume of anesthetic or a more concentrated solution because this increases the number of agent molecules in the region of the nerve. When a local anesthetic is injected in the epidural or intrathecal space, increased volume of the solution also influences the cranial spread of the agent.

SITE OF INJECTION

The shortest duration of action is usually seen after intrathecal administration, and the longest duration, after peripheral nerve blocks (e.g., brachial plexus and sciatic). This is generally independent of the agent used.

USE OF HYALURONIDASE

Addition of the mucolytic enzyme hyaluronidase is thought to enhance the diffusion of local anesthetic agents to the site of action (e.g., peripheral nerve). However, it may also enhance systemic absorption (and thus toxicity) and is currently not believed to be cost-effective.

USE OF VASOCONSTRICTORS

In vivo, the duration of action is influenced not only by the intrinsic action of the drug on nerves but also by the action on local blood vessels. At low concentrations, local anesthetics tend to cause vasoconstriction, whereas in clinical doses, vasodilation is usually present. Thus the duration of block may be shorter in vivo than that determined in vitro. Addition of a vasoconstrictor to the local anesthetic solution decreases local perfusion, delays the rate of vascular absorption of local anesthetic, and therefore prolongs anesthetic action. Epinephrine (5 µg/ml or 1:200,000) is the agent most commonly added to the local anesthetic. Phenylephrine and norepinephrine have no substantial clinical advantage over epinephrine. Lack of clinical benefit from the addition of epinephrine may be related to the low pH of the epinephrine preparation; this potentially decreases available free base for diffusion, thus delaying the onset of the local anesthetic block (Box 12-2).

CARBONATION AND pH ADJUSTMENT

In the isolated nerve preparation, addition of bicarbonate to the local anesthetic solution results in a more rapid onset of nerve blockade and at a reduced anesthetic concentration. This effect is likely due to an increase in the amount of drug in the uncharged base form. Controversy exists concerning the merits of this practice under clinical conditions.

BARICITY

Varying the baricity of local anesthetic solutions may influence the spread within the spinal cord. Hypobaric solutions (i.e., those with a specific gravity less than that of cerebrospinal fluid [CSF]) tend to migrate to nondependent areas, whereas hyperbaric solutions (i.e., those with a specific gravity greater than that of CSF) migrate from the site of injection to dependent areas. Baricity of a specific drug may vary with drug concentration or as a result of additives.

BOX 12-2

Effect of Addition of Epinephrine

Addition of epinephrine to lidocaine and bupivacaine delays local anesthetic absorption and prolongs anesthetic action.

Hyaluronidase is thought to enhance the diffusion of local anesthetic agents to the site of action

MIXTURES OF LOCAL ANESTHETICS

Although the clinical practice of mixing local anesthetics to enhance onset and prolong the duration of neural blockade is sometimes useful, it is not universally effective. Potentially beneficial effects are likely negated by drug interactions. For example, in isolated nerve studies, it has been suggested that when chloroprocaine (short onset and duration) and bupivacaine (long onset and duration) are mixed, metabolites of chloroprocaine may inhibit the binding of bupivacaine to receptor sites. Thus at present, mixing of local anesthetics remains controversial.

PREGNANCY

Duration of the ester local anesthetics may be prolonged in pregnant patients because plasma cholinesterase activity is reduced. The spread and depth of an epidural or spinal local anesthetic is also reported to be greater in pregnant patients. Mechanical factors (smaller epidural space) and hormonal changes (elevations in progesterone levels) associated with pregnancy have been implicated. Therefore, it is generally recommended that the dose of spinal or epidural local anesthetics be reduced during pregnancy.

TOXICITY

When administered at an appropriate dose, local anesthetic agents are relatively free of harmful side effects. Most potentially harmful reactions occur after accidental intravenous (IV) administration or following vascular absorption of large amounts of anesthetic after regional administration.

SYSTEMIC TOXICITY
Central Nervous System

◆ Low systemic doses of local anesthetic administered to awake, unmedicated human beings are reported to cause numbness of the tongue and oral cavity. Low systemic doses also likely contribute to reduced anesthetic requirement during general anesthesia.[5-7] As the plasma concentration of the drug increases, local anesthetics produce a predictable pattern of CNS excitement and then depression that may be accompanied by apnea and cardiovascular collapse.

BOX 12-3

Caution with Injections

Always aspirate before injection. Bupivacaine can cause cardiac dysrhythmias and ventricular fibrillation if injected intravenously.

◆ Plasma concentrations producing the various phases of overdose are drug-related (and perhaps species-related). For example, in cats, procaine is least potent in terms of CNS effects (convulsions at about 35 mg/kg), and bupivacaine is one of the most potent (convulsions beginning at about 5 mg/kg).[8] In dogs, the relative CNS toxicity of bupivacaine, etidocaine, and lidocaine is 4:2:1.[9]

Cardiovascular System

Local anesthetics can produce direct effects on the heart and peripheral vascular smooth muscle and indirect effects through influence on autonomic nervous activity.

◆ Direct effects on the heart may be electrophysiologic and mechanical. Both effects on the heart result in a decrease in cardiac output. Bupivacaine and etidocaine may produce severe cardiac dysrhythmias, including ventricular fibrillation[10,11] (Box 12-3).

◆ The effect of local anesthetics on peripheral vascular smooth muscle may be biphasic. When low concentrations are used, constriction may occur, especially in the pulmonary circulation, resulting in increases in pulmonary artery resistance and hypertension.[3] The more usual clinical response, especially with increasing concentrations, is relaxation resulting in vasodilation.

◆ The vasodilation and the decrease in cardiac output result in arterial hypotension. When a local anesthetic is administered via the epidural or intrathecal route, cardiovascular collapse may be further exacerbated by sympathetic nervous system blockade as the agent spreads cranially.

LOCAL TOXICITY
Neural Toxicity

Although local anesthetics are rarely neurotoxic at clinically administered concentrations, irreversible conduction blockade in isolated nerves has been reported.[3] Prolonged sensory and motor deficits reported after epidural or subarachnoid administration of chloroprocaine are now believed to be related to the antioxidant sodium bisulfite and not the parent drug itself.

Skeletal Muscle Toxicity

When properly used, local anesthetics rarely produce localized tissue damage. However, some reports indicate that even when clinical doses are used for local infiltration, skeletal muscle damage may be associated with the longer-acting agents.[12,13]

OTHER EFFECTS
Methemoglobinemia

Methemoglobinemia has been reported to develop after exposure to a number of local anesthetics, most notably prilocaine.[14,15] Breakdown products (e.g., o-toluidine) from the metabolism of the local anesthetic are likely responsible.

Allergies

Although allergic-type reactions to the amide local anesthetics are rare, it is possible for the aminoester local anesthetics such as procaine to cause hypersensitivity or anaphylactic responses. PABA, a product of ester metabolism, is most commonly implicated. Preservatives (e.g., methylparaben) contained in local anesthetic solutions may also result in allergic reactions.

Addiction

Although cocaine is rarely used in veterinary medicine, abuse directly (e.g., by human beings with access to the compound) and indirectly (e.g., administration to horses as a stimulant before a race) are possibilities.

CLINICAL APPLICATION OF LOCAL ANESTHETICS

Local anesthetics are most often used to produce regional anesthesia and analgesia (Table 12-2). *Regional anesthesia* is a term loosely used to refer to a variety of applications of local anesthetics for anesthetic purposes. The term implies that a region of the body is affected as opposed to the entire body as with general anesthesia. The region affected may be limited or broad. In terms of organization, regional anesthesia includes the following subcategories. These subcategories are discussed in depth in Chapter 15:

TABLE 12-2	Clinical Attributes of Selected Local Anesthetic Agents		
Drug	**Onset**	**Duration (Minutes)**	**Main Clinical Uses**
ESTERS			
Procaine	Slow	45-60	Local and perineural infiltration
Tetracaine	Slow	60-180	Topical application
AMIDES			
Lidocaine	Rapid	60-120	Local and perineural infiltration; intravenous regional, epidural, and subarachnoid administration
Mepivacaine	Intermediate	90-180	Local and perineural infiltration
Bupivacaine	Intermediate	180-480	Local and perineural infiltration; epidural and subarachnoid administration
Ropivacaine	Intermediate	180-480	Local and perineural infiltration; epidural and subarachnoid administration

◆ Topical anesthesia
◆ Local infiltration
◆ Peripheral nerve block
◆ Intraarticular administration
◆ IV block
◆ Epidural block
◆ Spinal (subarachnoid) block

Local anesthetics may also be used to supplement actions of IV and inhalation anesthetics, to treat neuropathic pain, or to prevent or treat cardiac dysrhythmias. In rare cases, lidocaine may be administered in low doses to suppress grand mal seizures and to prevent or treat increases in intracranial pressure.

LOCAL ANESTHETIC AGENTS

AMINO-ESTER LOCAL ANESTHETICS

Procaine Hydrochloride

◆ Procaine hydrochloride is a weak organic base, with a pK_a of 8.9. Procaine is nonirritant and promptly effective when injected subcutaneously. Procaine provides a relatively brief period of anesthesia (45 to 60 minutes), which may be prolonged by addition of a vasoconstrictor.

◆ The drug is rapidly hydrolyzed, in plasma (but not CSF) by nonspecific pseudocholinesterases. The plasma half-life is about 25 minutes.[16] The kidneys excrete procaine and PABA, a product of procaine degradation.

◆ Procaine is used in veterinary medicine for infiltration and nerve block. A concentration of 1% is used for small patients, and 2% is preferable for larger animals. Procaine is rarely used for surface anesthesia because it is not very effective with this route of administration.

Tetracaine Hydrochloride

◆ Tetracaine is 8 times as potent as procaine and has a pK_a of 8.5. Although the onset of drug action is slow, it is rapidly absorbed from mucosal surfaces to which it is applied. The duration of effect is intermediate (60 to 180 minutes).

◆ Because of rapid absorption and slower metabolism (than that for procaine) by plasma cholinesterases, there is an increase in the potential for systemic toxicity.

◆ Tetracaine is used to provide topical anesthesia of the eye, nose, and throat and for spinal anesthesia when sensory and motor blockade are desired. Tetracaine is a component of the topical local anesthetic mixture *Cetacaine*. Recently, a patch application system and a gel preparation have been evaluated as percutaneous analgesia with favorable results.[17]

Benzocaine

◆ Benzocaine is structurally similar to procaine except that it lacks a terminal diethyl amino group. Benzocaine is available as a dusting powder or as oil in an ointment for surface application.

◆ Benzocaine is relatively nonirritating to tissues, and after absorption, it is metabolized to PABA and acetyl PABA. Benzocaine has been reported to cause methemoglobinemia in some species (e.g., sheep), which may limit its widespread use in clinical practice.

◆ Benzocaine has been used to varying degrees in dentistry to provide anesthesia of the gums and buccal mucosa and for cutaneous analgesia. The low solubility of benzocaine allows it to remain localized in wounds to provide long-term pain relief. Benzocaine is also a component (as is tetracaine) in a topical local anesthetic mixture known as Cetacaine, which is commonly used as a spray to anesthetize the larynx before intubation.

Proparacaine Hydrochloride

◆ Proparacaine hydrochloride is about equal in potency to tetracaine. Proparacaine is chemically distinct from procaine and exhibits little cross-sensitivity.

♦ Unlike some topical anesthetics, it produces little or no tissue irritation.[18] Because proparacaine induces little discomfort on instillation into the human eye, it is widely used as an ophthalmic anesthetic.

AMINO-AMIDE LOCAL ANESTHETICS
Lidocaine Hydrochloride

♦ Lidocaine is one of the most versatile and most widely used local anesthetics in veterinary medicine. The compound has a pK_a of 7.9 and is considered twice as potent as procaine. The clinical use of lidocaine is associated with a rapid onset of action and short (60 to 120 minutes) duration of effect. Lidocaine is available as a sterile aqueous solution in concentrations of 0.5% to 5% with or without epinephrine and in a gel preparation in concentrations of 2.5% to 5%.

♦ Lidocaine is quickly absorbed from the gastrointestinal tract and after injection.[19] The kinetics and oral absorption rate of lidocaine have been determined in the dog; 78% of the administered dose reaches the general circulation.[20] Emesis occurs regularly at 2½ hours after administration. Mexiletine is an inexpensive and orally active lidocaine analog that has been used for treatment of ventricular ectopy in dogs. Although the usefulness of mexiletine as a systemic analgesic has not been evaluated in the dog, it warrants consideration especially for neuropathic pain where local anesthetics have been shown to have efficacy. Gastrointestinal side effects include progressive inappetence and anorexia.

♦ The rate of systemic absorption after parenteral administration is slowed, and the duration of action is prolonged when lidocaine is used with a vasoconstrictor. Lidocaine is metabolized in the liver by mixed-function oxidases at a rate nearly as rapid as that for procaine. The metabolites and 10% to 20% of the unchanged form are excreted in urine of the dog.

♦ Lidocaine is used for all forms of local anesthesia. The transdermal (Lidoderm patch) administration of lidocaine produces local tissue concentrations far below those capable of producing toxicity but high enough to produce clinically effective local analgesia for periods of up to 24 hours without complete sensory block. The patches have been used to provide analgesia for skin abrasions, lacerations, and severe local skin irritation and itching (hot spots). The patch is supplied as a 10×14-cm adhesive bandage that may be cut into smaller sizes with a scissors before removing the protective drug release liner. Care should be taken to avoid contact with the attendant's skin or eyes to prevent numbing of the fingers or irritation, respectively.

- A rapidly acting lidocaine cream, LMX 5 (anorectal cream), containing 5% lidocaine is also available for producing fast-acting local analgesic effects. LMX 5 can be used to relieve pain caused by minor cuts, minor burns, abrasions, sunburn, and minor surgical sites. Lidocaine preparations are also commonly used to numb the skin before performing minor surgery, insertion of IV lines, obtaining blood specimens, and other such procedures. LMX 5 should only be used externally.
- In addition to its use as a local anesthetic, lidocaine is used IV as an antidysrhythmic agent and also as a supplement to general anesthesia (25 to 50 μg/kg per minute). Lidocaine decreases the requirement for inhalation and injectable anesthetics.[5-7,21]

Prilocaine Hydrochloride

Prilocaine hydrochloride has pharmacologic properties resembling those of lidocaine. However, it causes significantly less vasodilation and hence may be used without the addition of epinephrine to prolong the duration of effect. Prilocaine is also reported to be the least toxic of the amide local anesthetics and thus best suited for IV anesthesia. Methemoglobinemia is a side effect of overdose and accounts for its declining use, especially for human patients.

Eutectic Mixture of Lidocaine and Prilocaine

- Eutectic mixture of lidocaine and prilocaine (EMLA), a 1:1 mixture of lidocaine and prilocaine, is available commercially for transcutaneous application. It has been shown that when the base forms of these two compounds are mixed, oil is formed at temperatures higher than 18° C.[22] This eutectic mixture is commercially available in a preparation containing arlacton as an emulsifier and carbapol as a thickening agent. Each gram (or milliliter) contains 25 mg of lidocaine and 25 mg of prilocaine. The reported bioavailability is 3% for lidocaine and 5% for prilocaine.[23] This may, however, vary with the site of application, skin pigmentation, and condition.
- The toxicity of EMLA is related primarily to the metabolism of prilocaine to *o*-toluidine, which can result in methemoglobinemia. Blanching or hyperemia may be noted in the area of application after removal of the occlusive bandage and is likely due to the relative vasoactivity of the two compounds.
- EMLA has been evaluated as a percutaneous analgesic before venipuncture in dogs, cats, rabbits, and rats.[24] The efficacy of EMLA after a 60-minute application was good in dogs, cats, and rabbits but questionable in study rats.

Mepivacaine Hydrochloride

♦ The pharmacologic properties of mepivacaine hydrochloride are similar to those of lidocaine. Although actual potency figures vary, mepivacaine is about equal (or slightly less) in local anesthetic potency to lidocaine. Mepivacaine has a slightly longer duration (90 to 180 minutes) of action, likely because of less intrinsic vasodilator activity compared with lidocaine.

♦ Although the use of mepivacaine in clinical practice is similar to that of lidocaine, mepivacaine is not recommended for obstetric anesthesia because its actions are greatly prolonged in the fetus. In the adult, the toxicity of mepivacaine is about 1.5 to 2 times that of procaine but slightly less than that of lidocaine.

Bupivacaine Hydrochloride

♦ Bupivacaine is a long-acting local anesthetic chemically related to mepivacaine and about 4 times more potent than lidocaine. The onset of action is slow to intermediate, and the duration of action ranges from 3 to 10 hours.

♦ Bupivacaine is most commonly used for regional and epidural nerve blocks and was the first local anesthetic agent to show significant separation of sensory and motor blockade, making it the drug of choice for obstetric anesthesia. CNS and cardiac toxicity result from lower doses and blood levels than those reported for lidocaine.

♦ Because of the cardiac toxicity associated with bupivacaine, levobupivacaine, the S-enantiomer was developed for clinical use. Previous studies of isomers of local anesthetics suggested that the systemic toxicity of the *S*-isomer of various compounds may be less than that of racemic preparations. Although there is no difference in the efficacy of two compounds, the lethal dose of levobupivacaine has been shown to be 1.3 to 1.6 times that of bupivacaine, and hence this product may offer a clinical advantage.

Ropivacaine Hydrochloride

♦ Ropivacaine, another long-acting aminoamide local anesthetic, is structurally related to mepivacaine and bupivacaine but as with levobupivacaine is an *S*-isomer, whereas the other agents are racemic mixtures. The physiochemical properties of ropivacaine are similar to those of bupivacaine with the exception of its lipid solubility (ropivacaine is substantially less lipid soluble).[25] At low concentrations, ropivacaine has intrinsic vasoconstricting properties, whereas higher concentrations result in vasodilation.

◆ Ropivacaine is used in a manner similar to bupivacaine, but may be less potent. Reports indicate that the motor block after epidural administration is less dense and of a shorter duration than for bupivacaine. This, along with the reduced cardiotoxic potential of ropivacaine compared with bupivacaine, offers advantages for clinical use when differential blockade is desired.[26,27] Ropivacaine also reportedly caused fewer CNS symptoms in human volunteers and was at least 25% less toxic than bupivacaine in regard to the dose tolerated.[28,29]

ACKNOWLEDGMENT

Portions of this chapter are reproduced with modification with permission from Mama KR, Steffey EP: Local anesthetics. In Richard AH, editor: *Veterinary pharmacology and therapeutics*, ed 8, Ames, 2001, Iowa State University Press.

REFERENCES

1. Guyton AC, Hall JE: *Textbook of medical physiology*, ed 9, Philadelphia, 1996, WB Saunders.
2. Butterworth JF, Strichartz GR: Molecular mechanisms of local anesthesia: a review, *Anesthesiology* 72:711-734, 1990.
3. Strichartz GR, Berde CB: Local anesthetics. In Miller RD, editor: *Anesthesia*, ed 4, New York, 1994, Churchill Livingstone.
4. Tucker GT: Pharmacokinetics of local anesthetics, *Br J Anaesth* 58:717-731, 1986.
5. Himes RS Jr, DiFazio CA, Burmey RC: Effects of lidocaine on the anesthetic requirements of nitrous oxide and halothane, *Anesthesiology* 47:437-440, 1977.
6. Himes RS Jr, Munson ES, Embro WJ: Enflurane requirement and ventilatory response to carbon dioxide during lidocaine infusion in dogs, *Anesthesiology* 51:131-134, 1979.
7. Doherty TJ, Frazier DL: Effect of intravenous lidocaine on halothane minimum alveolar concentration in ponies, *Equine Vet J* 30:300-303, 1998.
8. Englesson S: The influence of acid-base changes on central nervous system toxicity of local anesthetic agents. I. An experimental study in cats, *Acta Anaesthesiol Scand* 18:79-87, 1974.
9. Liu PL, Feldman HS Giasi R et al: Comparative CNS toxicity of lidocaine, etidocaine, bupivacaine and tetracaine in awake dogs following rapid IV administration, *Anesth Analg* 62:375-379, 1983.
10. Kotelko DM, Shnider SM, Dailey PA et al: Bupivacaine-induced cardiac arrhythmias in sheep, *Anesthesiology* 60:10-19, 1984.
11. Bruelle P, Lefrant J-Y, de La CoussayeJE et al: Comparative electrophysiologic and hemodynamic effects of several amide local anesthetic drugs in anesthetized dogs, *Anesth Analg* 82:648-656, 1996.
12. Basson MD, Carlson BM: Myotoxicity of single and repeated injections of mepivacaine (Carbocaine) in the rat, *Anesth Analg* 59:275-282, 1980.

13. Benoit PW, Belt WD: Destruction and regeneration of skeletal muscle after treatment with a local anesthetic, bupivacaine (Marcaine), *J Anat* 107:547, 1970.

14. Ferraro L, Zeichner SGG, Groeger JS: Cetacaine-induced acute methemoglobinemia, *Anesthesiology* 69:614-616, 1988.

15. Paddleford RR, Krahwinkel DJ, Fuhr JE, et al: Experimentally induced methemoglobinemia in the dog following exposure to topical benzocaine HCl. In Grandy J, Hildebrand S, McDonell W et al, editors: *Proceedings of the second International Congress of Veterinary Anesthesia,* Santa Barbara, 1985, Veterinary Practice Publishing.

16. Tobin T, Blake JW, Tai CY et al: Pharmacology of procaine in the horse: a preliminary report, *Am J Vet Res* 37:1107-1110, 1976.

17. McCafferty DF, Woolfson AD: New patch delivery system for percutaneous local anaesthesia, *Br J Anaesth* 71:370-374, 1993.

18. Ritchie JM, Greene NM: Local anesthetics. In Goodman AG, Goodman LS, Gilman A, editors: *The pharmacological basis of therapeutics,* ed 8, New York, 1990, Pergamon Press.

19. Keenaghan JB, Boyes RN: The tissue distribution, metabolism and excretion of lidocaine in rats, guinea pigs, dogs and man, *J Pharmacol Exp Ther* 180:454-463, 1972.

20. Boyes RN, Adams HJ, Duce BR: Oral absorption and deposition kinetics of lidocaine hydrochloride in dogs, *J Pharmacol Exp Ther* 174:1-8, 1970.

21. Kissin I, McGee T: Hypnotic effect of thiopental-lidocaine combination in the rat, *Anesthesiology* 57:311-313, 1982.

22. Brodin A, Nyqvist-Mayer A, Wadsten T et al: Phase diagram and aqueous solubility of the lidocaine-prilocaine binary system, *J Pharm Sci* 73:481-484, 1984.

23. Klein J, Fernandes D, Gazarian M et al: Simultaneous determination of lidocaine, prilocaine and the prilocaine metabolite *o*-toluidine in plasma by high-performance liquid chromatography, *J Chromatogr B Biomed Sci Appl* 655:83-88, 1994.

24. Flecknell PA, Liles JH, Williamson HA: The use of lidocaine-prilocaine local anesthetic cream for pain-free venepuncture in laboratory animals, *Lab Anim* 24:142-146, 1990.

25. Rosenberg PH, Heinonen E: Differential sensitivity of A and C nerve fibres to long-acting amide local anaesthetics, *Br J Anaesth* 55:163-167, 1983.

26. Feldman H, Arthur G, Covino B: Comparative systemic toxicity of convulsant and supraconvulsant doses of intravenous ropivacaine, bupivacaine, and lidocaine in the conscious dog, *Anesth Analg* 69:794-801, 1989.

27. Reiz S, Haggmark S, Johansson G, Nath S: Cardiotoxicity of ropivacaine: a new amide local anaesthetic agent, *Acta Anaesthesiol Scand* 33:93-98, 1989.

28. Scott DB, Lee A, Fagan D et al: Acute toxicity of ropivacaine compared with that of bupivacaine, *Anesth Analg* 69:563-569, 1989.

29. Wolfe TM, Muir WW: Local anesthetics: pharmacology and novel applications, *Compendium* 25:916-927, 2003.

13 GLUCOCORTICOIDS

MARY O. SMITH

Glucocorticoids can play a significant role in pain control under specific sets of circumstances. An understanding of how the varying members of this group differ from each other is important so that an individual drug can be used appropriately and safely.

PROTOTYPE[1,2]

♦ Cortisol is the major endogenous glucocorticoid in most mammals.
♦ Cortisol is synthesized from cholesterol in the adrenal gland (zona fasciculata and zona reticularis).
♦ Cortisol is released into the circulation under the influence of corticotropin, which is secreted by the pituitary gland.
♦ Corticotropin secretion is controlled by the hypothalamus through the action of corticotropin-releasing hormone (CRH).
♦ CRH is secreted in response to physiological stress (see Chapter 3).
♦ Negative feedback control exists at the pituitary and hypothalamic levels.
♦ Some studies suggest that there are diurnal variations in circulating cortisol levels in animals, whereas others do not support this.[3,4]
♦ Plasma cortisol is greater than 90% protein-bound:
  • Most is bound to cortisol-binding protein synthesized by the liver.
  • A small amount is loosely bound to albumin.
  • Ten percent is free in plasma and physiologically active.
  • Increased release of cortisol from the adrenal glands produces higher levels of free cortisol in plasma and greater effects on target cells.
  • Circulating synthetic glucocorticoids are mostly bound to albumin.
  • Most cortisol (>80%) is metabolized within and excreted by the liver: reduction and conjugation to glucuronides and sulfates.

- The half-life of circulating cortisol is approximately 90 minutes and is increased by stress, hypothyroidism, and hepatic disease.

EFFECTS

GLUCOCORTICOID RECEPTORS

1. Effects of glucocorticoids are mediated by a variety of glucocorticoid receptors on target cells.
2. Binding to the glucocorticoid receptor induces conformational changes in the receptor.
3. The glucocorticoid-receptor complex is actively transported to the cell nucleus, where it binds to glucocorticoid receptor elements, altering the regulation of gene transcription.
4. The precise effect of the hormone within the target cell depends on the type of receptor to which it binds and the target gene for that receptor.
5. A large number of different glucocorticoid receptors exist.
6. Target gene expression varies among cell types.
7. Both of these factors contribute to the wide diversity of action of glucocorticoids within target cells.
8. Activation of glucocorticoid receptors alters protein synthesis within the cell.
   - Adverse effects of glucocorticoid—Many of the effects of glucocorticoids may be adverse when supraphysiologic doses are administered.
   - Increased gluconeogenesis and glycogen synthesis occur.
   - Increases in lipolysis and lipogenesis produce a net increase in body fat.
   - Catabolism of fat, muscle, skin, bone, lymphoid tissue, and connective tissue occurs.
   - Antiinflammatory effects—Pain relief afforded by glucocorticoid administration is due to a reduction in inflammation.

MECHANISMS OF ACTION

- The main mechanism of the antiinflammatory effects of glucocorticoids is the inhibition of phospholipase A2, the precursor of arachidonic acid.[5]
- Phospholipase A2 inhibition decreases the production of prostaglandins and leukotrienes.
- Prostaglandins and leukotrienes lower the nociceptive threshold, increasing sensitivity to substances that cause pain, such as histamine and bradykinin.

◆ Glucocorticoids reduce levels of cyclooxygenase enzymes in inflammatory cells, further inhibiting the production of prostaglandins.[1]
◆ Glucocorticoids have significant effects on leukocyte activity and distribution.[1]
◆ Glucocorticoid administration induces neutrophilia and lymphopenia.
  • Neutrophils are recruited from the bone marrow into the systemic circulation.
  • Migration of neutrophils from the vascular system into tissues is decreased, thereby decreasing inflammation.
  • Lymphocytes and other circulating leukocytes are recruited into lymphoid tissues.
  • Glucocorticoids inhibit the activity of lymphocytes and tissue macrophages.
◆ Basal levels of endogenous glucocorticoids appear to be critical for facilitating certain mechanisms of analgesia, such as those mediated by endogenous opioids.[6]

EFFICACY AND USE

See Box 13-1.
◆ Glucocorticoids are most commonly administered by systemic routes, oral or injectable.
◆ Many indications for the use of this group of drugs exist, but only painful conditions are discussed.
◆ Dosages used for the alleviation of pain should be those that suppress inflammation and not those that are immunosuppressive.
◆ Shorter-acting drugs, such as prednisone, prednisolone, or methylprednisolone, are preferred for systemic administration. These drugs carry a lower risk of toxic side effects compared with drugs with long half-lives and durations of action.

BOX 13-1

Common Uses of Glucocorticoids

Most glucocorticoid dosage regimens are empirical or have been extrapolated from use in human beings. Common uses include the following:
• Intervertebral disk disease
• Intraarticular pain
• Lumbar pain via the epidural route
• Otitis externa
• Systemic inflammatory disease

INTERVERTEBRAL DISK DISEASE

- ◆ Prednisone 0.1 to 0.2 mg/kg, administered orally once or twice daily, has been used successfully in combination with strict cage rest to treat mild cases of intervertebral disk disease (pain only or pain and mild paresis).[7]
- ◆ Successful treatment of animals with severe clinical signs (paraplegia) has been reported, although surgery is preferred.[8]
- ◆ High-dose methylprednisolone sodium succinate treatment within 8 hours of spinal cord trauma (including acute disk extrusion), although controversial, is widely used in dogs and cats. The main rationale for this use is to reduce inflammation and improve neurologic function, but some analgesic benefits may also be derived. A single dose of 30 mg/kg by slow intravenous injection (over 2 to 5 minutes) should be followed by a constant infusion of 5.4 mg/kg per hour for 24 to 48 hours.[9,10]

SYSTEMIC INFLAMMATORY DISEASES

- ◆ A variety of systemic inflammatory diseases may cause pain. Examples include polymyositis, masticatory myositis, polyarthritis, meningitis, and systemic lupus erythematosus.
- ◆ Glucocorticoids are generally used at immunosuppressive doses (e.g., prednisone, 1.1 to 2.2 mg/kg twice daily) to treat these diseases.
- ◆ Alleviation of pain is secondary to the main goal of glucocorticoid therapy, which is to suppress the immune-mediated disorder that underlies these diseases.

OTITIS EXTERNA[11]

- ◆ Topical or systemic use of glucocorticoids is often indicated for the treatment of otitis externa to reduce inflammation and edema in the ear. A decrease in pain is another beneficial effect.
- ◆ A wide variety of otic preparations that contain glucocorticoids are available, including 0.1% dexamethasone, betamethasone, or triamcinolone and 1.0% to 2.5% hydrocortisone. These drugs are administered as sole constituents or in combination with other drugs such as antibiotics.
- ◆ Oral prednisone or prednisolone may be indicated when inflammation is severe, at an antiinflammatory dose of 0.1 to 0.5 mg/kg once or twice daily.

INTRAARTICULAR ADMINISTRATION

◆ The major route for intralesional use of glucocorticoids is intraarticular.
◆ Conflicting data exist on the effects of glucocorticoids on joint cartilage. One study demonstrated minimal or even beneficial effects, whereas others have demonstrated evidence of cartilage damage.[12-15]
◆ Methylprednisolone (20 to 40 mg) and, particularly, triamcinolone (1 to 3 mg) are the preferred drugs for intraarticular administration.[16]

PERINEURAL INJECTION

◆ Injection of glucocorticoids around spinal nerve roots or peripheral nerves has been shown to alleviate pain in persons with nerve root disease or peripheral neuropathies.[17]
◆ This use has not been described in veterinary medicine to date.

EPIDURAL ADMINISTRATION

◆ Epidural glucocorticoid administration often is used in human beings as a conservative treatment for lumbar pain.
◆ The procedure is generally considered safe with minor temporary side effects such as headache.[18,19]
◆ Efficacy is most likely due to reduction in nerve root and meningeal inflammation.[20]
◆ A recent study showed that wound irrigation with 20 or 40 mg of triamcinolone substantially reduced postoperative pain in human beings after lumbar spinal surgery.[21]
◆ Beneficial effects of epidural injection of betamethasone have been demonstrated in a rat model of lumbar nerve root disease.[22]
◆ No recommendations or dosages for epidural glucocorticoid administration have been developed for animals.
◆ Cervical epidural administration of a corticosteroid has a potential for severe deleterious effects if the drug is accidentally administered into the cervical spinal cord parenchyma.[23]

OTHER USES

◆ Methylprednisolone has been shown to be effective in controlling cancer pain in human beings when added to 0.5% bupivacaine and administered intrapleurally.[24]
◆ Glucocorticoids have been used to produce an analgesic-sparing effect in human beings for the treatment of cancer pain or during spinal surgery.[25,26]

TABLE 13-1	Characteristics of Glucocorticoids Commonly Used in Veterinary Medicine		
Glucocorticoid	Relative Antiinflammatory Effect	Duration of Action After IV or Oral Administration (Hours)[27]	Routes of Administration
Hydrocortisone	1	<12	PO, IV, IM
Prednisone	4	12-36	PO, IV, IM, SC
Prednisolone	5	12-36	PO, IV, IM, SC
Methylprednisolone	5	12-36	PO, IV, IM, SC
Triamcinolone	5	12-36 weeks	PO, IM, SC
Betamethasone	25-40	>48	PO, IM
Dexamethasone	30	>48	PO, IV, IM, SC

Veterinary-approved products are not necessarily available.
PO, By mouth (per os); *IV*, intravenous injection; *IM*, intramuscular injection; *SC*, subcutaneous injection.

RELEVANT PHARMACOLOGY

- Synthetic steroids are synthesized from bovine cholic acid or from plant sapogenins.
- Metabolism and excretion of synthetic glucocorticoids occur primarily within the liver and are similar to metabolism and excretion of endogenous glucocorticoids.
- Synthetic glucocorticoids have stronger antiinflammatory effects than do endogenous glucocorticoids (Table 13-1).
- Synthetic glucocorticoids generally have longer half-lives than the naturally occurring forms.
- Synthetic glucocorticoids have greater affinity for cellular glucocorticoid receptors than do endogenous glucocorticoids.

SIDE EFFECTS AND TOXICITY

See Box 13-2.
- Glucocorticoids have a high potential for diverse toxicities because of their effects on almost every tissue in the body.
- Toxicity depends on dose and treatment duration.
- Patient-dependent variations in toxicity also exist.
- Toxicity may result not only from systemic use of glucocorticoids but also from localized use (e.g., ophthalmic, intraarticular, or topical).

BOX 13-2

Potential Adverse Effects of Glucocorticoid Therapy

- Delayed wound healing
- Effects on electrolyte and fluid balance
- Gastric ulceration
- Glaucoma and cataracts
- Hypoadrenocorticism (Addison's disease)
- Iatrogenic bacterial and fungal infections
- Iatrogenic hyperadrenocorticism (Cushing's syndrome)
- Immunosuppression
- Insulin resistance
- Neuropathy and myopathy
- Polyphagia

- ◆ Concurrent medications may potentiate toxicity (e.g., nonsteroidal antiinflammatory agents).
- ◆ Some side effects are managed fairly readily (e.g., polyphagia), whereas others may be life-threatening (e.g., gastric ulceration).
- ◆ Use of glucocorticoids may not slow progression of the primary disease for which the drugs are being used and may mask the primary disease and development of intercurrent disease.[5]

IATROGENIC HYPERADRENOCORTICISM (CUSHING'S SYNDROME)

- ◆ Administration of glucocorticoids for a medium-term or longer period (weeks to months) often results in clinical signs that mimic Cushing's syndrome, including polydipsia, polyuria, skin thinning, and hair loss.

HYPOADRENOCORTICISM (ADDISON'S DISEASE)

- ◆ Prolonged use of exogenous glucocorticoids produces atrophy of the adrenal gland (zona fasciculata and zona reticularis), resulting in the decreased production of endogenous glucocorticoids. Sudden withdrawal of exogenous drugs may produce signs of adrenocortical insufficiency.

NEUROPATHY AND MYOPATHY

- ◆ Signs of myopathy and neuropathy may develop, particularly with chronic glucocorticoid use. Generalized weakness and muscle atrophy are the major clinical signs.

POLYPHAGIA

◆ Increased appetite is a common side effect of glucocorticoid use and appears to be mediated by central nervous system (CNS) centers. Obesity can develop when administration is prolonged for more than a few days to weeks.

EFFECTS ON ELECTROLYTE AND FLUID BALANCE

◆ Glucocorticoids play a key role in the maintenance of normal fluid balance and do have some mineralocorticoid activity. Glucocorticoids promote polydipsia and polyuria as a result of inhibition of antidiuretic hormone release. Glucocorticoid administration also results in excretion of calcium and potassium, sodium and chloride retention, and increased extracellular fluid volume. In rare cases, hypokalemia or hypocalcemia may result from chronic administration.

GLAUCOMA AND CATARACTS

◆ Chronic use of glucocorticoids in the eye can result in the development of glaucoma or cataracts.

GASTRIC ULCERATION

◆ Glucocorticoids promote acid secretion in the stomach and can result in life-threatening gastric and intestinal ulceration. Although experimental studies have suggested that steroid administration alone does not usually cause ulceration, other factors, such as stress, increased autonomic nervous system activity; or the concurrent administration of drugs such as nonsteroidal antiinflammatory drugs may collaborate to cause ulceration.[28]

DELAYED WOUND HEALING

◆ Use of glucocorticoids can result in delayed wound healing.

IMMUNOSUPPRESSION

◆ Prolonged administration of high doses of glucocorticoids can result in immunosuppression and an increased susceptibility to infections in almost any organ system.
◆ The antiinflammatory effects of glucocorticoids may mask the presence of infections until they are severe.

- Glucocorticoids are contraindicated in the presence of infection, except when adequate measures (e.g., antibiotics) are used to control the infection.
- Systemic fungal infections are a particular contraindication to glucocorticoid use.

INSULIN RESISTANCE

- Glucocorticoids antagonize insulin, resulting in increased gluconeogenesis and often hyperglycemia.
- An appetite increase resulting from prolonged glucocorticoid administration results in hyperinsulinism and may lead to diabetes mellitus.

HEPATOPATHY

- Prolonged or high-dose glucocorticoid administration in dogs, but not cats, results in a steroid-induced production of an isoenzyme of alkaline phosphatase by the liver. High levels of this isoenzyme are found in serum of most dogs receiving glucocorticoids and can result in a significant hepatopathy in some animals, even resulting in hepatic failure.

CENTRAL NERVOUS SYSTEM EFFECTS

- Glucocorticoids can cause changes in behavior, particularly restlessness and increased aggression.
- Experimental studies in the rat suggest that glucocorticoids may lower the seizure threshold in the brain.[29]

IATROGENIC BACTERIAL AND FUNGAL INFECTIONS

- Glucocorticoids have diverse effects that combine to induce immunosuppression, making patients susceptible to opportunistic local or systemic infections.
- Intralesional use of glucocorticoids may result in bacterial infections caused by contamination introduced during injection. This could become life-threatening after epidural injections that result in CNS infection.[30]

OTHER SIDE EFFECTS AND TOXICITIES

- Increased intracranial pressure resulting in blindness caused by retinal and vitreal hemorrhages has been reported in one person after epidural steroid injection.[31]

CONCLUSIONS

- ◆ Glucocorticoids reduce pain by decreasing inflammation.
- ◆ Glucocorticoids have diverse and often deleterious effects on many tissues. Glucocorticoid administration can mask progression of the specific disease being treated and can also mask the development of new diseases (e.g., opportunistic infections).
- ◆ Although glucocorticoids may play a role in the control of pain in some patients, they should be used sparingly and with caution.
- ◆ The role of glucocorticoids for adjunctive analgesia and their use by novel routes (e.g., epidural administration) has not yet been thoroughly investigated in veterinary medicine.

REFERENCES

1. Goldfien A: Adrenoglucocorticoids and adrenocortical antagonists. In Katzung BG, editor: *Basic and clinical pharmacology,* Stamford, Conn, 1998, Appleton & Lange.
2. Ferguson D, Hoenig M: Glucocorticoids, mineralocorticoids, and steroid synthesis inhibitors. In Adam HR, editor: *Veterinary pharmacology and therapeutics,* ed 7, Ames, 1995, Iowa State University Press.
3. Kempainnen RJ: Principles of glucocorticoid therapy in nonendocrine disease. In Kirk RW, editor: *Current veterinary therapy IX,* Philadelphia, 1986, WB Saunders.
4. Feldman EC, Nelson RW: *Canine and feline endocrinology and reproduction,* Philadelphia, 1987, WB Saunders.
5. Johnston SA, Fox SM: Mechanisms of action of anti-inflammatory drugs used for the treatment of osteoarthritis, *J Am Vet Med Assoc* 210:1486-1492, 1997.
6. Sutton LC, Fleshner M, Mazzeo R et al: A permissive role of corticosterone in an opioid form of stress-induced analgesia: blockade of opiate analgesia is not due to stress-induced hormone release, *Brain Res* 663:19-29, 1994.
7. Coates JR: Intervertebral disc disease, *Vet Clin North Am Small Anim Pract* 30:77-110, 2000.
8. Hoerlein BF: Further evaluation of the treatment of disc protrusion paraplegia in the dog, *J Am Vet Med Assoc* 129:495-502, 1956.
9. Bracken MB, Shephard MJ, Collins WF Jr et al: A randomized controlled study of methylprednisolone or naloxone in the treatment of acute spinal cord injury, *N Engl J Med* 322:1045, 1990.
10. Siemering GB: High dose methylprednisolone sodium succinate: an adjunct to surgery for canine intervertebral disc herniation, *Vet Surg* 21:406, 1992.
11. Logas D: Appropriate use of glucocorticoids in otitis externa. In Bonagura JD, editor: *Kirk's current veterinary therapy: small animal practice,* ed 13, Philadelphia, 2000, WB Saunders.
12. Pelletier JP, Martel-Pelletier J: Protective effects of glucocorticoids on cartilage lesions and osteophyte formation in the Pond-Nuki model of osteoarthritis, *Arthritis Rheum* 32:181-193, 1989.

13. Chunekamrai S, Krook LP, Lust G et al: Changes in articular cartilage after intra-lesional injections of methylprednisolone acetate in horses, *Am J Vet Res* 50:1733-1741, 1989.

14. Behrens F, Shepard N, Mitchell N: Alterations of rabbit articular cartilage by intra-articular injections of glucocorticoids, *J Bone Joint Surg Am* 57:70-76, 1975.

15. Miller SL, Wertheimer SJ: A comparison of the efficacy of injectable dexamethasone sodium phosphate versus placebo in postoperative podiatric analgesia, *J Foot Ankle Surg* 37:223-226, 1998.

16. Caldwell JR: Intra-articular corticosteroids: guide to selection and indications for use, *Drugs* 52:507-514, 1996.

17. Abram SE: Neural blockade for neuropathic pain, *Clin J Pain* 16:S56-S61, 2000.

18. Botwin KP, Gruber RD, Bouchlas CG, et al: Complications of fluoroscopically guided transforaminal lumbar epidural injections, *Arch Phys Med Rehabil* 81:1045-1050,2000.

19. Reale C, Turkiewicz AM, Reale CA, et al: Epidural steroids as a pharmacological approach, *Clin Exp Rheumatol* 18:S65-S66, 2000.

20. Cannon DT, Aprill CN: Lumbosacral epidural steroid injections, *Arch Phys Med Rehabil* 81:S87-S98, 2000.

21. Pobereskin LH, Sneyd JR: Does wound irrigation with triamcinolone reduce pain after surgery to the lumbar spine? *Br J Anaesth* 84:731-734, 2000.

22. Hayashi N, Weinstein JN, Meller ST et al: The effect of epidural injection of betamethasone or bupivacaine in a rat model of lumbar radiculopathy, *Spine* 23:877-885, 1998.

23. Hodges SD, Castleberg RL, Miller T et al: Cervical epidural steroid injection with intrinsic spinal cord damage: two case reports, *Spine* 23:2137-2142, 1998.

24. Klein DS, Klein PW: Intermittent interpleural injection of bupivacaine and methylprednisolone for analgesia in metastatic thoracic neoplasm, *Clin J Pain* 7:232-236, 1991.

25. Twycross R: The risks and benefits of corticosteroids in advanced cancer, *Drug Saf* 11:163-178, 1994.

26. Korman B, MacKay RJ: Steroids and postoperative analgesia, *Anaesth Intensive Care* 13:395-398, 1985.

27. Plumb DC, editor: *Veterinary drug handbook,* ed 3, Ames, 1999, Iowa State University Press.

28. Hanson SM, Bostwick DR, Twedt DC et al: Clinical evaluation of cimetidine, sucralfate, and misoprostol for prevention of gastrointestinal tract bleeding in dogs undergoing spinal surgery, *Am J Vet Res* 58:1320-1323, 1997.

29. Lee PH, Grimes L, Hong JS: Glucocorticoids potentiate kainic acid-induced seizures and wet dog shakes, *Brain Res* 480:322-325, 1989.

30. Cooper AB, Sharpe MD: Bacterial meningitis and cauda equina syndrome after epidural steroid injections, *Can J Anaesth* 43:471-474, 1996.

31. Victory RA, Hassett P, Morrison G: Transient blindness following epidural analgesia, *Anaesthesia* 46:940-941, 1991.

14 OTHER DRUGS USED TO TREAT PAIN

JAMES S. GAYNOR

This section outlines drugs that have demonstrated or have perceived analgesic efficacy but are not in the mainstream of veterinary practice. Many of these drugs are commonly used in management of human pain. Much of the evidence substantiating their use comes from laboratory animal research, clinical trials in humans, or anecdotal reports in humans and animals.

INJECTABLE DRUGS

KETAMINE

> Microdoses of ketamine intraoperatively can decrease analgesia requirements postoperatively.

Mechanism of Action

Ketamine has traditionally been considered a dissociative anesthetic. Recently, ketamine has been characterized as a nonspecific N-methyl-D-aspartate (NMDA) receptor antagonist.

Efficacy/Use

NMDA receptor stimulation has been associated with central neuronal sensitization, the windup phenomenon. Blockade of the NMDA receptor results in the ability to provide analgesia with potentially lower doses of opioids and less dysphoria.[1,2] NMDA antagonism is also helpful in preventing severe acute pain and potentially chronic pain.

- ◆ Microdoses of ketamine, much lower than those used for anesthesia or chemical restraint, are used as an adjunct to analgesia protocols.

- Initial dosing of ketamine is 0.5 mg/kg IV before surgical stimulation.
- An infusion, 10 μg/kg per minute, is administered during the procedure until the end of stimulation.
- A lower infusion rate, 2 μg/kg per minute, is administered for the next 24 hours.
- Some studies have advocated an additional lower infusion rate, 1 μg/kg per minute, for the next 24 hours postoperatively.
- In the absence of an infusion pump, 0.6 ml (60 mg) of ketamine can be added to a 1-L bag of crystalloid solutions to be administered at 10 ml/kg per hour to achieve the intraoperative dosing rate, 10 μg/kg per minute.
- For administration of ketamine at 2 μg/kg per minute without a syringe pump postoperatively, 0.6 ml (60 mg) of ketamine for every 20 kg of body mass can be added to a 1-L bag of crystalloid solutions to be administered at 2 ml/kg per hour, approximately normal maintenance fluid rate for an awake patient.

Pharmacology

The pharmacology of microdose ketamine dosing has not been well established. Even with the low dosing, it has been demonstrated that ketamine actually binds NMDA receptors in dogs.[3]

Side Effects and Toxicity

The microdose ketamine appears to have few if any side effects. Anecdotal accounts indicate that small numbers of patients develop tachycardia.

Special Issues

One must remember that microdose ketamine by itself does not induce analgesia. Ketamine must be used in conjunction with an analgesic such as an opioid.

MAGNESIUM
Mechanism of Action

Central sensitization, or windup, is mediated by a cascade of events, including neuronal depolarization and NMDA receptor phosphorylation, resulting in an increase in the excitability of a cell. Activation of the NMDA receptor involves removal of a magnesium block. Presumably, administration of magnesium may decrease windup and act independently to suppress calcium currents and neuronal excitability. Intrathecal magnesium administration may also potentiate the effect of morphine and delay the onset of opioid tolerance.[4]

Efficacy/Use

◆ Very little information is available concerning magnesium use or efficacy for animal pain. Magnesium has been used intravenously in humans for treatment of headache, postoperative pain, and neuropathic pain and subarachnoidally for allodynia and as an adjunct to intrathecal morphine administration.[5,6]

◆ A dose of 5 to 15 mg/kg IV has been extrapolated from humans. This dose is used for refractory cardiac dysrhythmias in dogs with no apparent side effects.

◆ Humans have been administered a 50 mg/kg IV bolus followed by 8 mg/kg per hour as an adjuvant to perioperative analgesia management with fentanyl.[7]

Pharmacology

Magnesium is predominantly an intracellular ion. The pharmacology of magnesium is under investigation in animals.

Side Effects and Toxicity

In humans, minor side effects include headache and internal heat sensation. Vasodilation may cause, or predispose to, hypotension.

Special Issues

Measurement of plasma magnesium may be misleading because it may not reflect the intracellular component.

KETOROLAC (TORADOL)
Mechanism of Action

Ketorolac is a potent nonsteroidal antiinflammatory drug (NSAID) that produces analgesia similar to an opioid μ-agonist such as morphine or oxymorphone for some types of pain. Ketorolac is available in oral and parenteral formulations. The mechanism of action is similar to other NSAIDs (see Chapter 10), and ketorolac should be used with caution because there may be a high incidence of side effects.

Efficacy/Use

◆ Ketorolac is indicated for the management of moderate to severe pain and is synergistic with opioids.

◆ Although the use of ketorolac is limited to 5 days in humans, dogs and cats should not receive more than two treatments because of the side effects.[8]

Ketorolac should be used with caution because of its high likelihood of inducing gastrointestinal adverse effects.

- Dogs
    1. Postsurgical pain: 0.3 to 0.6 mg/kg IV or IM every 8 to 12 hours[8,9]
    2. 0.6 mg/kg IM apparently equipotent to oxymorphone 0.1 mg/kg IM[10]
    3. Nonsurgical orthopedic pain: dogs greater than 30 kg, 10 mg/dog orally once daily for 2 to 3 days
- Cats: Postsurgical pain—0.25 mg/kg IM every 12 to 24 hours
- Misoprostol (2 to 5 µg/kg orally every 8 hours) can be used as prophylaxis against gastrointestinal ulcer in dogs receiving ketorolac (see Chapter 10).

Pharmacology

Ketorolac, like other NSAIDs, is metabolized by the liver. The pharmacology in dogs is similar to that in humans. Ketorolac has an elimination half-life of 4½ hours.[11] The pharmacology in cats is not well described.

Side Effects and Toxicity

- In humans ketorolac is not used for more than 5 days because of the high likelihood of developing severe side effects such as gastrointestinal bleeding, perforating ulcers, and coagulation disorders. Similar side effects can be expected in dogs.
- Ketorolac should not be used in conjunction with other NSAIDs, corticosteroids, or aspirin.

Special Issues

- Ketorolac should not be used as a preemptive analgesic because of the unpredictability of hypotension under anesthesia and the greater increased risk of renal damage.
- Ketorolac should not be used intraoperatively in patients that may hemorrhage because of the likelihood of inhibition of normal clotting function.
- Ketorolac is contraindicated in patients with renal disease and those at risk for renal impairment due to hypovolemia and hypotension.

CLONIDINE
Mechanism of Action

Clonidine is an α2-agonist that produces analgesia independently and when administered in combination with opioids. Clonidine blocks the conduction of nerve fibers and has also been demonstrated to induce enkephalin-like substance release at peripheral sites.

Efficacy/Use

- Clonidine has been administered intrathecally in dogs, cats, and humans.
- Studies conducted in humans have shown clonidine to provide analgesia for postoperative pain.
- Clonidine could have potential use as an alternative to opioids for chronic pain in animals that have developed a tolerance to opioids or that experience pain unresponsive to opioid treatment.

Pharmacology

A study conducted in humans found the following[12]:
- Clonidine had an elimination half-life of 20 to 25½ hours, which remained constant after single and multiple doses.
- Approximately 62% of a dose was excreted unchanged in the urine, regardless of dose, formulation, or route of administration.
- No overshoot was observed after stopping administration.

Side Effects and Toxicity

Bradycardia and hypotension are likely to occur after clonidine administration. Bradyarrhythmias and sedation have also been noted in animals. Humans have reported experiencing dry mouth after clonidine administration.

Special Issues

Clonidine is not antagonized by naloxone. Doses in dogs and cats are unclear.

ZICONOTIDE
Mechanism of Action

Ziconotide blocks neurotransmission by blocking calcium channels.

Efficacy/Use

Ziconotide is an intrathecal analgesic indicated for severe chronic pain that is unresponsive to opioid treatment.

Pharmacology

- In humans, the clearance is 0.38 ml/min.
- Ziconotide maintains its analgesic efficacy over months and does not cause tolerance, dependence, or respiratory depression in humans.

Side Effects and Toxicity

Side effects reported in humans include bradycardia, dizziness, nausea, and confusion. These side effects are mild to moderate in severity and resolve over time and reverse after drug discontinuation.

Special Issues

Ziconotide should be used with caution in dogs and cats because experience with use in these species is limited. Doses in dogs and cats are unclear.

ORAL DRUGS

TRAMADOL

Mechanism of Action

Tramadol is a synthetic, centrally acting analgesic that is not related to opioids.[13]
- Tramadol binds to μ-opioid receptors.
  1. The parent compound has weak binding affinity.
  2. The metabolites have 200 times the binding affinity for the μ-receptor.
- Tramadol inhibits reuptake of norepinephrine and serotonin, thus acting like an α2-agonist.
- The mixed mechanism of action helps explain why naloxone (an opioid antagonist) only partially reverses the analgesia.

Efficacy/Use

- Tramadol may be useful for moderate to severe pain. Tramadol has analgesic potency similar to meperidine.[14]
- In humans, tramadol has been used to alleviate pain associated with osteoarthritis, fibromyalgia, diabetic neuropathy, and neuropathic pain.

Tramadol can provide mild to moderate pain control and works especially well in conjunction with a nonsteroidal antiinflammatory drug.

- Tramadol may also be useful in patients with allodynia.[15]
- Humans dosed with 50 to 200 mg orally postoperatively or for chronic pain seem to experience good analgesia.
- Clinically, dogs respond to doses of 3 to 5 mg/kg PO bid to qid.
- Cats respond to doses of tramadol similar to dogs. Larger cats can be given portions of a tramadol tablet. If tramadol needs to be compounded, it may be difficult to mask the bitterness without compounding it into a capsule.
- Tramadol can be administered to dogs and cats at 2 to 4 mg/kg IV.

Pharmacology

- Oral dosing of tramadol in dogs results in rapid absorption with approximately 75% bioavailability. Dosing with or without food seems to make no difference.
- The biotransformation of tramadol is qualitatively similar between dogs and humans. Dogs metabolize approximately 99% of tramadol, whereas humans metabolize about 30%. The balance of the drug appears to be excreted unchanged by the kidneys.[16]

Side Effects and Toxicity

- Tramadol may cause respiratory depression when combined with other anesthetics, although this has not been documented in dogs and cats.
- Short-term administration of tramadol may cause some nausea and vomiting, although this is unlikely at recommended doses.
- Long-term administration may cause constipation or diarrhea. This occurs infrequently in dogs. The likelihood is unknown in cats.
- A small percentage of humans anecdotally have related seizures when taking tramadol. This has not been documented in dogs or cats.

Special Issues

Tramadol is less likely to induce tolerance in animals and humans compared with morphine because of its nonopioid mechanism of action.[17]

AMANTADINE

Amantadine was originally developed as an antiviral drug for use in humans. Amantadine has been shown to have efficacy for treatment of drug-induced extrapyramidal effects and for Parkinson's disease.

Amantadine may help with allodynia and opioid tolerance in patients with chronic pain.

Mechanism of Action

Amantadine has antagonist effects at the NMDA receptor.

Efficacy/Use

- In humans, amantadine has been used for neuropathic pain.[18,19]
- Amantadine is used in animals suffering from windup, allodynia, and opioid tolerance. Amantadine use may permit a lower dose of the opioid and helps increase analgesia provided by the opioid. Dogs with problem osteoarthritis often demonstrate increased efficacy of their primary NSAID when amantadine is administered for 21 days as needed. Amantadine also appears to be helpful in maintaining comfort in dogs with osteosarcoma.
- The dose for dogs and cats is approximately 3 to 5 mg/kg PO once daily. Amantadine is available in 100-mg capsules and a 10-mg/ml liquid.

Pharmacology

The pharmacology of amantadine in dogs and cats has not been well established, although the pharmacology of rimantadine, a similar drug, is known for dogs.[19] Amantadine is well absorbed in humans, is not metabolized, and is excreted in the urine.

Side Effects and Toxicity

- The feline toxic dose is 30 mg/kg.[19]
- Dogs may develop high anxiety, restlessness, and dry mouth as the daily dose approaches 6 mg/kg or if there is impaired renal excretion.
- Behavioral effects in dogs and cats[10] begin at 15 mg/kg orally.

Special Issues

The duration of action of amantadine may be prolonged in patients with renal insufficiency.

GABAPENTIN

Gabapentin is a structural analog of γ-aminobutyric acid (GABA).[20] Gabapentin was originally introduced as an antiepileptic drug.

Mechanism of Action

The mechanism of action of gabapentin is unclear and elusive.

◆ Although gabapentin is related to GABA, it does not appear to have any analgesic effect at GABA receptors.

◆ Gabapentin does not interact with NMDA receptors, and its analgesic effects are likely unrelated to blockade of sodium channels, binding of opioid receptors, alteration of cyclooxygenase activity, or inhibition of dopamine, serotonin, or norepinephrine uptake.

Efficacy/Use

> Gabapentin is useful for helping control pain related to neuropathic conditions, osteoarthritis, and cancer.

◆ A number of rat studies have investigated the effects of gabapentin on signs of neuropathic pain, such as hyperalgesia and allodynia. Other studies indicate a role for gabapentin in decreasing incisional pain and arthritis.[21]

◆ Gabapentin appears to be best suited for pain of nonnociceptive origin.

◆ Exact indications and efficacy for gabapentin have not yet been determined.

◆ Most information related to pain and gabapentin has been derived from anecdotal case reports in humans:

1. Neuralgia has occurred following herpes zoster infection.
2. Diabetic neuropathy: Whether veterinary patients develop this problem is unclear.
3. Neuropathic cancer pain: When gabapentin is added to an opioid regimen for patients who are only partially opioid responsive, the patients experience significantly better analgesia. These patients also experience less allodynia.
4. Burning and lancinating pain is more likely to respond to gabapentin compared with dull, aching pain.

◆ A number of animal studies, especially in rats, have been performed to generate more specific information regarding the uses for and effects of gabapentin.

1. Gabapentin does not alter nociceptive/pain thresholds; therefore, it does not produce analgesia when administered alone but assists other drugs in producing analgesia (adjunctive analgesic).

2. Gabapentin has different effects in normal patients compared with those with inflammatory pain states.
   a. In the absence of any pathologic pain, gabapentin may actually facilitate nociceptive responses in spinal cord dorsal horn neurons.
   b. Gabapentin dose-dependently inhibits dorsal horn responses to inflammation-induced pain.
3. Gabapentin decreases allodynia related to mechanical pressure and cold but does not affect nociceptive thresholds.
4. Gabapentin reduces hyperalgesia when given systemically or intrathecally.
5. Gabapentin, given prophylactically, can inhibit hyperalgesia related to incisional, peripheral nerve, and thermal injury.

◆ Dosing
1. Although dosing has not been established in dogs or cats, the following recommendations are extrapolations from humans. One must remember that there are no controlled or evidence-based studies in dogs and cats using gabapentin. Gabapentin has been investigated as an antiepileptic drug in dogs, with dosing between 800 and 1500 mg daily.
2. Initial doses range from 2.5 to 10 mg/kg PO bid.
3. Doses may be able to be increased up to 50 mg/kg PO bid to tid. Anecdotally, some practitioners have used even higher doses more frequently.

Pharmacology

Gabapentin is highly bioavailable in dogs. Gabapentin is metabolized by the liver and almost exclusively excreted by the kidneys. The pharmacokinetics of gabapentin are not changed by multiple dosing. The half-life is about 3 to 4 hours.

Side Effects

In human clinical trials the side effects occur in 25% or less of patients:
◆ Sleepiness
◆ Fatigue
◆ Weight gain with chronic administration

Special Issues

The use of gabapentin for analgesia has only been anecdotally reported in clinical veterinary patients, but gabapentin appears to be a useful adjunct to NSAIDs for the control of problem osteoarthritis pain. Gabapentin has also been used effectively as part of a multimodal approach for control of cancer pain.

PREGABALIN
Mechanism of Action

◆ Pregabalin binds with high affinity to the α2-delta site in the central nervous system. The exact mechanism of action is unclear, but this binding affinity is likely related to the antinociceptive and antiseizure effects of pregabalin in animal models.

◆ Pregabalin does not block sodium channels, bind opioid receptors, or alter cyclooxygenase activity, and it does not inhibit dopamine, serotonin, or norepinephrine uptake.

Efficacy/Use

Pregabalin is indicated for the relief of neuropathic pain related to diabetic neuropathy and postherpetic neuralgia, in addition to the control of epilepsy in humans.

◆ Pregabalin is likely useful for similar conditions in animals. A similar compound, PD-0200347, has been shown to decrease cartilage lesions in experimental studies of canine osteoarthritis.[22]

◆ The appropriate dose of pregabalin in domestic species is unknown. Extrapolating from humans, the dog dose would range from 0.3 to 4.0 mg/kg PO bid to tid. Caution should be exercised in dosing domestic animals because of the lack of information.

Pharmacology

Pregabalin is excreted almost entirely unchanged by the kidneys in humans, rats, and monkeys. The pharmacology in domestic species is unclear at this time.

Side Effects and Toxicity

The most common side effects of pregabalin in humans seem to be dizziness and somnolence. The side effect profile in dogs and cats is unknown.

Special Issues

Pregabalin is classified as schedule V controlled substance and should be handled with the appropriate considerations.

MEXILETINE
Mechanism of Action

Mexiletine inhibits nerve conduction by blocking sodium channels.

Efficacy/Use

Mexiletine has been used in humans for the treatment of peripheral neuropathic pain.

Pharmacology

- Mexiletine reduces the rate of rise of the action potential by inhibiting the inward sodium current.
- Mexiletine is relatively well absorbed from the gut and has a low first-pass effect.
- Mexiletine can be dosed in dogs at 5 to 8 mg/kg PO bid to tid. Mexiletine is contraindicated in cats.

Side Effects and Toxicity

Gastrointestinal disturbances are the most likely effect in animals. Central nervous system effects (tremors, dizziness), shortness of breath, premature ventricular contractions, and chest pain have been reported in humans. Seizures, agranulocytosis, and thrombocytopenia are rare but may occur.

Special Issues

Use with caution in animals with liver disease or heart dysfunction.

ALENDRONATE

Mechanism of Action

Alendronate is a bisphosphonate that inhibits osteoclast-mediated bone resorption.

Efficacy/Use

In human patients with osteosarcoma-related pain, alendronate has been used to reduce pain and pathologic fractures.

Pharmacology

Alendronate is excreted unchanged in humans and has a long half-life (measured in weeks).
- Alendronate should not be given with food. Feeding should be delayed for a minimum of 30 minutes after administration.
- Alendronate should not be administered with other medications that may contain calcium.

Dosing

Dogs can be administered 0.5 to 1.0 mg/kg orally *once* daily. No dose has been described in cats.

Side Effects and Toxicity

In humans, gastrointestinal effects are most common. Osteonecrosis of the jaw has also been reported.

Special Issues

Alendronate should not be used in patients with severe kidney disease.

NIMODIPINE
Mechanism of Action

Nimodipine enhances the antinociceptive properties of morphine by blocking calcium channels.

Efficacy/Use

Nimodipine has been administered perioperatively in humans to decrease postoperative morphine requirements.

Pharmacology

Nimodipine is an L-type dihydropyridine calcium channel blocker with relatively high blood-brain-barrier penetration.

Side Effects and Toxicity

Hypotension has been reported in humans.

Special Issues

Research of the use of nimodipine in dogs and cats is lacking.

NIFEDIPINE
Mechanism of Action

Nifedipine is a calcium channel blocker.

Efficacy/Use

Nifedipine has been administered sublingually with epidural morphine administration in humans to decrease morphine requirements and improve analgesia.

Pharmacology

A study conducted in rats showed that nifedipine has an inhibitory effect on morphine-induced corticosterone secretion.[23]

Side Effects and Toxicity

Hypotension has been reported in humans.

Special Issues

Research of the use of nifedipine in dogs and cats is lacking. Therefore, no good doses can be recommended.

NUTRACEUTICALS

Multiple nutraceuticals are available over the counter for use in animals. These include glucosamine sulfate, glucosamine hydrochloride, chondroitin sulfate, *Perna canaliculus,* methylsulfonylmethane, microlactin, and buffered vitamin C. Some doses and potential side effects have been determined (Table 14-1).

Nutraceutical formulations are not controlled by the Food and Drug Administration. Therefore, there is no oversight of quality or quantity in the various products available.

◆ Glucosamine/chondroitin
  • Many glucosamine/chondroitin supplements are available for humans and animals. There seem to be few formulations for which there are data for efficacy in pets.
  1. The combination of glucosamine hydrochloride, low-molecular-weight chondroitin, and manganese has been shown to induce biosynthetic activity in canine cartilage.
  2. This combination also has a protective effect when administered before an acute joint injury. Patients receiving this combination before joint injury heal more quickly than those administered the combination after injury.[24]
◆ Data support the supplementation of *P. canaliculus* based on the effects in a rat model[25] and in humans with arthritis.[26]
◆ No clinical data support the use of methylsulfonamethane or buffered vitamin C in animals in the relief of pain. These products may be beneficial, but well-controlled studies have not been performed to document this.
◆ Emerging data indicate that the combination of glucosamine hydrochloride, *P. canaliculus,* methylsulfonylmethane, and manganese may be effective at ameliorating the clinical signs of osteoarthritis in dogs.[27]
◆ Microlactin is thought to be a potent inhibitor of neutrophil adherence, migration, and participation in the immune response to musculoskeletal conditions including arthritis. Unpublished data show efficacy for pain relief in dogs with osteoarthritis.
◆ Buffered vitamin C is believed to have chondroprotective, antiinflammatory, and immunoresponsive effects that may provide pain control for animals with osteoarthritis. No documented evidence exists for its efficacy in veterinary patients.

TABLE 14-1	Concerns and Dosages Associated with Commonly Administered Nutraceuticals		
		Dosage	
Nutraceutical	**Concerns**	**Dogs**	**Cats**
Glucosamine sulfate Glucosamine hydrochloride	Minor gastrointestinal (GI) disturbance	Large dogs: up to 750 mg PO bid	250 mg PO bid
Glucosamine + chondroitin sulfate	Minor GI disturbance	13-15 mg/kg chondroitin PO sid	15-20 mg/kg chondroitin PO sid
Perna canaliculus	Allergic reactions, fluid retention, skin rash, and upset stomach. In addition, *Perna* mussel supplements should not be given to persons or animals with allergies to fish or shellfish.	*1-20 kg:* loading dose (10 days): 2 tablets per day; maintenance dose: 1 tablet per day *21-40 kg:* loading dose: 3 tablets per day; maintenance dose: 2 tablets per day *40 kg and over:* loading dose: 4 tablets per day; maintenance dose: 3 tablets per day (1 tablet = 600 mg)	
Methylsulfonylmethane	Sulfur toxicity at extreme doses	Large dogs: up to 2 g PO bid	100-250 mg PO bid
Microlactin	Vomiting, diarrhea	*Less than 40 lb:* 500 mg PO bid *40-80 lb:* 1000 mg PO bid *81-120 lb:* 1500 mg PO bid	*Up to 12 lb:* 200 mg PO bid *Over 12 lb:* 300 mg PO bid
Buffered vitamin C	Minor GI disturbance at high doses; should not be administered with anesthetics	Gradually increase dose to 250-1000 mg PO bid	Gradually increase dose to 250 mg PO bid

REFERENCES

1. Felsby S, Nielsen J, Arendt-Nielsen L et al: NMDA receptor blockade in chronic neuropathic pain: a comparison of ketamine and magnesium chloride, *Pain* 64:283-291, 1996.

2. Wilder-Smith OH, Arendt-Nielsen L, Gaumann D et al: Sensory changes and pain after abdominal hysterectomy: a comparison of anesthetic supplementation with fentanyl versus magnesium or ketamine, *Anesth Analg* 86:95-101, 1998.

3. Mama KR, Golden AE, Monnet E et al: Plasma and cerebrospinal fluid concentrations and NMDA receptor binding activity associated with intraoperative administration of low-dose ketamine. In *Proceedings 7th World Congress of Veterinary Anaesthesia, Berne* 2000 p 78, 2000 (abstract).

4. Ren K, Dubner R: Central nervous system plasticity and persistent pain, *J Orofac Pain* 13:155-163, 1999 (review; 68 refs; discussion, pp 164–171).

5. Crosby V, Wilcock A, Corcoran R: The safety and efficacy of a single dose (500 mg or 1 g) of intravenous magnesium sulfate in neuropathic pain poorly responsive to strong opioid analgesics in patients with cancer, *J Pain Symptom Manage* 19:35-39, 2000.

6. Kroin JS, McCarthy RJ, Von Roenn N et al: Magnesium sulfate potentiates morphine antinociception at the spinal level, *Anesth Analg* 90:913-917, 2000.

7. Koinig H, Wallner T, Marhofer P et al: Magnesium sulfate reduces intra- and postoperative analgesic requirements, *Anesth Analg* 87:206-210, 1998.

8. Mathews KA: Nonsteroidal anti-inflammatory analgesics: indications and contraindications for pain management in dogs and cats, *Vet Clin North Am Small Anim Pract* 30:783-804, 2000.

9. Mathews KA, Paley DM, Foster RA et al: A comparison of ketorolac with flunixin, butorphanol, and oxymorphone in controlling postoperative pain in dogs, *Can Vet J* 37:557-567, 1996.

10. Popilskis S, Jordan D, Laurent L et al: Comparison of ketorolac and oxymorphone on postoperative pain relief and neuroendocrine response in dogs, *6th ICVA* p 107, 1997.

11. Pasloske K, Renaud R, Burger J et al: Pharmacokinetics of ketorolac after intravenous and oral single dose administration in dogs, *J Vet Pharmacol Ther* 22:314-319, 1999.

12. De Kock M, Crochet B, Morimont C, Scholtes JL: Intravenous or epidural clonidine for intra- and postoperative analgesia, *Anesthesiology* 79:525-531, 1993.

13. Minto CF, Power I: New opioid analgesics: an update, *Int Anesthesiol Clin* 35:49-65 1997 (review; 95 refs).

14. Lehmann KA: Tramadol for the management of acute pain, *Drugs* 47(suppl 1):19-32, 1994 (review; 71 refs).

15. Sindrup SH, Anderson G, Madsen C et al: Tramadol relieves pain and allodynia in polyneuropathy: a randomised, double-blind, controlled trial, *Pain* 83:85-90, 1999.

16. Lintz W, Erlacin S, Frankus E et al: [Biotransformation of tramadol in man and animal] (author's translation from German), *Arzneimittelforschung* 31:1932-1943, 1981.

17. Miranda HF, Pinardi G: Antinociception, tolerance, and physical dependence comparison between morphine and tramadol, *Pharmacol Biochem Behav* 61:357-360, 1998.

18. Pud D, Eisenberg E, Spitzer A et al: The NMDA receptor antagonist amantidine reduces surgical neuropathic pain in cancer patients: a double blind, randomized, placebo controlled trial, *Pain* 75:349-354, 1998.

19. Eisenberg E, Pud D: Can patients with chronic neuropathic pain be cured by acute administration of the NMDA receptor antagonist amantidine, *Pain* 74:337-339, 1988.

20. Radulovic LL, Turck D, von Hodenberg A et al: Disposition of gabapentin (neurontin) in mice, rats, dogs, and monkeys, *Drug Metab Dispos* 23:441-448, 1995.

21. Mao J, Chen LL: Gabapentin in pain management, *Anesth Analg* 91:680-687, 2000.

22. Boileau C, Martel-Pelletier J, Brunet J et al: Oral treatment with PD-0200347, an alpha2delta ligand, reduces the development of experimental osteoarthritis by inhibiting metalloproteinases and inducible nitric oxide synthase gene expression and synthesis in cartilage chondrocytes, *Arthritis Rheum* 52:488-500, 2005.

23. Mahani SE, Motamedi F, Ahmadiani A: Involvement of hypothalamic adrenal axis on the nifedipine-induced antinociception and tolerance in rats, *Pharmacol Biochem Behav* 85:422-427, 2006.

24. Canapp SO, McLaughlin RM, Hoskinson JJ et al: Scintigraphic evaluation of glucosamine hydrochloride and chondroitin sulfate as a treatment for acute synovitis in dogs, *Am J Vet Res* 60:1552-1557, 1999.

25. Lawson BR, Belkowski SM, Whitesides JF et al: Immunomodulation of murine collagen-induced arthritis by N, N-dimethylglycine and a preparation of *Perna canaliculus*, *BMC Complement Altern Med* 7:20, 2007.

26. Hurley L: New research and clinical report on the use of Perna canaliculus in the management of arthritis, *Townsend Letter for Doctors and Patients* pp 99-111, 2000.

27. Martinez SA, McCormick DJ, Powers MY et al: The effect of Glyco-Flex III on a stable stifle osteoarthritis model in dogs: a pilot study. Presented at the Veterinary Orthopedic Society Annual Scientific Meeting, Sun Valley, Idaho, 2007.

5

LOCAL AND REGIONAL ANESTHETIC TECHNIQUES FOR ALLEVIATION OF PERIOPERATIVE PAIN

JAMES S. GAYNOR AND KHURSHEED R. MAMA

Regional anesthesia implies that a region of the body is desensitized as opposed to the entire body, as occurs with general anesthesia. The region affected may be limited or broad. Unlike most instances of general anesthesia, during which it is mainly the "perception of pain" that is blocked (by virtue of unconsciousness), local anesthetics block the "transmission of noxious impulses." Because the analgesic effects of local anesthetics do not depend on central depression (anesthesia), regional analgesic techniques may be used in a conscious patient.

TOPICAL ANESTHESIA

- Surface, or topical, anesthesia results when the drug is applied to the skin or mucous membrane to cause loss of sensation by paralyzing sensory nerve endings.
- Local anesthetics are widely used on the mucous membranes of the eye, nose, and mouth. Most are ineffective if used on unbroken skin because cornified epidermis limits penetration.
- The introduction of a combination of lidocaine and prilocaine in a eutectic mixture has overcome this problem and is now commonly used to provide dermal analgesia for venipuncture and catheterization. This drug combination may cause methemoglobinemia in cats and has decreased in popularity since its introduction.
- A rapidly acting lidocaine cream, LMX 5 (anorectal cream), containing 5% lidocaine, is also available for producing fast-acting local analgesic effects. LMX 5 can be used to relieve pain caused by minor cuts, minor burns, abrasions, sunburn, and minor surgical sites. Lidocaine preparations are also commonly used to numb the skin before performing minor surgery, insertion of intravenous (IV) lines, obtaining blood specimens, and other such procedures. LMX 5 should only be used externally.

◆ The 5% lidocaine patch preparation (Lidoderm patch) produces local tissue concentrations far below those capable of producing toxicity but high enough to produce clinically effective local analgesia for periods of up to 24 hours without complete sensory block. The patches have been used to provide analgesia for skin abrasions, lacerations, and severe local skin irritation and itching (hot spots). The patch is supplied as a 10 × 14-cm adhesive bandage that may be cut into smaller sizes with a scissors *before* removing the protective drug release liner. Care should be taken to avoid contact with the attendant's skin or eyes in order to prevent numbing of the fingers or irritation, respectively.

TECHNIQUE

1. Clip the fur over the site to be desensitized.
2. Liberally apply the cream, and cover it with an occlusive bandage.
3. Apply the lidocaine patch, or cut it to the appropriate size and use it as a bandage (Fig. 15-1).

ANESTHESIA BY INFILTRATION

◆ Infiltration anesthesia is perhaps the most common method of regional anesthesia and consists of making numerous subcutaneous injections of small volumes of local anesthetic solution into the tissues.

CAUTION WITH LOCAL ANESTHETIC
Always aspirate for blood before injecting any local anesthetic.

◆ The drug diffuses into surrounding tissue from the site of injection and anesthetizes nerve fibers and endings. Large amounts of relatively dilute solutions are often infiltrated into operative sites.
◆ Epinephrine (1:200,000) may be used in combination with infiltration of local anesthetic to reduce systemic absorption of the anesthetic agent and prolong the duration of analgesia.

EPINEPHRINE AND LOCAL ANESTHETIC
Epinephrine should be combined with a local anesthetic only for blocks that are not on the distal extremities. This prevents distal ischemia.

◆ Acute pain therapy can be continued by infiltration anesthesia for several days by using the PainBuster Soaker (PainBuster Post-Op Pain Relief System; I-Flow Corp, Lake Forest, California). The local

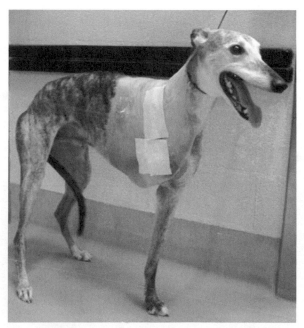

FIG. 15-1. Lidocaine patch applied to a dog.

anesthetic is delivered by an elastomeric reservoir (pump), which is filled with local anesthetic (e.g., lidocaine). The pump is attached to delivery tubing and a sterile multipore catheter that is placed at the surgical site. The elastomeric reservoir bulb delivers local anesthetic at a constant rate (0.5 to 5 ml/h) for up to 5 days (Fig. 15-2).

INCISIONAL LINE BLOCK

◆ Incisional line block is used before surgical incision or after the surgery before complete closure.

LINE BLOCK BEFORE INCISION
Needle

◆ 25-gauge, 2.5-cm (1-inch) or longer hypodermic or spinal needle

Technique

1. Insert the needle subcutaneously after a sterile prep.
2. Aspirate.
3. Inject enough local anesthetic to produce a noticeable bleb.

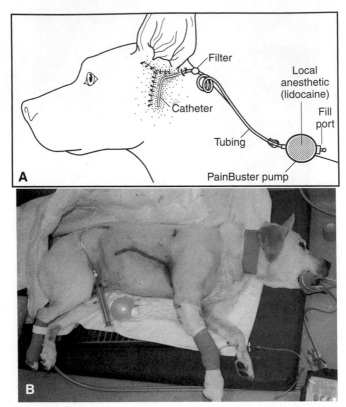

FIG. 15-2. A, Anesthesia by continuous infiltration of local anesthetic after total ear canal ablation. **B,** Anesthesia by continuous infiltration of local anesthetic of a large incision.

4. Remove the needle, and reinsert at the edge of the bleb.
5. After aspiration, inject more local anesthetic to extend the bleb.
6. Repeat the process until the length of the incision has been blocked.
   • Bupivacaine (0.5% = 5 mg/ml) with or without epinephrine or lidocaine (2% = 20 mg/ml) with or without epinephrine is often used at a dose of 1 to 2 mg/kg. This solution is then diluted with an equal amount of 0.9% saline to increase the injectate volume.

INCISIONAL BLOCK BEFORE CLOSING INCISION
Needle

◆ 25-gauge, 2.5-cm (1-inch) or longer hypodermic or spinal needle

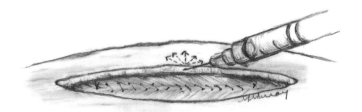

FIG. 15-3. Incisional block.

Technique (Fig. 15-3)

1. Incisional block is done in a sterile manner by the surgeon. Someone must pass the needle and syringe aseptically to the surgeon to prevent contamination.
2. Insert the needle at one end on the midline of the incision before closing the skin.
3. After aspiration for blood, inject local anesthetic in a fanlike manner to block subcutaneous and muscular tissues. If this is being performed on the abdominal body wall, inject local anesthetic down to the peritoneum.
4. Remove the needle and reinsert a slight distance away, reinjecting local anesthetic in a fanlike manner.
5. Repeat until the area under the whole incision has been infiltrated.

PERIPHERAL NERVE BLOCK

- The peripheral nerve block is a conduction block produced by injection of local anesthetic in the immediate vicinity of individual peripheral nerves or a nerve plexus.
- Paravertebral nerve blocks in cattle and horses, intercostal nerve blocks, and the brachial plexus block in dogs and cats may be considered examples of peripheral nerve blocks. Interpleural anesthesia is an alternative to multiple intercostal nerve blocks and may be considered a regional peripheral nerve block.

INTERPLEURAL BLOCK

- The interpleural block is used to provide analgesia and anesthesia related to thoracic and cranial abdominal pain, especially pain related to pancreatitis.

Needles

- 22-gauge butterfly catheter
- 20-gauge, 5-cm (2-inch) through-the-needle catheter
- Preexisting chest tube

Technique (Fig. 15-4)

1. Aseptically prepare the site of catheter insertion.
2. Place the catheter in the ninth intercostal space on the midlateral aspect of the thorax.
3. Aspirate.
4. Inject lidocaine (1.5 mg/kg) first. The patient may momentarily vocalize because the lidocaine may sting, but the onset of the lidocaine block is rapid.
5. Inject the bupivacaine (1.5 mg/kg) next. If bupivacaine is injected first, the patient will vocalize for 15 to 25 minutes, the amount of time it takes for onset.
6. This procedure can be repeated every 3 to 6 hours.
7. If injecting through a chest tube, a small amount of saline can be used to flush the local anesthetic into the chest.
8. The local anesthetic may be buffered with a small volume of sodium bicarbonate to minimize the initial stinging sensation. A volume of 0.3 ml per 9.7 ml of local anesthetic solution has been suggested.
9. Correct positioning of the patient after injection is unclear. There are several options:

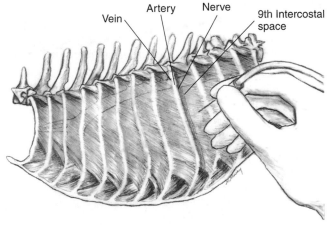

FIG. 15-4. Interpleural block.

- Roll the patient onto its back so the local anesthetic flows into the paravertebral gutters to block nerves before entering the spinal cord. This is most common in patients under anesthesia because they are easily moved.
- Place the patient in an upright position. This is most common in awake patients.
- Position the patient onto the affected side.
- Position the patient on the unaffected side.
- If interpleural anesthesia does not seem to work, attempt to alter the patient's position to change the distribution of the local anesthetic.

INTERCOSTAL BLOCK

◆ The intercostal block is useful for providing analgesia after intercostal thoracotomy and for desensitizing the area around isolated broken ribs.

Needle

◆ 22- to 25-gauge hypodermic needle

Technique

◆ This technique can be performed intraoperatively before closing the skin from an intercostal thoracotomy or percutaneously in a nonsurgical patient (Fig. 15-5).

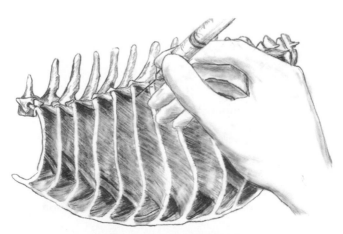

FIG. 15-5. Intercostal block.

1. Perform a sterile prep if performing the intercostal block percutaneously.
2. Blocks are performed two to three spaces cranial and caudal to the affected area.
3. The nerves are located on the caudal aspect of the rib behind the vein and artery.
4. Place the needle just caudal to the rib.
5. Aspirate for blood.
6. Inject local anesthetic.
7. Awake patients should be given a combination of lidocaine (1.5 mg/kg) combined with bupivacaine (1.5 mg/kg) to ensure a rapid onset of a block that should last 4 to 6 hours.
8. Patients who are receiving this block intraoperatively may receive only bupivacaine.
9. For chronic administration, a soaker catheter may be tunneled subcutaneously to facilitate continuous or intermittent delivery of local anesthetic.

INFRAORBITAL NERVE BLOCK

◆ The infraorbital block is used to provide anesthesia/analgesia to the upper lip and nose, dorsal aspect of the nasal cavity, and skin ventral to the infraorbital foramen.

Needle

◆ A 25-gauge, 2.5-cm (1-inch) hypodermic needle is adequate in virtually all dogs and cats.

Technique (Fig. 15-6)

1. Palpate the infraorbital foramen rostral and distal to the medial canthus of the eye.
2. Insert the needle into the foramen.
3. Aspirate for blood.
4. Deposit a small amount of local anesthetic (usually less than 1 ml).

MAXILLARY NERVE BLOCK

◆ The maxillary nerve block is used to provide anesthesia/analgesia to the ipsilateral maxilla, including the teeth, hard and soft palate, and nasal passage.

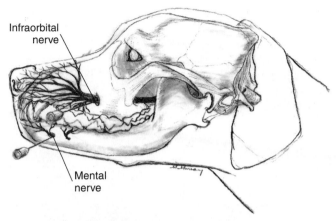

FIG. 15-6. Infraorbital and mental nerve blocks.

Needle

◆ A 25-gauge, 2.5-cm (1-inch) hypodermic needle is adequate in virtually all dogs and cats.

Technique (Figs. 15-7 and 15-8)

1. With the mouth open, palpate the edge of the hard palate just medial to the last cheek tooth on the desired side.
2. Insert the needle at this location.
3. Aspirate for blood.
4. Deposit a small amount of local anesthetic (usually less than 1 ml).

MENTAL NERVE BLOCK

◆ The mental nerve block provides analgesia to the lower lip and incisors on the ipsilateral side (see Fig. 15-6).

Needle

◆ A 25-gauge, 2.5-cm (1-inch) hypodermic needle is adequate in virtually all dogs and cats.

Technique (see Fig. 15-6)

1. Palpate the mental foramen on the lateral aspect of the mandible just caudal to the canine tooth.
2. Insert the needle into the mental foramen.
3. Aspirate for blood.
4. Inject a small amount of local anesthetic (usually less than 1 ml).

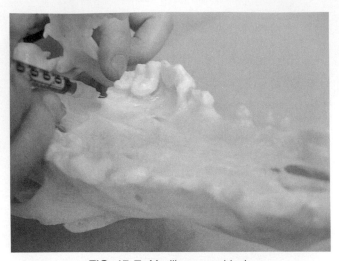

FIG. 15-7. Maxillary nerve block.

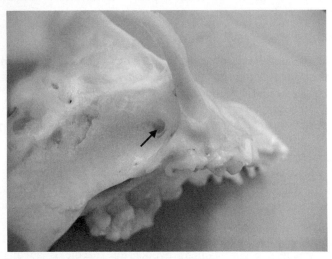

FIG. 15-8. Foramina (arrow) through which maxillary nerve passes.

MANDIBULAR NERVE BLOCK

◆ The mandibular nerve block provides anesthesia of the ipsilateral incisors, canine tooth, premolars, molars, and skin and mucosa of the chin and lower lip.

Needle

◆ 22-gauge, 2.5-cm (1-inch) hypodermic needle. Large dogs may require a 3.75-cm needle.

Technique (Fig. 15-9)

1. Aseptically prepare the site medial to the mandible.
2. Place an index finger in the patient's mouth. Palpate the mucosa on the medial aspect of the cheek for the mandibular nerve, which feels like a thin fibrous band.
3. Insert the needle with the other hand from the ventral-medial aspect of the mandible.
4. The index finger in the mouth guides the needle to placement next to the nerve.
5. Aspirate for blood.
6. Inject a small amount of local anesthetic (usually less than 1 ml).

FOREFOOT BLOCK

◆ This block is useful for declawing procedures in cats, toe amputations, or any surgery of the foot distal to the carpus.
◆ A combination of lidocaine (1.5 mg/kg) and bupivacaine (1.5 mg/kg) for dogs or cats is used. The total dose should be split between areas to be desensitized. This dose may be diluted if additional volume is necessary.

Needle

◆ 25-gauge hypodermic needle

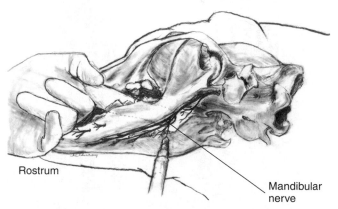

Rostrum

Mandibular nerve

FIG. 15-9. Mandibular nerve block; canine head in right lateral position.

Technique (Fig. 15-10)

1. Insert the needle just distal to the carpus on the proximal-medial aspect of the metacarpus.
2. Always aspirate before injection.
3. Inject a small amount of the combined local anesthetics to produce a small bleb.
4. Insert needle and repeat injections, continuing across the dorsum of the foot to the lateral aspect.
5. Complete the block by inserting the needle in the depression just distal to the accessory carpal pad, aspirating, and injecting a small amount of local anesthetic, ensuring a continuous infiltration from the medial aspect to the lateral aspect.

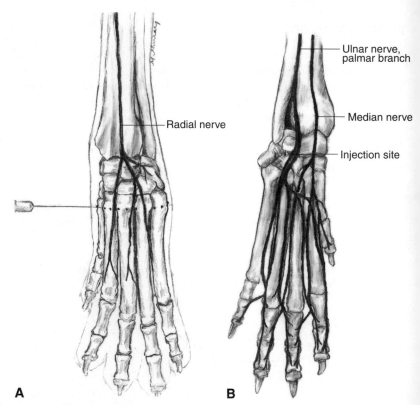

FIG. 15-10. A, Forefoot block, dorsal aspect. **B,** Forefoot block, palmar aspect.

BRACHIAL PLEXUS BLOCK

◆ A brachial plexus block is used to provide anesthesia distal to the elbow.

Needles

◆ 22-gauge and up to a 7.5-cm (3-inch) spinal needle for blind technique
◆ 22-gauge and up to a 7.5-cm (3-inch) insulated needle for guided technique

Nerve Locator–Guided Technique (Fig. 15-11)

◆ The guided technique is much more accurate and successful in obtaining a good brachial plexus block with a minimum of local anesthetic.
  1. Aseptically prepare the area medial to the scapulohumeral joint.
  2. Attach one electrode from the nerve locator to the skin; attach the other to the proximal portion of the needle.
  3. Insert the needle medial to the scapulohumeral joint, advancing toward the costochondral junction of the first palpable rib, medial to the scapula but outside the thorax.
  4. As the needle is inserted, turn on the nerve locator to the highest current setting.
  5. As the paw begins to twitch, precisely place the needle to obtain a maximal twitch with as little current as possible (0.3 mA is recommended, 0.1 millisecond and 2 Hz.
  6. Aspirate for blood.
  7. Inject a small amount of local anesthetic until the twitch disappears.
  8. Because the brachial plexus is diffuse, perform this technique two more times, fanning the needle dorsal and ventral from the initial placement.
  9. Inject a maximum of lidocaine 1.5 mg/kg or bupivacaine 1.5 mg/kg. Typically, considerably less drug is necessary because the local anesthetic is deposited directly on the nerves.
  10. Alternate application: When using the nerve locator, this block may also be done as a "paravertebral block" at C6, C7, and T1. This should effectively block the lower limb below the shoulder joint.

Blind Technique (Fig. 15-12)

◆ The blind technique only has a variable success rate even when using large volumes of local anesthetic.
  1. Aseptically prepare the area medial to the scapulohumeral joint.
  2. Insert the needle medial to the scapulohumeral joint, advancing

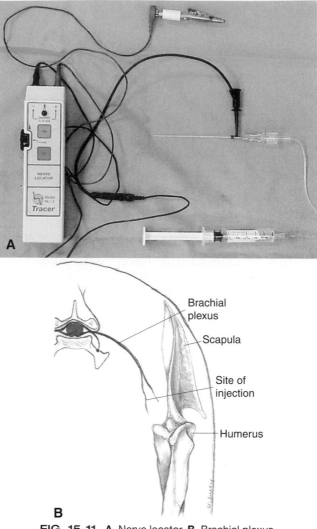

FIG. 15-11. A, Nerve locator. **B,** Brachial plexus.

toward the costochondral junction of the first palpable rib, medial to the scapula but outside the thorax.

3. Aspirate for blood.
4. Inject local anesthetic while withdrawing the needle 75% of the distance inserted.
5. Reinsert the needle two more times, approximately 30 degrees dorsal and 30 degrees ventral.

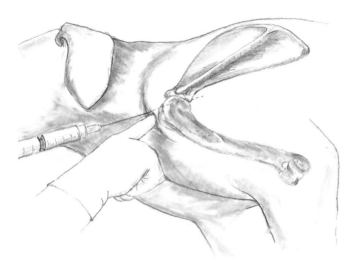

FIG. 15-12. Brachial plexus block.

6. Aspirate for blood after each insertion, and then inject local anesthetic while withdrawing.
7. Local anesthetic dose can be as high as lidocaine 1.5 mg/kg or bupivacaine 1.5 mg/kg.

FEMORAL (SAPHENOUS) NERVE BLOCK

◆ The femoral nerve block provides anesthesia of the medial part of the thigh, tibia, and tarsus and akinesia of quadriceps femoris muscle.

Needle

◆ 22-gauge insulated or 22-gauge, 1-inch hypodermic needle

Technique: Inguinal Approach

1. Aseptically prep site.
2. Insert needle just cranial to the femoral artery and below the inguinal ligament in a craniodorsal direction superficially.
3. Use of nerve locator induces a distal twitch to help ensure appropriate needle placement.
4. Insertion can also be performed in a blind manner without a nerve locator based on palpation.
5. Inject a small amount of local anesthetic. One should be able to use less than the calculated dose because the local anesthetic is being deposited directly over the nerve.

SCIATIC NERVE BLOCK

◆ The sciatic nerve block provides anesthesia of the caudal muscles of the thigh and surrounding tissues and skin.

Needle

◆ 22-gauge insulated or 22-gauge, 1-inch hypodermic needle

Technique

1. Aseptically prep site.
2. Draw a line between the greater trochanter and ischiatic tuberosity.
3. Introduce a 22-gauge needle directed cranially at about one third the distance between the two, and look for plantar dorsiflexion if using a nerve locator.
4. Insertion can also be performed in a blind manner.
5. Inject a small amount of local anesthetic. One should be able to use less than the calculated dose because the local anesthetic is being deposited directly over the nerve (Box 15-1).

INTRAARTICULAR ADMINISTRATION

The intraarticular route may be used to facilitate diagnosis of lameness as is commonly done in the horse. The technique may also be used to desensitize the affected joint before (preemptive analgesia) and after surgical intervention (e.g., arthroscopy). In small animals the stifle joint is most commonly injected, but this technique may be similarly applied to other joints, most commonly the hip, shoulder, and elbow.

STIFLE JOINT
Needle

◆ 22-gauge, 2.5-cm (1-inch) hypodermic needle

BOX 15-1

Joint Injections

Joints can be injected with a variety of substances, each for a different purpose:
- Local anesthetics for lameness diagnosis or perioperative anesthesia
- Morphine for analgesia of 18 to 24 hours' duration
- Corticosteroids for pain relief of severe osteoarthritis (This may last days to months.)
- Hyaluronic acid for increased joint lubrication in the presence of severe osteoarthritis (This effect may last days to months.)
- Autologous stem cells for potential cartilage regeneration and analgesia

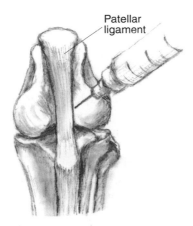

FIG. 15-13. Stifle joint, intraarticular injection.

Technique (Fig. 15-13)

1. Clip and aseptically prepare the joint.
2. Insert the needle lateral to the patellar ligament.
3. Aspirate to ensure that the needle is not in tissue. Joint fluid is likely to be aspirated in the stifle.
4. Inject local anesthetic:
   - Lidocaine 1 to 2 mg/kg
   - Bupivacaine 1 to 2 mg/kg
   - The stifle joint of most medium to large dogs holds approximately 5 ml of fluid.
5. Morphine 0.1 mg/kg can be injected into joints postoperatively to provide analgesia.
6. Alternative substances for injection:
   - Corticosteroids, such as methylprednisolone or triamcinolone can be injected to provide analgesia in the presence of severe arthritis. Caution should be taken with mild to moderate disease because corticosteroids hasten the degradation of cartilage within the joint.
   - Autologous stem cells, extracted from the patient's own adipose tissue, can be injected to help regenerate cartilage. These cells may also have antiinflammatory and pain-relieving effects.

ELBOW JOINT
Needle

- 22-gauge, 2.5-cm (1-inch) hypodermic needle

Technique (Fig. 15-14)

1. Clip and aseptically prepare the joint.
2. Use a medial approach.
3. Palpate the medial epicondyle of the humerus.
4. Slide a finger distal to the epicondyle to the approximate level of the joint.
5. Insert needle at that point or just caudal.
6. Aspirate for synovial fluid, which is not always possible.
7. Inject local anesthetic, about 0.5 to 1 ml.
8. Alternatively, corticosteroids, morphine, or autologous stem cells may be injected based on the indication.

HIP JOINT
Needle

◆ 20- to 22-gauge, 1½- to 3½-inch spinal needle with stylet

Technique

1. Clip and aseptically prepare the joint.
2. Flex hip slightly and position femur parallel to table to open up joint space.
3. Flex knee and use tibia as a handle to place traction on hip.
4. Palpate hip joint.
5. Insert needle at the midpoint of the proximal edge of the greater trochanter.

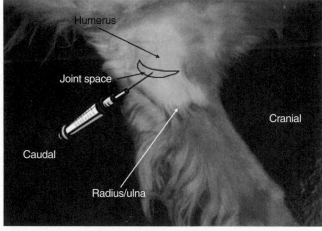

FIG. 15-14. Elbow injection.

6. Withdraw stylet.
7. Aspirate for synovial fluid, which is not always possible.
8. Inject local anesthetic, about 0.5 to 1 ml.
9. Alternative substances for injection:
   - Corticosteroids, such as methylprednisolone or triamcinolone can be injected to provide analgesia in the presence of severe arthritis. Caution should be taken with mild to moderate disease because corticosteroids hasten the degradation of cartilage within the joint.
   - Autologous stem cells, extracted from the patient's own adipose tissue, can be injected to help regenerate cartilage. These cells may also have antiinflammatory and pain-relieving effects.

INTRAVENOUS LOCAL OR REGIONAL ANESTHESIA

Local or regional anesthesia is also accomplished by IV injection of large volumes of dilute local anesthetic into an extremity isolated from the rest of the circulation by a tourniquet. The tissue distal to the tourniquet is blocked. This technique is also called a *Bier block*. The apparent mechanism of action is by diffusion of local anesthetic across blood vessels to local nerves. Normal nervous and muscle function returns quickly upon release of the tourniquet, which allows blood flow to dilute the regional local anesthetic concentration.

FORELIMB BLOCK
Needle

- 22-gauge, 2.5-cm (1-inch) hypodermic needle

Technique (Fig. 15-15)

1. Apply an occlusive bandage in a distal-to-proximal manner to remove blood from the limb.
2. Place a tourniquet proximal or distal to the elbow.
3. Remove the occlusive bandage.
4. Inject lidocaine into the cephalic vein. Onset of block is fast. Between 1 and 2 ml of 2% lidocaine can be diluted with an equal amount of 0.9% saline (producing 1% lidocaine). Of the dilute lidocaine, 2 to 4 ml can be injected.
5. Apply a second tourniquet (preferably pneumatic) in the blocked area distal to the first tourniquet. Remove the first tourniquet. This decreases tourniquet-induced pain.
6. The tourniquet must be removed within 90 minutes to avoid shock, endotoxemia, and potential death on tourniquet release.

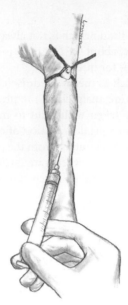

FIG. 15-15. Forelimb Bier block.

REAR LIMB BLOCK
Technique

1. This technique is performed similar to that of the IV regional fore-limb block.
2. Apply an occlusive bandage in a distal-to-proximal manner to remove blood from the limb.
3. Apply a tourniquet proximal to the tarsus.
4. Remove the occlusive bandage.
5. Inject lidocaine into the saphenous vein. Onset of block is fast. Between 1 and 2 ml of 2% lidocaine can be diluted with an equal amount of 0.9% saline (producing 1% lidocaine). Of the dilute lidocaine, 2 to 4 ml can be injected.
6. Apply a second tourniquet (preferably pneumatic) in the blocked area distal to the first tourniquet. Remove the first tourniquet. This decreases tourniquet-induced pain.
7. The tourniquet must be removed within 90 minutes to avoid shock, endotoxemia, and potential death on tourniquet release.

EPIDURAL ANESTHESIA AND ANALGESIA

Injecting local anesthetic solution into the epidural space generally at the lumbosacral space (for dogs and pigs) or the first or second intercoccygeal space (for horses and cows; sometimes referred to as *caudal anesthesia*) produces epidural or extradural anesthesia. The anesthetic acts on the posterior spinal nerves before they leave the vertebral column. The extent of anesthetic action depends on the spread of the drug and diffusion to neural tissues from the site of injection. Long-term administration of drugs is facilitated by placement of an epidural catheter. This technique also facilitates craniad distribution of the drug. Anesthesia can be produced by using a local anesthetic such as lidocaine or bupivacaine. Analgesia can be produced without loss of motor function with the use of an opioid such as morphine (Box 15-2). Regardless of the desired effect, the technique of epidural injection is the same. Most epidural injections in dogs and cats are performed at the LS space. The spinal cord usually ends at the last lumbar vertebra (L7) in dogs; thus there is less chance of obtaining cerebrospinal fluid (CSF) at this space. The spinal cord usually ends at the first sacral vertebra in cats, making it likely to obtain CSF if attempting an epidural injection at the LS space.

BOX 15-2

Epidural and Spinal Injections

The epidural and spinal (subarachnoid) spaces can be injected with a variety of substances, each for a different purpose:

- Local anesthetics for regional anesthesia (This will result in lack of sensation and motor paralysis.)
- Opioids, such as morphine, for analgesia of various durations (Motor function is still present, but the patient can have significant pain control.)

EPIDURAL INJECTION
Needles

- 18-, 20-, and 22-gauge beveled spinal needles of various lengths are commonly used.
- An alternative is an 18- or 20-gauge blunt-pointed Tuohy epidural needle.

Single Epidural Injection Technique

1. Place the patient in lateral or sternal recumbency.
2. Patients with rear limb trauma may not easily be placed in sternal recumbency because of the potential for worsening a fracture. An advantage of the sternal position is the ability to use the hanging drop technique (Fig. 15-16, *A*).

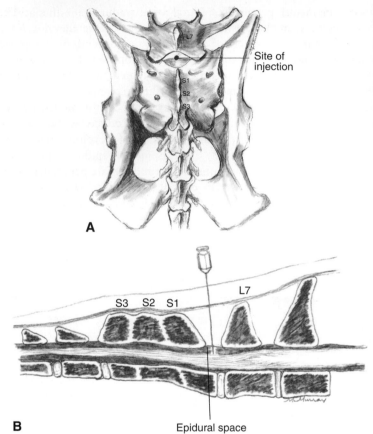

FIG. 15-16. A, Dorsal view of lumbosacral area of a dog. **B,** Lateral view of lumbosacral area of a dog.

3. Virtually all patients can be placed in lateral recumbency for this procedure (Fig. 15-16, *B*).

4. Clip and aseptically prepare an area of fur just cranial to wings of the ilium, caudal to the second sacral vertebra, and as wide as the lateral aspects of the ilium wings.

5. Locate the LS space by placing the thumb and smallest finger on opposite wings of the ilium. Palpating between these fingers, on midline, is the dorsal spinous process of the sixth lumbar vertebra (L6). A significant space can be felt just caudal to L6. Directly caudal to that space is the dorsal spinous process of L7. Further caudal is a large palpable depression, the LS space.

6. Place the needle perpendicular to the skin on midline in the middle of the space. Sometimes angling the needle tip slightly cranially is beneficial.
7. Insert the needle slowly. Often, resistance can be felt as the needle passes through the ligamentum flavum at the top of the vertebral canal. At this point, the needle is in the epidural space.
   - Remove the stylet of the needle. If blood comes from the needle, the needle should be removed. If CSF is encountered, use half the dose of local anesthetic. Opioid doses, in general, do not need to be changed.
   - Inject 1 ml of air with a glass syringe (or other epidural loss-of-resistance syringe) to verify placement. Minimal resistance occurs with a glass syringe plunger on a glass barrel. If the air stays in the space without pushing the syringe plunger back, the needle is likely to be in the correct place. If injection of air leads to resistance and pushing back of the plunger, the needle is not in the desired location.

Alternative Hanging Drop Technique

1. Place the patient in sternal recumbency.
2. Remove the stylet before puncturing the ligamentum flavum.
3. Place a drop of sterile saline in the hub of the needle.
4. As the needle passes through the ligamentum flavum into the epidural space, the negative pressure in the space sucks in the saline. This is a definitive sign of proper needle placement. Sometimes the movement of saline does not occur because of blockage of the needle from passing through tissue without the stylet in place.
5. Stabilize the needle and administer the drug slowly over a 1-minute period. Minimal resistance should be encountered on injection.

PLACEMENT OF AN EPIDURAL CATHETER
Technique

1. The technique is identical to placement of an epidural injection described previously except that a Tuohy needle is used.
2. Insert the catheter through the needle a distance that will stay in the epidural space and is equal to the depth of the needle in the skin plus approximately 1 to 3 inches.
3. Remove the needle by securing the catheter and needle together and withdrawing from the skin. This helps prevent shearing off the catheter in the epidural space.
4. The advantage of epidural catheter placement is the ability to provide epidural anesthesia or analgesia for days without the trauma of repeated epidural punctures.

DILUTION AND ADMINISTRATION OF MORPHINE AND BUPIVACAINE FOR CONTINUOUS EPIDURAL ADMINISTRATION
Technique

1. Dilute preservative-free morphine (1 mg/ml) with sterile preservative-free 0.9% saline to a concentration of 0.5 mg/ml by adding equal amounts of saline to the morphine.
2. Add 1 ml of bupivacaine (0.75%) to 5 ml of the dilute preservative-free morphine. This produces a solution of bupivacaine (1.25 mg/ml) and morphine (0.42 mg/ml).
3. The solution is administered at a rate of 0.03 to 0.05 ml/kg per hour. This delivers morphine at a rate of 0.3 to 0.5 mg/kg per 24 hours.
4. If rear limb motor paralysis occurs, the bupivacaine should be diluted into 11 ml of dilute morphine solution and administered at the rate described previously to deliver the same morphine dose but a considerably lower bupivacaine dose.

SPINAL ANESTHESIA

Spinal anesthesia is produced by injecting local anesthetic into the subarachnoid space. This can be accomplished at the LS space in cats or at L5 to L6 or L6 to L7 vertebral spaces in dogs. Because the vertebral level of termination of the spinal cord varies among animal species, this form of anesthesia is technically more difficult than epidural injection in other veterinary species.

◆ Local anesthetic doses for subarachnoid injection are usually 50% of doses for epidural injection.
◆ Opioid doses do not need to change for subarachnoid injection.

Suggested Readings

Muir WW, Hubbell JAE, Skarda RT et al: *Handbook of veterinary anesthesia*, ed 3, St Louis, 2000, Mosby.

Thurman JC, Tranquilli WJ, Benson GJ: *Lumb & Jones' veterinary anesthesia*, ed 3, Baltimore, 1996, Williams & Wilkins.

6

COMPLEMENTARY AND ALTERNATIVE MEDICINE FOR PAIN MANAGEMENT IN VETERINARY PATIENTS

NARDA G. ROBINSON*

Truly effective, long-lasting pain relief often requires an integrated, multidisciplinary approach.[1] Not all types of pain respond equally to one complementary and alternative medicine (CAM) approach. For example, certain physical ailments such as back pain may respond more quickly to those modalities (i.e., acupuncture and massage) that target the musculature as opposed to those focused on joints (i.e., chiropractic).

As evidence accumulates to justify the inclusion of CAM procedures in the management of animal pain, the matter of *not* informing clients about CAM options becomes less acceptable. However, treating an animal by CAM without adequate consideration of its risks and unknowns could lessen the value and relevance of CAM for a given animal in pain and even endanger the life and well-being of a patient.[2,3] Furthermore, prescribing alternative pain control measures based on a blind allegiance to and uncritical acceptance of CAM not only could compromise patient care but also could open one to medical malpractice liability.[2,4]

Thus, veterinarians considering CAM should apprise themselves of the latest evidence and scientifically based information pertaining to the modality in question. Although clients have ready access to the endless supply of Web-based (and usually profit-driven) health information, the responsibility of directing clients to meaningful and legitimate practices rests with the veterinarian.[5] Metaphysical or metaphorical explanations such as "releasing stuck energy" do little to inform clients or colleagues about the actual nature of the mechanism of action of a treatment and are usually inaccurate. Additional concerns arise when "holistic" practitioners offer consultations online, without ever seeing or examining the patient. This practice violates the requirement of securing a valid

---

*With contributions from Roman T. Skarda, Dr.MedVet, PhD, DACVA (1944-2005).

veterinarian-client-patient relationship before treatment and exposes the patient to potentially needless and harmful herbs or supplements.

The following pages provide a general overview of various techniques within the CAM domain that address pain. Unless otherwise specified, the CAM treatment applies to a wide variety of painful conditions, acute and chronic. The mechanisms of action, contraindications, and risks for each technique are provided when available. However, one should keep in mind that in addition to the treatment method itself, the education and proficiency of the practitioner factor into the relative safety and analgesic value of each CAM treatment.[6] Practitioner qualifications that include "certifications" may or may not indicate sufficient background and experience. At the time of this writing, all CAM certification programs were self-appointed, and none have received recognition by the American Veterinary Medical Association as legitimate and/or specialty certifications.

ACUPUNCTURE

Acupuncture ranks readily as the most deeply scrutinized and well-researched of all CAM modalities.[7] Scientific investigations have unveiled many of its mechanisms of action. This research allows veterinarians to provide acupuncture-based pain relief and to tailor treatment strategies built on a solid understanding of the nervous system and the generation of pain rather than to extract point prescriptions from the dim shadows of mystery and metaphor.

Acupuncture for Pain

- Acupuncture points and channels follow neurovascular pathways.
- Acupuncture treats pain by inducing neuromodulation along peripheral, central, and autonomic pathways.
- Successful acupuncture neuromodulation and acupuncture analgesia depends on accurate identification of the structures responsible for generating pain and adequate stimulation of these structures.
- Acupuncture treatments involve somatic afferent stimulation through a variety of means: needling, electroacupuncture, low-level laser, and manual pressure.

Acupuncture usually involves the insertion of thin, sterile needles into specific anatomic sites richly supplied with nerve endings (Figs. 16-1 to 16-3). Other forms of acupuncture point stimulation exist, such as low-level laser therapy (Fig. 16-4), heat, and electroacupuncture. Adding electrical stimulation to the acupuncture treatment (known as

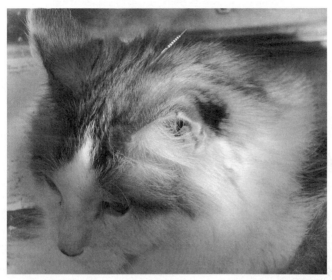

FIG. 16-1. Demonstration of an acupuncture needle at a calming point on the vertex of the scalp.

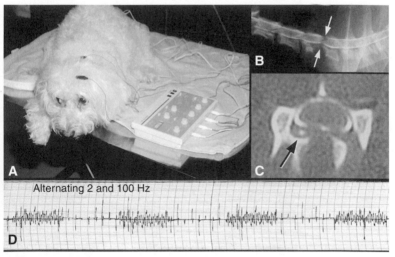

FIG. 16-2. A, Bichon Frise (11 years old) with relief from severe chronic neck pain during percutaneous electrical nerve stimulation (PENS). **B,** Myelographic radiograph of the lateral projection of the caudal cervical spine of the dog, indicating extradural spinal cord compression (as indicated by *arrows*) at the cervical vertebrae C5/C6. **C,** Axial computed tomographic image at the level of the C6 vertebra, indicating calcified disk material (*arrow*) displacing the spinal cord dorsally at the right side of the spine. The defect of vertebral body after vertebral decompression is visible. **D,** Biphasic stimulation with alternating 2-Hz and 100-Hz frequencies. Recorded at 25 mm/s and 5 mV/cm.

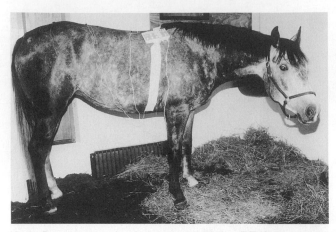

FIG. 16-3. Percutaneous electrical nerve stimulation (PENS) of an unrestrained horse (Warmblood mare, 610 kg, 5 years old, with fracture of transverse process of third cervical vertebra) in its stall. Acupuncture needles are placed at BL 18, BL 23, BL 25, and BL 28 bilaterally and are connected via paired leads to the electroacupuncture stimulator (ITO IC 4107), which is secured to the horse with a bandage.

"electroacupuncture") often augments analgesia conferred by acupuncture. As such, this form of stimulation provides the basis for much of the existing acupuncture research demonstrating effectiveness. In electroacupuncture treatments, clips attach the electrode leads to the needles, which then bring the electrical impulses deep into the tissues, bypassing the formidable electrical resistance of the skin. The term for electroacupuncture treatments in which the needle acts as an electrode, penetrating the skin, is "percutaneous electrical nerve stimulation," or "PENS." This contrasts with "transcutaneous electrical nerve stimulation," or "TENS," which delivers the electricity to surface electrode pads. In this case, the electrical stimulus must overcome the skin resistance that limits its access to underlying nerve fibers. Some electric point finders locate acupuncture points (as areas of reduced electrical resistance) and also deliver stimulation. Although one could rely on electric point finders to determine acupuncture point location, these machines are unreliable in human patients for whom they were designed and in non-humans (Fig. 16-5, *C*).

MECHANISM OF ACTION

Acupuncture works through neuromodulation; that is, introducing the needle into tissue at an acupuncture point incites a series of responses and reflexes within the peripheral, autonomic, and central nervous systems, some of which are involved in providing analgesia.[8] Neurohumoral and

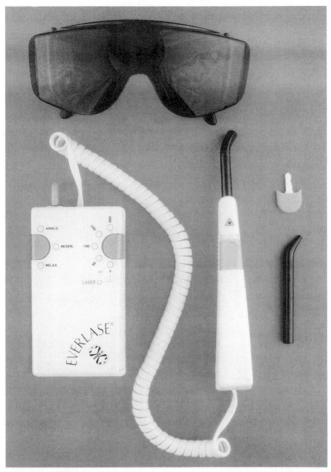

FIG. 16-4. Everlase medical laser (M.E.D. Servi-Systems Canada Ltd, Sittsville, Ontario, Canada) for pain relief, tissue regeneration, and muscle relaxation, with protective eyeglasses.

neuroendocrine changes alter pain transmission and augment intrinsic pain control mechanisms. Acupuncture attenuates inflammation in part by activating the hypothalamic-pituitary-adrenal axis.[9] Opioid peptides in the spinal cord and brain participate in endogenous pain control.[10] The reduction in central nervous system excitation helps dampen pain transmission and sympathetic tone. Acupuncture improves muscle blood flow, which benefits patients with chronic pain.[11] Sustained stimulation from manual acupuncture reduces muscle tension by reducing α-motoneuron excitability.[12,13]

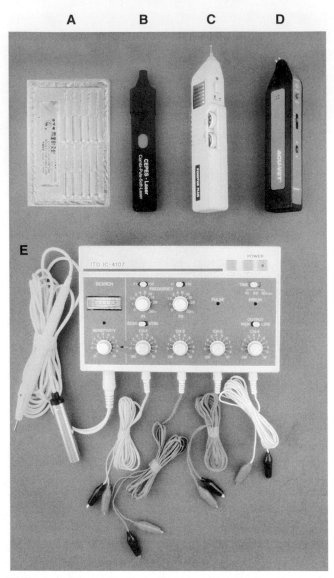

FIG. 16-5. A, Package with 10 sterile acupuncture needles (Hwato, size 0.3 × 25 mm) for single use. **B,** CEPES-laser Combi-Plus-Soft-Laser. **C,** Pointer-Plus handheld unit for locating and stimulating acupuncture points transcutaneously (transcutaneous electrical nerve stimulation, TENS). **D,** Acu-Vet handheld unit for locating and stimulating acupuncture points transcutaneously (TENS). **E,** Electro-Acupuncture Unit IC-4107 for locating and stimulating acupuncture points percutaneously (percutaneous electrical nerve stimulation). Further description can be found in the text.

Brain centers that participate in nociception and antinociception may become deactivated or activated as a consequence of acupuncture.[8] One can also target the frequency and location of stimulation delivered through electroacupuncture to the specific analgesic needs of the patient. A practitioner may select a low (2-Hz) or high (100-Hz) frequency, depending on whether a patient requires rapid-onset pain relief as in a postoperative state, long-lasting relief as for chronic conditions, or a mixture of both.[14] Furthermore, lead placement should follow neuroanatomic pathways involved in the production and perpetuation of the pain being addressed.

As opposed to what many claim, acupuncture does *not* work by moving invisible energy through invisible meridians. Although traditional Chinese medicine practitioners commonly explain its mechanisms in metaphorical and metaphysical terms, the ancient acupuncture doctors actually had a far greater appreciation of the anatomic and physiological aspects of acupuncture than many persons realize and even a more relevant conceptualization of its mechanisms of action than many practitioners hold today.[15,16] Furthermore, requiring practitioners to adopt an irrational belief system about acupuncture does little to teach veterinarian acupuncturists how to address animal pain successfully. What is required is a sophisticated understanding of the neurophysiological influences of acupuncture, highly developed myofascial palpation skills, and a cogent method of effectively providing analgesia based on the anatomic distribution of the pain and the most efficient and long-lasting delivery of acupuncture analgesia.

ACUPUNCTURE POINTS FOR PAIN

Acupuncture works best for the treatment of pain when carefully tailored to the patient's presentation. In other words, although point "recipes" for pain can provide the novice with a starting point (Figs. 16-6 to 16-8; Box 16-1), more refined and effective interventions require a comprehensive understanding of the sources of pain (i.e., muscle, bone, joint, and visceral) and the neuroanatomic pathways involved in mediating that pain and resultant analgesia. For example, see Tables 16-1 and 16-2.

INDICATIONS

Acupuncture works for a wide variety of acute and chronic painful conditions of somatic and visceral origin. See Table 16-1 for evidence related to the treatment of pain.

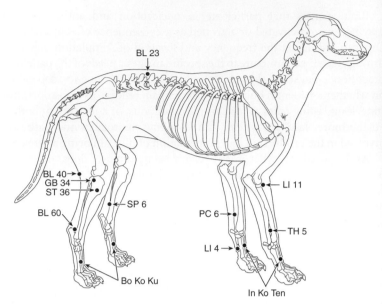

FIG. 16-6. Locations of various acupuncture points to induce analgesia in dogs.

CONTRAINDICATIONS

Few contraindications to acupuncture exist. Contraindications include excessive patient movement or aggression that prohibit safe and effective treatment, pregnancy, sepsis, severe bleeding abnormalities, spinal or joint instability local to the treatment site, and tumor or infection at the site of desired needling.

ADVERSE EFFECTS

Negative outcomes from acupuncture relate to the effects of inserting a long, sharp object into the body and include bleeding, inadvertent organ puncture, or infection, though severe adverse effects are rare.[30]

GOLD BEAD IMPLANTS

An odd technique of implanting tiny pieces of gold or other metals into periarticular or soft tissue locations has arisen within the veterinary profession.[31] Long abandoned in human acupuncture, this variant of needle fragment implantation has enjoyed a resurgence in veterinary

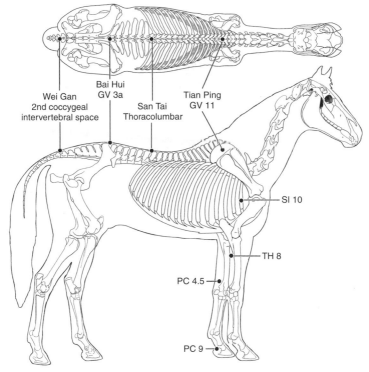

FIG. 16-7. Locations of various acupuncture points to induce analgesia in horses.

spheres. Although gold bead enthusiasts claim an 80% or greater success rate in treating pain from hip dysplasia,[32] two controlled, blinded studies evaluating the technique found that gold bead implantation was no more successful at relieving pain than a control method that differed by not leaving behind metal.[33,34] In addition, the potential for fragment migration and penetration into organs, viscera, nervous tissue, or the vasculature represents a significant risk factor.[35-37] Imaging artifacts on computed tomography and magnetic resonance imaging scans may severely lessen the diagnostic value of studies done on patients containing these permanent implants.[38]

Thus, because the mechanisms of action proposed for gold bead implantation (i.e., ongoing energy release or long-term ionization potentials) lack rationality or proof and because the procedure itself has

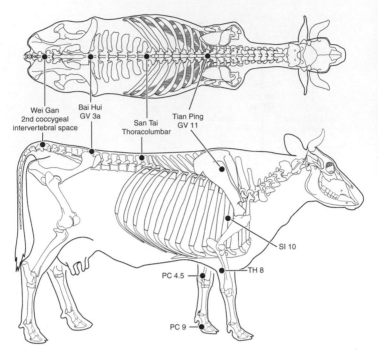

FIG. 16-8. Locations of various acupuncture points to induce analgesia in cattle.

been shown to be no better than a control procedure, the documented risks associated with needle implantation appear to outweigh the elusive benefits.

SPECIFIC ACUPUNCTURE APPROACHES FOR PAIN CONTROL
Spinal Pain

Controlled trials and systematic reviews in human research provide increasingly stronger evidence that acupuncture effectively treats chronic spinal pain.[19,39-46] Several uncontrolled studies have reported that acupuncture improves spinal pain of various causes in dogs and horses.[47-53] According to Adrian R. White, MD, the author of several systematic reviews on acupuncture, "Acupuncture treatment should be considered for anyone who has nonspecific mechanical back pain that has persisted for 6 weeks or more despite standard treatment."[20,54] In humans, 10 sessions of needle body acupuncture produced stable, long-term effects lasting at least 6 months according to a recently published prospective

---

BOX 16-1

Abbreviations and Anatomic Locations of Acupuncture Points in the Dog

1. LI 4 (Large Intestine point 4): Approximately midway along the shaft of second metacarpal bone on the radial side.
2. LI 11 (Large Intestine point 11): At the end of the lateral cubital crease, found with the elbow flexed.
3. PC 6 (Pericardium point 6): Two rib-widths above the carpal joint, between the tendons of the flexor digitorum superficialis and flexor carpi radialis.
4. TH 5 (Triple Heater 5): Two rib-widths above the carpus, on the cranial aspect of the interosseous space between the radius and ulna.
5. In Ko Ten: Between metacarpal bones 2 and 3.
6. BL 23 (Bladder point 23): One and a half rib-widths lateral to midline, level with the caudal border of spinous process of the second lumbar vertebra.
7. ST 36 (Stomach point 36): One finger-breadth from the anterior crest of the tibia, in the belly of the cranial tibialis muscle.
8. GB 34 (Gallbladder point 34): In the depression cranial and distal to the fibular head.
9. BL 40 (Bladder point 40): In the center of the popliteal crease.
10. SP 6 (Spleen point 6): Three rib-widths directly above the tip of the medial malleolus, on the caudal border of the tibia.
11. BL 60 (Bladder point 60): In the depression between the lateral malleolus and calcaneal tendon, level with the tip of the lateral malleolus.
12. Bo Ko Ku: Between metatarsal bones 2 and 3.

---

cohort study.[55] A 2005 paper systematically reviewing acupuncture for chronic low back pain echoed the findings of earlier work, concluding that adding acupuncture to conventional treatment produced better analgesia and functional improvement than conventional treatments alone.[17,56] However, not all acupuncture treatments are equal. Deeper acupuncture stimulation in humans with lumbar myofascial pain provides greater pain reduction than does superficial needling, although it causes more posttreatment soreness.[57-59] Neuroanatomically focused acupuncture addresses spine-related pain by treating the nerves mediating pain from spinal structures.[60,61] Stimulation of paravertebral somatic afferent fibers at acupuncture points along the spine suppresses activity in spinal nociceptive neurons.[62]

A commonly overlooked source of spinal pain resides within the musculature itself and its enveloping fascia. Myofascial pain syndrome can sometimes mimic radicular pain or internal organ disease.[63] Identifying this type of pain entails palpating for taut bands and trigger points encased within the myofascial fabric. Once identified, myofascial pain can readily respond to physical medicine approaches such as acupuncture, even after medication has failed.[64,65]

TABLE 16-1	**Studies Concerning Acupuncture for Pain**
Condition Studied	**Outcome**
Low back pain	Acupuncture done with dry needling is useful for chronic low back pain.[17-20]
Knee osteoarthritis	Acupuncture improves pain and function in patients with knee osteoarthritis.[21]
Chronic visceral hyperalgesia	Electroacupuncture effectively treats visceral pain in rats subjected to colorectal distention as an irritable bowel syndrome model.[22]
Perioperative analgesia	Acupuncture was found to be a useful adjunct to conventional anesthesia for patients receiving maxillofacial surgery and helped stabilize pulse rate and blood pressure during surgery.[23]
Lateral epicondyle pain	Acupuncture provides short-term relief for lateral epicondyle pain.[24]
Chronic orofacial pain	Acupuncture provides significant short-term relief for patients with chronic orofacial pain.[25]
Migraine	Real and sham acupuncture benefited patients with migraines more than a waiting list control, raising the issue that the question about proper selection of sham points because both demonstrated physiological impact and benefit.[26] Ear acupuncture to tender points in the ear-aborted migraines.[27]
Pain during shock wave lithotripsy	Electroacupuncture provided analgesia comparable to sedoanalgesics during shock wave lithotripsy.[28]
Pain after knee arthroscopy	Auricular acupuncture reduced postoperative analgesic requirements after ambulatory knee arthroscopy.[29]

Table 16-2 lists various structures pertaining to the spine that can generate back or neck pain in small animals.[66] Inflammation, compression, developmental anomalies, or degeneration of these tissues can lead to spinal discomfort. The table includes mention of particular acupuncture point groupings that most directly influence pain transmission in the affected nerves.

Treatment of Other Pain Problems with Acupuncture

Table 16-3 provides acupuncture point suggestions for additional regional pain problems. As with spine-related pain, one should first palpate the body for areas of tension, taut bands, tissue warmth, and tenderness. Whether these sites constitute "conventional" acupuncture points matters little when isolating "local" points for needling, that is, involved regions that are causing spontaneous pain or tenderness upon palpation. Additional points to consider are those that influence autonomic function

TABLE 16-2	Potential Sources of Neck and Back Pain in Dogs and Cats	
Structural Source of Back Pain	**Related Neural Elements**	**Acupuncture Points Influencing Nerves Related to the Pain Source**
Intervertebral disk	The periphery of intervertebral disks in dogs contains nociceptors and mechanoreceptors; the sinuvertebral nerve supplies sensory innervation.	Huatojiaji points, "facet joint points"
Facet joint capsule	The joint capsule is richly innervated by proprioceptors and nociceptors.	Huatojiaji points, "facet joint points"
Dorsal root ganglion (DRG)	Mechanically sensitive nociceptors (i.e., mechanonociceptors) in the nervi nervorum of the epineuria surrounding the DRG may contribute to pain if compression or tension affects the DRG.	Points along the inner Bladder channel
Spinal ligaments: (1) Dorsal longitudinal ligament (2) Supraspinal ligaments (3) Interspinous ligaments	These ligaments contain free nerve endings that have been implicated as potential contributors to back pain.	Points along the Governor Vessel channel
Vertebral periosteum	The periosteum contains an extensive plexus of nerve fibers that exhibits the lowest pain threshold of any of the deep tissues.	Huatojiaji points or points along the Governor Vessel channel
Meninges	The dura is sensitive to mechanical and noxious stimulation; meningeal irritation may contribute to back and neck pain in dogs and cats.	Points along the Bladder channel
Muscles attaching or referring to the back or neck	Myofascial pain is characterized by palpable, taut bands occurring lengthwise along muscles that contain exquisitely tender regions. Myofascial pain is often mistaken for radicular pain and may be accompanied by visceral pain syndromes including bowel irritability and cystitis.	Local, direct needling into the taut band or trigger point

Continued

TABLE 16-2	Potential Sources of Neck and Back Pain in Dogs and Cats—*cont'd*	
Structural Source of Back Pain	**Related Neural Elements**	**Acupuncture Points Influencing Nerves Related to the Pain Source**
Thoracolumbar fascia	Cutaneous branches from dorsal rami of lumbar spinal nerves innervate the thoracolumbar fascia. Nerves supplying the thoracolumbar fascia in humans with chronic mechanical back pain may undergo degeneration because of ischemia or inflammation.	Points along the Governor Vessel, Bladder, or Gallbladder channels, depending on the area affected by pain, as determined by palpation

Data from Wong JY: *A manual of neuro-anatomical acupuncture,* vol 1, *Musculo-skeletal disorders,* Toronto, 1999, Toronto Pain and Stress Clinic; Webb AA: *Vet J* 165(3):193-213, 2003.

TABLE 16-3	Acupuncture Points to Consider for Pain on the Head
Painful Region	**Acupuncture Points**
General head pain	Palpate for myofascial restrictions in the neck (especially the suboccipital region) and the head (especially the temporalis muscle). GB 14, GB 20 BL 7, BL 8, BL 10 GV 14, GV 20 LI 4, ST 44
Eye	TH 23, BL 2, LR 3 GB 2, GB 14, GB 20, BL 10 Yintang (GV 24.5), GV 14
Nose	LI 20, LI 4, LU 7 ST 2, ST 3, ST 4 Yintang (GV 24.5)
Mouth, teeth	LI 4, LU 7 ST 2, ST 4, ST 6 SI 18, SI 19
Neck	Palpate for myofascial restrictions in the neck (especially the suboccipital, cervicothoracic, and lateral regions).

(especially sympathetic pathways) and thereby counteract windup. These points include LI 4, ST 36, LR 3, GV 20, and all of the midline and paravertebral points along the thoracolumbar region on the back.

ACUPUNCTURE COURSES AND SUPPLY COMPANIES

For information on veterinary acupuncture courses, consult Appendix 1. A list of acupuncture equipment suppliers appears in Appendix 2. Internet chat sites on acupuncture appear in Appendix 3.

HERBS

Some phytopharmaceuticals, as the predecessors to many modern medications for pain, possess potent analgesic activity. In addition, certain herbs confer antiinflammatory effects. Herbs such as yucca appear frequently in supplement formulations for pain (Fig. 16-9). However, unlike synthetic drugs, certain botanical pain relievers provide significant benefits without dangerous side effects, at least in humans. Because many of these products lack the centuries of empirical evidence in nonhuman species, extrapolating aspects of safety and effectiveness from humans to dogs and cats may be risky. Species- and breed-specific metabolic idiosyncrasies may turn an otherwise safe herbal product

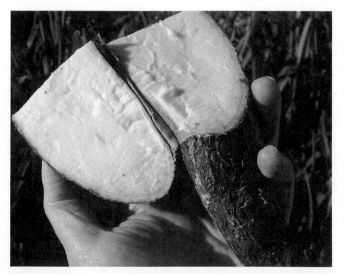

FIG. 16-9. Fresh yucca root. Yucca often appears in antipain arthritis formulations.

TABLE 16-4	Herbs for Pain		
Herb	**Mechanism of Action**	**Pain-Related Use and Advantages**	**Contraindications, Drug-Herb Interactions, Precautions, and Side Effects**[68]
Arnica gel	Sesquiterpene lactones provide antiinflammatory activity.[69] Topical counterirritant	May be effective for osteoarthritis[70]	Toxic if injected. May cause severe liver and kidney damage when taken internally Interacts with antihypertensive medication
Boswellia	Inhibits leukotriene synthesis[71,72]	Effective for dogs with arthritis[73]	Side effects are usually minor and involve minor gastrointestinal changes such as diarrhea or flatulence[74]
Capsaicin	May alter with neuropeptide metabolism and influence nociceptive afferents[68]	Topical application for analgesia appears to be relatively safe and effective in humans.[68]	Internal usage may lead to gastric irritation. May interfere with acid-inhibiting and antihypertensive medication May accentuate the effects of sedating psychoactive medications and platelet inhibitors
Chamomile	The antiinflammatory effect of apigenin, one of the flavonoids in chamomile, involves interfering with leukocyte adhesion and adhesion protein up-regulation in human endothelial cells. Apigenin also inhibits interleukin-1α (IL-1α) induced prostaglandin synthesis and tumor necrosis factor-α–induced IL-6 and IL-8 formation.[75]	May ameliorate skin and mucosal irritations and inflammation	Generally regarded as safe, but large doses combined with anticoagulants may increase bleeding risk Theoretically, may confer additive sedating effects when combined with benzodiazepines Those allergic to plants in the daisy family may exhibit strong allergic responses to chamomile.

Clove gel	The oily liquid eugenol, contained in clove, confers analgesic properties.	Topical anesthetic, especially before dental procedures May reduce local anesthetic requirements Less expensive than topical anesthetics Shown to be equal to benzocaine in effectiveness as a topical agent[76]	May cause aphthouslike ulcers in the area of application; eugenol can cause tissue irritation in high concentrations[76] Has antiplatelet activity May lead to contact dermatitis in susceptible individuals applying it often
Comfrey	Various constituents contribute to antiinflammatory effects: allantoin, choline, and rosmarinic acid.[77]	May ease muscle and joint pain when applied topically[77,78]	Hepatotoxicity is due to pyrrolizidine alkaloids.[79] Cultivars devoid of alkaloids in aerial parts may reduce this concern.[78]
Corydalis	Reduces vascular permeability and inhibits histamine release[80]	Possible benefits for inflammation and pain[81]	None found
Devil's claw	Reduces the synthesis of two inducible, proinflammatory enzymes: cyclo-oxygenase-2 (COX-2) and inducible nitric oxide synthase[82]	Effective in treating pain from muscular and/or joint disease[68]	Hypoglycemic effects in diabetic persons Promotes bile production in patients with cholelithiasis May interfere with acid-inhibiting, antihypertensive, and cardiac medications
Ginger	COX-1 inhibition[83] COX-2 inhibition[84]	Possible pain-relieving benefits for arthritis	Theoretical interactions with anticoagulant, antidiabetic, antacid, and cardiac medication; otherwise, generally regarded as safe
White willow bark	COX-1 inhibitor, similar to aspirin because of salicylate content	Possible effectiveness for pain	Unsafe for cats because of salicylates
Yucca (Fig. 16-2)	Yucca polyphenols have potent antioxidant, antiplatelet aggregation, and free-radical scavenging activity.[85]	Pain and inflammation from arthritis[85]	None found

---

Herbs for Pain

- Botanical compounds are appearing with increasing regularity in supplement formulae for pain and arthritis.
- Many plant compounds offer effective and proven antiinflammatory and analgesic benefits, alone or in combination.
- Despite the promising results from research and anecdotal evidence, concerns with herbs for animals remain. These concerns include lack of regulatory oversight and enforced manufacturing guidelines, underreporting of adverse effects, contaminants, undisclosed adulteration with pharmaceuticals, and unknowns regarding differences in metabolism of these products between human and nonhuman animals.

---

into an unsafe approach. Table 16-4 provides a short overview of various herbs with putative analgesic properties; their mechanisms of action, if known; and their analgesic applications, contraindications, interactions, and side effects. When introducing herbs into an animal's pain-reduction plan, one should consider additive or counteractive properties when mixing herbs with drugs. For example, psychoactive botanicals such as kava kava, St. John's wort, and valerian can cause excessive sedation and confusion, especially when combined with pharmaceuticals.[67]

VETERINARY MANUAL THERAPY

Veterinary manual therapy serves as an umbrella term for several disciplines, including animal or veterinary chiropractic, manipulative approaches derived from osteopathic medicine, and massage therapy. Essentially, any healing modality performed with the hands by a veterinarian qualifies as veterinary manual therapy.

Veterinary Manual Therapy

- Veterinary manual therapy includes a variety of manipulative techniques, ranging from high-velocity, low-amplitude chiropractic thrusts to less invasive measures such as massage and soft tissue therapy.
- Evidence concerning the safety and effectiveness of manual therapy approaches for non–humans is largely lacking. However, the literature on humans offers substantial evidence for the benefits of manipulative therapy for certain types of pain, most notably for functional spinal pain.

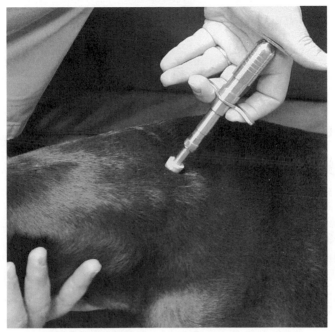

FIG. 16-10. A handheld device known as an "Activator."

MECHANISM OF ACTION

High-velocity, low-amplitude thrusting techniques work to promote restoration of healthy joint motion and mechanical functions. High-velocity, low-amplitude methods can be applied manually or with the aid of an instrument called an "Activator" (Fig. 16-10). Low-force techniques may also focus on joint mobility or instead on the musculature and fascia itself, by stretching and lengthening the soft tissues.

INDICATIONS

Evidence suggests that manual therapy delivers a certain degree of relief for human patients with low back pain.[86,87] Some evidence documents the benefits of manual therapy for other types of pain, although there is practically no research indicating long-lasting and clinically meaningful analgesia from manual therapy in veterinary patients.

CONTRAINDICATIONS

Several contraindications exist for veterinary manual therapy, including lack of a clear diagnosis to justify treatment, evidence of spinal cord compression, joint instability, and lack of evidence of clear advantages from its inclusion that outweigh the potential risks.[3]

ADVERSE EFFECTS

A recent report from the University of California—Los Angeles concerning the frequency and clinical predictors of adverse reactions to chiropractic manipulation in human patients with neck pain revealed that 25% of participants reported increased pain and stiffness after treatment.[88] High-velocity treatments caused more problems than less forceful techniques.

Injuries following chiropractic in humans include paraplegia, vertebral artery dissection and cerebellar infarction, and spinal fluid leak.[89-91]

MAGNET THERAPY

Magnets exist in two forms. One type, called "static" or "permanent," frequently contains iron, steel, rare-earth elements, or alloys. Its magnetic field remains constant. Static magnets must touch or be near the body to deliver maximal effects because even though the gauss (strength) ratings of a static magnet may range in the hundreds, the magnetic field strength merely an inch away may fall into the low double digits. The other type of magnet requires electricity to generate the magnetic field that pulses on and off. This latter version creates a pulsed electromagnetic field.

Research on magnet therapy yields mixed results; some suggest that the hype surrounding magnets far outweighs the evidence.[92] Others insist that the true potential of magnets is as yet untapped.[93]

MECHANISM OF ACTION

Static magnet suppliers may claim that their products are uniquely effective because of a certain arrangement of magnetic polarity, that is, in concentric circles, checkerboard patterns, or stripes. If one accepts the idea that magnets improve circulation maximally when placed perpendicular to vessels, then when polarities lay in varying directions, the resultant fields will be perpendicular to at least some vessels.

Research shows that magnets affect circulation in a bidirectional fashion; that is, researchers evaluating cutaneous microcirculation in

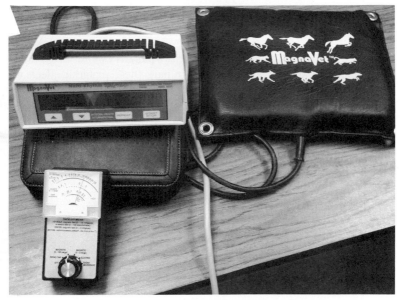

FIG. 16-11. A pulsed electromagnetic field generator designed for animals.

rabbits have shown that static magnetic fields not only cause vasodilation but also can promote vasoconstriction. The outcome depends on the pretreatment neurotransmitter-driven tone of the vessels.

More research is available for pulsed electromagnetic field (PEMF) therapy than for static magnets (Fig. 16-11). PEMF instruments create magnetic fields as electrical current flows through coils of metal wire; more turns of the coil or number of coils can create stronger magnetic fields. Unlike static magnets that produce a permanent magnetic field, PEMF generators only establish a magnetic field when current flows through the coils. The on-off frequency of the PEMF generator determines the rate of pulsation.

Magnet Therapy for Pain

- Magnet therapy devices come in two types: static magnets and pulse electromagnetic field (PEMF) generators.
- Research suggests that PEMF provides analgesia largely through opioid-mediated effects, although other mechanisms are likely involved as well, which may include changes in blood flow to the affected area.

INDICATIONS

The main application of PEMF therapy is for the treatment of pain, including neuropathic pain. PEMF increases pain thresholds in a manner consistent with an analgesic response. In part, these analgesic effects are opioid-mediated, for naloxone attenuates, but does not ablate, PEMF-induced analgesia. Although critics claim that the pain-relieving effects of magnets are placebo-driven, evidence from well-designed studies demonstrating analgesia benefits is beginning to appear. Furthermore, magnets appear to deliver statistically significant benefits for chronic skin ulcer healing, which broadens the potential for the inclusion of magnets in chronic disability cases.[94]

ADVERSE EFFECTS

If an animal ingests multiple magnets, and if these pass beyond the stomach, they may attract each other across thin-walled intestinal loops, leading to ischemia, necrosis, and perforation.[95]

HOMEOPATHY

MECHANISM OF ACTION

The diluted substances in homeopathic remedies supposedly improve the ability of the body to recover from or stave off illness or pain in an unknown and unproven manner. The idea underlying homeopathy rests on the premise that administering a small quantity of an illness- or symptom-producing substance causes the body to fight this illness or provocative substance in a preventive or curative manner. Although the concept resembles vaccination, the dilutions of homeopathic remedies are extremely small and may consist of plant, animal, or mineral substances.

Homeopathy is conceptually difficult for scientifically oriented practitioners to grasp. In addition to the nearly water-strength potencies,

---

Homeopathy for Pain

- The evidence of effectiveness of homeopathic medicine for pain is mixed. The most commonly recommended homeopathic remedy for pain is arnica, which is usually applied presurgically to limit bruising or following trauma or surgery to encourage healing.
- Safety concerns with homeopathic remedies are limited because of their diluted contents.

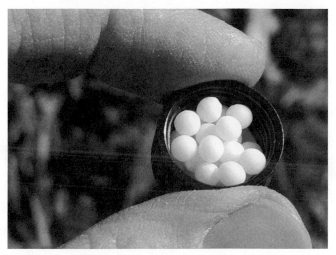

FIG. 16-12. Homeopathic pellets.

another premise of homeopathy is that more dilute remedies confer stronger healing properties and must be used carefully.

As difficult as homeopathic theory is to swallow, the remedies are as easy to administer as sugar pills because, for many remedies, the pills are just that: lactose tablets impregnated on the outer surface with the diluted homeopathic mixture (Fig. 16-12).

INDICATIONS

Homeopathic use of arnica is one of the most common remedies for pain. However, evidence is mixed regarding its value for muscle soreness and pain and bruising following surgery.[96,97]

The lack of sufficient evidence in support of homeopathy in the published literature—across the board and specifically for cancer pain—suggests that homeopathy cannot, and should not, replace standard or other effective analgesic measures.[98]

ADVERSE EFFECTS

Homeopathy maintains a low-risk profile because of the dilute nature of most homeopathic products. However, injectable homeopathic products may contain some risk, including severe adverse reactions such as anaphylaxis, feverish symptoms, and asthma.[99]

CONCLUSION

Many CAM options exist that putatively lessen veterinary patients' pain. Ascertaining the source of pain (musculoskeletal, neuropathic, inflammatory) helps determine which, if any, of the CAM modalities would be most suitable for a given patient and which should be avoided (such as chiropractic for an unstable spine).

REFERENCES

1. Ernst E: Musculoskeletal conditions and complementary/alternative medicine, *Best Pract Res Clin Rheumatol* 18(4):539-556, 2004.
2. Cohen MH: Legal and ethical issues relating to use of complementary therapies in pediatric hematology/oncology, *J Pediatr Hematol Oncol* 28(3):190-193, 2006.
3. Ernst E: The complexity of complementary medicine: chiropractic for back pain, *Clin Rheumatol* 24:445-446, 2005.
4. Hektoen L: Review of the current involvement of homeopathy in veterinary practice and research, *Vet Rec* 157:224-229, 2005.
5. Suarez-Almazor ME, Kendall CJ, Dorgan M: Surfing the Net: information on the World Wide Web for persons with arthritis—patient empowerment or patient deceit? *J Rheumatol* 28:185-191, 2001.
6. Cummings M, Reid F: BMAS policy statements in some controversial areas of acupuncture practice, *Acupunct Med* 22(3):134-136, 2004.
7. Pascoe PJ: Alternative methods for the control of pain, *J Am Vet Med Assoc* 221(2):222-229, 2002.
8. Staud R, Price DD: Mechanisms of acupuncture analgesia for clinical and experimental pain, *Expert Rev Neurother* 6(5):661-667, 2006.
9. Zhang R-X, Lao L, Wang X et al: Electroacupuncture attenuates inflammation in a rat model, *J Altern Complement Med* 11(1):135-142, 2005.
10. Han J-S: Acupuncture and endorphins, *Neurosci Lett* 361:258-261, 2004.
11. Sandberg M, Larsson B, Lindberg L-G, Gerdle B: Different patterns of blood flow response in the trapezius muscle following needle stimulation (acupuncture) between healthy subjects and patients with fibromyalgia and work-related trapezius myalgia, *Eur J Pain* 9:497-510, 2005.
12. Chan AK, Vujnovich A, Bradnam-Roberts L: The effect of acupuncture on alpha-motoneuron excitability, *Acupunct Electrother Res* 29(1-2):53-72, 2004.
13. Yu YH, Wang HC, Wang ZJ: The effect of acupuncture on spinal motor neuron excitability in stroke patients, *Zhonghua Yi Xue Za Zhi* 56(4):258-263, 1995.
14. Somers DL, Clemente FR: Transcutaneous electrical nerve stimulation for the management of neuropathic pain: the effects of frequency and electrode position on prevention of allodynia in a rat model of complex regional pain syndrome type II, *Phys Ther* 86(5):698-709, 2006.
15. Xie H: How to use acupuncture for treatment of osteoarthritis in dogs and cats. In Proceedings of the North American Veterinary Conference, Orlando, Fla Jan 17-21, 2004.

16. Kendall DE: Early understanding of physiology. In *Dao of Chinese medicine: understanding an ancient healing art*, Hong Kong, 2002, Oxford University Press.

17. Furlan AD, van Tulder M, Cherkin D et al: Acupuncture and dry-needling for low back pain: an updated systematic review within the framework of the Cochrane Collaboration, *Spine* 30:944-963, 2005.

18. Furlan AD, van Tulder MW, Cherkin DC et al: Acupuncture and dry-needling for low back pain, *Cochrane Database Syst Rev* Jan 25, 2005; 1:CD-1351.

19. Molsberger AF, Mau J, Pawalec DB, Winkler J: Does acupuncture improve the orthopedic management of chronic low back pain: a randomized, blinded, controlled trial with 3 months follow up, *Pain* 99:579-587, 2002.

20. Manheimer E, White A, Berman B et al: Meta-analysis: acupuncture for low back pain, *Ann Intern Med* 142:651-663, 2005.

21. Berman BM, Lao L, Langenberg P et al: Effectiveness of acupuncture as adjunctive therapy in osteoarthritis of the knee: a randomized, controlled trial, *Ann Intern Med* 141:901-910, 2004.

22. Cui KM, Li WM, Gao X et al: Electro-acupuncture relieves chronic visceral hyperalgesia in rats, *Neurosci Lett* 376:20-23, 2005.

23. Pohodneko-Chudakova IO: Acupuncture analgesia and its application in cranio-maxillofacial surgical procedures, *J Craniomaxillofac Surg* 33:118-122, 2005.

24. Trinh KV, Phillips SD, Ho E, Damsma K: Acupuncture for the alleviation of lateral epicondyle pain: a systematic review, *Rheumatology* 43:1085-1090, 2004.

25. Goddard G: Short term pain reduction with acupuncture treatment for chronic orofacial pain patients, *Med Sci Monit* 11(2):CR71-CR74, 2005.

26. Linde K, Streng A, Jürgens S et al: Acupuncture for patients with migraine: a randomized controlled trial, *JAMA* 293(17):2118-2125, 2005.

27. Romoli M, Allais G, Airola G, Benedetto C: Ear acupuncture in the control of migraine pain: selecting the right acupoints by the "needle contact test" *Neurol Sci* 26:S158-S161, 2005.

28. Resim S, Gumusalan Y, Ekerbicer HC et al: Effectiveness of electro-acupuncture compared to sedo-analgesics in relieving pain during shockwave lithotripsy, *Urol Res* 33(4):285-290, 2005 (Epub June 22, 2005).

29. Usichenko TI, Hermsen M, Witstruck T et al: Auricular acupuncture for pain relief after ambulatory knee arthroscopy: a pilot study, *Evid Based Complement Altern Med* 2(2):185-189, 2005.

30. Ernst E: Acupuncture: a critical analysis, *J Intern Med* 259:125-137, 2006.

31. Durkes TE: Gold bead implants, *Probl Vet Med* 4(1):207-211, 1992.

32. Durkes TE: Gold bead implants. In Schoen AM, editor: *Veterinary acupuncture: ancient art to modern medicine*, St Louis, 2001, Mosby.

33. Hielm-Bjorkman A, Raekallio M, Kuusela E et al: Double-blind evaluation of implants of gold wire at acupuncture points in the dog as a treatment for osteoarthritis induced by hip dysplasia, *Vet Rec* 149(15):452-456, 2001.

34. Bolliger C, DeCamp CE, Stajich M et al: Gait analysis of dogs with hip dysplasia treated with gold bead implantation acupuncture, *Vet Comp Orthop Traumatol* 15(2):116-122, 2002.

35. Hama Y, Kaji T: A migrated acupuncture needle in the medulla oblongata, *Arch Neurol* 61(10):1608, 2004.
36. Patrick BS: Acupuncture complication: a case report, *J Miss State Med Assoc* 46(7):195-197, 2005.
37. Vassiou K, Kelekis NL, Fezoulidis IV: Multiple retained acupuncture needle fragments, *Eur Radiol* 13:1188-1189, 2003 (letter).
38. Gerard PS, Wilck E, Schiano T: Imaging implications in the evaluation of permanent needle acupuncture, *Clin Imaging* 17(1):36-40, 1993.
39. Ernst E, White AR: Acupuncture for back pain, *Arch Intern Med* 158: 2235-2241, 1998.
40. Irnich D, Behrens J, Gleditsch JM et al: Immediate effects of dry needling and acupuncture at distant points in chronic neck pain: results of a randomized, double-blind, sham-controlled crossover trial, *Pain* 99:83-89, 2002.
41. Irnich D, Behrens N, Molzen H et al: Randomised trial of acupuncture compared with conventional massage and "sham" laser acupuncture for treatment of chronic neck pain, *BMJ* 322:1574-1578, 2001.
42. Ghoname EA, Craig WF, White PF et al: Percutaneous electrical nerve stimulation for low back pain: a randomized crossover study, *JAMA* 281(9):818-823, 1999.
43. Carlsson CPO, Sjölund BH: Acupuncture for chronic low back pain: a randomized placebo-controlled study with long-term follow-up, *Clin J Pain* 17:296-305, 2001.
44. White P, Lewith G, Prescott P, Conway J: Acupuncture versus placebo for the treatment of chronic mechanical neck pain, *Ann Intern Med* 141: 911-919, 2004.
45. Blossfeldt P: Acupuncture for chronic neck pain: a cohort study in an NHS pain clinic, *Acupunct Med* 22(3):146-151, 2004.
46. Leibing E, Leonhardt U, Köster G et al: Acupuncture treatment of chronic low-back pain: a randomized, blinded, placebo-controlled trial with 9-month follow-up, *Pain* 96:189-196, 2002.
47. Han HJ, Jeong SW, Kim JY et al: The effect of conservative therapy on thoracolumbar intervertebral disc disease on 15 dogs, *Journal of Veterinary Clinics* 20(10):52-58, 2003.
48. Graw U: Acupuncture as the standard therapy for discopathy with ataxia of the hind legs, *Ganzheitliche Tiermedizin* 17(1):9-13, 2003.
49. Kim MS, Kim SY, Seo KM, Nam TC: Acupuncture treatment for acute torticollis (wry neck) in a dog, *Journal of Veterinary Clinics* 21(4):395-397, 2004.
50. Jeong SM, Park SW: Application of traditional acupuncture on canine intervertebral disc disease, *Journal of Veterinary Clinics* 21(1):49-51, 2004.
51. Janssens LAA: Trigger points in 48 dogs with myofascial pain syndromes, *Vet Surg* 20(4):274-278, 1991.
52. Kim M-S, Xie H, Seo K-M, Nam T-C: The effect of electro-acupuncture treatment for chronic back pain in horses, *Journal of Veterinary Clinics* 22(2):144-147, 2005.
53. Klide AM, Martin BB: Methods of stimulating acupuncture points for treatment of chronic back pain in horses, *J Am Vet Med Assoc* 195(10): 1375-1379, 1989.

54. White AR: Interview, *Mod Med* 67:46, 1999.
55. Kukuk P, Lungenhausen M, Molsberger A, Endres HG: Long-term improvement in pain coping for cLBP and gonarthrosis patients following body needle acupuncture: a prospective cohort study, *Eur J Med Res* 10:263-272, 2005.
56. Longworth W, McCarthy PW: A review of research on acupuncture for the treatment of lumbar disk protrusions and associated neurological symptomatology, *J Altern Complement Med* 3(1):55-76, 1997.
57. Ceccherelli F, Rigoni MT, Gagliardi G, Ruzzante L: Comparison of superficial and deep acupuncture in the treatment of lumbar myofascial pain: a double-blind randomized controlled study, *Clin J Pain* 18(3):149-153, 2002.
58. Itoh K, Katsumi Y, Kitakoji H: Trigger point acupuncture treatment of chronic low back pain in elderly patients: a blinded RCT, *Acupunct Med* 22(4):170-177, 2004.
59. Baldry P: Superficial versus deep dry needling, *Acupunct Med* 20(2-3):78-81, 2002.
60. Wong JY: *A manual of neuro-anatomical acupuncture*, vol 1, *Musculo-skeletal disorders*, Toronto, 1999, Toronto Pain and Stress Clinic.
61. Gunn CC, Milbrandt WE, Little AS, Mason KE: Dry needling of muscle motor points for chronic low-back pain: a randomized trial with long-term follow-up, *Spine* 5(3):279-291, 1980.
62. Gillette RG, Kramis RC, Roberts WJ: Suppression of activity in spinal nocireceptive 'low back' neurons by paravertebral somatic stimuli in the cat, *Neurosci Lett* 241:45-48, 1998.
63. Facco E, Ceccherelli F: Myofascial pain mimicking radicular syndromes, *Acta Neurochir Suppl* 92:147-150, 2005.
64. Gerwin RD: A review of myofascial pain and fibromyalgia: factors that promote their persistence, *Acupunct Med* 23(3):121-134, 2005.
65. Lundeberg T, Hurtig T, Lundeberg S, Thomas M: Long-term results of acupuncture in chronic head and neck pain, *Pain Clinic* 2(1):15-31, 1988.
66. Webb AA: Potential sources of neck and back pain in clinical conditions of dogs and cats: a review, *Vet J* 165(3):193-213, 2003.
67. Rubin D, McGovern B, Kopelman RI: Back to basics, *Am J Med* 119:482-483, 2006.
68. Wirth JH, Hudgins JC, Paice JA: Use of herbal therapies to relieve pain: a review of efficacy and adverse effects, *Pain Manag Nurs* 6(4):145-167, 2005.
69. Wagner S, Suter A, Merfort I: Skin penetration studies of *Arnica* preparations and of their sesquiterpene lactones, *Planta Med* 70(10):897-903, 2004.
70. Knuesel O, Weber M, Suter A: *Arnica montana gel* in osteoarthritis of the knee: an open, multicenter clinical trial, *Adv Ther* 19(5):209-218, 2002.
71. Hostanska K, Daum G, Saller R: Cytostatic and apoptosis-inducing activity of boswellic acids toward malignant cell lines in vitro, *Anticancer Res* 22(5):2853-2862, 2002.
72. Roy S, Khanna S, Krishnaraju AV et al: Regulation of vascular responses to inflammation: inducible matrix metalloproteinase-3 expression in human microvascular endothelial cells is sensitive to anti-inflammatory *Boswellia*, *Antioxid Redox Signal* 8(3-4):653-660, 2006.

73. Reichling J, Schmokel H, Fitzi J et al: Dietary support with *Boswellia* resin in canine inflammatory joint and spinal disease, *Schweiz Arch Tierheilkd* 146(2):71-79, 2004.

74. Kimmatkar N, Thawani V, Hingorani L et al: Efficacy and tolerability of *Boswellia serrata* extract in treatment of osteoarthritis of knee: a randomized double-blind placebo controlled trial, *Phytomedicine* 10:3-7, 2003.

75. McKay DL, Blumberg JB: A review of the bioactivity and potential health benefits of chamomile tea (*Matricaria recutita* L.), *Phytother Res* 20(7): 519-530, 2006.

76. Alqareer A, Alyahya A, Andersson L: The effect of clove and benzocaine versus placebo as topical anesthetics, *J Dent* 34(10):747-750, 2006.

77. Kucera M, Barna M, Horacek O et al: Efficacy and safety of topically applied *Symphytum* herb extract cream in the treatment of ankle distortion: results of a randomized controlled clinical double blind study, *Wien Med Wochenschr* 154(21-22):498-507, 2004.

78. Kucera M, Barna M, Horacek O et al: Topical *Symphytum* herb concentrate cream against myalgia: a randomized controlled double-blind clinical study, *Adv Ther* 22(6):681-692, 2005.

79. Stickel F, Seitz HK: The efficacy and safety of comfrey, *Public Health Nutr* 3(4A):501-508, 2000.

80. Kubo M, Matsuda H, Tokuoka K et al: Anti-inflammatory activities of methanolic extract and alkaloidal components from *Corydalis* tuber, *Biol Pharm Bull* 17(2):262-265, 1994.

81. Wei F, Zou S, Young A et al: Effects of four herbal extracts on adjuvant-induced inflammation and hyperalgesia in rats, *J Altern Complement Med* 5(5):429-436, 1999.

82. Huang TH-W, Tran VH, Duke RK et al: Harpagoside suppresses lipopolysaccharide-induced iNOS and COX-2 expression through inhibition of NK-kappaB activation, *J Ethnopharmacol* 104:149-155, 2006.

83. Nurtjahja-Tjendraputra E, Ammit AJ, Roufogalis BE et al: Effective anti-platelet and COX-1 enzyme inhibitors from pungent constituents of ginger, *Thromb Res* 111:259-265, 2003.

84. Tjendraputra E, Tran VH, Liu-Brennan D et al: Effect of ginger constituents and synthetic analogues on cyclooxygenase-2 enzyme in intact cells, *Bioorg Chem* 29:156-163, 2001.

85. Cheeke PR, Piacente S, Oleszek W: Anti-inflammatory and anti-arthritic effects of *Yucca schidigera*: a review, *J Inflamm* 3:6, 2006.

86. Hurwitz EL, Morgenstern H, Kominski GR et al: A randomized trial of chiropractic and medical care for patients with low back pain, *Spine* 31(6):611-621, 2006.

87. Santilli V, Beghi E, Finucci S: Chiropractic manipulation in the treatment of acute back pain and sciatica with disc protrusion: a randomized double-blind clinical trial of active and simulated spinal manipulations, *Spine J* 6:131-137, 2006.

88. Hurwitz EL, Morgenstern H, Vassilaki M et al: Frequency and clinical predictors of adverse reactions to chiropractic care in the UCLA neck pain study, *Spine* 30(13):1477-1484, 2005.

89. Wang C-C, Kuo J-R, Chio C-C et al: Acute paraplegia following chiropractic therapy, *J Clin Neurosci* 13:578-581, 2006.

90. Chen W-L, Chern C-H, Wu Y-L et al: Vertebral artery dissection and cerebellar infarction following chiropractic manipulation, *Emerg Med J* 23:e1, 2006.

91. Mathews MK, Frohman L, Lee H-J et al: Spinal fluid leak after chiropractic manipulation of the cervical spine, *Arch Ophthalmol* 124:283, 2006.

92. Finegold L, Flamm BL: Magnet therapy, *BMJ* 332(7532):4, 2006.

93. Teo JT: Don't discount magnet therapy, *BMJ* 332(7534):180, 2006.

94. Eccles NK, Hollinworth H: A pilot study to determine whether a static magnetic device can promote chronic leg ulcer healing, *J Wound Care* 14(2):64-67, 2005.

95. Oestreich AE: Danger of multiple magnets beyond the stomach in children, *J Natl Med Assoc* 98(2):277-279, 2006.

96. Tveiten D, Bruset S: Effect of arnica D30 in marathon runners: pooled results from two double-blind placebo controlled studies, *Homeopathy* 92:187-189, 2003.

97. Stevinson C, Devaraj VS, Fountain-Barber A et al: Homeopathic arnica for prevention of pain and bruising: randomized placebo-controlled trial in hand surgery, *J R Soc Med* 96:60-65, 2003.

98. Milazzo S, Russell N, Ernst E: Review: efficacy of homeopathic therapy in cancer treatment, *Eur J Cancer* 42:282-289, 2006.

99. Baars EW, Adriaansen-Tennekes R, Eikmans KJL: Safety of homeopathic injectables for subcutaneous administration: a documentation of the experience of prescribing practitioners, *J Altern Complement Med* 11(4): 609-616, 2005.

APPENDIX 1
ACUPUNCTURE SUPPLIERS

LHASA OMS, INC.

230 Libbey Parkway
Weymouth, MA 02189
Order toll free: 1-800-722-8775
Information: 781-340-1071
Fax: 781-335-5779
E-mail: *info@lhasaoms.com*
www.lhasaoms.com

THE SUPPLY CENTER

6829 Canoga Ave., Suite 5
Canoga Park, CA 91303
818-710-6868
Fax: 818-710-6855
E-mail: *info@thesupplycenter.com*
www.thesupplycenter.com

HELIO MEDICAL SUPPLIES, INC.

606 Charcot Ave.
San Jose, CA 95131
1-800-946-9264 (1-800-YIN-YANG)
Fax: 408-433-5566
E-mail: *sales@heliomed.com*
www.heliomed.com

M.E.D. SERVI-SYSTEMS CANADA LTD.

EASTERN BRANCH

120 Iber Road, Unit 105
Stittsville (Ottawa), ON K2S 1E9
1-800-267-6868 (North America)
613-836-3004 (worldwide)
Fax: 613-831-9356

WESTERN BRANCH (HEAD OFFICE)

9109 Shaughnessy St.
Vancouver, BC V6P 6R9
1-800-667-6866 (North America)
604-263-5042 (worldwide)
Fax: 877-660-6866
Fax: 604-263-8781
www.easterncurrents.ca or *www.acupuncturesupplies.com/*

APPENDIX 2

VETERINARY ACUPUNCTURE COURSES

MEDICAL ACUPUNCTURE FOR VETERINARIANS: OFFERED CONJOINTLY THROUGH COLORADO STATE UNIVERSITY, COLORADO VETERINARY MEDICAL ASSOCIATION, AND THE AMERICAN ACADEMY OF VETERINARY MEDICAL ACUPUNCTURE

Contact:
Narda G. Robinson, DO, DVM, MS, FAAMA
Shipley Professor of Complementary and Alternative Medicine
Director, CSU Center for Comparative and Integrative Pain Medicine
Colorado State University College of Veterinary Medicine and Biomedical Sciences
Department of Clinical Sciences
300 W. Drake Road
Fort Collins, CO 80523
970-221-4535
Fax: 970-297-1275
E-mail: *Narda.Robinson@colostate.edu*

THE INTERNATIONAL VETERINARY ACUPUNCTURE SOCIETY

P.O. Box 271395
Fort Collins, CO 80527-1395
970-266-0666
Fax: 970-266-0777
E-mail: *office@ivas.org*

CHI INSTITUTE

9700 West Hwy. 318
Reddick, FL 32686
1-800-891-1986
Fax: 1-866-700-8772
E-mail: *Barbara@tcvm.com*

APPENDIX 3

Professional Veterinary Acupuncture Archives, Tips, and Chat Rooms on the Internet

PVA-L ARCHIVES

www.listquest.com/secure/pvalist/lq/search.htm?In=pvalist
Username: pva-l
Password: vetacupuncture

PVA-L TIPS

http://users.med.auth.gr/~karanik/english/pva-l/pvaltips.html

PVA-L CHAT ROOM

http://users.med.auth.gr/~karanik/english/vetchatp.html

FOUR

ACUTE AND CHRONIC PAIN MANAGEMENT

17 | Selecting Analgesic Drugs and Routes of Drug Administration

WILLIAM W. MUIR III

CHOICE OF ANALGESIC THERAPY

The choice of analgesic therapy, whether pharmacologic or nonpharmacologic, should be tailored to each animal's needs with the following goals:

- Eliminating or suppressing pain
- Eliminating or suppressing pain behavior and promoting normal behavior
- Making the animal more comfortable
- Returning the animal to maximum function despite residual pain
- Removing stress or distress
- Improving quality of life

The pain experience is often multifaceted and always multidimensional. Pain experience incorporates physiologic (nociception, autonomic, endocrine), sensory (location, intensity, quality), postural (stance, gait), and behavioral (activity, mood, appetite) responses. Pharmacologic approaches to the treatment of pain should be carefully considered, given the diverse effects, metabolism, and toxicity of the drugs that are used to treat pain and the potential for human abuse if opioid analgesics are used. Determining the cause, location, severity, and duration of pain are the three most important factors in the design of a therapeutic plan. The choice of analgesic drugs for treatment of pain produced by a simple elective surgical procedure, for example, may be considerably different from that prescribed for the treatment of osteoarthritis from hip dysplasia. Similarly, the treatment of pain caused by acute inflammatory conditions (abscesses) or abrasions is different from therapy designed to obtund or eliminate pain caused by severe trauma with nerve damage. The choice of drug and dosage recommendations must be individualized to the patient and patient's needs because serum levels are poor guides to analgesic efficacy and do little more than confirm that the drug is present in the animal's body. The patient's physical status, medical history, and behavior pattern, in addition to the pet owner's compliance with and understanding of therapy, are also factors that must be considered when pain therapy is prescribed. Ultimately, the treatment of pain is only as good as one's understanding of its causes and the use of therapeutic approaches that target these causes. Research in the basic sciences is currently unraveling many of the mechanisms responsible for pain and will continue to suggest the design and manufacture of safer, more efficacious therapeutic alternatives.

ANAMNESIS

The dog's or cat's age, weight, sex, breed, and physical status are important determinants of drug selection and dose (Box 17-1).

Age

Young (less than 12 weeks) and older animals generally require lower dosages of drugs. Drug metabolism and elimination pathways may not be fully developed in the very young or may be impaired because of normal aging or concurrent disease (reduced renal, hepatic function) in older animals. Similarly, young and older animals generally demonstrate a more pronounced central nervous system (CNS) response to analgesic drugs that also produce calming or sedative effects.

Weight

Weight should be used only as a guide for determining dose. Animals that are obviously overweight or underweight generally require lower dosages than are recommended. Overweight cats are particularly susceptible to

---

BOX 17-1

Factors to Consider Before Prescribing Analgesic Drugs

- Patient: age, weight, sex, breed, physical status, medical behavior, drug history, and environment
- Mechanism of pain (inflammatory, neuropathic, cancer, other)
- Location and severity of pain
- Consequences of pain
- Duration of pain
- Route of administration (drug delivery)
- Drug efficacy/safety
- Potential for drug toxicity
- Potential for drug interactions
- Clinical experiences

drug overdose because it may be more difficult to estimate their true lean body weight compared with estimation of lean body weight in overweight dogs. Regardless, all animals, particularly the smaller ones, should be weighed as accurately as possible before initiating drug therapy.

Sex

Scientific studies have demonstrated sex-related differences in drug dose-response characteristics. Clinically, however, drug dosages are rarely affected by sex differences other than by the effects of sex hormones on behavior. More aggressive animals usually require a larger dose.

Breed

Breed differences can have a significant impact on drug selection and dose. Veterinary textbooks should be consulted, and the package insert for veterinary-approved drugs should be carefully read before any drug is prescribed. Doberman pinschers, for example, are predisposed to the extrapyramidal side effects produced by opioid drugs. Some boxers have demonstrated pronounced side effects and may have died after administration of acepromazine as an adjuvant to opioid analgesia. Himalayan cats frequently demonstrate increased locomotor activity and hyperexcitability when administered standard doses of opioids for pain control.

Physical Status

The patient's physical status is a major determinant of drug dosage and the technique selected to produce analgesia. Sick, depressed, or debilitated dogs and cats may derive more benefit and demonstrate fewer side effects from analgesic techniques (preemptive, constant rate infusion [CRI]) and nonconventional routes (epidural, transcutaneous) for drug administration. Close patient monitoring must be provided to all dogs and cats that are unconscious or demonstrate signs of cardiorespiratory compromise and are administered intravenous (IV), intramuscular (IM), or subcutaneous (SC) analgesic drugs.

HISTORY

The patient's medical, pharmacologic, and pain history provides valuable information regarding the choice of analgesic therapies and the development of short- and long-term analgesic plans (see Chapter 5). Although typically not emphasized, nonpharmacologic approaches should always be considered as an alternative or in addition to the use of drugs for the treatment of acute and chronic pain (see Chapter 16).

Medical History

The patient's medical history rarely alters drug selection but does significantly affect drug dosage. Dogs or cats with a history of significant CNS or behavioral disorders (seizures, aggression, separation anxiety) may demonstrate pronounced CNS or behavioral changes when administered drugs that are known to produce CNS effects in addition to analgesia. The administration of relatively low dosages of opioids to older dogs that have become less social, for example, may produce depression, periods of disorientation, or episodes of aggression lasting for several weeks. Similarly, dogs or cats with diseases that affect drug metabolism and elimination (liver, renal) may demonstrate drug-related side effects if administered standard dosages of drugs.

Pharmacologic History

The patient's response to previous drug therapy, particularly the response to analgesic and sedative drugs, should be determined. Drug dosages are published as guidelines and should be used only as a starting point. Many animals experience one or more side effects (e.g., vomiting, nervousness, or urine retention) when drugs are first administered. Dogs or cats that are being administered nonsteroidal antiinflammatory drugs (NSAIDs) or behavior-modifying drugs (tricyclic antidepressants), for example, are more likely to demonstrate exaggerated drug-related effects, side effects, and toxicity than animals that are not receiving medications. Ultimately, analgesic therapy must be tailored to meet the animal's needs, and knowledge of the animal's response to previous analgesic therapies can be helpful in this regard.

Pain History/Behavior

The choice of analgesic and the development of an analgesic plan depend on the duration of the pain (transient, acute, chronic), its severity, and the animal's response to pain. The dog's or cat's pain history may be important in the initial design of an analgesic plan. Some dogs and cats, for example, seem to overreact to mild noxious events, demonstrating exaggerated signs or responses to what would otherwise be considered minimal or moderately painful events. Other dogs and cats demonstrate little or no response to painful stimuli for several days or until they are examined. Insight as to how the dog or cat responds to painful events helps determine whether the patient is hypersensitive or a stoic and suggests the types and dosages of drugs needed to restore a more normal behavior and reduce stress. Nervous, hyperexcitable, small-breed dogs that have lived the majority of their lives indoors, for example, generally demonstrate exaggerated responses to minor traumatic events, including physical manipulation, compared with larger, more sedentary outside dogs. Although a generalization, the last statement emphasizes the importance of knowing the animal's history and response (e.g., aggressive when hurt) to pain. Hyperexcitable, hypersensitive dogs or cats, for example, may benefit more from drugs that produce not only analgesia but also mild sedation.

Environment

The patient's environment may provide clues to the factors responsible for initiating pain and pain-associated behaviors. One must know whether there are children in the house and how they interact with the pets. Older osteoarthritic dogs, for example, that are required to go up or down stairs may refuse to move and become agitated when coerced. Similarly, younger animals (dogs or cats) that are in pain may become aggressive if disturbed or forced to play.

Owner Expectations

The owners' opinions and expectations regarding pain and pain therapies should be determined. Their ability to administer medications or perform nonpharmacologic therapeutic techniques must be determined. The advantages, disadvantages, and cost of the pain therapy chosen should be explained to every owner. Owners who are unfamiliar with or unsure of the drugs and techniques used for the treatment of pain are much less likely to comply with therapeutic recommendations.

CAUSE, SEVERITY, AND DURATION OF PAIN

General guidelines regarding the cause (inflammatory, mechanical, neuropathic), severity (mild, moderate, severe), and duration (transient, acute, chronic) of pain should be developed and serve as major determinants of the therapeutic plan (see Chapter 6).

Cause

Pain can be caused by tissue trauma and inflammation, nerve damage or irritation, cancer, or unknown factors (idiopathic). Knowing or determining the cause of pain provides insight into its severity and duration, thereby suggesting potential therapeutic approaches. Gastric distention (visceral pain) with or without displacement ("bloat"), for example, may require gastric decompression, the administration of potent opioids, surgical intervention, and long-term (days) use of analgesics. Similarly, the severe visceral pain and respiratory distress caused by thoracic trauma with pneumothorax cannot be effectively treated by analgesics alone; antiinflammatory medications, chest tubes, and possibly surgical reconstruction are required when there are fractured or displaced ribs. Dogs with cervical disk disease (neuropathic pain) may temporarily and repeatedly benefit from antiinflammatory (glucocorticosteroids) and analgesic (opioids) drugs but eventually require surgery for long-term relief of pain. Determining the cause of pain therefore helps determine the importance of the mechanical, inflammatory, and neuropathic components and suggests appropriate remedies (surgery, antiinflammatory medications, analgesics).

Severity

Animals demonstrating signs of severe pain attract attention. It can be safely assumed, regardless of individual animal variability, that the more pronounced the signs, the more pronounced the pain. With this in mind, an obvious conclusion is that severe pain requires the administration of drugs and the use of techniques that provide immediate, potent, and sustained analgesic effects. In other words, the severity of the pain determines which and to what extent various analgesic drugs and techniques are used. Toward this end, many pain scoring systems and variations of these systems have been developed to quantitate, categorize, and evaluate pain and the severity of pain in animals (see Chapter 6). Pain scoring systems are an integral part of patient evaluation and serve as the basis for drug selection, dose determination, and choice of route of administration. A dog or cat with severe pain resulting from tissue trauma caused by an automobile accident, for example, generally requires the IV administration of a potent opioid (hydromorphone) and/or NSAID for immediate-onset, short-term analgesia. Oral antiinflammatory drugs (firocoxib, carprofen, deracoxib, etodolac, tepoxalin) are administered for long-term analgesia. In contrast, a dog or cat subjected to intense transient pain associated with the placement of a large-gauge IV needle (jugular catheter) or the placement of a chest tube may benefit more from the administration of a local or topical local anesthetic (lidocaine). Less severe forms of pain generally respond to weaker analgesic drugs administered at lower dosages, thereby decreasing the potential for drug-related side effects and toxicity.

Duration

The duration of pain helps to determine drug(s), drug dose, and duration of therapy. The injection of a local anesthetic may suffice as analgesic therapy for an otherwise normal, healthy dog or cat subjected to acute, transient pain. Animals that have experienced moderate to severe pain for extended periods, however, usually require potent analgesic drugs administered in larger dosages because of the plasticity and upregulation of the sensory nervous system. Chronic pain can be responsible for the production of "windup," central sensitization, and allodynia (see Chapter 2). Patients with chronic pain often derive more benefit from a combination of analgesic drugs that act by different mechanisms than from larger doses of a single drug. Drug combinations, although potentially more cumbersome to administer and more expensive, may offer the advantage of drug synergism and a reduction in drug-related side effects and toxicity (see Chapter 7). The choice of drug, drug dosage, and therapeutic plan (pharmacologic and nonpharmacologic) may need to be periodically modified or changed to maintain adequate analgesia, prevent development of drug tolerance, and minimize the potential for drug toxicity.

DEVELOPING A TREATMENT PLAN

The development and periodic reassessment of a therapeutic plan is essential for producing adequate and effective short- or long-term analgesia in dogs and cats (Box 17-2). A rational approach to the treatment of pain is most logically based on a clinical appreciation of the various mechanisms responsible for producing pain and a knowledge of which mechanisms are important in the production of clinical pain.

Similar to an understanding of the mechanisms responsible for causing pain, there must be a conceptual and working understanding of the various types of pain (e.g., inflammatory, neuropathic, and cancer) and their severity. The treatment of severe pain with drugs that are capable of producing only mild analgesic effects not only is ineffective but also makes pain harder to treat and increases the likelihood for drug failure or toxicity.

Several different therapeutic approaches should be designed for the treatment of mild, moderate, and severe pain. From a practical standpoint, the cost of therapy should be integrated into these plans. Nonpharmacologic therapies should be considered and suggested

---

BOX 17-2

Key Components of Analgesic Drug Therapy

- Drug or method for alleviating pain
- Pain prevention program
- Analgesic technique
- Outcome goals
- Methods of assessing analgesia
- Documentation of success/failure
- Pain diary
- Education of staff/pet owner

whenever appropriate. Educational materials describing the harmful consequences of pain, the advantages of pain therapy, and the advantages and disadvantages of different therapeutic approaches should be made available to help educate pet owners.

DRUGS

Drug selection and therapeutic technique should be based on the cause, severity, and duration of pain (see Chapters 6 and 8). Drugs should be thought of and categorized based on their mechanism of action, analgesic potency, and potential to produce unwanted side effects (Box 17-3). A pain scoring combined with quality of life rating system should be developed or adopted and used for assessing the severity of pain and the success or failure of therapy (see Chapter 6). Clinical experience and familiarity with a select group of drugs is important in achieving a beneficial drug effect.

Opioids

Opioids (e.g., morphine, oxymorphone, butorphanol, and codeine) produce mild to excellent analgesia with minimal to moderate behavior modification or depression. The efficacy of oral opioid administration has not been substantiated in dogs and cats, although oral opioid elixirs (morphine) may be useful. Transdermal and epidural routes of drug administration offer an alternative to parenteral administration.

α_2-Agonists

α_2-Agonists (e.g., xylazine, medetomidine, romifidine, and clonidine) produce good to excellent analgesia and moderate to profound sedation. Orally administered α_2-agonists have not been developed for animals. Epidural administration offers an alternative to parenteral routes and is less likely to produce sedation. Clonidine patches are available for transdermal delivery.

BOX 17-3

Key Drug Issues

- Mechanism of action
- Analgesic potency
- Duration of effect
- Central nervous system depression
- Antiinflammatory effects
- Side effects/toxicity
- Drug interactions
- Cost

Nonsteroidal Antiinflammatory Drugs

NSAIDs (e.g., firocoxib, carprofen, deracoxib, etodolac, meloxicam, tepoxalin) produce mild to moderate analgesia and antiinflammatory effects. Oral and parenteral preparations are available. Although NSAIDs are frequently prescribed for chronic use, liver and renal function should be periodically evaluated in animals receiving these drugs.

Local Anesthetics

Local anesthetics produce excellent analgesia but must be administered by injection, and they block sensory and motor nerve fibers. Some administration techniques (e.g., lidocaine CRI) enhance the anesthetic and analgesic effects of concurrently administered drugs.

Other Drugs and Techniques

Many drugs, although not noted for their analgesic effects, can produce mild analgesia (e.g., mexiletine and diltiazem) or enhance the analgesic effects of drugs that do (e.g., acepromazine and droperidol). These drugs are often combined with more traditional analgesic therapies (acepromazine-hydromorphone) to enhance or prolong analgesic drug effects.

ROUTES OF DRUG ADMINISTRATION

Choosing the appropriate route for drug administration and the administration technique can be the deciding factor in producing adequate analgesia while avoiding drug-related side effects or toxicities (Fig. 17-1). The concept of minimal effective concentration, for example, is of limited value in the clinical administration of analgesics, given the wide variation in response to analgesic drugs, despite similar plasma concentrations. Dogs or cats that are sick or that demonstrate signs of CNS depression or cardiovascular or respiratory compromise may not accept or adequately absorb oral medications or may not tolerate the high plasma concentrations produced by IV, IM, or even SC drug administration compared with alternate routes (e.g., epidural or transcutaneous). The route of drug administration may be more important than the drug administered (Box 17-4).

Oral

The oral administration of drugs is preferred for the treatment of most types of chronic and many types of acute pain. Analgesic drugs (NSAIDs) can be administered orally as preemptive analgesia or in conjunction

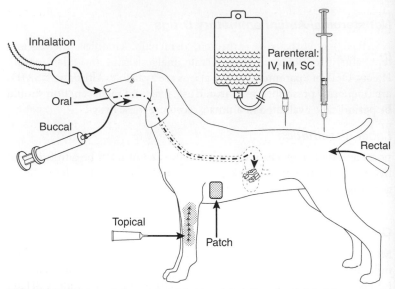

FIG. 17-1. Routes of drug administration. Inhalation, buccal (sublinqual), oral (PO), IV, IM, SQ, topical (cream, patch) and rectal.

BOX 17-4

Routes of Analgesic Drug Administration

- Oral
- Intravenous
- Intramuscular/subcutaneous
- Epidural/subarachnoid
- Transcutaneous/topical
- Sublingual/buccal/transmucosal
- Intranasal/inhalational
- Transdermal
- Rectal

---

with injectable analgesics to produce additive or synergistic effects. Oral administration of drugs can be accomplished in the hospital or at home with minimal to no supervision. Drug effects are relatively prolonged after oral administration, and drug side effects and toxicities are comparatively minimal. Orally administered drugs are subject to first-pass metabolism in the liver, which limits their bioavailability and clinical efficacy. Diet, eating behavior, drug formulation, and concurrent diseases can produce prolonged absorption from the gastrointestinal tract and erratic absorption patterns, leading to an inadequate analgesic response. Finally, the owner must comply with dosage schedules for therapy to be effective.

Intravenous

IV administration of drugs provides the most rapid and predictable effects. Drugs can be administered IV as a bolus, slow injection, or CRI. Drugs that are administered IV must be closely monitored for immediate or delayed adverse drug effects. Drug plasma concentrations are at their highest immediately after IV drug administration, increasing the potential for drug-related side effects and toxicity. Sites of venous access in dogs or cats receiving CRI must be evaluated for signs of extravasation, thrombophlebitis, and generalized inflammation.

Intramuscular and Subcutaneous

IM and SC drug administration are easily performed and provide relatively rapid (5 to 20 minutes) onset of effects. SC drug administration is relatively painless if small needles are used. Analgesic drugs can be administered less frequently than required for IV injections, and plasma concentrations are not as high, reducing the potential for side effects and drug-related toxicity. The IM administration of drugs can be painful, particularly when larger volumes are administered. Drug absorption is occasionally erratic after IM or SC drug administration, producing more variable drug effects than after IV administration. Erratic drug absorption is more likely to occur in dogs and cats with poor peripheral circulation (dehydration, hypovolemia, hypothermia).

Epidural/Subarachnoid (Spinal)

More and more drugs are being investigated for epidural or subarachnoid administration in dogs and cats. Although the epidural route was originally used only for administration of local anesthetics (lidocaine) and opioids (morphine), recent clinical trials have investigated the analgesic effects of epidural administration of NSAIDs (ketoprofen), dissociative anesthetics (ketamine), and α_2-agonists (xylazine, medetomidine). Epidural drug administration produces good to excellent analgesia for extended periods (hours) with relatively small drug doses, thereby limiting the potential for side effects and toxicity. The epidural administration of opioids, α_2-agonists, and NSAIDs also avoids the loss of motor control associated with the epidural administration of local anesthetic drugs. Epidurally administered drugs should be sterile and preservative-free and should have a relatively poor lipid solubility to limit absorption and prolong effects. The epidural or subarachnoid administration of drugs must be performed by appropriately trained and skilled personnel and requires sterile technique.

Transdermal and Topical

Analgesic drugs are available for transdermal (fentanyl, clonidine) delivery or topical administration. A eutectic mixture of local anesthetics (lidocaine-prilocaine [EMLA] cream) and multiple concentrations of lidocaine cream (4% or 5% lidocaine [LMX]) are available. Transdermally delivered drugs are easy to administer with minimal training. The drug is absorbed into the blood, bypassing liver metabolism (first-pass elimination), and effects persist for as long as the patch contains drug and remains in contact with the skin. Transdermal drug delivery is an excellent method for providing preemptive analgesia or "background" analgesia before major surgery and as adjunct analgesia after a major traumatic event. The potential for drug-related side effects and toxicity is low because of slow drug absorption. Slow drug absorption also prolongs the time to produce analgesia, making it difficult to predict drug effects and titrate drug dosage. Skin irritation develops in some dogs and cats.

Sublingual, Buccal, and Transmucosal

Like transdermal drug delivery, the sublingual, buccal, and transmucosal routes of drug delivery depend on drug absorption from the body surface, in this case the mucous membranes. The absorbed drug is not subjected to first-pass liver metabolism. Although potentially having the same advantages as transdermal drug delivery, the sublingual and buccal routes of drug administration to dogs and cats requires patient cooperation. The influence of saliva on drug absorption and the unfamiliar taste produced by many drugs can be problematic. Regardless, the oral administration of various opioid-containing syrups (e.g., codeine, morphine, and buprenorphine) and dextromethorphan results in absorption of drug through the mucous membranes, producing analgesic effects that last for several hours in dogs and cats. The buccal absorption of opioids depends on pH and may be limited by an acidic environment.

Intranasal or Inhalational

Intranasal and inhalational drug delivery are similar to sublingual and buccal administration but do not require patient cooperation. Drug absorption is rapid, producing almost immediate drug effects. Few analgesic drugs other than butorphanol have been investigated for intranasal administration.

Rectal

The rectal administration of drugs to dogs and cats is rarely used. Although rectal administration of drugs can be performed, the bioavailability of rectally administered drugs to dogs and cats is poor. Furthermore, rectally administered drugs are generally absorbed slowly, and drug absorption can be interrupted by defecation or straining to defecate.

TECHNIQUES FOR ANALGESIC DRUG ADMINISTRATION

The medical philosophy adopted for drug administration can be as important as the drug selected in determining the therapeutic efficacy of analgesic drug therapy (Box 17-5). The efficacy of butorphanol, for example, for the treatment of severe pain in dogs and cats is unsubstantiated. Similarly, the analgesic effects of more potent opioids (e.g., morphine and fentanyl) are generally enhanced by the concurrent administration of NSAIDs and frequently reduce the total amount of opioid required to produce effective analgesia.

Local and Regional Anesthetic Nerve Blocks

Local and regional anesthetic nerve blocks (e.g., infiltration, epidural, and intercostal) are valuable adjuncts to the administration of parenteral analgesic medications. Performed properly, these techniques provide excellent analgesia that lasts for several hours with a low potential for serious side effects (see Chapter 15).

Preemptive Analgesia

Preemptive (i.e., treatment before pain occurs) analgesic drugs and techniques should be used whenever possible. The earlier pain is treated, the sooner patient well-being and homeostasis can be reestablished. The use of preemptive techniques to treat pain generally reduces drug dosages and the total amount of drug required to maintain analgesia.

Constant Rate Infusion

A CRI can be used to provide continuous titratable analgesia for extended periods (Fig. 17-2). The use of a CRI to produce a steady-state plasma concentration of drug avoids the peaks (potential toxicity)

BOX 17-5

Drug Administration Techniques

- Local/regional anesthesia
- Preemptive analgesia
- Constant rate infusion
- Multimodal
- Drug rotation schedules

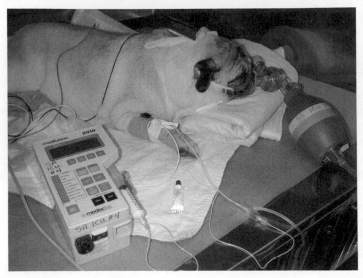

FIG. 17-2. The quantitative and accurate infusion of drugs (analgesics, anesthetics) is markedly facilitated by programmable syringe infusion pumps.

and troughs (potential loss of drug effect) associated with repeated injectable or oral drug administration. Opioids, local anesthetics, and some anesthetic drugs (e.g., ketamine and tiletamine-zolazepam [Telazol]) can be administered by CRI to provide excellent analgesia for hours or days. One or two IV bolus drug doses (loading dose plus CRI) are usually administered in conjunction with the initiation of CRI to help establish and sustain therapeutic plasma drug concentrations until steady-state drug concentrations are reached (see Chapter 7).

Multiple Low Dosing

The administration of multiple low doses of analgesic drugs by IV or IM injection is similar to CRI because a lower dose of drug is administered more frequently, thus minimizing peak and trough drug concentrations and the potential for toxicity and ineffective drug plasma concentrations, respectively. This technique can be used when CRI cannot be used or is technically difficult to perform and is well suited for high-risk patients in which higher-dose bolus administration is more likely to produce unwanted side effects. This technique, however, is labor intensive and more disturbing to the patient than CRI.

Multiple Routes

The same or different analgesic drugs can be administered by multiple routes to produce immediate and sustained drug effects. The IV administration of a drug in conjunction with its IM or SC administration produces immediate drug effects, which are sustained for a longer duration, depending on the rate of absorption and pharmacokinetics of the drug administered. This technique is particularly useful for drugs that have intermediate (1 to 2 hours) to short (<30 minutes) half-lives. Repeated IM administration of morphine in conjunction with the placement of a fentanyl patch (transcutaneous drug delivery), for example, can be used to initiate opioid analgesia (morphine) until effective plasma concentrations of fentanyl are reached, which may take 6 to 12 hours (see Chapter 9).

Multiple Drug Administration

The administration of two or more analgesic drugs (multimodal therapy), sequentially or together in solution (compounding), is an effective method of improving and enhancing analgesic drug effects. Generally speaking, drugs that act by different mechanisms of action are additive and frequently supraadditive (synergistic) when administered at the same time. Synergism allows lower doses of each drug to be administered, decreasing the potential for the development of drug-related side effects or toxicity.

Drug Rotation Schedules

The rotation of drugs that act by the same general mechanism or different mechanisms (e.g., opioids and NSAIDS) may help prevent the development of drug tolerance and drug-related toxicities. Intermittent dosage schedules (3 days on, 2 days off) and alternate administration of carprofen with etodolac or codeine, for example, may help to sustain analgesic drug effects and avoid toxicities unique to single-drug therapy.

WHAT TO DO WHEN THE THERAPEUTIC PLAN DOES NOT WORK

Anyone who has treated dogs, cats, or any animals in pain is familiar with therapeutic failure. Many causes for pain exist and many factors influence the patient's response to painful sensations and the effects of analgesic therapies (Box 17-6). Behavior-modifying drugs or techniques and changes in the animal's environment may be required to treat pain effectively in some animals. Lack of owner compliance with prescribed recommendations should be considered as one possible cause of therapeutic failure.

BOX 17-6

How to Respond to Therapeutic Failure

- Reevaluate patient.
- Reevaluate treatment plan: drug, dose, technique.
- Reevaluate owner compliance.
- Reevaluate patient environment.
- Reevaluate nonpharmacologic treatments.
- Consider alternative or adjunctive therapies.
- Consider drug tolerance/interactions.
- Consider behavioral modification.

SUGGESTED READINGS

Asburn MA, Lipman AG: Management of pain in the cancer patient, *Anesth Analg* 76:402-416, 1993.

Beckman BW: Pathophysiology and management of surgical and chronic oral pain in dogs and cats, *J Vet Dent* 23(1):50-60, 2006.

Bushnell TG, Justins DM: Choosing the right analgesic, *Drugs* 46(3):394-408, 1993.

Clark TP: The clinical pharmacology of cyclooxygenase-2-selective and dual inhibitors, *Vet Clin North Am Small Anim Pract* 36(5):1061-1085, 2006.

Giuliano EA: Nonsteroidal anti-inflammatory drugs in veterinary ophthalmology, *Vet Clin North Am Small Anim Pract* 34(3):707-723, 2004.

Henrotin Y, Sanchez C, Balligand M: Pharmaceutical and nutraceutical management of canine osteoarthritis: present and future perspectives, *Vet J* 170(1):113-123, 2005.

Lascelles BD, McFarland JM, Swann H: Guidelines for safe and effective use of NSAIDs in dogs, *Vet Ther* 6(3):237-251, 2005.

Mathews KA, Dyson DH: Analgesia and chemical restraint for the emergent patient, *Vet Clin North Am Small Anim Pract* 35(2):481-515, 2005.

Muir WW, Woolf CJ: Mechanisms of pain and their therapeutic implications, *J Am Vet Med Assoc* 219:1346-1356, 2001.

Practice guidelines for acute pain management in the perioperative setting: a report by the American Society of Anesthesiologists Task Force on Pain Management, Acute Pain Section, *Anesthesia* 85:1071-1081, 1995.

Robertson SA: Managing pain in feline patients, *Vet Clin North Am Small Anim Pract* 35(1):129-146, 2005.

Robertson SA, Taylor PM: Pain management in cats: past, present and future. 2. Treatment of pain: clinical pharmacology, *J Feline Med Surg* 6(5):321-333, 2004.

Taylor PM, Robertson SA: Pain management in cats: past, present and future. 1. The cat is unique, *J Feline Med Surg* 6(5):313-320, 2004.

Woolf CJ: Pain: moving from symptom control towards mechanism-specific pharmacologic management, *Ann Intern Med* 140:441-451, 2004.

8

ACUTE PAIN MANAGEMENT:

A Case-Based Approach

JAMES S. GAYNOR AND WILLIAM W. MUIR III

The following are specific cases of painful animals. The cause for pain and the rationale for specific treatment are described in detail. Each case presents a unique aspect or challenge as it relates to pain management. Various drugs and procedures are mentioned, including the doses of drugs administered. More detail on each drug and procedure is provided in other portions of the *Handbook*. All patients should be considered healthy unless otherwise noted.

CASE 1	CANINE OVARIOHYSTERECTOMY (BOX 18-1)

Analgesic management was for a dog undergoing ovariohysterectomy (OHE) in a practice that discharges patients the same day as surgery.

Signalment: 6-month-old female mixed-breed dog weighing 20 kg

Challenge: Most owners do not like to take their pet home sedate. The veterinarian is likely to be called if an animal remains sedate into the evening. The challenge is to provide adequate analgesia without sedation for 24 hours.

Source of Pain: The pain from an OHE is multifold. Abdominal wall pain from the incision definitely occurs. Visceral pain from manipulation of the uterus and ovaries and from stretching of associated ligaments also occurs.

BOX 18-1 | CASE 1: CANINE OVARIOHYSTERECTOMY— DESCRIPTION OF PAIN

- Somatic and visceral pain
- Mild to moderate
- Inflammatory and surgically induced tissue trauma
- Acute onset; short duration

TREATMENT AND RATIONALE

Many dogs do not exhibit signs of pain in the presence of humans. Therefore, like any other surgical procedure, it is best to treat pain preemptively and then follow up with the appropriate postoperative evaluation and therapy.

Preemptive Analgesia

Appropriate preemptive analgesic therapy should include an opioid agonist such as morphine or oxymorphone. This dog received morphine 0.5 mg/kg SC combined with acepromazine 0.02 mg/kg and atropine 0.04 mg/kg. The acepromazine was added to the premedication for tranquilization. The atropine was added to offset vagal-induced bradycardia associated with the morphine.

Immediate Postoperative Analgesia

Morphine has a duration of action of approximately 4 to 6 hours when administered at this dose subcutaneously. Because most OHEs are short (20 to 40 minutes), most dogs do not require additional drugs upon recovery from anesthesia. If the OHE is performed in the morning, an additional dose of morphine at 0.5 mg/kg SC should be administered to provide analgesia for the rest of the day. Morphine provides maximal analgesia for the immediate postoperative period.

Analgesia at the End of the Day

Dogs are treated with nalbuphine at 1.0 mg/kg SC as the dog leaves the hospital to ensure several more hours of analgesia with minimal or no sedation.

24-Hour Analgesia

Mild to moderate pain can be treated with a nonsteroidal antiinflammatory drug (NSAID) such as injectable carprofen 4 mg/kg SC followed by oral carprofen 4 mg/kg PO sid the next day. Carprofen can be administered before surgery, after sedation, if the patient will receive intravenous (IV) fluid administration and will have arterial blood pressure monitored to ensure adequate perfusion of the kidney. Alternatively, carprofen should be administered after the procedure during recovery to increase and extend the period of analgesia. This helps to avoid NSAID-related renal toxic effects in animals that are not administered IV fluids or are not having their blood pressure monitored.

4-Day Analgesia

Some practices like to provide approximately 3 days of analgesia after performing an OHE.

1. Carprofen 4.4 mg/kg PO sid. Carprofen should not be administered orally if another NSAID was originally administered parenterally. This particular dog received this protocol.
2. Oral tramadol 2 to 3 mg/kg PO bid
3. Transdermal fentanyl patch 2 to 3 µg/kg per hour (Box 18-2)

**BOX 18-2 | CASE 1: CANINE OVARIOHYSTERECTOMY—
THERAPEUTIC OPTIONS**

- Preemptive analgesia: Morphine 1 mg/kg SC
- Postoperative analgesia: Morphine at 0.5 to 1.0 mg/kg SC
- Analgesia at the end of the day: Nalbuphine at 1.0 mg/kg SC
- 24-hour analgesia: Carprofen 4.4 mg/kg SC
- 3-day analgesia: Carprofen 4 mg/kg PO sid or
  Oral tramadol 2 to 3 mg/kg PO bid or
  Transdermal fentanyl patch 2 to 3 µg/kg per hour

CASE 2	CANINE OVARIOHYSTERECTOMY 2 (BOX 18-3)

This case is an example of an analgesic protocol used for dogs that stay one night in the hospital after OHE.

Signalment: 6-month-old female mixed-breed dog weighing 8 kg

Challenge: The goal is to provide analgesia for 24 hours. The challenge is that the facility is not staffed in the evening to provide redosing of analgesics.

Source of Pain: The pain from an OHE is multifold. Abdominal wall pain from the incision definitely occurs. Visceral pain from manipulation of the uterus and ovaries and from stretching of associated ligaments also occurs.

TREATMENT AND RATIONALE

OHEs, like other surgical procedures, are painful. Patients should receive preemptive and postoperative analgesics.

**BOX 18-3 | CASE 2: CANINE OVARIOHYSTERECTOMY—
DESCRIPTION OF PAIN**

- Somatic and visceral pain
- Mild to moderate
- Inflammatory and surgically induced tissue trauma
- Acute onset; short duration

Preemptive Analgesia

The dog received morphine 7.5 mg SC (approximately 1 mg/kg) 30 minutes before anesthesia. Morphine has a duration of action of approximately 4 to 6 hours when administered at this dose subcutaneously. The dog also received acepromazine 0.02 mg/kg and atropine 0.04 mg/kg combined with the morphine and given subcutaneously. The acepromazine was added to the premedication for tranquilization. The atropine was added to offset any potential for vagal-induced bradycardia associated with the morphine.

Immediate Postoperative Analgesia

Because most OHEs are short (20 to 40 minutes), most dogs do not require additional drugs during recovery from anesthesia. This OHE was performed in the morning, so an additional dose of morphine at 1.0 mg/kg SC was administered 4 hours after the first dose to provide analgesia for the rest of the day. Morphine provides maximal analgesia for the immediate postoperative period.

Analgesia at the End of the Day

Because no one is available to redose morphine after 6 PM, this dog received buprenorphine 0.01 mg/kg SC. The advantage of buprenorphine is that it has a long duration of action, approximately 4 to 12 hours. The analgesia is not as good as that produced by morphine, but it should be adequate, especially if an NSAID is administered postoperatively.

24-Hour Analgesia

Analgesia can be maintained with an NSAID such as meloxicam or carprofen. The NSAID, in the form carprofen 4 mg/kg SC, should be administered after the procedure during recovery to avoid any potential complications produced by anesthetic-associated hypotension (Box 18-4).

**BOX 18-4 | CASE 2: CANINE OVARIOHYSTERECTOMY—
THERAPEUTIC OPTIONS**
- Preemptive analgesia: Morphine 1 mg/kg SC
- Postoperative analgesia: Morphine 1.0 mg/kg SC
- Analgesia at the end of the day: Buprenorphine 0.01 mg/kg SC
- 24-hour analgesia: Carprofen 4 mg/kg SC

CASE 3   CANINE CASTRATION (BOX 18-5)

Signalment: 10-month-old 30-kg male dog
Challenge: To provide analgesia that will extend for 24 hours.

Source of Pain: Castration causes mild to moderate somatic and visceral pain.

BOX 18-5 | CASE 3: CANINE CASTRATION—DESCRIPTION OF PAIN
- Visceral pain
- Mild to moderate
- Inflammatory and surgically induced tissue trauma
- Acute onset; short duration

TREATMENT AND RATIONALE

Preemptive Analgesia

This dog was premedicated with acepromazine 0.04 mg/kg for tranquilization, atropine 0.04 mg/kg to prevent vagal-induced bradycardia, and hydromorphone 0.1 mg/kg for analgesia, all combined and administered subcutaneously.

Immediate Postoperative and 24-Hour Analgesia

Because the pain from castration is believed to be mild to moderate, it can be treated with carprofen 4.4 mg/kg SC. This should be administered during recovery from anesthesia (Box 18-6).

BOX 18-6 | CASE 3: CANINE CASTRATION—THERAPEUTIC OPTIONS
- Preemptive analgesia: Hydromorphone 0.1 mg/kg SC
- Immediate postoperative and 24-hour analgesia: Carprofen 4.4 mg/kg SC

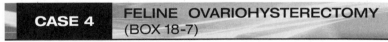

CASE 4 — FELINE OVARIOHYSTERECTOMY (BOX 18-7)

This is a case of a cat that will go home the same day as surgery.

Signalment: 6-month-old female domestic shorthair cat weighing 3 kg
Challenge: To provide analgesia that will extend throughout the night
Source of Pain: The source of pain is a combination of surgical trauma to the abdominal wall and visceral pain from stretching of ligaments.

BOX 18-7 | CASE 4: FELINE OVARIOHYSTERECTOMY—
DESCRIPTION OF PAIN
- Somatic and visceral pain
- Mild to moderate
- Inflammatory and surgically induced tissue trauma
- Acute onset; short duration

TREATMENT AND RATIONALE

Preemptive Analgesia

This cat was premedicated with buprenorphine 0.01 mg/kg SC for analgesia combined with medetomidine 0.02 mg/kg for additional analgesia and sedation, and atropine to prevent bradycardia induced by the other two drugs. The effects of buprenorphine should last 4 to 8 hours in cats.

Postoperative Analgesia

Meloxicam 0.2 mg/kg SC was administered at the end of the procedure and should persist for 24 hours (Box 18-8).

**BOX 18-8 | CASE 4: FELINE OVARIOHYSTERECTOMY—
THERAPEUTIC OPTIONS**
- Preemptive analgesia: Buprenorphine 0.01 mg/kg and medetomidine 0.02 mg/kg SC
- Postoperative analgesia: Meloxicam 0.2 mg/kg SC

CASE 5   FELINE CASTRATION (BOX 18-9)

Signalment: 8-month-old male Abyssinian cat weighing 3 kg
Challenge: Providing analgesia without sedation so the owner can take the cat home the same day as surgery
Source of Pain: Visceral pain related to spermatic cord and cremaster muscle tension. This pain is probably mild to moderate.

BOX 18-9 | CASE 5: FELINE CASTRATION—DESCRIPTION OF PAIN
- Visceral pain
- Mild to moderate
- Inflammatory and surgically induced tissue trauma
- Acute onset; short duration

TREATMENT AND RATIONALE

Preemptive Analgesia

This cat was premedicated with hydromorphone 0.1 mg/kg SC for analgesia combined with medetomidine 0.02 mg/kg for analgesia and sedation, and atropine to prevent bradycardia induced by the other two drugs. The hydromorphone should last 3 to 4 hours in a cat.

Postoperative Analgesia

Carprofen 3 mg/kg SC was administered at the end of the procedure. This should last 24 to 72 hours (Box 18-10).

**BOX 18-10 | CASE 5: FELINE CASTRATION—
              THERAPEUTIC OPTIONS**

- Preemptive analgesia: Hydromorphone 0.1 mg/kg and medetomidine 0.02 mg/kg SC
- Postoperative analgesia: Carprofen 3 mg/kg SC

CASE 6   DECLAW—FRONT FEET (BOX 18-11)

Signalment: 1½-year-old castrated male domestic longhair cat weighing 5.5 kg

Challenge: Pain from declaw procedure is one of the most difficult sources of pain to treat. Anecdotally, some owners believe their cats are much meaner after being declawed, presumably from the intense pain experienced.

Source of Pain: Severe pain originating from severed ligaments, tendons, and potentially traumatized bone and periosteum

---

**BOX 18-11 | CASE 6: DECLAW—FRONT FEET—
              DESCRIPTION OF PAIN**

- Somatic pain
- Severe
- Inflammatory and surgically induced tissue trauma
- Neuropathic; nerve damage
- Acute onset; short duration

TREATMENT AND RATIONALE

Preemptive Analgesia

1. This cat was premedicated with methadone 0.5 mg/kg SC for analgesia combined with medetomidine 0.02 mg/kg for additional analgesia and sedation, and atropine to prevent bradycardia induced by the other two drugs. Methadone was specifically chosen because of its μ-receptor–induced analgesia and its potential to block N-methyl-D-aspartate (NMDA) receptors, thus helping to prevent windup and the development of chronic pain. The dose of methadone was considerably higher than that used for most other procedures in cats because of the pain intensity. Methadone lasts 3 to 5 hours in cats.

2. Before surgery, a declaw local anesthetic block was performed using bupivacaine (0.75%) 1.5 mg/kg split between both front paws. This block lasts approximately 3 to 6 hours. Bupivacaine without epinephrine should be used in peripheral blocks like this. The epinephrine component causes vasoconstriction and decreased perfusion to the periphery, potentially resulting in tissue ischemia.

Postoperative Analgesia

A multimodal approach to analgesia is crucial because of the potential for severe pain.

1. Meloxicam 0.2 mg/kg SC was administered at the end of the procedure. This should provide analgesia for up to 24 hours.
2. Four hours after the initial methadone dose, another dose of methadone 0.5 mg/kg SC was administered. This analgesia was present as the bupivacaine effect subsided.
3. Buprenorphine 0.01 mg/kg SC was administered 3½ hours after the last methadone dose. Buprenorphine has a longer duration of action than methadone and should help keep the cat comfortable throughout the night, along with the meloxicam.
4. Butorphanol was specifically not used in this case because of the intensity of pain. Butorphanol only provides mild to moderate analgesic effects (see Chapter 9). Methadone produces excellent analgesia in cats (Box 18-12).

BOX 18-12 | CASE 6: DECLAW—FRONT FEET— THERAPEUTIC OPTIONS

- Preemptive analgesia: Methadone 0.5 mg/kg and medetomidine 0.02 mg/kg SC; bupivacaine declaw block
- Postoperative analgesia: Meloxicam 0.2 mg/kg SC; methadone 0.5 mg/kg SC 4 hours after local anesthetic infiltration
- Overnight analgesia: Buprenorphine 0.01 mg/kg SC 3½ hours after the last morphine administration
- Analgesia to go home: Buprenorphine 0.01 mg/kg buccally bid for 2 days and meloxicam 0.05 mg/kg PO sid for 4 days

---

Analgesia to Go Home

Although technically easy to perform, onychectomy is a surgical procedure that requires analgesia for 4 to 7 days.

1. Buprenorphine 0.01 mg/kg buccally bid for 2 days. Administration of buccal buprenorphine for longer periods is likely to induce inappetence and lethargy.
2. Meloxicam 0.05 mg/kg PO sid for 4 days
3. Transdermal fentanyl patch 25 µg/h; leave on for 5 days.

CASE 7 | INCISOR EXTRACTION (BOX 18-13)

Signalment: 12-year-old spayed female miniature poodle, weighing 9 kg, with periodontitis requiring extraction of two left lower incisors. This dog also has mitral regurgitation with a 2/6 systolic murmur. There are no apparent signs of heart failure, and the dog is not being administered any medications.

Challenge: To provide analgesia for several days following tooth extraction

Source of Pain: Mild to moderate pain arising from the tooth root and surrounding soft tissue

---

BOX 18-13 | **CASE 7: INCISOR EXTRACTION—DESCRIPTION OF PAIN**
- Somatic pain
- Mild to moderate
- Inflammatory and surgically induced tissue trauma
- Acute onset; short duration

TREATMENT AND RATIONALE

Preemptive Analgesia

A multimodal therapeutic approach was taken for this dog.

1. This dog was premedicated with oxymorphone 0.1 mg/kg SC for analgesia, along with glycopyrrolate 0.01 mg/kg to prevent oxymorphone-induced bradycardia.
2. A left mental nerve block was performed using 0.5 ml of bupivacaine (0.75%). The dose was approximately 0.4 mg/kg. A low dose can be used because the nerve being blocked requires only a small volume of local anesthetic.

Postoperative Analgesia

1. The dentistry procedure took only 30 minutes. Therefore the oxymorphone lasted approximately another 4 hours. The dog was then given nalbuphine 1.0 mg/kg SC to provide several hours of analgesia without sedation so that it could be discharged to go home.
2. This dog was prescribed oral morphine elixir (4 mg/ml) 0.5 mg/kg PO tid to qid. This was to provide analgesia for mild pain for several days (Box 18-14).

BOX 18-14 | **CASE 7: INCISOR EXTRACTION— THERAPEUTIC OPTIONS**
- Preemptive analgesia: Oxymorphone 0.1 mg/kg SC; bupivacaine mental nerve block
- Postoperative analgesia: Nalbuphine 1.0 mg/kg SC; oral morphine elixir (4 mg/ml) 0.5 mg/kg PO tid to qid

---

CASE 8   IMAXILLECTOMY (BOX 18-15)

Signalment: 8-year-old spayed female terrier mix dog weighing 9 kg
Challenge: Mass just behind right upper canine tooth requiring a partial maxillectomy
Source of Pain: Bone and soft tissue surgical trauma

BOX 18-15 | CASE 8: MAXILLECTOMY—DESCRIPTION OF PAIN

- Somatic pain
- Moderate to severe
- Inflammatory and surgically induced tissue trauma
- Acute onset; short duration

TREATMENT AND RATIONALE

Preoperative Analgesia

1. This dog was premedicated with oxymorphone 0.1 mg/kg SC to provide precmptive analgesia and atropine 0.04 mg/kg SC to prevent vagal-induced bradycardia.
2. An infraorbital nerve block was performed using 2.5 mg of 0.5% (0.5 ml) bupivacaine. This provided regional anesthesia to the nose, which was being partially resected.

Postoperative Analgesia

This dog received a fentanyl bolus 2 µg/kg IV followed by a fentanyl infusion of 3 to 5 µg/kg per hour IV. Occasionally, the dog appeared dysphoric. As a result, acepromazine 0.01 mg/kg IV was administered (Box 18-16).

BOX 18-16 | CASE 8: MAXILLECTOMY—THERAPEUTIC OPTIONS

- Preemptive analgesia: Oxymorphone 0.1 mg/kg SC; bupivacaine infraorbital block
- Postoperative analgesia: Fentanyl bolus 2 µg/kg IV followed by fentanyl infusion 3 to 5 µg/kg per hour IV

CASE 9   MANDIBULECTOMY (BOX 18-17)

Signalment: 8-year-old FS golden retriever weighing 25 kg
Challenge: This dog had a mass under the left lower canine tooth, diagnosed as osteosarcoma by previous biopsy. The surgical procedure included a complete rostral mandibulectomy, resecting 2.5 cm of mandible. The extensive bone cutting results in significant pain.
Source of Pain: The pain originates from cut bone and periosteum along with some severed nerves. The potential for severe pain exists.

BOX 18-17 | CASE 9: MANDIBULECTOMY—DESCRIPTION OF PAIN
- Somatic pain
- Moderate to severe intensity
- Inflammatory and surgically induced tissue trauma
- Neuropathic; nerve damage
- Acute onset; short duration

TREATMENT AND RATIONALE

Preemptive Analgesia

Mandibulectomies can be very painful and difficult to treat. This case, like most cases of potential severe pain, warrants a multimodal approach to pain control.

1. Parenteral analgesia: This dog received morphine 1.0 mg/kg SC as premedication, along with acepromazine 0.025 mg/kg SC and atropine 0.01 mg/kg SC.
2. Local anesthesia: Local anesthetic blocks are effective when administered with opioids to help prevent windup resulting from the surgical insult. This results in a patient that may be easier to keep comfortable postoperatively.
   a. Mental nerve blocks are useful for cranial mandibulectomies. This dog's mandibulectomy resected bone caudal to the mental nerve. As a result, a mental nerve block was not used.
   b. Mandibular nerve blocks are useful for providing local anesthesia to the ramus of the mandible. This dog received bilateral mandibular nerve blocks using 7.5 mg of (0.5%; 1.5 ml) bupivacaine at each site. This low dose of local anesthetic is possible because the local anesthetic is deposited directly over the nerve.
   c. Ketamine was administered as a bolus 0.5 mg/kg IV, immediately before surgical stimulation followed by a ketamine infusion, 10 µg/kg per minute, to help prevent windup and help prevent pain-induced dysphoria postoperatively.

Postoperative Analgesia

1. This dog was started on a fentanyl infusion, 3 µg/kg per hour following a fentanyl bolus of 2 µg/kg IV, immediately after induction to anesthesia. The infusion was adjusted as needed throughout the night. The infusion was discontinued 24 hours after surgery.
2. The ketamine infusion was lowered to 2 µg/kg per minute for the next 24 hours.
3. This dog became anxious 12 hours after surgery. Acepromazine 0.01 mg/kg IV was administered. This calmed the dog and presumably potentiated analgesic drug effects.

Multiday Analgesia

This dog was discharged from the hospital approximately 24 hours after surgery. Sustained-release morphine at approximately 1.0 mg/kg PO bid was prescribed for 4 days. The owners discontinued the morphine after 3 days and replaced it with carprofen 50 mg PO bid for another 3 days. The dog exhibited normal behavior at home (Box 18-18).

BOX 18-18 | CASE 9: MANDIBULECTOMY—THERAPEUTIC OPTIONS

- Preemptive analgesia: Morphine 1.0 mg/kg SC; bupivacaine mandibular nerve block; ketamine low-dose infusion
- Immediate postoperative analgesia: Fentanyl bolus 2 µg/kg IV followed by fentanyl infusion 3 µg/kg per hour IV
- Multiday analgesia: Sustained-release morphine 1 mg/kg PO bid; carprofen 50 mg PO bid

---

CASE 10   NASAL BIOPSY (BOX 18-19)

Signalment: 12-year-old spayed female mixed-breed dog weighing 7 kg
Challenge: This dog had a 4-month history of epistaxis requiring rhinoscopy and potential biopsy.
Source of Pain: Stimulation of nasal mucosa produced moderate to severe pain.

BOX 18-19 | CASE 10: NASAL BIOPSY—DESCRIPTION OF PAIN

- Visceral pain
- Mild to moderate
- Inflammatory and surgically induced tissue trauma
- Acute onset; short duration

TREATMENT AND RATIONALE

Preemptive Analgesia

This dog was very calm and required little premedication for restraint purposes. Nonetheless, the dog was administered oxymorphone 0.05 mg/kg SC for basal analgesia and to produce an anesthetic-sparing effect. Atropine 0.02 mg/kg SC was administered to prevent opioid-induced vagal bradycardia.

◆ This dose of oxymorphone may not be adequate analgesia to prevent movement as the rhinoscope approaches the back of the nasal passage. Increasing concentrations of isoflurane and xylazine 0.1 mg/kg IV were administered when the scoping procedure and biopsy became very stimulating. Low doses of xylazine provide good analgesia, especially when administered in conjunction with an opioid, with which it is synergistic (see Chapter 11). Xylazine administration decreased movement and allowed completion of the procedure.

Postoperative Analgesia

Postoperative pain is mild to moderate following rhinoscopy and nasal biopsy. As such, analgesics are administered based on the dog's attitude and clinical signs (Box 18-20).

BOX 18-20 | CASE 10: NASAL BIOPSY—THERAPEUTIC OPTIONS
- Preemptive analgesia: Oxymorphone 0.05 mg/kg SC
- Intraoperative analgesia: Xylazine 0.1 mg/kg IV
- Postoperative analgesia: None

CASE 11	SHOULDER SURGERY (BOX 18-21)

Signalment: 2-year-old castrated male Labrador retriever mixed-bred dog weighing 41 kg
Challenge: Osteochondritis dissecans (OCD) of the left shoulder
Source of Pain: Articular cartilage defect and surgical trauma producing moderate to severe pain

---

**BOX 18-21 | CASE 11: SHOULDER SURGERY—
DESCRIPTION OF PAIN**
- Somatic pain
- Moderate
- Inflammatory and surgically induced tissue trauma
- Acute onset; 3 to 5 days' duration

TREATMENT AND RATIONALE

Preemptive Analgesia

This dog was premedicated with buprenorphine 0.01 mg/kg SC for analgesia along with acepromazine 0.02 mg/kg SC for calming and atropine 0.02 mg/kg SC to offset vagal-induced bradycardia. All drugs were combined in one syringe. Buprenorphine was administered with the intent of providing a long duration of analgesia.

Postoperative Analgesia

The dog had a very rough recovery from anesthesia and surgery. Pain was thought to contribute to the recovery. A test dose of IV fentanyl (2 μg/kg) was administered. Fentanyl administration did not improve the dog's demeanor, possibly because of buprenorphine antagonism of fentanyl effects. The dog was then administered medetomidine 1 μg/kg IV, which calmed the dog considerably. Carprofen 4 mg/kg SC was also administered. Medetomidine was repeated approximately every 90 minutes for 4 hours. Four hours after surgery, morphine 1.0 mg/kg was administered SC and then repeated every 5 hours until the next morning (Box 18-22).

**BOX 18-22 | CASE 11: SHOULDER SURGERY—
THERAPEUTIC OPTIONS**
- Preemptive analgesia: Buprenorphine 0.01 mg/kg SC
- Postoperative analgesia: Medetomidine 1 μg/kg IV; carprofen 4 mg/kg SC; morphine 1 mg/kg SC

CASE 12   ELBOW SURGERY (BOX 18-23)

Signalment: 24-month-old female Newfoundland dog weighing 56 kg
Challenge: This dog had OCD of the right elbow joint.
Source of Pain: Articular cartilage defect and surgical trauma producing moderate to severe pain

---

**BOX 18-23 | CASE 12: ELBOW SURGERY—
DESCRIPTION OF PAIN**
- Somatic pain
- Moderate to severe
- Inflammatory and surgically induced tissue trauma
- Acute onset; 3 to 5 days' duration

TREATMENT AND RATIONALE

Preemptive Analgesia

The dog was premedicated with hydromorphone 0.1 mg/kg for analgesia along with acepromazine 0.015 mg/kg for calming and glycopyrrolate 0.01 mg/kg to help prevent hydromorphone-induced bradycardia. All drugs were combined in one syringe and administered SC.

Postoperative Analgesia: Multimodal Approach

1. A dose of 2.5 mg morphine and 7.5 mg bupivacaine was injected into the joint at the termination of surgery.
   a. Morphine should activate articular opioid receptors and provide some degree of analgesia.
   b. Bupivacaine should block sodium channels and provide good analgesia for 4 to 8 hours.

2. This dog woke up very comfortable. Oral tramadol 150 mg 3 times daily was initiated 6 hours after surgery. Carprofen 4 mg/kg PO sid was started the morning after surgery.

3. The dog remained comfortable for the 4 days it received the tramadol and carprofen (Box 18-24).

BOX 18-24 | CASE 12: ELBOW SURGERY—THERAPEUTIC OPTIONS
- Preemptive analgesia: Hydromorphone 0.1 mg/kg SC
- Postoperative analgesia: Morphine 2.5 mg and bupivacaine 7.5 mg intraarticular injection
- Multiday analgesia: Tramadol 3 mg/kg PO tid; carprofen 4.0 mg/kg PO cid

---

CASE 13	**RADIUS/ULNAR FRACTURE REPAIR (BOX 18-25)**

Signalment: 10-year-old castrated male mixed-breed dog weighing 30 kg
Challenge: This dog jumped from the back of a truck and fractured its left radius and ulna 3 days before presentation for anesthesia and surgery. It had been hemodynamically stabilized before presentation.
Source of Pain: Fractured bones producing severe pain

**BOX 18-25 | CASE 13: RADIUS/ULNAR FRACTURE REPAIR—
DESCRIPTION OF PAIN**
- Visceral and somatic pain
- Moderate to severe
- Inflammatory and trauma-induced tissue trauma
- Acute onset

TREATMENT AND RATIONALE

Preemptive Analgesia: Multimodal Approach

1. This dog was premedicated with morphine 1.0 mg/kg for analgesia along with atropine 0.01 mg/kg SC to prevent bradycardia. No sedative or tranquilizer was used because this dog was very calm.

2. A brachial plexus block was performed using 5 ml of bupivacaine (0.75%), equivalent to approximately 1.3 mg/kg after surgical preparation of the left forelimb.

Postoperative Analgesia

1. This dog was administered morphine 1.0 mg/kg SC during recovery from anesthesia.

2. Two hours later this dog was administered another dose of morphine 1.0 mg/kg SC.

3. The dog was uncomfortable to palpation and was unable to rest comfortably. Electroacupuncture treatment was administered.
   a. Small intestine meridian 3 to 9
   b. Large intestine meridian 4 to 15
   c. Pericardium meridian 6 to 3
   d. 2.5-Hz alternating current continuous stimulation for 20 minutes
   e. This dog was comfortable throughout the night and did not require any additional analgesics or sedation (Box 18-26).

**BOX 18-26 | CASE 13: RADIUS/ULNAR FRACTURE REPAIR—
THERAPEUTIC OPTIONS**

• Preemptive analgesia: Morphine 1.0 mg/kg SC; bupivacaine brachial plexus block
• Postoperative analgesia: Morphine 1.0 mg/kg SC; electroacupuncture

---

CASE 14   FORELIMB AMPUTATION (BOX 18-27)

Signalment: 12-year-old male golden retriever weighing 38 kg
Challenge: Osteosarcoma of the right forelimb
Source of Pain: Cancer and soft tissue surgical trauma resulting from scapulectomy and forelimb removal producing moderate to severe pain

---

**BOX 18-27 | CASE 14: FORELIMB AMPUTATION—
DESCRIPTION OF PAIN**

• Visceral and somatic pain
• Moderate to severe
• Inflammatory and surgically induced tissue trauma
• Acute onset

TREATMENT AND RATIONALE

Preemptive Analgesia

1. The dog was premedicated with morphine 1.0 mg/kg SC to provide preemptive analgesia and atropine 0.04 mg/kg SC to prevent morphine-induced bradycardia.
2. Low-dose ketamine was administered as 0.5 mg/kg bolus followed by 10 µg/kg per minute infusion. Ketamine was infused throughout surgery. Ketamine blocks NMDA receptors and should help decrease postoperative pain and dysphoria.

Postoperative Analgesia

1. Morphine 0.1 mg/kg per hour was infused after administering a morphine bolus of 0.1 mg/kg IV.
2. The low ketamine infusion was decreased to 2 µg/kg per minute for the first 24 hours after surgery.
3. The dog remained comfortable while in the hospital (Box 18-28).

**BOX 18-28 | CASE 14: FORELIMB AMPUTATION—
THERAPEUTIC OPTIONS**

- Preemptive analgesia: Morphine 1.0 mg/kg SC; low-dose ketamine IV
- Postoperative analgesia: Morphine bolus 0.1 mg/kg IV followed by morphine infusion 0.1 mg/kg per hour; microdose ketamine

---

CASE 15	**THORACOTOMY—STERNOTOMY** (BOX 18-29)

Signalment: 11-year-old spayed female domestic shorthair cat weighing 3.2 kg

Challenge: Pulmonary tumor

Source of Pain: Sternotomy and stretching of associated tissues producing moderate to severe pain

---

**BOX 18-29 | CASE 15: THORACOTOMY—STERNOTOMY—
DESCRIPTION OF PAIN**

- Visceral and somatic pain
- Severe
- Inflammatory and surgically induced tissue trauma
- Acute onset

TREATMENT AND RATIONALE

Premedication

The cat was very fractious. High doses of ketamine or a potent sedative would need to be administered to achieve adequate chemical restraint. In addition, this cat required excessive physical restraint that would have produced an excessive amount of stress. As a result, this cat was box-induced with sevoflurane.

Intraoperative Analgesia

The cat was administered fentanyl 2 µg/kg IV bolus followed by 5 µg/kg per hour IV infusion before and during surgery to provide analgesia.

Postoperative Analgesia

The cat was administered lidocaine 1.5 mg/kg and bupivacaine 1.5 mg/kg mixed together interpleurally and administered through the chest tube before waking up. This drug combination was administered every 3 to 6 hours. Fentanyl was infused, 2 to 4 µg/kg per hour (Box 18-30).

**BOX 18-30 | CASE 15: THORACOTOMY—STERNOTOMY—
THERAPEUTIC OPTIONS**

- Preemptive and intraoperative analgesia: Fentanyl 2 µg/kg IV followed by fentanyl 5 µg/kg per hour IV
- Postoperative analgesia: Lidocaine and bupivacaine interpleural block; fentanyl infusion 2 to 4 µg/kg per hour IV

CASE 16 | THORACOTOMY—INTERCOSTAL (BOX 18-31)

Signalment: 5-month-old female Labrador retriever weighing 15 kg
Challenge: Patent ductus arteriosus
Source of Pain: Soft tissue surgical trauma plus displacement and stretching of soft tissue, cartilage, and bone, producing moderate to severe pain

---

**BOX 18-31 | CASE 16: THORACOTOMY—INTERCOSTAL—
DESCRIPTION OF PAIN**

- Visceral and somatic pain
- Moderate to severe
- Inflammatory and surgically induced tissue trauma
- Acute onset

TREATMENT AND RATIONALE

Premedication

This dog was premedicated with methadone 1.0 mg/kg SC along with atropine 0.02 mg/kg to counter increases in vagal tone, and acepromazine 0.02 mg/kg for calming. Methadone provides excellent intraoperative analgesia in addition to blocking NMDA receptors, thereby helping to prevent windup and central sensitization.

◆ Bupivacaine 2 mg/kg was divided and injected two intercostal spaces cranial and caudal to the surgical site at the time of closure.

Postoperative Analgesia

The dog received methadone 0.05 mg/kg IV upon recovery from anesthesia followed by methadone 0.1 mg/kg per hour. The combination of local anesthetic and opioid provided excellent analgesia (Box 18-32).

**BOX 18-32 | CASE 16: THORACOTOMY—INTERCOSTAL—
THERAPEUTIC OPTIONS**

- Preemptive analgesia: Methadone 1.0 mg/kg SC
- Postoperative analgesia: Bupivacaine intercostal nerve block; methadone bolus 0.05 mg/kg IV followed by methadone infusion 0.1 mg/kg per hour IV

CASE 17 | LAPAROTOMY—INTESTINAL RESECTION AND ANASTOMOSIS (BOX 18-33)

Signalment: 6-year-old castrated male Labrador retriever weighing 47 kg
Challenge: Intestinal foreign body requiring resection and anastomosis

Source of Pain: Body wall incisional trauma and abdominal ligament stretching, producing moderate to severe somatic and visceral pain

---

BOX 18-33 | CASE 17: LAPAROTOMY—INTESTINAL RESECTION AND ANASTOMOSIS—DESCRIPTION OF PAIN

- Somatic and visceral pain
- Moderate to severe
- Inflammatory and surgically induced tissue trauma
- Acute onset

TREATMENT AND RATIONALE

Premedication

The dog was premedicated with morphine approximately 1.0 mg/kg SC as preemptive analgesia, along with acepromazine 0.01 mg/kg SC for calming, and atropine 0.04 mg/kg SC to prevent bradycardia.

♦ An epidural injection of morphine 0.1 mg/kg combined with bupivacaine 0.1 mg/kg was unsuccessfully attempted at the lumbosacral vertebral space before surgery. A subarachnoid injection was performed at the lumbar 6-7 intervertebral space. The low dose of bupivacaine permitted no alterations in dose, despite injecting in the cerebrospinal fluid instead of epidurally.

  1. Epidural morphine administration provides analgesia, but not anesthesia, for 12 to 24 hours. Typically, no change in morphine dose is necessary, regardless of epidural or subarachnoid injection. Epidural morphine administration may cause urinary retention. Bladder expression or a urinary catheter postoperatively may be required.

  2. Epidural bupivacaine administration can produce dose-dependent effects. Larger doses produce motor and sensory blockade. The doses used in this dog were small with the intent of blocking sensory nerve transmission without motor blockade or paralysis. Doses intended for epidural injection should be halved for subarachnoid injection.

Postoperative Analgesia

The skin was desensitized using 40 mg of 0.5% bupivacaine in 1:200,000 epinephrine, diluted in half with sterile normal saline. The combination of subarachnoid drugs and the incisional block produced excellent analgesia. This dog did not experience urinary retention (Box 18-34).

BOX 18-34 | CASE 17: LAPAROTOMY—INTESTINAL RESECTION AND ANASTOMOSIS—THERAPEUTIC OPTIONS

- Preemptive analgesia: Morphine 1.0 mg/kg SC; epidural morphine and bupivacaine administration
- Postoperative analgesia: Bupivacaine incisional block

CASE 18	LAPAROTOMY—CYSTOTOMY (BOX 18-35)

Signalment: 4-year-old male cocker spaniel mixed-breed dog weighing 12 kg
Challenge: Urinary calculi requiring laparotomy and cystotomy
Source of Pain: Body wall incisional trauma and abdominal ligament stretching, producing moderate to severe pain

---

BOX 18-35 | CASE 18: LAPAROTOMY—CYSTOTOMY— DESCRIPTION OF PAIN

- Somatic and visceral pain
- Moderate to severe
- Inflammatory and surgically induced tissue trauma
- Acute onset

TREATMENT AND RATIONALE

Premedication

This dog had a history of idiopathic epilepsy and was extremely nervous and active. The dog was premedicated with morphine 1.0 mg/kg SC for preemptive analgesia. Acepromazine was avoided because of a history of seizures. Xylazine 0.4 mg/kg SC was administered with the morphine. Xylazine has synergistic effects with opioids to produce better sedation and analgesia. Atropine 0.04 mg/kg SC was added to the mixture because both drugs increase vagal tone and can cause bradycardia.

Postoperative Analgesia

1. This dog was not administered epidural morphine or local anesthetic even though this would likely produce good postoperative analgesia. The dog's behavior made it extremely difficult to maintain a urinary catheter without him chewing at it. Because epidural morphine administration can cause urinary retention and this patient was undergoing bladder surgery, it was believed best to not subject the cystotomy incision to excess intraluminal pressure.
2. An incisional block was performed before skin closure using 15 mg of 0.5% bupivacaine with 1:200,000 epinephrine diluted in half with 0.9% saline. This provided good body wall analgesia for approximately 8 hours.
3. Fentanyl 2 to 5 µg/kg per hour was administered to provide good abdominal analgesia.
4. The dog became dysphoric and was administered xylazine 0.05 mg/kg IV as needed.

5. This dog was discharged from the hospital the following day with no other analgesics (Box 18-36).

BOX 18-36 | CASE 18: LAPAROTOMY—CYSTOTOMY— THERAPEUTIC OPTIONS

- Preemptive analgesia: Morphine 1.0 mg/kg and xylazine 0.4 mg/kg SC
- Postoperative analgesia: Bupivacaine incisional block; fentanyl bolus 2 µg/kg IV followed by fentanyl infusion 2 to 5 µg/kg per hour

---

CASE 19   PANCREATITIS (BOX 18-37)

Signalment: 12-year-old spayed female miniature schnauzer dog
Challenge: History of vomiting and lethargy for 3 days; abdominal pain; no abdominal obstruction; blood work consistent with pancreatitis
Source of Pain: Severe visceral pain associated with pancreatitis

---

BOX 18-37 | CASE 19: PANCREATITIS—DESCRIPTION OF PAIN

- Visceral pain
- Moderate to severe
- Inflammatory
- Acute onset

TREATMENT AND RATIONALE

◆ This dog was initially unsuccessfully treated with continuous infusion of fentanyl 3 to 6 µg/kg per hour after a bolus of 2 µg/kg. The dog was still unable to rest comfortably.

◆ Interpleural local anesthetic administration can provide analgesia for thoracic and cranial abdominal pain. The nerves from the cranial abdomen enter the spinal cord in the thorax.

1. Lidocaine 1.5 mg/kg was injected in the sixth intercostal space through a 22-gauge butterfly catheter. Lidocaine was injected initially to produce an immediate block.

2. Bupivacaine 1.5 mg/kg was injected following the lidocaine. Bupivacaine has a 15- to 20-minute duration until the onset of analgesia and can cause stinging. The lidocaine prevents the bupivacaine from stinging.

3. This technique produced comfort, allowing this dog to sleep. The local anesthetic technique was repeated every 4 hours. The fentanyl was continued at 2 µg/kg per hour (Box 18-38).

BOX 18-38 | CASE 19: PANCREATITIS—THERAPEUTIC OPTIONS

- Analgesia: Lidocaine and bupivacaine interpleural block

CASE 20   LUMBOSACRAL DISK SURGERY (BOX 18-39)

Signalment: 7-year-old spayed female miniature dachshund dog weighing 8 kg
Challenge: Lumbosacral disk protrusion
Source of Pain: Spinal cord swelling and disk entrapment of nerve roots causes severe pain.

BOX 18-39 | CASE 20: LUMBOSACRAL DISK SURGERY—DESCRIPTION OF PAIN

- Somatic and visceral pain
- Moderate to severe
- Inflammatory and surgically induced tissue trauma and underlying disease
- Acute onset

TREATMENT AND RATIONALE

Premedication

This dog was premedicated with morphine 0.75 mg/kg SC to provide analgesia, along with glycopyrrolate 0.01 mg/kg to help prevent bradycardia.

Intraoperative Analgesia

This dog received fentanyl 2 µg/kg IV followed by fentanyl 10 µg/kg per hour to provide good intraoperative analgesia and decrease the concentration of inhalant anesthetic, thereby helping to maintain cardiac output and arterial blood pressure. The fentanyl infusion was discontinued 30 minutes before the anticipated completion of surgery to facilitate a timely extubation.

Postoperative Analgesia

This dog had a smooth recovery. He remained sedate. The fentanyl infusion was restarted at 3 µg/kg per hour. This dog remained comfortable for the next 36 hours before it was discharged from the critical care unit (Box 18-40).

BOX 18-40 | CASE 20: LUMBOSACRAL DISK SURGERY—THERAPEUTIC OPTIONS

- Preemptive analgesia: Morphine 0.75 mg/kg SC
- Intraoperative analgesia: Fentanyl bolus 2 µg/kg IV followed by fentanyl infusion 10 µg/kg per hour IV
- Postoperative analgesia: Fentanyl infusion 3 µg/kg per hour IV

CASE 21   TAIL AMPUTATION (BOX 18-41)

Signalment: 2-year-old castrated male domestic shorthair cat

Challenge: The cat's tail got caught in a radiator fan, causing a degloving injury and a fracture distal to coccygeal bone 5.

Source of Pain: Bone fracture and soft tissue trauma, producing severe localized pain

---

BOX 18-41 | CASE 21: TAIL AMPUTATION—DESCRIPTION OF PAIN

- Somatic pain
- Moderate
- Inflammatory and surgically induced tissue trauma and underlying disease
- Acute onset

TREATMENT AND RATIONALE

Preemptive Analgesia

1. This cat received medetomidine 0.02 mg/kg and hydromorphone 0.1 mg/kg administered together SC for analgesia and sedation. Atropine 0.02 mg/kg SC was also administered to prevent bradycardia.
2. Bupivacaine 0.75 mg/kg was injected epidurally between coccygeal bones 1 and 2 after induction of anesthesia.

Postoperative Analgesia

1. Meloxicam 0.2 mg/kg SC was injected in recovery to provide analgesia and to reduce inflammation.
2. The cat received hydromorphone 0.1 mg/kg SC 4 hours after the initial hydromorphone injections (Box 18-42).

BOX 18-42 | CASE 21: TAIL AMPUTATION— THERAPEUTIC OPTIONS

- Preemptive analgesia: Hydromorphone 0.1 mg/kg SC and medetomidine 0.02 mg/kg SC; bupivacaine epidural
- Postoperative analgesia: meloxicam 0.2 mg/kg SC and hydromorphone 0.1 mg/kg SC

CASE 22   REAR LIMB AMPUTATION (BOX 18-43)

Signalment: 7-year-old spayed female rottweiler dog weighing 42 kg

Challenge: Osteosarcoma of the left rear limb, requiring amputation

Source of Pain: Cancer surgical trauma producing severe pain

BOX 18-43 | CASE 22: REAR LIMB AMPUTATION— DESCRIPTION OF PAIN

- Somatic pain
- Moderate to severe
- Inflammatory and surgically induced tissue trauma
- Acute onset

TREATMENT AND RATIONALE

Preoperative Analgesia

1. The dog was administered morphine 1.0 mg/kg SC for preemptive analgesia and atropine 0.05 mg/kg SC. No other tranquilizer or sedative was administered.
2. Morphine 0.1 mg/kg and bupivacaine 0.3 mg/kg were combined and administered epidurally to provide supplemental intraoperative and postoperative analgesia of 12 to 24 hours' duration.

Postoperative Analgesia

The dog was administered fentanyl 4 to 6 mg/kg per hour IV over the next 24 hours to maintain analgesia. This was followed by sustained-release morphine 30 mg PO twice daily for the next 4 days (Box 18-44).

BOX 18-44 | CASE 22: REAR LIMB AMPUTATION— THERAPEUTIC OPTIONS

- Preemptive analgesia: Morphine 1.0 mg/kg SC; morphine and bupivacaine epidural
- Postoperative analgesia: Fentanyl bolus 2 µg/kg IV followed by fentanyl infusion 4 to 6 mg/kg per hour IV
- Multiday analgesia: Sustained-release morphine 30 mg PO bid

---

CASE 23 | **BILATERAL FEMORAL FRACTURE REPAIR (BOX 18-45)**

Signalment: 6-year-old spayed female Australian shepherd mixed-breed dog weighing 26 kg
Challenge: This dog slipped off an icy deck under construction and fell 25 feet; radiographs revealed bilateral comminuted femoral fractures.
Source of Pain: Broken bones and soft tissue trauma producing severe pain

---

BOX 18-45 | CASE 23: BILATERAL FEMORAL FRACTURE REPAIR—DESCRIPTION OF PAIN

- Somatic pain
- Severe
- Inflammatory, surgically, and traumatically induced tissue trauma
- Acute onset

TREATMENT AND RATIONALE

Preemptive Analgesia

Femoral fracture repairs can be very painful and difficult to treat. This case, like most cases of potential severe pain, warrants a multimodal approach.

1. Parenteral analgesia: This dog received morphine 1.0 mg/kg SC as premedication, along with acepromazine 0.025 mg/kg SC and atropine 0.01 mg/kg SC.
2. An epidural catheter was inserted in the lumbosacral space and advanced three disk spaces cranially after inducing anesthesia. Morphine 0.1 mg/kg along with bupivacaine 0.1 mg/kg was injected through the catheter before surgery. This catheter allowed redosing of epidural analgesics for several days. Placing morphine in the epidural space provided good analgesia for 12 to 24 hours with minimal central nervous system side effects. The low dose of bupivacaine blocked sensory nerve transmission with minimal effect on motor nerve transmission. This approach allowed the dog to feel its legs in recovery, preventing self-trauma and mutilation, which sometimes occurs with epidural regional anesthesia. This dog underwent uneventful anesthesia and surgery.

The dog recovered from anesthesia very painful and agitated.

1. Morphine 0.1 mg/kg was administered IV and infused, 0.1 mg/kg per hour, to provide analgesia in addition to the epidural morphine. The infusion was continued for 16 hours.
2. Acepromazine 0.25 mg IV was administered in recovery because of agitation. It was redosed 3½ hours later.
3. Epidural morphine 0.1 mg/kg was redosed 12 hours after the initial dose and then at 24-hour intervals for 3 days, at which time the epidural catheter was removed (Box 18-46).

**BOX 18-46 | CASE 23: BILATERAL FEMORAL FRACTURE REPAIR—
THERAPEUTIC OPTIONS**

- Preemptive analgesia: Morphine 1.0 mg/kg SC; morphine and bupivacaine via epidural catheter
- Postoperative analgesia: Morphine bolus 0.1 mg/kg IV followed by morphine infusion 0.1 mg/kg per hour IV; epidural morphine administration

---

| CASE 24 | GENERAL TRAUMA (BOX 18-47) |

Signalment: 7-year-old castrated male domestic shorthair cat weighing 3 kg

Challenge: The cat was recently hit by a car and suffered head trauma, a broken left humerus, and general soft tissue trauma.

Source of Pain: General soft tissue trauma and fractured bone, producing severe pain

---

BOX 18-47 | CASE 24: GENERAL TRAUMA—DESCRIPTION OF PAIN
- Somatic pain
- Moderate to severe
- Inflammatory and trauma-induced tissue trauma
- Acute onset

TREATMENT AND RATIONALE

◆ The immediate goal was to provide good analgesia overnight but be able to assess mentation periodically in order to determine the status of the head trauma.

◆ Fentanyl was considered for pain control but rejected because it would make it difficult to assess mentation.

◆ Remifentanil does not require liver metabolism but is cleared via nonspecific esterases throughout the body. Remifentanil has a duration of action of 8 to 10 minutes regardless of infusion time. Remifentanil was administered 6 μg/kg per hour, which kept the cat very comfortable. The remifentanil infusion was discontinued when neurologic assessment was desired. Neurologic assessment was performed 10 minutes later. Analgesia was rapidly reestablished by administering a bolus of remifentanil 4 μg/kg and restarting the infusion (Box 18-48).

BOX 18-48 | CASE 24: GENERAL TRAUMA—THERAPEUTIC OPTIONS
- Continuous analgesia: Remifentanil 6 μg/kg per hour

| CASE 25 | EXERCISE-INDUCED TRAUMA (BOX 18-49) |

Signalment: 4-year-old spayed female mixed-breed dog weighing 25 kg
Challenge: Limping on right rear limb after a long hike in the mountains
Source of Pain: The dog has mild hip dysplasia of the right coxofemoral joint resulting in moderate osteoarthritic pain. He has some muscle soreness also.

BOX 18-49 | CASE 25: EXERCISE-INDUCED TRAUMA— DESCRIPTION OF PAIN
- Somatic pain
- Mild to moderate
- Inflammatory and exercise-induced tissue trauma
- Acute onset

TREATMENT AND RATIONALE

The dog was successfully treated with carprofen 50 mg orally twice daily for 7 days (Box 18-50).

BOX 18-50 | CASE 25: EXERCISE-INDUCED TRAUMA— THERAPEUTIC OPTIONS
- Analgesia: Carprofen 2.2 mg/kg PO bid

---

9 CHRONIC PAIN MANAGEMENT:

A Case-Based Approach

JAMES S. GAYNOR AND WILLIAM W. MUIR III

Following are specific cases of animals with chronic pain. The nature of the case and rationale for specific treatment are described. Each case presents a unique aspect or problem as it relates to pain management. Because the animals were evaluated and treated by different veterinarians, diverse therapeutic protocols were used. Various drugs, procedures, and drug doses are detailed. The selection of drugs and response to therapy should be considered anecdotal because patient well-being was subjectively assessed and primarily determined by improvement of the animal's quality of life. More detailed information on each drug and procedure can be found in various portions of the *Handbook*. All patients should be considered systemically healthy unless otherwise noted.

Please note the abbreviations for frequency of dosing as recognized within the pharmacy profession:

bid = Twice daily
qd = Once daily
qid = 4 times daily
qod = Every other day
sid = once a day
tid = 3 times daily

CASE 1	HIP DYSPLASIA (BOX 19-1)

Pain control was provided for a dog with degenerative disease of both hip joints.

Signalment: 12-year-old female spayed German shepherd weighing 36 kg with bilateral hip dysplasia, left worse than right

Challenge: This dog has had chronic osteoarthritis pain for 8 years. The pain continues to worsen with age.

Cause of Pain: Osteoarthritis of the coxofemoral joints

BOX 19-1 | CASE 1: HIP DYSPLASIA—DESCRIPTION OF PAIN

- Coxofemoral osteoarthritis
- Moderate to severe intensity
- Somatic: inflammatory
- Long term to lifelong

TREATMENT AND RATIONALE

◆ This dog was initially receiving aspirin as needed on bad days for several years. The owner and the veterinarian became concerned with the possibility of gastrointestinal side effects (ulcers, hemorrhage).

◆ The dog began receiving carprofen 25 mg PO bid. This dose was low, but the dog was much more comfortable within 1 day.

◆ The hip-associated pain worsened, and the dose of carprofen was increased to 50 mg PO bid. This made the dog more comfortable for approximately 6 months.

◆ The dog was in pain again after 6 months. Rather than increasing the dose of carprofen and risking side effects, the veterinarian recommended switching from carprofen to etodolac.

  • It is reasonable to expect that if one drug does not work well for an individual, another might work better.

  • Considerable risk is present when immediately switching from one non-steroidal antiinflammatory drug (NSAID) to another. It is possible to get additive side effects, such as gastrointestinal ulceration or renal toxicity.

  • It is advisable to have a washout period between ending one NSAID and starting another. A period of 10 days is considered safe or at least five half-lives of the drug being discontinued.

  • If a washout period is not possible, administering a gastrointestinal protectant, such as misoprostol or omeprazole, for approximately 4 to 10 days is advisable. For example, end one NSAID on the evening of one day and start misoprostol 2 to 5 µg/kg PO bid. Start the new NSAID the following day.

  • To keep a dog comfortable during the washout period, opioids can be administered orally.

◆ Carprofen was discontinued for 10 days, during which time this dog became very uncomfortable. Etodolac 450 mg PO daily was then administered. The dog did not experience a great improvement in quality of life compared with carprofen.

- The veterinarian and owner then discussed the potential of acupuncture for relief of pain.
- Electroacupuncture was instituted twice weekly for 3 weeks, alternating hips at each treatment using the following protocol.
  1. GB 29 to GB 30
  2. BL 40 to BL 54
  3. GB 34
  4. Bilateral BL 11
  5. Alternating current, 2 5 Hz, continuous for 20 minutes
- The dog became much more comfortable. During the fourth week of acupuncture the dog received only one treatment.
- Acupuncture was spread out to one treatment every 4 to 6 weeks. After 2 months the etodolac dose was decreased to 300 mg PO daily. The dog remained comfortable (Box 19-2)

BOX 19-2 | CASE 1: HIP DYSPLASIA—THERAPEUTIC OPTIONS
- *First therapy:* Carprofen 25 to 50 mg PO bid
- *Second therapy:* Etodolac 450 mg PO qd
- *Final therapy:* Electroacupuncture

CASE 2   HIP OSTEOARTHRITIS (BOX 19-3)

Signalment: 5-year-old female spayed 40-kg Old English sheepdog with bilateral degenerative joint disease of the coxofemoral joints
Challenge: This dog has had chronic osteoarthritis pain for 3 years. She has been taking deracoxib 50 mg PO qd for 3 years. The deracoxib became less effective for controlling pain recently. The dog was switched to carprofen 150 mg PO qd, which maintained her comfort for several months before its efficacy began to decrease.
Cause of Pain: Osteoarthritis of the coxofemoral joints

BOX 19-3 | CASE 2: HIP OSTEOARTHRITIS—DESCRIPTION OF PAIN
- Moderate intensity
- Somatic and central: inflammatory and neuropathic
- Long term to lifelong

TREATMENT AND RATIONALE

- Amantadine 3 mg/kg PO qd for 21 days to treat potential central neuronal hyperexcitability (windup). Windup occurs because of a prolonged low-medium–grade constant noxious stimulus bombarding the spinal cord. This case typifies the clinical presentation. When treating patients with osteoarthritis and windup, NSAID administration can be maintained.

◆ Carprofen 150 mg PO qd. This dog became comfortable on the third day of treatment and remained comfortable for months on carprofen alone (Box 19-4).

BOX 19-4 | CASE 2: HIP OSTEOARTHRITIS—THERAPEUTIC OPTIONS

• *First therapy:* Amantadine 3 mg/kg PO qd for 21 days
• *Concurrent therapy:* Carprofen 150 mg PO qd

| CASE 3 | RADIATION-INDUCED PAIN (BOX 19-5) |

Signalment: 9-year-old spayed female Labrador retriever weighing 31 kg

Challenge: This dog had a mast cell tumor removed from the lateral aspect of her mid left thigh and has been treated with radiation therapy for 14 treatments over a 3-week period. The dog has developed progressively more pain than could be managed at home with oral morphine and will not stand up.

Cause of Pain: Radiation-induced soft tissue damage and inflammation.

BOX 19-5 | CASE 3: RADIATION-INDUCED PAIN— DESCRIPTION OF PAIN

• Radiation therapy
• Severe intensity
• *Somatic:* inflammatory
• Days to weeks

TREATMENT AND RATIONALE

The dog has developed severe pain that has affected her quality of life and the ability of the owner to cope with her.

Initial Therapy

The initial goal of therapy for this dog was to gain control of her pain.

◆ The dog was hospitalized, and a peripheral catheter was placed in her cephalic vein. Ketamine was diluted and administered as a bolus of 0.5 mg/kg IV followed by 1 µg/kg per minute. Ketamine was used as an N-methyl-D-aspartate (NMDA) receptor antagonist to help decrease central neuronal hyperexcitability and reduce the chronic pain.

♦ Fentanyl was administered concurrently, initially as a 2-µg/kg bolus followed by a 5-µg/kg per hour infusion. Within 1 hour, this dog was willing and able to stand and walk.

♦ Fentanyl and ketamine were administered for approximately 48 hours, decreasing the fentanyl to 2 µg/kg per hour during the last 12 hours.

Continued Therapy

This dog was hospitalized for an additional 48 hours to make the transition to oral drug therapy before releasing her back to the owner's care.

♦ Oral sustained-release morphine was started, 30 mg PO bid for 10 days. It was believed that this dose of morphine would control the pain based on the low dose of fentanyl on which the dog had been maintained during her initial therapy. This is the same dose of morphine she was receiving before admission to the hospital. After 10 days, she was weaned to sustained-release morphine 30 mg PO qd for 5 days. Morphine was then discontinued completely.

♦ Amantadine was started, 100 mg PO qd for 5 days, to block the NMDA receptors and prevent central neuronal excitability.

♦ This dog was released from the hospital comfortable and remained comfortable at home (Box 19-6).

**BOX 19-6 | CASE 3: RADIATION-INDUCED PAIN—
THERAPEUTIC OPTIONS**

- *First therapy:* Sustained-release oral morphine 30 mg PO bid
- *Second therapy:* Ketamine 0.5 mg/kg IV followed by 1 µg/kg per min concurrent fentanyl 2 µg/kg bolus followed by 5 µg/kg/hr; 2 µg/kg per hour over 48 hours
- *Final therapy:* Sustained-release oral morphine 30 mg PO bid for 10 days and amantadine 100 mg PO qd for 5 days

---

CASE 4	FORELIMB AMPUTATION PAIN (BOX 19-7)

Signalment: 7-year-old spayed female husky weighing 25 kg

Challenge: The dog had osteosarcoma of the right front limb culminating in an uneventful forelimb amputation. The dog was presented with a complaint of intermittently crying out. The dog has been receiving codeine 30 mg with acetaminophen 300 mg orally twice daily for 5 days. Upon physical examination the dog was hypersensitive to touch and cried when lightly touched across her lateral thorax and abdomen. The dog had no neck or back pain. Allodynia was diagnosed.

Source of Pain: The source of pain was unclear but was considered to be diffuse.

BOX 19-7 | CASE 4: FORELIMB AMPUTATION PAIN—
DESCRIPTION OF PAIN

- Moderate intensity
- *Somatic:* inflammatory and neuropathic
- Long-term duration if not treatable

TREATMENT AND RATIONALE

Current analgesic therapy was ineffective. Chronic refractory pain with allodynia is difficult to treat with a single drug (opioids) and generally requires a multimodal approach.

◆ Amantadine 100 mg PO qd for 5 days was initiated to block NMDA receptors and decrease central neuronal excitability, with the intent of decreasing her allodynia.

◆ Sustained-release morphine 30 mg PO bid was started for 10 days to provide analgesia from the chronic pain.

◆ The owner reported that the dog was comfortable within 2 days. The seventh day after her new analgesic protocol had started (2 days after discontinuing the amantadine), she started developing allodynia again. Amantadine 100 mg PO qd was started for another 10 days, and the sustained-release morphine for another 5 days. The owner did not report any more pain at the end of 10 days (Box 19-8).

BOX 19-8 | CASE 4: FORELIMB AMPUTATION PAIN—
THERAPEUTIC OPTIONS

- *First therapy:* Acetaminophen 300 mg and codeine 30 mg PO bid
- *Second therapy:* Amantadine 100 mg PO qd for 5 days concurrent with sustained-release morphine 30 mg PO bid for 10 days
- *Final therapy:* Amantadine 100 mg PO qd for 10 days concurrent with sustained-release morphine 30 mg PO bid for 10 days

---

| CASE 5 | BILATERAL HIP OSTEOARTHRITIS (BOX 19-9) |

Signalment: 11-year-old female spayed 4-kg Himalayan

Challenge: This cat cannot jump or play as she has in the past. The owner believed this change in behavior was due to old age.

Source of Pain: Cartilage damage in coxofemoral joints

BOX 19-9 | CASE 5: BILATERAL HIP OSTEOARTHRITIS—
DESCRIPTION OF PAIN

- Moderate to severe intensity
- Somatic: inflammatory
- Long term to lifelong

TREATMENT AND RATIONALE

◆ Meloxicam was administered with progressively decreasing doses. Doses decrease because of most cats' inability to metabolize meloxicam adequately. The concept behind this dosing regimen is to maintain effective blood levels of meloxicam without causing any toxicity.
  1. 0.05 mg/kg (1 drop from the dosing syringe) PO qd for 5 days
  2. 0.05 mg/2 kg (1 drop/2 kg) PO qd for 5 days
  3. 0.05 mg/cat PO qd for 5 days
  4. 0.05 mg/kg PO qod for three treatments
  5. Discontinue meloxicam for 7 days and then restart at the high dose (Box 19-10)

**BOX 19-10 | CASE 5: BILATERAL HIP OSTEOARTHRITIS—
THERAPEUTIC OPTIONS**

• *First therapy:* 0.05 mg/kg (1 drop from the dosing syringe) PO qd for 5 days
• *Second therapy:* 0.05 mg/2 kg (1 drop/2 kg) PO qd for 5 days
• *Third therapy:* 0.05 mg/cat PO qd for 5 days
• *Fourth therapy:* 0.05 mg/kg PO qd for three treatments
• *Fifth therapy:* Discontinue meloxicam for 7 days and then restart at the high dose

---

◆ If a cat develops pain during the step-down dosing, this likely signifies a reasonable level of metabolic activity. The cat is then administered the previously higher dose.
◆ Complete blood count and blood chemistries focusing on renal function are analyzed before treatment, 2 to 3 weeks after starting treatment, and then every 3 to 6 months. Cat kidneys seem to be particularly susceptible to the cyclooxygenase inhibitory effects of NSAIDs.

CASE 6   **BILATERAL STIFLE
OSTEOARTHRITIS (BOX 19-11)**

Signalment: 15-year-old female spayed 3.5-kg domestic longhair cat
Challenge: This cat no longer jumps and plays and is being treated for chronic renal failure.
Source of Pain: Damaged cartilage in both stifles

**BOX 19-11 | CASE 6: BILATERAL STIFLE OSTEOARTHRITIS—
DESCRIPTION OF PAIN**

• Moderate to severe intensity
• Somatic: inflammatory
• Long term to lifelong

TREATMENT AND RATIONALE

- The challenge is that the cat has compromised kidneys and should not receive NSAIDs.
- A reasonable alternative to NSAID therapy is Microlactin, a milk-based protein that has antiinflammatory and pain-relieving effects. Microlactin is a biological response modifier, but not a drug. A brand is chosen that has documented efficacy because production is not regulated by the U.S. Food and Drug Administration. The cat should receive 200 mg orally twice daily.
- A combination of glucosamine hydrochloride and chondroitin sulfate can be administered. Manganese acts as a catalyst for these two compounds to increase their bioactivity. The cat received 125 mg of glucosamine, 100 mg of chondroitin, and 1 mg of manganese as a powder on food twice daily. A brand is chosen that has documented efficacy because nutraceutical production is not regulated by the U.S. Food and Drug Administration (Box 19-12).

**BOX 19-12 | CASE 6: BILATERAL STIFLE OSTEOARTHRITIS—
        THERAPEUTIC OPTIONS**

- *First therapy:* 200 mg MicroLactin PO bid
- *Second therapy:* 125 mg glucosamine sulfate, 100 mg chondroitin sulfate, and 1 mg manganese PO bid

---

CASE 7   BILATERAL ELBOW DYSPLASIA (BOX 19-13)

Signalment: 7-year-old female spayed Chow-Labrador mix weighing 32 kg

Challenge: To attain adequate relief from elbow pain is usually difficult. The dog has severe osteoarthritis resulting from elbow dysplasia. She has been treated with multiple NSAIDs, including carprofen, deracoxib, meloxicam, etodolac, and tepoxalin. Tepoxalin 300 mg daily seems to have provided a small amount of pain relief.

Source of Pain: Cartilage damage in both elbows

**BOX 19-13 | CASE 7: BILATERAL ELBOW DYSPLASIA—
        DESCRIPTION OF PAIN**

- Severe intensity
- Somatic: inflammatory
- Long term to lifelong

TREATMENT AND RATIONALE

◆ Tepoxalin 300 mg PO daily was maintained for inflammatory pain.

◆ Amantadine 100 mg PO daily was added with the rationale that the dog likely had some degree of centrally mediated hyperexcitability. The dog became more comfortable after 3 days.

◆ Tramadol 100 mg PO bid was added to improve pain relief. Tramadol immediately induced drowsiness. Tramadol was decreased to 75 mg PO once daily, the highest dose that did not cause drowsiness, but there was no pain relief.

◆ Low-level therapeutic laser was initiated twice weekly for 2 weeks. A continuously pulsing signal was applied at four sites surrounding each elbow, 30 seconds per site with an energy level of 1 J/s. The dog responded to this therapy, walking and playing much more vigorously. The low-level laser therapy was applied at progressively increasing treatment intervals.

◆ This dog's reasonable level of comfort was maintained with tepoxalin 300 mg PO sid qd and low-level therapeutic laser therapy once every 12 to 14 weeks (Box 19-14).

**BOX 19-14 | CASE 7: BILATERAL ELBOW DYSPLASIA—
THERAPEUTIC OPTIONS**

• *First therapy:* Tepoxalin 300 mg PO qd
• *Second therapy:* Amantadine 100 mg PO qd for 21 days
• *Third therapy:* Tramadol 75 to 100 mg PO qd to bid
• *Fourth therapy:* Low-level therapeutic laser

CASE 8	**BILATERAL ELBOW OSTEOARTHRITIS (BOX 19-15)**

Signalment: 4-year-old female spayed Newfoundland weighing 58 kg

Challenge: This dog has had elbow dysplasia and secondary osteoarthritis since puppyhood. The dog has received multiple therapies. Like many other dogs, she has received multiple sequential NSAIDs, with meloxicam 6.0 mg PO daily providing the best but minimal pain relief. Amantadine 200 mg PO qd for 21 days and tramadol 200 mg PO qid had been administered before admission with no obvious effect.

Source of Pain: Damaged cartilage resulting from elbow dysplasia

---

**BOX 19-15 | CASE 8: BILATERAL ELBOW OSTEOARTHRITIS—
DESCRIPTION OF PAIN**

• Severe intensity
• Somatic: inflammatory
• Long term to lifelong

TREATMENT AND RATIONALE

- ◆ Meloxicam 6.0 mg PO daily was continued as the base for inflammatory pain.
- ◆ Gabapentin bid was started in an escalating dose scale in an attempt to provide multimodal analgesia. The dog was initially administered 300 mg PO of gabapentin bid for 14 days and demonstrated minimal pain relief. The dose of gabapentin was increased to 600 mg PO bid, which improved pain relief. The dose of gabapentin was increased to 900 mg PO bid. The dog became intermittently drowsy, so the dose was decreased to 600 mg PO bid.
- ◆ The owner was interested in attempting an alternative multimodal approach to pain control. Clomipramine, a tricyclic antidepressant, 80 mg PO qd, was initiated. The dog's pain relief increased significantly over the next 7 days (Box 19-16).

**BOX 19-16 | CASE 8: BILATERAL ELBOW OSTEOARTHRITIS—
          THERAPEUTIC OPTIONS**

- • *First therapy:* Meloxicam 5.0 mg PO qd
- • *Second therapy:* Gabapentin 600 mg PO qd
- • *Third therapy:* Clomipramine 80 mg PO qd

CASE 9	UNILATERAL HIP PAIN WITH SECONDARY LUMBAR PAIN (BOX 19-17)

Signalment: 3-year-old female spayed mixed-breed dog weighing 2 kg
Challenge: This dog had pain associated with documented moderate hip dysplasia of the left coxofemoral joint that was unsuccessfully treated with carprofen 75 mg PO sid before referral. The dog's hips were not painful during physical examination, but the dog demonstrated moderate to severe pain of her epaxial muscles between the thoracolumbar and lumbosacral junctions. This was likely caused by an abnormal gait and the clinical manifestations of pain including trouble standing and jumping into the car. Muscular pain is difficult to treat, especially when it is not responsive to antiinflammatory drug therapy.
Source of Pain: Damaged cartilage and skeletal muscle tension and stress

---

**BOX 19-17 | CASE 9: UNILATERAL HIP DYSPLASIA WITH
          SECONDARY LUMBAR PAIN—DESCRIPTION OF PAIN**

- • Moderate intensity
- • Somatic: inflammatory
- • Long term to lifelong

TREATMENT AND RATIONALE

◆ Carprofen 75 mg PO qd was continued, and tramadol 75 mg PO bid was added. This was determined to be unsuccessful after 2 weeks.

◆ Acupuncture therapy was initiated twice weekly for 2 weeks, then at progressively increasing intervals. Acupuncture induces local antiinflammatory effects and centrally mediated analgesic effects and can relieve muscle spasms. The acupuncture points used were bilateral BL 19, BL 21, BL 23, and BL 40. The dog responded after the first treatment and continued to improve during the first four treatments. Carprofen therapy was maintained, and acupuncture therapy was applied as needed (Box 19-18).

**BOX 19-18 | CASE 9: UNILATERAL HIP DYSPLASIA WITH
SECONDARY LUMBAR PAIN—THERAPEUTIC OPTIONS**

- *First therapy:* Carprofen 75 mg PO qd
- *Second therapy:* Tramadol 75 mg PO bid
- *Third therapy:* Acupuncture

CASE 10   OSTEOSARCOMA (BOX 19-19)

Signalment: 7-year-old female spayed Great Dane weighing 49 kg
Challenge: The dog had been limping for several weeks with pain localized to the distal right humerus. Radiographs and subsequent biopsy indicate osteosarcoma. The owner elected palliative pain control rather than amputation or radiation/chemotherapy. Pain control in this patient required an aggressive multimodal approach.
Source of Pain: Disruption of bone and periosteum, with swelling and inflammation of the surrounding soft tissues

---

**BOX 19-19 | CASE 10: OSTEOSARCOMA—
DESCRIPTION OF PAIN**

- Moderate to severe intensity
- Somatic: inflammatory
- Long term to lifelong until euthanasia

TREATMENT AND RATIONALE

◆ Carprofen 200 mg PO qd was initiated for inflammatory pain.

◆ Amantadine 200 mg PO qd was added into the NSAID therapy to help prevent centrally mediated hypersensitization, which can persist for the life of the patient.

♦ Tramadol 150 to 200 mg PO bid to qid was administered. Tramadol produces analgesia by an alternative mechanism, thereby providing a more comprehensive multimodal approach.

♦ Pamidronate 60 mg IV was infused every 3 to 4 weeks. As a bisphosphonate, pamidronate inhibits osteoclast activity of the tumor, potentially decreasing bony and periosteal pain. The tumor tends to expand outward and has less invasive effects.

♦ Oxycodone 5 to 15 mg PO bid to tid was administered. Tramadol was replaced with oxycodone, a potent μ-opioid agonist, as the pain became more severe (Box 19-20).

BOX 19-20 | CASE 10: OSTEOSARCOMA—THERAPEUTIC OPTIONS

- *First therapy:* Carprofen 200 mg PO qd
- *Second therapy:* Amantadine 200 mg PO qd
- *Third therapy:* Tramadol 150 to 200 mg PO bid to qid
- *Fourth therapy:* Pamidronate 60 mg IV infusion every 3 to 4 weeks
- *Fifth therapy:* Oxycodone 5 to 15 mg PO bid to tid

♦ Acetaminophen 500 mg PO bid was administered. Acetaminophen has been used in conjunction with NSAIDs for breakthrough pain for 1 to 5 days at a time. Acetaminophen should only be used when absolutely necessary at low doses and for short periods in animals with normal hepatic and renal function.

♦ The dog's quality of life, as defined by the owner, remained good. This included eating regularly, walking daily, and playing with the other dogs in the house. The dog was euthanized because of dyspnea resulting from pulmonary metastases 5½ months after her original diagnosis.

20

DRUG ANTAGONISM AND ANTAGONISTS

WILLIAM W. MUIR III

Drug-related side effects and toxicity are common consequences of drug administration, even when recommended drug dosages and dosing schedules are followed. Some side effects are easily eliminated (e.g., opioid-induced bradycardia and depression), whereas others may be irreversible and fatal (e.g., nonsteroidal antiinflammatory drug–induced acute renal failure). Acute onset of life-threatening side effects (e.g., apnea) is particularly problematic because of the potential consequences. Many of the drugs used to produce analgesia (e.g., opioids, α_2-agonists, and local anesthetics) have the potential to produce a wide variety of side effects and toxicity. Opioids are notorious for their ability to induce vomiting, bradycardia, and augmentation of the respiratory depressant effects of anesthetics. α_2-Agonists can produce bradycardia, respiratory depression, and excessive central nervous system (CNS) depression in otherwise normal healthy dogs or cats, even when low dosages are administered. The intravenous (IV) bolus administration of benzodiazepines (e.g., diazepam and midazolam), drugs usually considered to be relatively free of side effects or toxicity, can induce acute collapse, bradycardia, and unconsciousness. The initial response to a drug-related side effect, once identified, should be focused on its elimination. Fortunately, a variety of drugs and pharmacologic techniques can be used to antagonize or eliminate unwanted drug side effects. This chapter focuses on mechanisms of drug antagonism that can be used to reduce or eliminate the side effects and toxicities produced by analgesic drugs. Receptor blockade and physiologic drug antagonism are emphasized after a brief discussion of other methods for drug antagonism (Box 20-1).

BOX 20-1

Drug Antagonism

- Change in method of drug administration (reduce dose or rate of administration, or discontinue)
- Pharmacokinetic antagonism (prevent absorption; hasten metabolism and elimination)
- Competitive antagonism (bind or inactive receptors)
- Physiologic antagonism (counteract adverse effect)

DISCONTINUING DRUG ADMINISTRATION

Stopping the administration of a drug, slowing the rate of drug administration, or decreasing the frequency of drug administration are simple and effective methods for minimizing unwanted drug-related side effects or toxicity. Patients that are receiving drugs chronically (nonsteroidal antiinflammatory drugs) should be monitored periodically for signs of toxicity (e.g., gastric ulcers and abnormal renal and liver function test results). These procedures, however, are not effective for the immediate termination of acute drug-related side effects.

DRUG ADMINISTRATION

The dose, rate of drug administration, and frequency and route of drug administration can be changed to help decrease the possibility of drug-related side effects. Decreasing the drug dosage, or rate of administration or incrementally administering the dose decreases peak plasma drug concentrations, thereby decreasing the potential for the development of drug-related side effects.

ROUTE OF ADMINISTRATION

Administering drugs by routes that delay drug absorption (e.g., oral or transdermal) prolongs the onset to peak drug effect but decreases peak plasma drug concentrations, thereby decreasing the potential for the development of drug-related side effects.

PHARMACOKINETIC ANTAGONISM

Pharmacokinetic antagonism is the use of therapies and techniques that decrease the plasma concentration of the drug. Toward this end, therapies that decrease or inhibit drug absorption or increase drug elimination should be considered.

DECREASING DRUG ABSORPTION

The absorption of orally administered drugs can be decreased or inhibited by the administration of substances that interfere with drug absorption from the gastrointestinal tract (kaolin, pectin). Alternatively, drugs that induce vomiting (apomorphine) can be administered to limit the amount of drug that is absorbed from the gastrointestinal tract. Local anesthetics are frequently administered with epinephrine to decrease the local blood supply, thereby decreasing their systemic absorption and intensifying their local analgesic actions. Their delayed entry into the blood supply also minimizes their plasma concentration and the potential for systemic side effects.

INCREASING DRUG ELIMINATION

Drug elimination can be enhanced by improving or ensuring adequate blood supply to the major organs of elimination (liver, kidneys, lungs) for the drug in question. This may require subcutaneous or IV administration of fluids and cardiovascular stimulants (dopamine, dobutamine). The renal excretion of drugs can be increased by administering fluids, optimizing pH (e.g., alkaline urine pH), and promoting diuresis (furosemide).

RECEPTOR BLOCKADE (DRUG ANTAGONISTS)

Opioids and α_2-agonists produce their effects by combining with and activating receptors (agonists). Drugs that combine with receptors and produce less than the expected maximal response are referred to as *partial agonists* (e.g., buprenorphine). Furthermore, two drugs with the same ability to combine (affinity) with a receptor could produce different degrees of analgesia (activity). The drug that produces the maximal effect is termed *a full agonist,* whereas the drug that produces less than the maximal effect is termed *a partial agonist.* Pure drug antagonists combine with receptors without causing their activation, thereby preventing the effects of agonists. The affinity of the drug antagonist for the receptor determines how much drug is necessary to produce an antagonistic effect (high affinity = low amounts of drug). Some drugs combine with, activate, and inhibit the receptor occupation of other drugs. These drugs are called *agonists-antagonists.* Some drug antagonists and agonist-antagonists compete for receptors with the agonist or partial agonist, implying that the receptor binds to one drug at a time and that the effects of the antagonist or agonist-antagonist are surmountable if enough agonist or partial agonist is administered (see Chapter 7). Butorphanol, for example, is an opioid agonist-antagonist that is additive with full opioid agonists when administered at low dosages. Larger dosages (greater than 0.2 mg/kg) of butorphanol can be used to antagonize the effects of the pure opioid agonists morphine and hydromorphone. Low doses of the opioid antagonist naltrexone have been administered in conjunction with hydromorphone to humans in order to minimize opioid-related side effects (delirium, depression, vomiting, constipation) without interfering with opioid agonist–induced analgesia. Most drug antagonists are generally administered in doses far in excess of what is required to overcome agonist effects. This is an important point, considering the administration of a drug antagonist reverses toxic and analgesic effects of another drug. Special consideration should be given to the antagonist selected, its dose, and route of administration. Unless a life or death situation, drug antagonists should be administered incrementally (titrated) to achieve the desired effect whenever possible. Finally, caution is advised whenever a drug antagonist is administered to reverse CNS depression because the return to consciousness may produce excitement, agitation, and aggression.

OPIOID ANTAGONISTS

Naloxone and naltrexone are pure opioid antagonists (i.e., produce no opioid effects) that have high affinity for μ-, κ-, and δ-opioid receptors. Relatively small doses of either drug can be used to rapidly reverse unwanted or lingering CNS, respiratory, and cardiac (bradycardia) effects produced by opioid agonists or partial agonists. Naloxone is rapidly metabolized and eliminated in dogs and cats, producing relatively short-lived (10 to 20 minutes) effects and predisposing to renarcotization and respiratory depression. Naltrexone produces effects similar to those of naloxone but has a much longer duration of action (several hours). Both drugs produce few direct, drug-related effects when administered IV. Naloxone and naltrexone will reverse the analgesic effects of systemic and parenteral opioid administration and inhibit acupuncture analgesia. The IV administration of large doses of naloxone or naltrexone may produce a state of hyperalgesia in dogs and cats because these drugs interfere with the protective effect of endogenous opioids (e.g., endorphin and enkephalin). IV bolus administration of naloxone generally produces rapid reversal of opioid-related side effects but may cause some animals to become excited, delirious, or aggressive. Unless an emergency situation exists, small doses of either drug should be incrementally administered to produce the desired effect (e.g., consciousness; Table 20-1).

TABLE 20-1	Opioid Antagonists	
Drug	**Recommended Use**	**Emergency Use**
Naloxone*	5-15 µg/kg IV	50-100 µg/kg IV
Naltrexone*	50-100 µg/kg SQ	—
Nalorphine*	0.05-0.1 mg/kg IV	—
Flumazenil	0.2 mg total dose IV	—
Butorphanol	0.05-1.0 mg/kg IV	—
Pentazocine	0.1-0.5 mg/kg IV	—
Buprenorphine†	5-10 µg/kg IV	—

*Repeat as necessary.
†Monitor for respiratory depression; drug is a partial agonist.

OPIOID PARTIAL OR MIXED AGONISTS-ANTAGONISTS

Nalorphine, nalbuphine, pentazocine, butorphanol, and buprenorphine are opioids classified as partial agonists (i.e., buprenorphine; produce less than the maximal response) or agonist-antagonists (i.e., butorphanol; activate and block opioid receptors), depending on the opioid receptor in question (see Chapters 8 and 9). These drugs are used clinically to produce analgesia and, on occasion, to reverse the unwanted effects (e.g., prolonged sedation) of pure opioid agonists (e.g., morphine and hydromorphone). Butorphanol, for example, can be administered during recovery from anesthesia to antagonize prolonged recovery produced by the preanesthetic administration of hydromorphone. Butorphanol administration, if necessary, increases the level of consciousness, thereby helping prevent respiratory depression in the unstimulated postsurgical patient and produces mild to moderate opioid receptor–mediated analgesia. Evidence also exists that the administration of small doses of opioid agonist-antagonists (e.g., nalorphine, pentazocine, or butorphanol) in conjunction with or after the administration of a pure opioid agonist (e.g., morphine or hydromorphone) may produce additive analgesia. This suggests that analgesia is improved in the postoperative patient in which the sedative effects of morphine are partially antagonized. Care must be taken in the selection of partial agonists or agonist-antagonists to antagonize the effects of a pure opioid agonist (morphine, hydromorphone) because some partial agonists (buprenorphine) are known to exaggerate the respiratory depressant effects of pure opioid agonists. This effect could become problematic in animals that do not regain consciousness after the administration of buprenorphine.

α_2-AGONISTS

Yohimbine, tolazoline, and atipamezole are α_2-receptor antagonists that can antagonize central and peripheral α-receptors (Table 20-2). Yohimbine ($\alpha_2/\alpha_1 = 40/1$) and tolazoline ($\alpha_2/\alpha_1 = 4/1$) are relatively nonspecific α_2-antagonists compared with atipamezole ($\alpha_2/\alpha_1 = 8500/1$) and occasionally produce hypotension (α_1 blockade) and reflex tachycardia. Tolazoline is also noted for producing histamine release, which may contribute to hypotension. All three drugs are recommended for the reversal of α_2-agonist–induced (xylazine, medetomidine, detomidine, romifidine) side effects, including sedation, respiratory depression, and bradycardia. The intramuscular (IM) administration of atipamezole produces rapid and complete reversal of α_2-agonist effects, including the elimination of analgesia. The IV bolus administration of manufacturer-recommended dosages of α_2-agonists should be reserved for emergency or life-threatening situations. α_2-Agonist administration can initiate involuntary muscle twitching (jactitations), excitement, delirium, and aggression associated with vomiting, urination, and defecation. Clinically, the IM or subcutaneous administration of atipamezole produces rapid uneventful recovery from α_2-agonist sedation and respiratory depression without significant untoward effects.

BENZODIAZEPINE ANTAGONISTS

Diazepam and midazolam are centrally acting muscle relaxants that are frequently combined with opioids to produce calming and muscle relaxation before surgery. Diazepam and midazolam can induce disorientation, delirium, and on rare occasions profound CNS and associated respiratory depression. On rare occasions, the IV bolus administration of diazepam can also produce bradycardia and hypotension. Flumazenil is a rapidly acting and specific competitive antagonist of diazepam- and midazolam-induced CNS and respiratory

TABLE 20-2	α_2-Antagonists
Drug	**Dose**
Yohimbine	0.1-0.3 mg/kg IV
	0.3-0.5 mg/kg IM
Tolazoline	0.5-1.0 mg/kg IV
	2-5 mg/kg IM
Atipamezole	0.05-0.2 mg/kg IV
	2-5 times medetomidine dose

depression. Flumazenil is also capable of producing partial reversal of inhalant anesthetic–induced CNS depression. Clinical dosages range from 0.1 mg/kg IV to 0.3 mg/kg IM. IV administration is rarely associated with emergence delirium or signs of excitement. Larger doses (>3 mg/kg IV plus infusion) of flumazenil antagonize platelet-activating factor and have been shown to be beneficial in the treatment of hemorrhagic shock.

PHYSIOLOGIC ANTAGONISM

Physiologic antagonism refers to the administration of drugs that do not act as specific receptor antagonists but are administered to produce effects that oppose or cancel the effects of the problem drug (Table 20-3). The administration of fluids or dopamine to oppose the hypotensive effects of inhalant anesthesia is one example of physiologic antagonism.

TABLE 20-3	Therapy for Analgesic Drug-Related Side Effects	
Problem	**Therapy**	**Dose**
Sedation/depression	Analeptics	
	Doxapram	0.2-0.5 mg/kg IV
	Aminophylline	2-10 mg/kg IV
Excitement/seizures	Tranquilizers/muscle relaxants	
	Acepromazine	0.01-0.1 mg/kg IV, IM
	Droperidol	0.1-1.0 mg/kg IV, IM
	Medetomidine	0.02-0.05 mg/kg IV, IM
	Diazepam	0.1-0.5 mg/kg IV, CRI
	Phenobarbital	1-3 mg/kg IV
	Propofol	1-3 mg/kg IV; 0.1-0.2 mg/kg per minute
Vomiting	Antiemetics	
	Ondansetron	0.5 mg/kg IV
	Metoclopramide	0.1-0.3 mg/kg IV
Bradycardia	Anticholinergics	
	Atropine	0.01-0.02 mg/kg IV, IM
	Glycopyrrolate	0.005-0.01 mg/kg IV, IM
Respiratory depression	Respiratory stimulants	
	Doxapram	0.2-0.5 mg/kg IV
	Ventilation	
Hypotension	Catecholamines	
	Dopamine	0.001-0.005 mg/kg per minute IV
	Dobutamine	0.001-0.010 mg/kg per minute IV
	Ephedrine	0.1-0.5 mg/kg IM

The administration of atropine or glycopyrrolate to treat opioid or α_2-agonist bradycardia is another example of physiologic antagonism. The wide variety of drugs acting by diverse mechanisms, which are used as analgesics in dogs and cats, have the potential to produce many unwanted side effects. CNS depression or excitement, respiratory depression, bradycardia, hypotension, and muscle twitching are among the most commonly encountered side effects associated with the administration of analgesic drugs. Behavioral changes are also common side effects of opioids, α_2-agonists, and benzodiazepines and are best treated by changing or discontinuing medication.

ANALEPTICS

Sedation and depression are common side effects of many analgesic drugs. Excessive sedation or depression can produce an unresponsive, listless pet, a reduction in appetite, and the potential for significant respiratory depression during sleep. This type of response to centrally acting analgesic drugs is best treated by reducing the analgesic drug dose or selecting an analgesic that does not produce CNS effects. Clinically, many postoperative patients demonstrate good analgesia but significant CNS depression, requiring semicontinuous monitoring. A decision may need to be made whether the patient should be administered a specific drug antagonist (if appropriate) with the risk of reducing or eliminating analgesia. Low doses of a specific antagonist can be titrated to effect with the hope of producing increased consciousness and little or no loss of analgesia. In some instances, agonist-antagonists (e.g., butorphanol) can be administered to counteract unwanted CNS depression and produce analgesia. An alternative approach would be to administer a specific antagonist, a CNS stimulant or analeptic. Doxapram is a respiratory stimulant that increases CNS activity in dogs and cats. Although not a specific antagonist, doxapram can counteract the CNS depressant effects of low to moderate doses of α_2-agonists, opioids, and injectable or inhalant anesthetics. Once conscious, most animals remain conscious, but because of the relatively short half-life of doxapram, animals administered this drug should be closely monitored to avoid a relapse to CNS and respiratory depression. Aminophylline, although noted for its bronchodilatory effects, also stimulates the CNS. The IV or IM administration of aminophylline to dogs and cats can shorten recovery from anesthesia, increase alertness, and counteract mild to moderate sedation without antagonizing the effects of analgesic drugs. Aminophylline has a much longer duration of action than doxapram.

TRANQUILIZERS/MUSCLE RELAXANTS

Nervousness, apprehension, agitation, seizures, and involuntary muscle twitching are potential side effects associated with the use of traditional centrally acting analgesic medications. These side effects are more frequent when large doses are administered or when analgesic drugs are given to animals with preexisting CNS disorders. Acepromazine is an excellent tranquilizer that produces adjunctive analgesic and antiemetic effects when combined with opioids. Relatively low IV or IM doses (0.01 mg/kg) can be used to calm nervous or agitated dogs and cats. Although acepromazine is effective, the dose may be difficult to titrate, frequently producing more sedation than needed. Droperidol and haloperidol are butyrophenone tranquilizers noted for their mild calming and antiemetic effects and can be used as alternatives to acepromazine. Droperidol and haloperidol are frequently used as behavior modifiers, and either drug can be used to reduce or eliminate apprehension and agitation in dogs and cats. Drug dose should be titrated to the desired effect, and initial dosages of droperidol should not exceed 0.1 mg/kg IV or IM. Diazepam and midazolam are excellent centrally acting neuromuscular blocking drugs that can be used to control involuntary muscle twitching or spasms and seizures. Repeated IV administration (0.1 mg/kg) or infusion (0.1 to 0.5 mg/kg per hour) may be required to control involuntary muscle spasms or seizures in some animals. Dogs and cats with seizures that do not respond to diazepam or midazolam therapy should be administered phenobarbital (1 to 3 mg/kg IV) or anesthetized with propofol (1 to 3 mg/kg IV; 0.1 to 0.2 mg/kg per minute).

ANTIEMETICS

Nausea and vomiting are common but self-limiting side effects associated with the use of opioid and α_2-agonist drugs. Occasionally, vomiting may persist and result in dyspnea, bradycardia, and potentially aspiration. Vomiting is particularly problematic when it occurs in association with the induction, maintenance, or recovery from anesthesia. As noted previously, acepromazine or droperidol can be used before or in combination with opioids or α_2-agonists to reduce vomiting. Ondansetron (0.5 mg/kg IV) or metoclopramide (0.2 to 0.5 mg/kg IM) can be used to prevent or eliminate vomiting without producing sedation. Persistent vomiting in dogs should be treated by infusing metoclopramide (0.01 to 0.02 mg/kg per hour).

ANTICHOLINERGICS

Sinus bradycardia, first- and second-degree atrioventricular block with ventricular escape beats, and rarely, third-degree atrioventricular block may occur after the administration of opioids and particularly α_2-agonists. Cardiac rhythm disturbances can occur, although they are less common. Opioid-induced bradyarrhythmias are generally caused by increases in parasympathetic tone and are readily responsive to treatment with atropine (0.01 to 0.02 mg/kg IV) or glycopyrrolate (0.005 to 0.01 mg/kg IV). α_2-Agonist–induced bradyarrhythmias may also be due to increases in parasympathetic tone but can be augmented by decreases in sympathetic tone. Regardless, initial therapy is identical to that for opioids.

RESPIRATORY STIMULANTS

Respiratory depression is an underappreciated and significant side effect associated with IV or long-term analgesic drug administration; it is most common when opioids and α_2-agonists are administered in conjunction with injectable or inhalant anesthetics. Signs of respiratory depression are often subtle, unless significant decreases in respiratory rate or apnea are observed. Respiratory rate and depth should be closely monitored after the IV administration of opioids, α_2-agonists, and benzodiazepines. Doxapram is an excellent CNS and respiratory stimulant but is not a specific drug antagonist and produces only short-term effects. Significant respiratory depression may follow a period of transient respiratory stimulation if consciousness does not improve, for carbon dioxide concentrations (the principal drive to breathing) may have been significantly reduced. Respiratory depression therefore is best treated by careful patient monitoring, oxygen supplementation, nursing care, and techniques that hasten drug elimination. If necessary, assisted or mechanical ventilation should be used to maintain breathing and normal pH and blood gas values.

CATECHOLAMINES

Arterial blood pressure should be determined in any patient in which hypotension is suspected. Hypotension and poor tissue perfusion may occur as a consequence of loss of consciousness, bradyarrhythmias, vasodilation, and low cardiac output. Clinically, hypotension may result in lethargy, depression, muscle weakness, and considerable delays in recovery from anesthesia. Acute hypotension should be treated with appropriate fluids (10 to 20 ml/kg IV lactated Ringer's solution; 5 to 10 ml/kg IV hetastarch) and the administration of dopamine (1 to 4 µg/kg per minute), dobutamine (1 to 10 µg/kg per minute), or ephedrine (0.1 to 0.5 mg/kg IV to effect).

SUGGESTED READINGS

Heniff MS, Moore G, Trout A et al: Comparison of routes of flumazenil administration to reverse midazolam-induced respiratory depression in a canine model, *Acad Emerg Med* 4:1115-1118, 1997.

Muir WW, Hubbell JAE: Drugs used for preanesthetic medication. In Muir WW, Hubbell JAE, editors: *Handbook of veterinary anesthesia,* ed 3, St Louis, 1999, Mosby.

Salonen S, Vuorilehto L, Vainio O et al: Atipamezole increases medetomidine clearance in the dog: an agonist-antagonist interaction, *J Vet Pharmacol Ther* 18:328-332, 1995.

Schaffer DD, Hsu WH, Hopper DL: Antagonism of xylazine-induced depression of shuttle-avoidance responses in dogs by administration of 4-aminopyridine, doxapram, or yohimbine, *Am J Vet Res* 47(10):2116-2121, 1986.

Thurman JC, Tranquilli WJ, Benson GJ: Preanesthetics and anesthetic adjuncts. In Thurman JC, Tranquilli WJ, Benson GJ, editors: *Lumb & Jones' veterinary anesthesia,* ed 3, Baltimore, 1996, Williams & Wilkins.

21 CANCER PAIN MANAGEMENT

JAMES S. GAYNOR

- The treatment of cancer has become commonplace in veterinary practice as knowledge, drugs, and therapeutic techniques evolve. Although some cancers still are not effectively treated, many owners want palliative pain control in order to maintain a good quality of life.
- An attempt to alleviate the pet's pain is vitally important. Cancer pain is estimated to be effectively managed in 90% of humans with currently available drugs and techniques.

CANCER PAIN
Most cancer pain is controllable.

The four main steps in ensuring that pain management is optimized in veterinary patients are as follows.

FOUR STEPS TO OPTIMIZE CANCER PAIN CONTROL
1. Educate yourself on the assessment and alleviation of cancer pain.
2. Create real client expectations.
3. Assess pet pain regularly.
4. Use opioids as part of a *multimodal* approach.

---

1. Educate and train staff concerning the importance of alleviation of pain, assessment of pain, available drugs and potential complications, and interventional techniques.
2. Educate the client concerning realistic expectations surrounding pain control. Convey the idea that most of the patient's pain can be managed. This involves letting the client know that owner involvement in evaluating the pet and providing feedback on therapy is crucial to success. The veterinarian and owner should participate in developing

effective strategies to alleviate pain. Owner involvement also helps decrease the potential feeling of helplessness.

3. The third step is to assess the pet's pain and quality of life thoroughly (see Chapter 29) at the start and throughout the course of therapy, not just when pain gets severe.

4. Provide excellent support for the use of opioids and other controlled substances (be available!).

DRUGS AND TECHNIQUES FOR ALLEVIATION OF PAIN

◆ A good starting point for the management of cancer pain is to follow the World Health Organization ladder, which is a three-step hierarchy (Fig. 21-1).

1. Drugs within the same category can have different side effects. Therefore, if possible, it may be best to substitute drugs within a category before switching therapies. It is always best to try to keep dosage scheduling as simple as possible. The more complicated the regimen, the more likely that noncompliance will occur.

2. Mild to moderate pain should be treated with a nonsteroidal antiinflammatory drug (NSAID).

3. As pain increases, opioids or opioid-like drugs should be added to the regimen. As pain becomes more severe, increase the dose of the medication. Drugs should be dosed on a regular basis, not just as

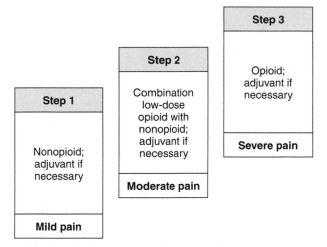

FIG. 21-1. World Health Organization analgesia ladder. (Used by permission of the World Health Organization, Geneva, Switzerland.)

needed, as pain becomes moderate to severe. Continuous analgesia facilitates maintenance of patient comfort. Additional doses of analgesics can then be administered as pain is intermittently more severe.

4. Adjuvant drugs should be administered to help with specific types of pain and anxiety (e.g., gabapentin and alendronate [Fosamax]).

NONOPIOIDS

◆ Nonopioid analgesics include drugs such as NSAIDs and acetaminophen. Use of an NSAID that is approved for use in the intended species is desirable because these drugs have been more thoroughly studied and generally have significantly fewer side effects than nonapproved drugs (see Chapter 10).

◆ All nonopioids except acetaminophen are considered NSAIDs. Despite the low antiinflammatory activity of acetaminophen, it possesses beneficial analgesic effects, minimal risk of bleeding in thrombocytopenic patients, decreased gastrointestinal side effects, and synergism with opioid analgesics, such as codeine. Acetaminophen should not be used in cats because of inadequate cytochrome P_{450}–dependent hydroxylation.

1. Mild to moderate pain—especially that caused by intrathoracic masses, intraabdominal masses, and bone metastases—generally responds to NSAID therapy. NSAIDs have an opioid-sparing effect so that better analgesia can be achieved with lower doses of opioids when needed.

2. NSAIDs have central analgesic and peripheral antiinflammatory effects mediated via inhibition of cyclooxygenase. The choice of NSAID ultimately depends on available species information, clinical response, and tolerance of side effects (see Chapter 10).

3. The most common side effect of NSAID administration in dogs is gastric irritation and bleeding because of loss of gastric acid inhibition and of cytoprotective mucous production normally promoted by prostaglandins.

   a. Other side effects include renal failure and hepatic dysfunction that may lead to failure.

   b. NSAIDs that are more selective for inhibition of cyclooxygenase-2 (COX-2) seem to have fewer gastrointestinal effects and potentially fewer renal effects.

   c. Selective COX-2 inhibitors—such as carprofen, deracoxib, meloxicam, firocoxib, and the dual inhibitor tepoxalin—should be considered priority NSAIDs in cancer patients.

A blood chemistry panel should be performed before initiating NSAID therapy.

d. If there is evidence of liver or renal disease, dehydration, or hypotension, another approach to therapy should be considered. Therapy with NSAIDs may also inhibit platelet function leading to bleeding and oozing of blood from incision sites. Therapy with NSAIDs should be stopped if this occurs.

e. If clinical effectiveness is not achieved with one NSAID, it should be discontinued and another started 7 days later to avoid additive or synergistic COX inhibition effects.

f. Aspirin should be avoided in dogs because of the increased possibility of gastrointestinal bleeding, even with buffered formulations.

g. Administration of misoprostol or omeprazole can help provide gastrointestinal protection during the switch-over period. All cancer patients should be closely monitored for gastrointestinal bleeding during NSAID therapy because chemotherapy may induce thrombocytopenia.

OPIOIDS

◆ Opioids are extremely effective therapy for cancer pain (see Chapter 9). Tramadol, an opioid-like drug, can provide excellent adjunctive therapy (see Chapter 14).

◆ Opioids are the major class of analgesics used in the management of moderate to severe cancer pain. Opioids are the most effective and predictable and have a low risk of side effects.

◆ The required dose of opioid increases as a patient's pain increases.

OPIOIDS
- Opioids are the most effective, predictable analgesics.
- Do not be afraid to increase dose as duration and intensity of pain increase.

---

1. Veterinarians have an ethical obligation to alleviate animal pain.

2. Opioids can be administered while managing side effects to maximally help the patient. Side effects of opioid administration include diarrhea and vomiting initially and constipation with long-term use. Sedation and dysphoria may also occur. The initial gastrointestinal effects occur most frequently with the first injection (first-dose effect) in the perioperative period and usually do not occur with subsequent dosing. These effects usually do not, but may, occur with oral dosing.

3. Discussion of dosing schedules is important when sending a patient home with oral medications.
   a. The prescribed dose may be perfect, may not provide enough analgesia, may induce sedation, or may induce dysphoria or excitement.
   b. Adjustment of the dose requires excellent doctor-client interaction.
   c. Bradycardia is a potential side effect associated with opioid administration but is most common if opioids are administered parenterally. If bradycardia occurs, an anticholinergic, such as atropine or glycopyrrolate, can be administered, rather than discontinuing the opioid.

♦ μ-Agonists, such as morphine, produce dose-dependent analgesia and are not limited by a ceiling effect. As pain increases, larger doses may be administered.

♦ Morphine is an extremely effective and versatile opioid for cancer-related pain. Morphine is available in multiple injectable and oral formulations, including short-duration tablets and liquids and sustained-release tablets.

♦ Oral morphine is effective for providing long-term analgesia in dogs and cats with moderate to severe pain. Patients receiving analgesics at set dosing intervals should be provided with a short-duration opioid for breakthrough pain.

♦ Oxymorphone is only available as an injectable analgesic and can induce panting by changing the temperature set-point in the brain. This usually is not an issue, except when attempting thoracic or abdominal radiography.

♦ Meperidine is very short-acting in animals, limiting its use as an analgesic in cancer patients.

♦ Codeine is available alone or with acetaminophen, allowing some flexibility in choice of oral medications.

♦ Fentanyl is an injectable drug that is potent and effective. Fentanyl can be infused because it is short acting. This trait also enables the dose to be changed rapidly if necessary in order to achieve good analgesia and minimal sedation.

♦ Buprenorphine is a partial μ-agonist. Buprenorphine does not produce the same degree of analgesia as does morphine and has a ceiling effect. Cats seem to develop a greater degree of analgesia than do dogs. The advantage of buprenorphine is that it has a very long duration of action, 6 to 12 hours. Buprenorphine also has a long time to onset of effect, approximately 40 minutes, even when given intravenously. Buprenorphine should only be used for mild to moderate cancer pain because of the inherent lack of maximal analgesia compared with morphine.

◆ Oral oxycodone is currently being used more and more frequently for severe pain in dogs. Oxycodone seems to induce less sedation and dysphoria than oral morphine and provides a greater degree of pain control than oral codeine.

◆ Butorphanol is a κ-agonist/μ-antagonist. The analgesia is not as good as that produced by morphine. Even in large parenteral doses, butorphanol produces analgesia of very short duration in dogs and may be of limited value for the treatment of moderate to severe cancer pain.

Transdermal fentanyl patches are an alternative to oral morphine, providing multiple-day analgesia. Fentanyl patches require 12 to 24 hours to take effect and last 2 to 4 days.

1. Additional analgesia must be provided during the first half to 1 day after patch placement.
2. Failure of appropriate patch application or inappropriate dosing can result in unreliable plasma concentrations in dogs.
3. Fentanyl patches may not provide enough analgesia for severe pain but allow lower doses of adjunctive drugs.
4. Fentanyl patches are expensive and should not be the first approach to chronic therapy.
5. Transdermal fentanyl administration is most appropriate in those patients that do not tolerate oral medication.

◆ Epidural opioid administration, especially of morphine, has been used as a method for providing perioperative analgesia. Opioids can be administered epidurally for days to weeks following placement of an epidural catheter (see Chapter 16).

◆ Opioid dose is selected to produce analgesia and minimize side effects.
1. The need for increased doses often reflects progression of disease.
2. Long-term use of opioids can produce tolerance.
3. Veterinarians should not be afraid of increasing opioid doses in patients that continue to show signs of pain. A distinct advantage of using opioids for pain control is that they are reversible with naloxone or nalmefene if unacceptable side effects occur. Prolonged use may produce constipation. Oral laxatives can help alleviate this problem.

α_2-AGONISTS

◆ Xylazine and medetomidine are two α_2-agonists approved for use in small animals in the United States. They are noncontrolled parenteral drugs and provide excellent visceral analgesia, but only for 20 minutes to 2 hours.

◆ Xylazine and medetomidine should not be the first or only choice for providing analgesia perioperatively to cancer patients because of cardiovascular side effects.

◆ Xylazine and medetomidine are synergistic with opioids. This effect is useful postoperatively for enhancing analgesia and alleviating dysphoria (see Chapter 11).

NMDA RECEPTOR ANTAGONIST

◆ Ketamine has been identified as an N-methyl-D-aspartate (NMDA) receptor antagonist. NMDA receptors are believed to be important in the processes leading up to central sensitization and windup.

◆ As an NMDA receptor antagonist, ketamine reduces postoperative pain and opioid requirements for a variety of procedures in humans.

◆ Ketamine doses are much smaller than those for anesthesia.
  1. Patients do not develop behavioral or cardiovascular effects.
  2. Microdose ketamine may decrease the incidence of opioid-induced dysphoria postoperatively.

◆ Microdose ketamine has been demonstrated to be effective for pain control in the perioperative period and after the dog has been sent home. Specific studies have not been completed to document efficacy in other situations. Presumably, other intense painful procedures and ailments would benefit from ketamine administration.

◆ Ketamine should be administered as a bolus (0.5 mg/kg IV) followed by an infusion (10 µg/kg per minute) before and during surgical stimulation. A lower infusion rate (2 µg/kg per minute) may be beneficial for the first 24 hours postoperatively and an even lower rate (1 µg/kg per minute) for the next 24 hours.

◆ Ketamine can be mixed in a bag of crystalloid solutions for administration during anesthesia in the absence of an infusion pump. Adding 60 mg (0.6 ml) of ketamine to a 1-L bag of crystalloid fluids will deliver ketamine at 10 µg/kg per minute when the administration rate is 10 ml/kg per hour.

◆ Amantadine can be administered at 3 mg/kg PO once daily to prevent windup. Amantadine should be part of the early intervention in patients with osteosarcoma.

TRANQUILIZERS

◆ A concern that frequently arises with pain management is concurrent tranquilization and sedation. Many drugs produce concurrent sedation. As mentioned previously, opioids can produce dysphoria instead of sedation.

◆ Dysphoria becomes more likely when cats are administered dog doses of opioids and when a patient is already experiencing high anxiety.
1. Dysphoric patients sometimes can be treated by petting and soothing or by changes in position.
2. Low-dose acepromazine (Table 21-1), both intravenously (IV) and/or intramuscularly (IM), is reasonable drug therapy for dysphoria. Although acepromazine does not alleviate pain, it calms anxious patients and makes them care less about their pain. Acepromazine can also be given orally, especially in the evening for animals that have trouble sleeping.
3. Alprazolam, 0.1 to 0.5 mg/kg PO daily, can be administered as an anxiolytic.
4. The benzodiazepines diazepam and midazolam can be administered as alternative therapy for animals in which acepromazine is contraindicated and those with bleeding and seizure disorders.
   a. Benzodiazepines should not be used by themselves in most alert patients because they frequently cause apprehension and excitement. Sedation usually occurs when combined with opioids.
   b. A low dose of xylazine, IV or IM, also can decrease dysphoria and increase analgesia in patients that are hemodynamically stable.
5. Patients that develop dysphoria after oral analgesic medications often respond well to oral acepromazine or diazepam. To determine whether the opioid is effective is important before changing the analgesia regimen.

TABLE 21-1	Commonly Used Adjuvant Drugs for Patients with Cancer Pain	
Drug	**Route**	**Dose**
Acepromazine	IV	0.005-0.03 mg/kg
Acepromazine	SQ, IM	0.02-0.05 mg/kg
	PO	0.05-0.1 mg/kg
Diazepam/midazolam (Versed)	IV	0.1-0.2 mg/kg
Xylazine	IV	0.05-0.1 mg/kg
Xylazine	IM	0.2 mg/kg
Medetomidine (Domitor)	IV	0.001 mg/kg
Medetomidine	IM	0.002 mg/kg
Amitriptyline (Elavil)	PO	Dog: 1-2 mg/kg q12-24h
		Cat: 2.5-12.5 mg per cat q24h
Imipramine (Tofranil)	PO	Dog: 0.5-1.0 mg/kg q8h
		Cat: 2.5-5 mg/kg q12h

Doses are the same for dogs and cats unless otherwise described.

TRICYCLIC ANTIDEPRESSANTS

◆ Tricyclic antidepressants, such as amitriptyline and imipramine, block the reuptake of serotonin and norepinephrine in the central nervous system. They also have antihistamine effects.

◆ These drugs have been used in humans for the treatment of chronic and neuropathic pain at doses considerably lower than those used to treat depression. Presumably, they have similar analgesic properties and enhance opioid analgesia.

LOCAL ANESTHETICS

◆ Local anesthetic techniques can be used instead of general anesthesia in selected patients or more commonly in combination with injectable analgesics (see Chapters 12 and 15).

EPIDURAL ANALGESIA

◆ A catheter can be placed in the epidural space. Maintenance of this catheter requires veterinarian and client vigilance to ensure cleanliness and prevent infection migrating to the spinal cord. With proper care, an epidural catheter can remain in place for days to weeks.

LOCAL OR WHOLE BODY RADIATION

◆ Local or whole body radiation can enhance analgesic drug effectiveness by reducing metastatic or primary tumor bulk.

◆ Radiation dose should be adjusted to the amount necessary to kill tumor cells and that which would affect normal cells.

◆ Mucositis of the oral cavity and pharynx can develop after radiation of the neck, head, or oral cavities, resulting in impaired ability to eat and drink.

◆ Mucositis therapy includes analgesics, sucralfate, 2% viscous lidocaine, and green tea rinses.

BISPHOSPHANATES

◆ Bony metastases are one of the most common causes of pain in advanced cancer. Some tumors cause osteoblastic metastases, but most cause osteolytic lesions.

◆ Administration of bisphosphonates, such as pamidronate or alendronate (Fosamax), reduces pain and pathologic fractures in humans.

- Bisphosphonates accumulate on bone surfaces and inhibit osteoclast-induced resorption, favoring bone formation. This therapy may be expensive but has been shown to be useful in patients with osteosarcoma-related pain.

STRONTIUM-89

- Intravenous administration of strontium-89 has also been shown to provide analgesia related to bony metastases in approximately 50% of humans, but its use is uncommon in veterinary patients.

ACUPUNCTURE

- Acupuncture can be used as a pain-relieving modality, often when conventional therapy does not work.
- Acupuncture is useful in conjunction with other therapy to allow lower doses of drugs that may have side effects (see Chapter 17).
- In general, acupuncture analgesia is extremely useful for pelvic, radial/ulnar, and femoral bone pain and cutaneous discomfort resulting from radiation therapy.
- Acupuncture helps alleviate nausea associated with chemotherapy and opioid analgesics and promotes general well-being.

APPROACH TO PAIN IN THE CANCER PATIENT

- The first principle is to practice a multimodal approach to analgesia. Use drugs in combination that work by different mechanisms of action to allow optimal analgesia at the lowest dose possible.
- A simple flowchart (Table 21-2) can help with the sequence of activities related to pain assessment and management. This flowchart emphasizes the use of multiple modalities, beginning therapy with the least invasive methods and advancing treatment to meet the patient's needs.
- Pain control should be achievable by following these simple ABCs:

ABCs OF CANCER PAIN CONTROL
A—Assess pain.
B—Believe owner.
C—Choose appropriate therapy.
D—Deliver therapy in a logical manner.
E—Empower clients to participate.
F—Facilitate combination therapy.

---

1. Assess the pain. Ask for the owner's perceptions.
2. Believe the owner. The owner sees the pet everyday in its own environment.
3. Choose appropriate therapy following the World Health Organization ladder and other more specific paradigms.
4. Deliver therapy in a logical, coordinated manner.
5. Combine pain therapy programs and regimens with recommendations for managing and improving the animal's quality of life (see Chapter 29).
6. Empower the clients to participate actively in their pet's well-being.

SURGICAL CASE EXAMPLES

◆ The following generic examples, in conjunction with the flowchart, present useful approaches to specific types of pain encountered in

TABLE 21-2	Management of Surgical Pain	
Time	**Drugs**	**Rationale**
Preoperative	Morphine	Preemptive, long-lasting analgesia
	±Acepromazine	Tranquilization, calming, anxiolysis
	Atropine/glycopyrrolate	Prevent bradycardia associated with opioids
	Appropriate nerve blocks	Preemptive analgesia, prevent windup
	Epidural anesthesia if applicable	Preemptive analgesia, prevent windup
Intraoperative	Fentanyl continuous infusion	Decrease cardiovascular effects of inhalant agents; additional analgesia
	Microdose ketamine	Prevent windup
	Morphine-lidocaine-ketamine	Decrease cardiovascular effects of inhalant agents; additional analgesia
		Prevent windup
Acute postoperative	Appropriate nerve blocks	Analgesia
	Fentanyl continuous infusion	Analgesia adjustable to patient needs
	Microdose ketamine	Prevent windup, dysphoria
Postoperative adjuncts	Acepromazine	Anxiolysis, dysphoria
	Alprazolam	Anxiolysis
	Diazepam/midazolam	Dysphoria
	Xylazine/medetomidine	Additional analgesia, dysphoria

oncology practice. The examples recommend specific techniques for the procedure rather than a complete analgesia program.

- Lateral thoracotomy
  1. Intercostal nerve block
  2. Interpleural local anesthetic
  3. Opioid epidural
- Sternotomy
  1. Interpleural local anesthetic
  2. Opioid epidural
- Forelimb amputation
  1. Brachial plexus nerve block
  2. Opioid epidural
- Rear limb amputation: opioid epidural
- Cranial mandibular surgery
  1. Mandibular nerve block
  2. Mental nerve block
- Upper lip and nose procedure: infraorbital nerve block
- Maxillary surgery: maxillary nerve block
- Midcaudal abdominal surgery: opioid epidural (local anesthetic also if in caudal abdomen)
- Cranial abdominal surgery
  1. Interpleural local anesthetic
  2. Opioid epidural
- Although not all types of pain can be addressed, pain relief should be considered achievable by following recommendations and paradigms in this manuscript.

OUTPATIENT CASE EXAMPLES

- Osteosarcoma—assuming the patient does not have an amputation
  1. Initial therapy with an approved NSAID for mild to moderate pain
  2. Continuous therapy with amantadine to treat and prevent windup
  3. Pamidronate, a bisphosphonate, every 3 to 4 weeks to decrease osteoclast function
  4. Tramadol with the NSAID for moderate to severe pain
  5. Oxycodone to replace tramadol as the pain gets worse
- Chondrosarcoma
  1. Initial therapy with an approved NSAID for mild to moderate pain
  2. Gabapentin in progressively increasing doses for analgesia and to help prevent windup

- Transitional cell carcinoma
  1. This is the only tumor that has been identified definitively as being responsive to piroxicam. Hence, piroxicam should be administered for anticancer effects and for analgesia. The patient's packed cell volume should be monitored closely because piroxicam is a nonspecific COX-1/COX-2 inhibitor, predisposing to moderate to severe ulceration and the potential for gastrointestinal bleeding.
  2. Administer tramadol with piroxicam for more severe pain.

SUMMARY

- Most animals with cancer have pain that can be treated.
- Engage the owners as fully as possible.
- Practice multimodal analgesia.
- If a specific regimen is not working, increase the dose or change protocols.

SUGGESTED READINGS

Cancer pain relief, ed 2, Geneva, 1996, World Health Organization.

Friedland J: Local and systemic radiation for palliation of metastatic disease, *Urol Clin North Am* 26:391-402, 1999.

Fu ES, Miguel R, Scharf JE: Preemptive ketamine decreases postoperative narcotic requirements in patients undergoing abdominal surgery, *Anesth Analg* 84:1086-1090, 1997.

Goisis A, Gorini M, Ratti R, et al: Application of a WHO protocol on medical therapy for oncologic pain in an internal medicine hospital, *Tumori* 75:470-472, 1989.

Golden BD, Abramson SB: Selective cyclooxygenase-2 inhibitors, *Rheum Dis Clin North Am* 25:359-378, 1999.

Jacox A, Carr DB, Payne R, et al: *Management of cancer pain*, Rockville, Md, 1994, Agency for Health Care Policy and Research.

Kasalicky J, Krajska V: The effect of repeated strontium-89 chloride therapy on bone pain palliation in patients with skeletal cancer metastases, *Eur J Nucl Med* 25:1362-1367, 1998.

Merskey H: Pharmacologic approaches other than opioids in chronic non-cancer pain management, *Acta Anaesthesiol Scand* 41:187-190, 1997.

Nair N: Relative efficacy of 32P and 89Sr in palliation of skeletal metastases, *J Nucl Med* 40:256-261, 1999.

Sawyer DC, Rech RH, Durham RA, et al: Dose response to butorphanol administered subcutaneously to increase visceral nociceptive threshold in dogs, *Am J Vet Res* 52:1826-1830, 1991.

Shaw N, Burrows CF, King RR: Massive gastric hemorrhage induced by buffered aspirin in a greyhound, *J Am Anim Hosp Assoc* 33:215-219, 1999.

22

PAIN MANAGEMENT IN THE CAT

SHEILAH A. ROBERTSON

Cats now outnumber dogs as pets in many countries, including the United States and the United Kingdom. Most cats will undergo at least one surgery in their life span, usually elective neutering, that is associated with the potential for them to experience acute pain. Until recently, there was little awareness of chronic pain in cats, and it is likely this has been greatly underestimated. New studies suggest that many senior cats (>10 years of age) have radiographic or clinical evidence of degenerative joint disease and that the clinical signs are different from those seen in dogs. The incidence of other long-term pain conditions such as cancer, intervertebral disk disease, and oral and ocular pain is unknown but undoubtedly significant.

Alleviation of pain in cats historically has lagged behind that in other companion animals, but this is rapidly changing. The challenges of treating pain in cats are unique but not insurmountable (Box 22-1).

The drugs discussed elsewhere in this book can be used in a pain management plan for cats and include opioids (Chapter 9), nonsteroidal antiinflammatory drugs (NSAIDs; Chapter 10), α_2-agonists (Chapter 11), local anesthetics (Chapter 12), and many of the drugs listed under "other

---

BOX 22-1

Challenges of Treating Pain in Cats

- Difficulty in recognizing pain in cats
- Lack of species-specific information
- Unique metabolism of drugs (e.g., low capacity for hepatic glucuronidation)
- Risk of adverse side effects (e.g., toxicity with long-term use of nonsteroidal antiinflammatory drugs)
- Paucity of drugs with market authorization
- Difficulty in administration of medications to cats

---

drugs used to treat pain" (Chapter 14). In addition, complementary therapies are applicable to cats (Chapter 16). This chapter discusses the unique features of these drugs and modalities when used in cats and also provides practical information for managing common pain conditions in the feline patient.

RECOGNITION OF PAIN IN CATS

No validated gold standard pain scoring systems exist for use in animals, but specific pain behaviors are now recognized (Chapters 5 and 6). Studies that have tried to correlate objective physiological data such as heart rate, temperature, respiratory rate, plasma cortisol, and β-endorphins with pain in cats have been unsuccessful because these are influenced by many factors other than pain. Therefore, observation of behavior is the best means of assessing the presence and degree of pain experienced by a cat. Knowing a cat's personality before onset of pain is important, and often veterinarians must rely on information from the owner. Pain may turn a previously friendly cat into an aggressive one or a social cat into a solitary one. Loss of normal behavior may also occur; for example, a cat with degenerative joint disease no longer jumping up onto its favorite resting spots, or adoption of a new strategy such as standing to urinate rather than squatting because of hip or spinal pain.

ACUTE PAIN

Because even pain-free cats change their behavior in a veterinary clinic because of fear, this can make assessing pain very difficult. However, cats in acute pain following surgery or trauma are often depressed, immobile, and tense and try to hide. These cats do not respond positively to human interaction such as stroking. The painful cat that is immobile and hiding at the back of the cage is often overlooked and goes untreated. In some cats the response to pain is different and exhibited by manic and aggressive behavior, growling, hissing, and rolling around their cage. The latter behavior is often a response to restrictive bandages regardless of their pain, but the two must be differentiated: often if the bandage can be removed, the cat calms down; if not, then pain should be suspected. Cats with abdominal pain frequently adopt a sternal posture, with their head down, elbows drawn back, stifles forward, abdominal muscles tensed, and back arched, and their eyes are often half-shut or "squinting" (Fig. 22-1).

Limb pain prevents weight bearing; however, pain is often bilateral in cats (forelimb declaw) and therefore easily overlooked. One of the many commonly reported problems following onychectomy is excessive

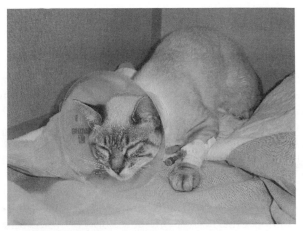

FIG. 22-1. The typical features suggestive of abdominal pain are seen in this cat: note the sternal posture, with head down, elbows drawn back, stifles forward, and arched back with half-shut or "squinting" eyes.

licking and chewing of the feet. If possible, one should assess the response to palpation on or around the source of pain, for example; a cat that has been given appropriate analgesic agents should tolerate gentle pressure around a surgical incision.

It is important that pain does not go untreated just because one is unsure of its presence or severity. If in doubt, administer an analgesic agent and observe for a positive improvement in behavior or demeanor.

Pain should always be assessed and recorded in hospitalized patients. A pain scoring system that suits the individual clinic should be adopted; this must be user friendly and not too time consuming; for examples, see Chapter 6.

CHRONIC PAIN

The most common cause of chronic pain in cats is osteoarthritis (OA), but cancer or oral, ocular, and long-standing skin diseases or wounds are also important causes.

Because of their small size and their innate agility, cats can cope with severe orthopedic disease and because of a pet cat's lifestyle, lameness or exercise intolerance are not common owner complaints. In addition, bilateral involvement—for example, both elbow or hip joints—is common, and this makes lameness difficult to detect. To elicit pain on clinical examination of some cats is also notoriously difficult.

Clinical experience suggests that the behavioral changes that accompany OA are insidious and easily missed or are assumed to be inevitable with advancing age; therefore the owner does not seek veterinary advice. Changes in behavior including decreased grooming, reluctance to jump up on favorite places, inability to jump as high as before, and soiling outside the litter box should prompt the veterinarian to look for sources of chronic pain. Other changes that owners report are altered sleeping habits (an increase or decrease), withdrawing from human interaction, hiding and dislike of being stroked or brushed. Inactivity, which may result from chronic joint pain, is much more difficult to determine in cats because they naturally sleep a lot and are often solitary, and in many cases the owners are not home all day to monitor their cat's activity level.

Analgesic trials may sometimes be the only way to confirm that chronic pain was present. For example, after intervention with an NSAID in cats with a presumptive diagnosis of OA, the majority of owners believed that their cats made an improvement, and the most common clinical sign that improved was the unwillingness to jump, the height of the jump, and a noticeably less stiff gait.[1]

METABOLISM OF DRUGS

Compared with other mammals, cats have a very low capacity for hepatic glucuronidation of exogenously administered drugs.[2] Cats may lack these metabolic pathways because of their all-meat diet and lack of exposure and therefore need to metabolize plants containing phytoalexins.

These metabolic differences can lead to toxic side effects if doses and dosing intervals are not adjusted. Alternatively, if the parent compound must be metabolized to an active component via this pathway, the drug may be less effective. The deficiency of the glucuronidation pathway in cats explains their susceptibility to the toxic side effects of phenolic drugs such as acetaminophen (paracetamol) and long half-lives of other drugs such as carprofen and aspirin. Only small amounts of morphine-6-glucuronide (M-6-G) are produced after administration of morphine in cats, and because this metabolite contributes to the overall analgesic profile of morphine in other species, morphine may be less effective in cats.

Armed with a better understanding of feline drug metabolism, one can understand why the response to some drugs is unpredictable and different from other species, and this allows clinicians to make more appropriate choices, for example, choosing a drug that relies more on oxidative pathways, such as meloxicam, and using pharmacokinetic data such as half-life from research studies to devise dosing intervals.

ANALGESIC DRUGS

OPIOIDS

Opioids are the most versatile, reliable, and efficacious drugs for the treatment of pain and have an excellent safety record. In cats, opioids should be the foundation of most acute pain analgesic plans. As veterinarians study cats more, it is becoming clear that as in other species, there are genetic differences between individuals in their response to opioids. This may be correlated with individual differences in metabolism and with the number, type, and distribution of opioid receptors. For these reasons, one should not expect all cats to respond equally to a set dose of a specific opioid, emphasizing the need for careful pain assessment and individually tailored treatment protocols.

Timing of Administration

Opioids have distinct advantages when given before surgery; this is termed *preemptive analgesia.* Opioids can decrease but not fully prevent central sensitization, and animals that receive opioids before surgery have lower pain scores and higher pain thresholds for a longer period compared with those receiving them after surgery. When opioids are on board during a surgical procedure, heart rate and blood pressure tend to remain stable because they are not influenced by noxious stimuli.

Another advantage of using opioids before anesthesia in many species is their anesthetic-sparing effect; for example, less inhalant agent is required, often resulting in less cardiopulmonary depression. In cats this effect is less apparent than in dogs[3] but is still clinically useful.

Side Effects

Many opioids can be used successfully in cats. The notion that cats are likely to become "manic" (so-called morphine mania) is a myth based on studies using doses far in excess of those needed to alleviate pain. The opioids and doses suggested in this chapter often result in sedation and euphoric behavior (rubbing against the cage or a person, purring and kneading with the forepaws). Dysphoria is an unusual response to opioid administration in painful cats or when used in combination with drugs such as acetylpromazine or medetomidine that provide sedation.

In contrast to many other species, opioids cause mydriasis in cats rather than miosis, but the analgesic effects can wear off before pupil size returns to normal, so pupil size should not be relied on as an indicator that analgesia is still present. Mydriasis, inability to focus, and poor depth perception may lead to cats becoming startled when approached quickly, bumping into objects, and showing aversion to bright light.

Nausea (licking of the lips, apprehension, and salivation) and vomiting are features of opioid administration in many species. In research and clinical settings the incidence of these side effects varies with the drug and the route of administration. Vomiting and nausea is most often associated with morphine and hydromorphone in cats and is rarely seen after administration of butorphanol, buprenorphine, fentanyl, meperidine, methadone, or oxymorphone. Vomiting is much more likely after subcutaneous injection than after intravenous dosing, with intramuscular administration lying in between. These side effects are also more likely to be seen in a pain-free cat (for example, when opioids are used as a preemptive analgesic in an elective case) and if they are not coadministered with acetylpromazine. Vomiting should be avoided in cats that are obtunded and may not have adequate airway protection and in those with a suspected increase in intracranial or intraocular pressure or with a corneal foreign body because the act of vomiting increases intracranial and intraocular pressure.

Long-term use of opioids is common in humans with chronic pain. However, in cats, inappetence is common after 2 to 3 days of opioid use and is likely associated with decreased gastrointestinal motility.

Route of administration also affects time to onset, intensity, and duration of action. In an experimental model using hydromorphone, onset time was shortest and intensity of effect and duration greatest after intravenous (IV) dosing. Time to peak effect was slowest after subcutaneous (SC) administration, and the duration and intensity of effect after intramuscular (IM) and SC administration were less than after IV dosing. When an IV catheter is available, this is the recommended route of administration. This avoids repeated SC or IM injections, which can be painful and stressful for cats and more difficult for nursing personnel to perform.

Opioid-Related Hyperthermia.   Hyperthermia can occur after opioid administration in cats. Hyperthermia is reported with meperidine and morphine, but only at high doses and not at those commonly used clinically. However, in a clinical setting using recommended doses (0.1 mg/kg) of hydromorphone, more than 60% of cats had temperatures greater than 40° C (104° F) at some time during recovery, with one cat reaching 42.5° C (108.5° F).[4] Hyperthermia was not alleviated by NSAID administration. These cats were treated with fans, bathing with cool water or alcohol, and administration of acepromazine to promote vasodilation; in two cases, naloxone was used after palliative measures failed. Mildly elevated rectal temperatures have been reported in association with transdermal fentanyl patches but rarely require treatment.

Cardiovascular depression, including bradycardia, is not a common side effect of opioids in clinical situations. If this does occur, it can be treated with atropine or glycopyrrolate (see Chapter 9). Respiratory depression is also uncommon, and during anesthesia it is often a result of other anesthetic agents and can easily be managed by providing ventilatory support. In conscious cats, hypoventilation after opioid use is rare and usually only seen after an overdose or if there is underlying pathologic condition such as head trauma. In these situations, naloxone can be given *to effect* until respiratory rate increases; by doing this, only respiratory depression is reversed and not all the analgesia. Naloxone (0.4 mg/ml) should be diluted in a 1:10 ratio with normal saline and given by slow IV injection until a response is seen. Alternatively, butorphanol (0.1 to 0.2 mg/kg) can be given to reverse μ-opioid agonists.

Clinical Use of Opioids

Buprenorphine. Buprenorphine is a partial μ-agonist that is widely used in cats. Buprenorphine is a popular choice in practice because it is versatile and is a less highly scheduled controlled drug than the pure μ-agonist agents. Onset of analgesia is faster than previously believed but dependent on route of administration; there is significant analgesia within 30 minutes after IV or transmucosal administration, but onset of effect can take up to 45 minutes to 1 hour after SC and IM dosing. Peak effect occurs 90 minutes after IV or transmucosal administration.

Transmucosal absorption through oral mucous membranes is effective in cats with almost 100% bioavailability by this route, likely a result of their alkaline saliva. Transmucosal administration has proved to be effective and acceptable in cats and can be mastered by owners for at-home treatment. The commercially available preparation for injection is used for transmucosal dosing and the small volume (0.3 ml at a dose of 0.02 mg/kg in a 5-kg cat) can easily be placed on any oral mucous membrane such as under the tongue or in the cheek pouch. Buprenorphine (0.02 mg/kg) was equally effective by the IV and transmucosal route and may provide analgesia for up to 6 hours. Buprenorphine rarely causes vomiting or dysphoria in cats and is suitable for perioperative pain management because it is easily administered, highly effective, and long acting.

A transdermal matrix patch delivery system for buprenorphine is now available for use in humans. Preliminary work in cats shows that absorption is good, but it has not yet been used or evaluated in a clinical setting.

Butorphanol. Butorphanol is an agonist-antagonist opioid and exhibits a "ceiling" effect after which increasing the dose does not produce any further analgesia. In cats, this ceiling dose may be as low as

0.1 mg/kg.[5] Butorphanol appears to be an effective visceral but poor somatic analgesic and so may be a good choice for temporary relief of visceral pain syndromes such as interstitial cystitis. Clinical and experimental investigations indicate that butorphanol is short acting in most cats (<2 hours) and requires frequent dosing to be effective. Some recent research studies show that some cats do respond well to butorphanol and for longer (>6 hours) periods after IM injection. This is likely due to intercat genetic variability in opioid receptors. Again this means that each cat must be individually assessed.

Nalbuphine. Nalbuphine is another agonist-antagonist, similar to butorphanol, but is currently not scheduled by the U.S. Food and Drug Administration (FDA). Nalbuphine also has a ceiling effect and is adequate for mild to moderate degrees of pain. Nalbuphine seems to provide good visceral and somatic analgesia, but well-designed studies are lacking. The recommended doses of nalbuphine in cats are 0.1 to 0.2 mg/kg IV and up to 0.5 mg/kg IM or SC.

Fentanyl. Fentanyl is a potent, short-acting pure μ-agonist that is used most commonly to supplement general anesthesia during which it can be given as intermittent boluses or by infusion (see Constant Rate Infusions).

Transdermal fentanyl patches that release fentanyl over several days have been used for alleviation of acute perioperative pain in cats. These patches provide a "hands-off" approach to pain management that is especially attractive in cats that are difficult to medicate. Plasma fentanyl concentrations are variable after patch placement in cats, and in some cats uptake is limited and does not reach an effective steady-state plasma concentration (>1 ng/ml); therefore, if patches are used, each cat must be assessed carefully for comfort. The variability may be related to the size of the patch compared with the weight of the cat, skin permeability, placement site, skin perfusion, subcutaneous fat, and body temperature. When effective, cats achieve steady-state plasma concentration faster than dogs (6 to 12 hours compared with 18 to 24 hours), and plasma levels take longer to decline after patch removal in cats (up to 18 to 20 hours). Transdermal fentanyl patches have proved useful in a clinical setting for routine ovariohysterectomy and onychectomy. Significantly elevated temperatures (1.0° C above baseline) 4 to 12 hours after transdermal fentanyl patch application are reported.

Meperidine (Pethidine, Demerol). Meperidine (pethidine, Demerol), should *only be given IM or SC* because IV injection can produce excitement. Meperidine rarely causes vomiting in cats. The main drawback of meperidine is its short duration of action. In clinical practice, meperidine performs as predicted in experimental studies, producing good analgesia for little more than 1 to 2 hours. This drug is a reasonable choice for minor procedures of short duration but is not ideal for cats that require longer treatment because repeated IM injections can be painful, and cats quickly become resentful of this.

Hydromorphone.   Doses of less than 0.05 mg/kg hydromorphone did not produce antinociception in a research model, whereas a dose of 0.1 mg/kg IV was effective for 3.5 to 7 hours, with considerable inter-cat variability on duration of effect. When combined with acepromazine (0.05 to 0 1 mg/kg), hydromorphone provides good analgesia and seda-tion. Hydromorphone can be associated with hyperthermia, nausea, and vomiting (see Side Effects).

Methadone.   Methadone has been used in cats at doses ranging from 0.1 to 0.6 mg/kg, normally by the IM or SC route, but IV dosing is also commonly performed. Nausea and vomiting are rare after administration. In a clinical setting when used for ovariohysterectomy, methadone was effective and produced no undesirable behavioral, cardiovascular, or respiratory effects. In addition to its μ-agonist actions, methadone may also contribute to analgesia via antagonism of N-methyl-D-aspartate receptors. Methadone shows great potential as a versatile analgesic agent for cats.[6,7]

Morphine.   Morphine has been widely used in cats and does not pro-duce excitation at doses of 0.1 to 0.2 mg/kg, which has provided clinically useful analgesia. After IM or SC administration, onset of analgesic action may take 45 to 60 minutes; so if morphine is used as a preemptive agent, timing of administration should be taken into account. In research cats, no M-6-G, the active analgesic metabolite, was detected after IM administra-tion. After IV dosing, M-6-G was detected in 50% of cats; therefore, if IV access is available, this may be a more effective route of administration.

Oxymorphone.   Oxymorphone been a popular analgesic for many years in the United States, where it is licensed for use in the cat. Oxymor-phone produces few undesirable side effects but is more expensive than other μ-opioid agonists.

Mixing of Opioids

It has been proposed that mixing of different classes of opioids may result in added benefits. However, the outcome seems variable; a combination of hydromorphone and butorphanol did not have additive effects but did produce a longer lasting (up to 9 hours) but less intense effect than hydromorphone alone. Low doses of oxymorphone and butorphanol in combination produced greater levels of antinociception than when used individually, but combining butorphanol and buprenorphine provided no added benefits over either drug used alone.

Constant Rate Infusions

Fentanyl. Fentanyl is suitable for constant rate infusion in cats but should be titrated to effect to reduce accumulation. Fentanyl is most commonly used during anesthesia so that less inhalant agents are required, and it also allows the anesthetist to alter the level of analgesia rapidly. Fentanyl infusion can be continued into the postoperative period, when again it is easily titrated to individual patient needs. A loading dose of 5 to 10 μg/kg IV is suggested, followed by 10 to 45 μg/kg per hour during anesthesia, reducing the dose postoperatively to 2 to 5 μg/kg hour, depending on the individual cat's needs.

Alfentanil. Alfentanil is a short-acting opioid that is suitable for infusion. Alfentanil reduced isoflurane requirements and improved some cardiovascular variables, but at effective doses hyperthermia and metabolic acidosis were reported.

Remifentanil. Remifentanil has an ideal pharmacokinetic profile for infusion and has been used successfully in dogs; early clinical reports of its intraoperative use in cats are promising using doses similar to those in dogs (0.1 to 1.0 μg/kg per minute).

Epidural Opioid Administration

Morphine, fentanyl, pethidine, methadone, and buprenorphine have been given via the epidural route in cats. Epidural injection is technically more challenging in cats because of their small size, and because the spinal cord ends more caudally, entering the subarachnoid space is more likely, even at the lumbosacral junction. Clinical reports suggest that this route is effective in cats, but more recent studies show that epidurally administered opioids may be less effective than previously believed,[8] so it is recommended that if the epidural route is chosen, a local anesthetic also be used (Chapter 15).

Each opioid drug is described in detail in Chapter 9, and recommended doses and routes of administration for cats are shown in Table 22-1.

NONSTEROIDAL ANTIINFLAMMATORY AGENTS

Until recently, NSAIDs have not been widely used in cats largely because of the fear of toxicity. Considerable species variation exists in cyclooxygenase (COX) expression, so safety in one species cannot be assumed in another. In addition, for many NSAIDs pharmacokinetic data are only available for single doses in cats. It is only recently that studies have examined the metabolism or safety of chronic administration. The deficiency of glucuronidation pathways in cats results in slow metabolism of several NSAIDs, particularly the phenolic compounds. However, drug metabolism

TABLE 22-1   Commonly Used Opioid Drugs and Doses for Cats

Opioid	Dose	Route of Administration	Comments
Butorphanol	0.1-0.8 mg/kg	IV, IM, SC	Little benefit to giving doses >0.2 mg/kg (ceiling effect) Short-acting in some cats
Buprenorphine	0.01-0.03 mg/kg	IV, IM, transmucosal	Not associated with vomiting or hyperthermia. Licensed for use in cats in UK (Vetergesic)
	35 μg/hour patch	Transdermal	Uptake occurs but dosing regimens and efficacy in clinical settings not established
Fentanyl			
Bolus	2-10 μg/kg	IV	All CRIs should be preceded with a bolus to achieve effective plasma concen-
CRI intraoperative	10-45 μg/kg /hour	IV	tration. Infusion rate can be adjusted to rapidly change degree of analgesia
CRI postoperative	5-10 μg/kg /hour	IV	
TDF patch	25 μg/hr, 2.5 mg	Transdermal (over shaved skin)	May take up to 12 hours to reach effective plasma concentrations. Elevated body temperature reported in some cats
Hydromorphone	0.05-0.1 mg/kg	IV, IM, SC	Doses of 0.1 mg/kg regardless of route may be associated with hyperthermia
Meperidine (pethidine, Demerol)	5-10 mg/kg	IM, SC	Not to be given IV
Methadone	0.1-0.6 mg/kg	IV, IM, SC	Also has NMDA antagonist properties. Not associated with vomiting or hyper- thermia
Morphine	0.2-0.5 mg/kg	IV, IM, SC	Active metabolites reported only in low concentration; therefore may be less effective than in other species
Oxymorphone	0.05-0.1 mg/kg	IV, IM, SC	Hyperthermia not reported
Tramadol	1-4 mg/kg	IV, IM	Has opioid actions but is not a scheduled drug.
Tramadol*	2 mg/kg	Oral (capsules, tablets, liquid)	

*The human product Ultracet contains acetaminophen and must not be used in cats.

CRI, Constant rate infusion; *TDF,* transdermal fentanyl.

and excretion pathways other than glucuronidation such as oxidation, sulfation, and active drug transport do not appear to be deficient in cats compared with other species. In recent years, a number of newer NSAIDs have become licensed for use in cats in several countries. NSAIDs have the advantage of being long acting, providing up to 24 hours of analgesia, and they are not subject to the purchase and storage restrictions of the opioids.

Side Effects

The adverse side effects of the newer NSAIDs are not yet well documented in cats but are similar to those described for other species (Chapter 10) and include renal, hepatic, and gastrointestinal toxicity. NSAIDs should not be used if there is preexisting renal or hepatic disease, if corticosteroids are being used, or in the face of hypovolemia, dehydration, or hypotension or if substantial blood loss is anticipated. A complete blood count and chemistry panel drawn before use may detect animals unsuitable for NSAID treatment (e.g., those with renal disease or significant liver disease) and provide baseline data if there is an unexpected complication following administration.

Clinically Useful NSAIDs

Carprofen. Carprofen (2 to 4 mg/kg SC or IV) provides good postoperative analgesia for at least 24 hours in cats following soft tissue surgery. Anecdotal reports of toxicity have been made, usually associated with concurrent disease and prolonged administration of the oral formulations. Carprofen undergoes glucuronidation, and problems with repeated dosing may be a result of variable intercat pharmacokinetics; for example, in one study the half-life of carprofen after IV administration to healthy adult cats ranged from 9 to 49 hours. Repeat dosing is not recommended.

Ketoprofen. Ketoprofen has proved to be an effective analgesic for use in cats; 2 mg/kg provided postoperative analgesia for at least 18 hours and was comparable to carprofen, meloxicam, and tolfenamic acid after neutering. Ketoprofen can alter platelet function and increase bleeding; therefore, it is usually given after surgery. Oral formulations (1 mg/kg once daily) have been used for longer periods to treat musculoskeletal disorders.

Meloxicam. Meloxicam is a COX-2 selective NSAID, and the injectable formulation is licensed for preoperative use in many countries (up to 0.3 mg/kg SC). Meloxicam is clinically effective for surgical procedures including ovariohysterectomy, castration, and orthopedic surgery.

The sweet-flavored oral formulation seems palatable to most cats, and in one study it was voted by owners as easier to administer than ketoprofen. The liquid formulation also allows for accurate dosing, which is important when this drug is used long term. Meloxicam has been used for long-term treatment of OA in cats, with owners reporting considerable improvement. Meloxicam does not have a prolonged half-life in cats because it is metabolized by hepatic oxidative pathways, and this may be why it has achieved success for long-term use. In 2007, meloxicam oral suspension (0.5 mg/ml) received market authorization for the treatment of OA in cats in several European countries. The suggested dose is 0.1 mg/kg on day one followed by a maintenance dose of 0.05 mg/kg once daily. The daily dose can be given on food or directly into the mouth using the drop dispenser of the bottle or the measuring syringe provided. Some cats may require lower maintenance doses, and this can be decided by the owner.

If NSAIDs are used off-label (e.g., oral meloxicam suspension in the United States), the owner should be made aware of this. In all cases the owner should be informed of the possible side effects verbally and in writing. This should include what clinical signs to look for (e.g., vomiting, inappetence, and bloody stool) that would warrant calling the veterinarian and stopping treatment.

Although there are no standard guidelines for monitoring cats receiving NSAIDs over prolonged periods, the veterinarian should follow the cats carefully. It is suggested that the packed cell volume, total protein, blood urea nitrogen, creatinine, and liver enzymes be measured in addition to urine analysis before and after 1 week of treatment and then at three monthly intervals. Liver enzymes may rise with chronic drug administration but do not reflect hepatic function; an increase of more than 200% should prompt running liver function tests such as a bile acid assay.

Clinical Choices

Little difference in the efficacy of the NSAIDs described previously is apparent in the acute perioperative setting, and all provide good analgesia in the majority of cats for up to 24 hours. Choice of agent depends on personal preference, convenience of dosing, and duration of use. For long-term use, meloxicam is currently the best choice and the only NSAID labeled for treatment of chronic musculoskeletal disorders in cats, at least in same countries. Once a NSAID has been chosen, the cat should not be placed on a different one without a period of "wash out," which is arbitrarily said to be 5 to 7 days (Chapter 10).

With the availability of newer NSAIDs the efficacy and safety of which are established, there appears to be little justification for use of the older NSAIDs such as aspirin, flunixin, and phenylbutazone to provide analgesia in cats. Paracetamol, ibuprofen, indomethacin, and naproxen are extremely toxic in cats and should never be used.

α₂-ADRENOCEPTOR AGONISTS

The α_2-adrenoceptor agonists, which include xylazine, medetomidine, and dexmedetomidine, provide sedation, muscle relaxation, and analgesia in cats. Medetomidine is labeled for use in cats in some countries. These drugs are not commonly used for their analgesic effect alone because of the profound sedation and cardiovascular depression that accompanies their use. The vasoconstriction and decrease in cardiac output associated with α_2-agonists preclude their use in cats with cardiovascular disease or preexisting hypovolemia.

Medetomidine can be used alone for chemical restraint so that minor painful procedures can be performed (cleaning wounds, lancing abscesses) or fractious cats can be examined. Published doses range from 5 to 150 μg/kg IM, and the effects of medetomidine are dose dependent. In most cases, doses of 30 to 50 μg/kg are sufficient. Duration of effect is also dose dependent, with a dose of 50 μg/kg lasting up to 3 hours. Much lower doses (5 to 20 μg/kg IM) can be used in combination with buprenorphine, methadone, or morphine to provide sedation and analgesia.

Low-dose constant rate IV infusions can be used in cats; this is a good technique for fractious cats; often 1 to 2 μg/kg per hour facilitates nursing care, and the dose can be titrated up or down depending on what interventions are required.

Medetomidine can be antagonized with atipamezole, but this will reverse analgesia in addition to sedation. The reversal dose (in micrograms) is 2.5 times the dose of medetomidine administered.

In painful and fractious cats, oral administration of medetomidine (up to 200 μg/kg), which likely results in transmucosal uptake, can be a useful technique for chemical restraint, but the responses can be variable, and excessive salivation occurs in some cats.[9]

Epidural administration of medetomidine (10 μg/kg) was found to be effective in cats, but the duration of effect was only 4 hours, and although cardiopulmonary variables were not considerably affected, most cats vomited after administration. Based on the variable results of epidural morphine administration, medetomidine may be a viable option for cats undergoing abdominal or hind limb surgery.

LOCAL ANESTHETICS

The local anesthetic techniques described in Chapter 12 can be adapted for use in the cat. One of the most commonly used local anesthetic techniques in cats is a digital nerve block before onychectomy (Fig. 22-2).

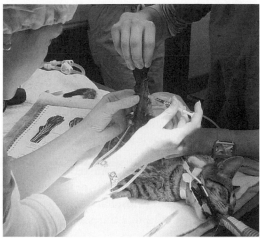

FIG. 22-2. Local anesthetic blocks are very effective for blocking nociceptive impulses during surgery. This image shows a digital nerve block being administered before onychectomy.

Bupivacaine (total dose 2 to 3 mg/kg) *without* epinephrine is often used, but longer-acting agents would be more beneficial. Cats do not lose motor function with this technique but may have proprioceptive deficits.

Implantable wound catheters that can remain in situ for several days have been used in cats after major surgery including limb amputations and extensive fibrosarcoma resection. Injection of local anesthetic agents (mepivacaine [Carbocaine], lidocaine, and bupivacaine) at 4- to 6-hour intervals maintains excellent analgesia, and in most cases the use of systemically administered opioids and NSAIDs can be reduced.

A topical liposome-encapsulated formulation of lidocaine is available (ELA-Max, over the counter), and a eutectic mixture of lidocaine and prilocaine (EMLA cream, prescription required) can be applied to shaved skin to provide analgesia in advance of venipuncture, catheter placement, and skin biopsies. Transdermal absorption did occur after application of 15 mg/kg of ELA-Max, but plasma concentrations remained significantly below toxic values.

IV infusions of lidocaine decrease inhalant anesthetic requirements in dogs and may provide analgesia. At plasma concentrations that reduce isoflurane requirements in cats, there is significant cardiovascular depression and impaired diffusion,[10] and therefore *this technique is not recommended in cats.*

OTHER DRUGS
Tramadol

Although not classified as an opioid, tramadol has weak binding affinity at μ-receptors and is also thought to act at adrenergic and serotonin receptors. Clinical experience shows that in cats, opioid-like effects such as dilated pupils and euphoria can be significant, depending on the dose. Tramadol has been used to treat acute pain in cats; preliminary data in research cats suggest that the effective injectable dose is greater than 1 mg/kg, and in the clinical setting, 2 to 5 mg/kg has provided analgesia for soft tissue surgery.

Oral bioavailability in cats is approximately 60% and peak concentration is reached within 45 minutes, making oral administration useful for postoperative pain control after hospital discharge and also for chronic pain in cats; 5 to 10 mg/kg PO 2 to 3 times a day has been suggested.

Gabapentin

Gabapentin is most appropriate for neuropathic pain and therefore could play an important role in cats that undergo limb amputation or declaw surgery or are diagnosed with cauda equina syndrome or intervertebral disk disease. Recommended starting doses are 10 mg/kg PO 2 times daily; doses may be increased or decreased based on the response. At higher doses, some cats become sedate.

Amitriptyline

Amitriptyline at doses ranging from 2.5 to 12.5 mg/kg PO q24h has provided relief of pain associated with interstitial cystitis in some cats, and anecdotal reports indicate some success with other chronic pain conditions.

Amantadine

Amantadine acts at central N-methyl-D-aspartate receptors and is recommended as an *adjunct* therapy for chronic pain. Doses have not been critically evaluated in cats, but 3 to 5 mg/kg PO 1 to 2 times a day is reported to be helpful in some cats; amantadine is often used with NSAIDs or gabapentin.

COMPLEMENTARY METHODS FOR TREATING FELINE PAIN

In recent years the popularity of more "holistic" or "natural" approaches to medicine for humans and pets has increased. Complementary, alternative, or integrative veterinary medicine is challenging to define, but the American Veterinary Medical Association states that this approach to medicine includes aromatherapy; Bach flower remedy therapy; energy therapy; low-energy photon therapy; magnetic field therapy; orthomolecular therapy; veterinary acupuncture, acutherapy, and acupressure; veterinary homeopathy; veterinary manual or manipulative therapy (similar to osteopathy, chiropractic, or physical medicine and therapy); veterinary nutraceutical therapy; and veterinary phytotherapy.

Of these modalities, acupuncture is the best studied, with enough evidence for it to be endorsed by the National Institutes of Health for humans with chronic OA. Contrary to popular belief, many cats are tolerant of acupuncture therapy, and it should be considered a viable choice for analgesic therapy, alone or in combination with drug therapy. Some cats that are painful will not eat, and acupuncture can be effective for appetite stimulation. The classic or traditional point that is often used is called Shan-gen, which is similar to GV-25 (GV means governor vessel), which is on the midline of the boundary between the hair and nonhair part of the nose.

ACUTE PAIN CASE STUDIES (Boxes 22-2 to 22-4)

TREATMENT OF CHRONIC PAIN

Osteoarthritis

As in dogs, weight control should be addressed in cats with OA. If there are no contraindications for use, meloxicam is effective in many cats.[1] In some cats, this alone is not sufficient, or preexisting renal or hepatic disease precludes its use. In these cases, tramadol, gabapentin, and amantadine or various combinations of these can make many cats comfortable. Many veterinarians and owners report that chondroprotective agents, nutraceuticals, and acupuncture are beneficial.

Chondroprotective and Nutraceutical Agents. Animal nutritional supplements typically are not subject to premarketing evaluation by licensing authorities for purity, safety, or efficacy and may contain active pharmacologic agents or unknown substances. The mechanism of action of many of the proposed compounds is not known, and no well-controlled prospective clinical trial using this approach to alleviation of pain related to OA in cats has been published.

Chondroprotectants are available as oral nutraceuticals and as injectable (IM, IV, or intraarticular) pharmaceuticals, but their modes of action are poorly understood and their efficacy is controversial. Mixtures of chondroitin sulfate, glucosamine hydrochloride, and manganese are commercially available in flavored powders and capsules specifically aimed at cats. Polysulfated glycosaminoglycans can be given to cats but

---

BOX 22-2

Ovariohysterectomy and Forelimb Declaw Pain

- Somatic and visceral pain
- Large inflammatory component to pain
- Moderate to severe intensity
- Potential to develop neuropathic pain (digits)
- Pain acute in onset
- Duration of several days or even weeks if complications arise

---

BOX 22-3

Ovariohysterectomy and Forelimb Declaw Analgesia

- Premedication: acetylpromazine 0.05 mg/kg IM or SC
                              buprenorphine 0.02 mg/kg transmucosally
- Induction: ketamine 5 mg/kg and diazepam 0.25 mg/kg IV
- Local anesthetic block: 2 mg/kg bupivacaine, digital nerve block
- Postoperatively (in clinic): meloxicam 0.2 mg/kg SC
                              buprenorphine 0.01 to 0.02 mg/kg every 6 to 8 hours
- Postoperatively (at home): meloxicam 0.1 mg/kg PO once daily for 4 days
                              buprenorphine 0.01 mg/kg transmucosally every 8 hours
                                 for three doses

BOX 22-4

Hind Limb Amputation Analgesia

- Premedication: medetomidine 5 µg/kg IM
                     methadone 0.3 mg/kg IM
                     meloxicam 0.2 mg/kg SC
- Induction: ketamine 5 mg/kg and diazepam 2.5 mg/kg IV
- Postoperatively: methadone 0.3 mg/kg IV q4-6h for 24 hours
                     lidocaine 3 mg/kg infused into wound catheter, every 4 to 6 hours
                        (3 days); remove catheter on fourth postoperative day (send
                        patient home)
                     gabapentin 10 mg/kg bid for 2 weeks (start on day of surgery)
                     meloxicam 0.1 mg/kg PO q24h for 4 days and then 0.025 to
                        0.05 mg/kg every other day for another four doses

are only licensed by the FDA for use in dogs in the United States. Adequan (polysulfated glycosaminoglycan) at 4.4 mg/kg IM every 3 to 5 days for a total of eight injections is reported in cats.[11]

Cancer Pain

COX-2 has been identified in many human and dog carcinomas, and there is growing evidence from experimental, epidemiologic, and clinical trials that NSAIDs and in particular the COX-2 selective drugs may have a role in the prevention and treatment of some types of cancer. NSAIDs are thought to inhibit tumor growth by several different mechanisms including restoration of apoptosis (programmed cell death) and inhibition of angiogenesis.[12]

Immunocytochemistry studies have been performed on a variety of feline neoplasms to determine COX-2 expression.[13] In contrast to canine studies in which COX-2 can be demonstrated in between 47% and 100% of squamous cell carcinomas, transitional cell carcinomas, and prostatic adenocarcinomas, COX-2 expression was found in only 37% of feline transitional cell carcinomas and 9% of oral squamous cell carcinomas. No COX-2 immunoreactivity could be found in feline cutaneous squamous cell carcinomas, several adenocarcinomas (intestinal and pulmonary), or vaccine-related sarcomas.[13] However, in one study 96% of invasive feline mammary carcinomas were positive for COX-2, supporting the role of COX-2 inhibitors in the treatment of these tumors.[14] Based on this species difference in COX-2 expression between canine and feline cancers, NSAIDs may have less of a role as anticancer agents in some feline cancers but may be beneficial to alleviate cancer-related pain. Opioids, tramadol, amantadine, and gabapentin have been used individually or in combination to provide comfort to cats with cancer in a similar fashion to that described for OA.

Oral Pain

Stomatitis, gingivitis, oral cancer, and dental disease are common medical conditions in cats and are accompanied by pain that can be severe and long-standing. In addition to specific surgical or medical intervention to treat the primary problem, pain must also be addressed. These cats resent any attempts to administer pills by mouth, but buprenorphine can often be dropped into the corner of the mouth, and the liquid formulation of meloxicam can be mixed with soft food.

Administration of Drugs

IV, IM, and SC administration of drugs may be possible in a hospital setting; however, it is notoriously difficult for owners to medicate cats successfully in a home environment, resulting in poor compliance and thus failure of the treatment plan. Oral administration of pills, caplets, or capsules requires physical restraint, often by more than one person, and in most cats this quickly becomes an aversive procedure. Many drugs have an unpleasant taste and because of their keen sense of smell, cats are suspicious of drugs placed in their food. Analgesics can be disguised or hidden in treats, "pill pockets," or strongly flavored cat food or be compounded in a liquid that the cat finds palatable. Little data exist on the stability of individual drugs after compounding, and if done, one must adhere to all laws on compounding.

Transdermal fentanyl patches are a "hands-off" approach, but as noted previously, effective uptake is not achieved in all cats. Compounding of drugs in transdermal creams has become popular but is based on empirical information. Fentanyl compounded in pluronic lecithin organogel cream failed to be absorbed through the skin of the inner pinnae or dorsum of the shaved neck in cats even after a dose of 30 µg/kg. The American Veterinary Medical Association has stated that "no published scientific data exist to document the proper regimen of a gel product necessary to deliver a safe, yet effective, dose of any drug in any species."

Transmucosal administration of buprenorphine for short-term pain control at home is reported to be simple by most owners because it is a tasteless and odorless liquid. The oral formulation of meloxicam is accepted by most cats, and only very small volumes are required.

SUMMARY

In the past 10 years, great strides have been made in the field of feline analgesia. A better understanding of cat's unique metabolism has shown that extrapolation across species boundaries is unwise and has prompted valuable cat-specific studies. The opioids are now used more commonly in cats with good analgesic effect and few side effects. Excellent acute pain management is achievable in cats by using opioids, NSAIDs, α_2-agonists, and local anesthetics. Although many studies use single drugs, a multimodal approach using agents that work at different parts of the pain pathway is commonly used in clinical settings with added benefit. Compared with dogs, few pain scoring systems have been developed for cats, and this remains an important goal.

Management of chronic pain in cats is a challenge because of the potential problems with long-term NSAID use; however, recent approval of long-term use of meloxicam (in some countries) and the success of long-term treatment is encouraging. As veterinarians gain experience with less traditional analgesics such as amitriptyline, amantadine, and gabapentin and critically evaluate complementary therapies, the ability to provide comfort to this population of cats will improve.

REFERENCES

1. Clarke SP, Bennett D: Feline osteoarthritis: a prospective study of 28 cases, *J Small Anim Pract* 47(8):439-445, 2006.
2. Court MH, Greenblatt DJ: Molecular genetic basis for deficient acetaminophen glucuronidation by cats: UGT1A6 is a pseudogene, and evidence for reduced diversity of expressed hepatic UGT1A isoforms, *Pharmacogenetics* 10(4):355-369, 2000.
3. Ilkiw JE, Pascoe PJ, Tripp LD: Effects of morphine, butorphanol, buprenorphine, and U50488H on the minimum alveolar concentration of isoflurane in cats, *Am J Vet Res* 63(8):1198-1202, 2002.
4. Niedfeldt RL, Robertson SA: Postanesthetic hyperthermia in cats: a retrospective comparison between hydromorphone and buprenorphine, *Vet Anaesth Analg* 33(6):381-389, 2006.
5. Lascelles BD, Robertson SA: Use of thermal threshold response to evaluate the antinociceptive effects of butorphanol in cats, *Am J Vet Res* 65(8):1085-1089, 2004.
6. Rohrer Bley C, Neiger-Aeschbacher G, Busato A, Schatzmann U: Comparison of perioperative racemic methadone, levo-methadone and dextromoramide in cats using indicators of post-operative pain, *Vet Anaesth Analg* 31(3):175-182, 2004.
7. Steagall PV, Carnicelli P, Taylor PM et al: Effects of subcutaneous methadone, morphine, buprenorphine or saline on thermal and pressure thresholds in cats, *J Vet Pharmacol Ther* 29(6):531-537, 2006.
8. Pypendop BH, Pascoe PJ, Ilkiw JE: Effects of epidural administration of morphine and buprenorphine on the minimum alveolar concentration of isoflurane in cats, *Am J Vet Res* 67(9):1471-1475, 2006.
9. Ansah OB, Raekallio M, Vainio O: Comparing oral and intramuscular administration of medetomidine in cats, *Journal of Veterinary Anaesthesia* 25(1):41-46, 1998.
10. Pypendop BH, Ilkiw JE: Assessment of the hemodynamic effects of lidocaine administered IV in isoflurane-anesthetized cats, *Am J Vet Res* 66(4):661-668, 2005.
11. Beale BS: Use of nutraceuticals and chondroprotectants in osteoarthritic dogs and cats, *Vet Clin North Am Small Anim Pract* 34(1):271-289, 2004.
12. de Groot DJ, de Vries EG, Groen HJ, de Jong S: Non-steroidal anti-inflammatory drugs to potentiate chemotherapy effects: from lab to clinic, *Crit Rev Oncol Hematol* 61(1):52-69, 2007.
13. Beam SL, Rassnick KM, Moore AS, McDonough SP: An immunohistochemical study of cyclooxygenase-2 expression in various feline neoplasms, *Vet Pathol* 40(5):496-500, 2003.
14. Millanta F, Citi S, Della Santa D, et al: COX-2 expression in canine and feline invasive mammary carcinomas: correlation with clinicopathological features and prognostic molecular markers, *Breast Cancer Res Treat* 98:115-120, 2006.

Suggested Readings

Beckman BW: Pathophysiology and management of surgical and chronic oral pain in dogs and cats, *J Vet Dent* 23(1):50-60, 2006.

Carroll GL, Howe LB, Peterson KD: Analgesic efficacy of preoperative administration of meloxicam or butorphanol in onychectomized cats, *J Am Vet Med Assoc* 226(6):913-919, 2005.

Lamont LA: Feline perioperative pain management, *Vet Clin North Am Small Anim Pract* 32(4):747-763, 2002.

Robertson SA: Managing pain in feline patients, *Vet Clin North Am Small Anim Pract* 35(1):129-146, 2005.

Robertson SA, Taylor PM: Pain management in cats: past, present and future. 2. Treatment of pain: clinical pharmacology, *J Feline Med Surg* 6(5):321-333, 2004.

Robertson SA, Taylor PM, Sear JW, Keuhnel G: Relationship between plasma concentrations and analgesia after intravenous fentanyl and disposition after other routes of administration in cats, *J Vet Pharmacol Ther* 28:1-7, 2005.

Taylor PM, Robertson SA: Pain management in cats: past, present and future. 1. The cat is unique, *J Feline Med Surg* 6(5):313-320, 2004.

Taylor PM, Robertson SA, Dixon MJ et al: Morphine, pethidine and buprenorphine disposition in the cat, *J Vet Pharmacol Ther* 24(6):391-398, 2001.

23

Pain Management in Horses and Cattle

PHILLIP LERCHE AND WILLIAM W. MUIR III

P ain is generally one of the first and most dominant signs of injury or disease (e.g., colic) in most horses. Furthermore, the inflammatory responses induced by surgical procedures and anesthesia (e.g., hypotension and ischemia) produce a series of behavioral, neurophysiologic, endocrine, metabolic, and cellular responses (stress response) that can initiate, maintain, and amplify pain.

PAIN PERCEPTION

Nociception (noxious stimulus perception) can be considered to involve five primary processes: transduction, transmission, modulation, projection, and perception (Fig. 23-1). Pain is normally produced by noxious mechanical, chemical, or thermal activation of small-diameter, high-threshold Aδ and C sensory nerve fibers. Noxious stimuli are transduced into electrical impulses by peripheral pain receptors and subsequently transmitted throughout the sensory nervous system. These electrical impulses are modulated by a variety of endogenous systems (e.g., opioid, serotonergic, and noradrenergic) in the dorsal horn of the spinal cord before being transmitted to the brain, where emotional, behavioral, and physiologic responses are initiated.

PHYSIOLOGIC PAIN

Pain is considered physiologic when it operates to protect the body by warning of contact with tissue-damaging stimuli. This type of pain is produced by stimulation of nociceptors innervated by high-threshold Aδ (group III) and unmyelinated C (group IV) fibers.

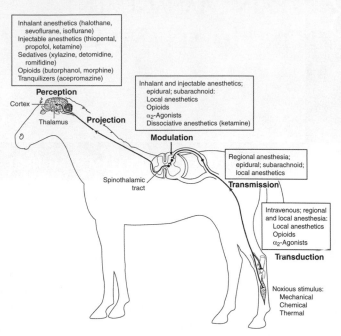

FIG. 23-1. Nociception involves transduction, transmission, modulation, projection, and perception. Various drugs and drug delivery techniques are used to inhibit these processes.

CLINICAL PAIN

"Clinical" pain, by contrast, is produced by peripheral tissue injury or nerve damage. Clinical pain therefore is categorized as inflammatory or neuropathic pain. The term *idiopathic pain* is used to describe pain of unknown origin.

Inflammatory Pain

Inflammatory pain is somatic (skin, joints, muscles, or periosteum) or visceral (thoracic and abdominal viscera).

- Somatic pain is easily localized; is aching, stabbing, or throbbing; and generally is acute. Somatic pain includes cutaneous or incisional pain after operation. Somatic pain is frequently identified as superficial (skin) or deep (joints, muscle, and periosteum).
- Visceral pain is poorly localized, cramping or gnawing, and crescendo/decrescendo and may be referred to cutaneous sites far from the site of injury.

Neuropathic Pain

Neuropathic pain occurs as a direct result of damage to peripheral nerves or the spinal cord; is described as burning, stabbing, and intermittent; and is often unresponsive to treatment.

Inflammatory and neuropathic pain can produce allodynia, hyperalgesia (primary and secondary), and central nervous system (CNS) and peripheral sensitization to external stimuli (see Chapter 2).

CHEMICAL MEDIATORS OF PAIN

Chemical mediators of pain and inflammation include histamine, serotonin, bradykinin, leukotrienes, prostaglandins (E_2), interleukins (IL-1, IL-6), neutrophil-chemotactic peptides, nerve growth factor, and neuropeptides, including substance P. These substances enhance the excitability of sensory nerves and postganglionic sympathetic nerve fiber activity, leading to peripheral sensitization, hyperalgesia, and allodynia (see Chapter 2).

Inflammation increases the sensitivity of Aδ and C fibers; causes some Aβ fibers to express substance P; stimulates the synthesis and release of nerve growth factor, a peptide that increases the synthesis of substance P and calcitonin gene-related peptide (CGRP); stimulates the release of histamine and leukotrienes; and is associated with the development of sensory hyperexcitability and hyperalgesia (Fig. 23-2). The net result of these inflammatory and tissue chemical responses is the development of diverse yet interrelated positive feedback loops, which enhance neural sensitivity and intensify pain.

Once transduced, the electrical impulses are transmitted to C-fiber terminals in the dorsal horn, where the excitatory neuropeptides (tachykinins), substance P, neurokinin A, CGRP, and the amino acid glutamate are released to activate postsynaptic tachykinin (NK1, NK2), CGRP, and glutamate (e.g., N-methyl-D-aspartate [NMDA]; amino-hydroxy-methyl-isoxazolepropionate, kainate) receptors.

Cumulative increases in the number of electrical impulses produced in dorsal horn cells caused by increased C-fiber stimulus frequency result in increases in excitability of spinal cord neurons and CNS "windup." Windup contributes to central sensitization, hyperalgesia, and allodynia. A similar phenomenon in the hippocampus has been termed *long-term potentiation* and is thought to be the basis for the acquisition of new information and certain forms of short-term memory.

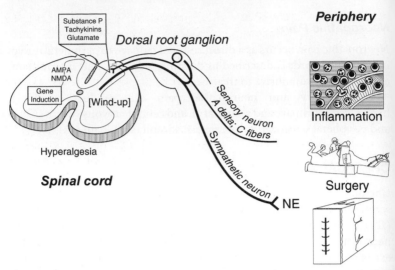

FIG. 23-2. Central sensitization: high-intensity chronic painful stimuli lead to activation of amino-hydroxy-methyl-isoxazolepropionate/kainate and N-methyl-D-aspartate receptors. The resulting activation of signaling pathways alters gene expression and increases the responsiveness of the central nervous system to further input ("windup").

EFFECTS OF PAIN

Pain is exaggerated by the inflammatory response, which in turn increases the production of pain neurotransmitters (e.g., substance P and CGRP) and increases the excitability of sensory neurons.

◆ Pain produces a catabolic state, suppresses the immune response, and promotes inflammation, which delays wound healing and predisposes the patient to infection and intensified medical care (see Chapter 3).
◆ Pain increases patient risk during anesthesia because more drugs are required to maintain a stable plane of anesthesia.
◆ Pain increases morbidity and the cost of patient care and occupies time better spent on other endeavors. These points justify the treatment of pain in all circumstances, which in turn produces a general feeling of mental satisfaction in hospital personnel and owners that patients are not needlessly suffering.

ASSESSMENT OF PAINFUL BEHAVIOR

Pain recognition relies on a sound understanding of normal equine or bovine physiology and behavior and of stress-related or behavioral changes (e.g., flank watching and decreased feed intake) that may indicate painful conditions. Also important to recognize are the behavioral changes that may occur when a patient is introduced to a new environment, which occurs when an animal is hospitalized. A thorough, detailed history may also be helpful in assessing pain because the owner or handler is more likely to be aware of behaviors that may be masked during an examination by a veterinarian.

Pain is a complex multidimensional experience, and no single measured parameter is a pathognomonic indicator. The behavioral response to pain depends on species, breed, age, disease or surgical process, and duration. Additionally, pain is an individual experience and is thus different for each animal. Although some behaviors are similar, horses and ruminants respond differently to pain (Table 23-1). Cattle are generally considered to have a higher tolerance for pain than horses. A draft horse is less likely to demonstrate overtly painful behavior compared with a highly excitable Thoroughbred. Older horses and cows are generally more stoic than foals and calves. One must recognize that nonspecific behavioral indicators may be present with painful and nonpainful conditions. Abdominal and limb pain exhibit relatively specific behaviors and postures in horses and cattle (Figs. 23-3 to 23-6).

Assessment of painful behavior is often best achieved by using a staged process. When possible, the animal should be observed when it cannot see the observer or other persons, for many animals change or mask their painful behavior in the presence of humans because of a protective response to avoid looking like "prey" or socialization instincts. Distant observation may require the use of a remote video camera. Following this, interaction with the silent observer, verbal response to the observer, and finally interaction through touch can be assessed. Painful animals are less likely to interact with humans, to explore their environment, and to spend time at the front of the stall, and they are more likely to ignore their environment and spend time at the back of the stall or avoid contact. Finally, direct palpation or manipulation of a painful area or limb usually elicits responses such as escape, avoidance, withdrawal, vocalization, kicking, or biting. This approach to assessing pain-related behavior is time-consuming but results in a better evaluation of otherwise unrecognized painful conditions.

PAIN ASSESSMENT TOOLS

The development of pain assessment tools (verbal rating, simple descriptive, numerical rating and visual analog scales) for horses and cattle lags behind that seen in dogs and cats. Recent studies have begun to develop and assess pain scales for specific types of pain in horses. As an example, evaluation

TABLE 23-1	Behavioral Indicators of Pain in Horses and Cattle	
Behavioral Indicator	**Equine**	**Ruminant**
NONSPECIFIC BEHAVIORAL INDICATORS		
Considerable restlessness, agitation, and anxiety	✓	✓
Rigid stance and reluctance to move	✓	✓
Lowered head carriage	✓	✓
Fixed stare and dilated nostrils, clenched jaw	✓	
Aggression toward own foal	✓	
Aggression toward handlers, horses, objects, and self	✓	
Tail wagging		✓
Foot stamping, kicking		✓
Bruxism (teeth grinding)		✓
Abnormal grazing pattern		✓
Lip curling		✓
BEHAVIORAL INDICATORS OF ABDOMINAL PAIN		
Vocalization (deep groaning, grunting)	✓	✓
Rolling	✓	✓
Kicking at abdomen	✓	✓
Flank watching	✓	
Stretching	✓	✓
Dullness and depression	✓	✓
BEHAVIORAL INDICATORS OF LIMB AND FOOT PAIN		
Weight-shifting between limbs	✓	
Limb guarding	✓	
Abnormal weight distribution	✓	✓
Pointing, hanging, and rotating limbs	✓	
Abnormal movement	✓	✓
Reluctance to move	✓	✓
Arched back		✓
BEHAVIORAL INDICATORS OF HEAD AND DENTAL PAIN		
Head shaking	✓	
Abnormal bit behavior	✓	
Altered eating; anorexia, quidding, food pocketing	✓	

of behavioral changes after arthroscopy showed that horses spent less time eating and less time at the front of the stall and demonstrated more abnormal (predefined) behaviors such as groaning and atypical postures in the first 48 hours after surgery. Validated numerical and descriptive pain scales are likely to be developed in the near future, although they will most likely be focused on colic pain or pain following arthroscopy. Use of visual analog scales to monitor trends may be useful in situations in which pain scales have not been validated. Pain scales are more accurate with observer training and experience. (See Table 23-2 and Figures 23-3 to 23-6 for behaviors associated with pain.)

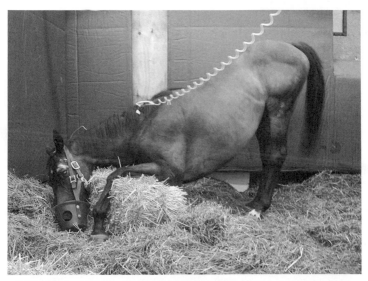

FIG. 23-3. Abnormal posture. This horse had abdominal pain (colic).

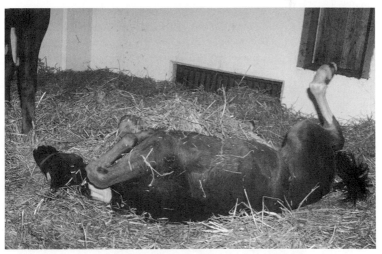

FIG. 23-4. Rolling. This foal had severe colic.

Response to therapy can also be used to assess pain and the effectiveness of analgesic therapy. The gradual return of normal behavior and the cessation of abnormal behavior after therapy would indicate that a patient is more comfortable.

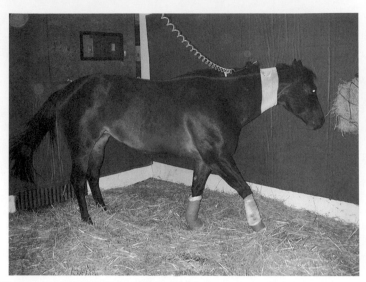

FIG. 23-5. Pointing. Postoperatively, this horse was reluctant to bear weight on the operated limb.

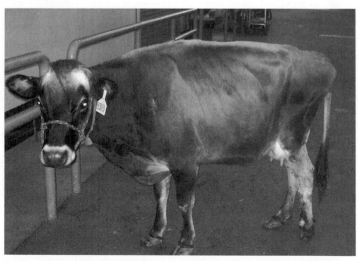

FIG. 23-6. Holding limb off the ground. This cow had an extensive hock wound and would alternate between barely toe-touching the ground and standing on three legs.

BOX 23-1

Drugs Used to Produce Analgesia in Horses and Cattle

Local and Regional Anesthesia
Local anesthetics (lidocaine)
Opioids, α_2-agonists, dissociative drugs (ketamine)*

Systemic Drugs
Nonsteroidal antiinflammatory drugs (phenylbutazone, flunixin meglumine, ketoprofen)
Opioids (morphine, butorphanol)
α_2-Agonists (xylazine, detomidine, romifidine)†
Dissociative drugs (ketamine)
Local anesthetics (lidocaine, mexiletine, infusion)

Analgesic Adjuncts‡
Phenothiazines (acepromazine)
Benzodiazepines (diazepam, midazolam)
Electrolytes (magnesium-26 salts)
Calcium blockers (diltiazem)

---

*Administered in the epidural or subarachnoid space.
†Not recommended in cattle.
‡Drugs that produce little or no analgesia when administered alone.

SYSTEMIC DRUG THERAPY

The magnitude of nociceptive input may vary considerably for different injuries or surgical procedures, resulting in a variety of physiologic responses (e.g., heart rate, blood pressure, and sympathetic outflow) that require multiple analgesic drugs used in combination (multimodal therapy) and additional adjunctive pain therapy. A wide variety of drug therapies is available for the treatment of pain in horses (Box 23-1; Table 23-2). Importantly, sedatives, tranquilizers, and opioids modulate CNS processing and the development of hyperalgesia and allodynia. The administration of drugs in cattle must always take into account drug withdrawal times, which may decrease the use of analgesics and adjuncts in cattle compared with horses and small animal species (Table 23-3; Box 23-1). Furthermore, side effects from systemic drug administration differ (e.g., significant respiratory depression with xylazine), limiting the use of some classes of analgesics in cattle.

Occasionally, analgesic drugs are deliberately administered 12 to 24 hours before extensive soft tissue or orthopedic surgery to preempt (minimize) the response to pain and to prevent the development of CNS hypersensitivity and resultant hyperalgesia and allodynia. This is termed *preemptive analgesia.*

TABLE 23-2 Drugs Used to Produce Analgesia in Horses

Drugs	Intravenous Dose (mg/kg)	Effects	Concerns/Comments
CORTICOSTEROIDS			
Hydrocortisone Sodium succinate	1.0-4.0	Antiinflammatory, analgesic	Laminitis, immune suppression
Dexamethasone Isonicotinate	0.015-0.050	Antiinflammatory, analgesic	Laminitis, immune suppression
Methylprednisolone	0.1-0.5	Antiinflammatory, analgesic	Laminitis, immune suppression
Prednisolone	0.25-1.0	Antiinflammatory, analgesic	Laminitis, immune suppression Tablets: 0.25-1.0 mg/kg PO
NONSTEROIDAL ANTIINFLAMMATORY DRUGS			
Dipyrone	5-22	Antiinflammatory, analgesic	Potential for gastrointestinal (GI) ulceration and renal toxicity
Phenylbutazone	2-4	Antiinflammatory, analgesic	Potential for GI ulceration and renal toxicity
Flunixin meglumine	0.2-1.1	Antiinflammatory, analgesic	Potential for GI ulceration and renal toxicity
Ketoprofen	1.1-2.2	Antiinflammatory, analgesic	Potential for GI ulceration and renal toxicity
Carprofen	0.5-1.1	Antiinflammatory, analgesic	Potential for GI ulceration and renal toxicity
OPIOIDS			
Butorphanol	0.01-0.04	Analgesia (0.5)	Potential for ataxia and disorientation
Pentazocine	0.5-1.0	Analgesia (0.5)	Potential for excitement and increased locomotor activity
Buprenorphine	0.01-0.04	Analgesia (3)	Potential for ataxia and disorientation
Morphine	0.05-0.1	Analgesia (1)	Potential for excitement and increased locomotor activity

Meperidine	0.2-1.0	Analgesia (0.5)	Potential for excitement and increased locomotor activity
Oxymorphone	0.001-0.02	Analgesia (10)	Potential for excitement and increased locomotor activity
Fentanyl	0.01-0.02; two 100-µg/h patches per 450 kg	Analgesia (100)	Potential for excitement and increased locomotor activity
α₂-AGONISTS			
Xylazine	0.5-1.0	Sedation, analgesia, and muscle relaxation	Potential for bradycardia, hypoventilation, and ataxia
Detomidine	0.01-0.02	Sedation, analgesia, and muscle relaxation	Potential for bradycardia, hypoventilation, and ataxia
Medetomidine	0.01-0.02	Sedation, analgesia, and muscle relaxation	Potential for bradycardia, hypoventilation, and ataxia
Romifidine	0.04-0.08	Sedation, analgesia, and muscle relaxation	Potential for bradycardia and hypoventilation

Numbers in parentheses indicate the analgesic potency of the drug. Higher numbers indicate greater potency.

TABLE 23-3	Drugs Used to Produce Analgesia in Cattle		
Drugs	Intravenous Dose (mg/kg)	Effects	Concerns/Comments
NONSTEROIDAL ANTIINFLAMMATORY DRUGS			
Flunixin meglumine	1.0	Antiinflammatory, analgesic	Potential for gastrointestinal ulceration and renal toxicity
Ketoprofen	2.0	Antiinflammatory, analgesic	Potential for gastrointestinal ulceration and renal toxicity
OPIOIDS			
Morphine	0.1-0.5	Analgesic	
Butorphanol	0.05-0.1	Analgesic	

MULTIMODAL THERAPY

The combination or sequential administration of analgesics that act by different mechanisms (multimodal therapy) is often advocated to maximize analgesic drug effects (Table 23-4). The administration of two major analgesics (nonsteroidal antiinflammatory drug [NSAID]–opioid, opioid–α_2-agonist) frequently produces supraadditive or synergistic analgesic effects that permit the reduction of individual drug doses and potentially a subsequent reduction in drug-related adverse side effects.

DRUG SYNERGISM

Many analgesic drugs are additive or synergistic (supraadditive) when administered together. Synergism or supraadditivity implies that the combination of two or more products produces more than additive effects. In more qualitative terms, the combination of two drugs produces a better effect (analgesia) than expected. Drug synergism usually allows the dose of most drugs to be reduced, thereby reducing the potential for side effects. Drug combinations that are likely to be synergistic are produced when drugs that act by different and distinct mechanisms of action are combined.

- Synergism or supraadditivity has been demonstrated when local anesthetics are combined with opioids or dissociative anesthetics and when NSAIDs are combined with opioids.
- The combination of α_2-agonists with opioids produces excellent clinical analgesia in horses (Table 23-4). The transdermal delivery of opioids (fentanyl patch; 100-μg/h patch per 200 to 250 kg) with low

TABLE 23-4	Analgesic Drug Combinations in the Horse	
Drug Combination	**Intravenous Dose (mg/kg)**	**Concerns**
Acepromazine	0.02-0.05	Hypotension
Butorphanol	0.02-0.05	
Acepromazine	0.02-0.05	Hypotension
Buprenorphine	0.005-0.01	
Acepromazine	0.02-0.05	Bradycardia, hypotension
Xylazine	0.2-0.5	
Xylazine*	0.3-0.5	Bradycardia, ataxia
Butorphanol	0.01-0.05	
Xylazine*	0.3-0.5	Bradycardia
Meperidine	0.5-1.0	
Xylazine*	0.5-1.0	Bradycardia, ataxia
Morphine	0.1-0.5	
Xylazine*	0.5-1.0	Bradycardia
Fentanyl	0.01-0.02	

*Detomidine or medetomidine (0.01-0.02 mg/kg) or romifidine (0.04-0.08 mg/kg) can be substituted for xylazine.

doses of α_2-agonists (e.g., xylazine or detomidine) as needed, provides excellent analgesia for extended periods (12 hours). α_2-Agonists are not used systemically to provide analgesia in cattle primarily because of their tendency to cause potent respiratory depression. Cattle are exquisitely sensitive to the respiratory depressant effects of xylazine.

◆ The administration of adjunctive drugs (tranquilizers) in conjunction with major analgesic drugs may potentiate analgesic effects and produces additional calming effects. The simultaneous or sequential administration of acepromazine and meperidine (neuroleptanalgesia) or acepromazine and xylazine potentiates analgesia. Several of the major analgesics (e.g., opioids and α_2-agonists) have the added benefit of being reversible (Table 23-4).

PREEMPTIVE ANALGESIA

Preemptive analgesia reduces the number and amount of anesthetics required to produce and maintain surgical anesthesia, helps to stabilize the maintenance phase of anesthesia, reduces the total amount of analgesic drugs required to control pain intraoperatively and postoperatively, and decreases overall patient morbidity associated with surgery and anesthesia. Local anesthetics or NSAIDs combined with low doses of opioids or α_2-agonists are the most routinely administered systemic major analgesic drugs used to provide analgesia for short-term pain therapy (Table 23-3).

COMBINATION OF OPIOID AGONISTS
WITH AGONIST-ANTAGONISTS

Reversing or antagonizing adverse effects may antagonize the drug's analgesic activity. Interestingly and surprisingly, however, the combination of opioid agonists with agonist-antagonists or "pure" antagonists has shown unexpected analgesic effects. The μ-opioid agonist morphine and κ-agonist butorphanol, the μ-agonist oxymorphone and κ-agonist butorphanol, and the μ-agonist morphine and the pure μ-receptor antagonist naloxone produced additive and synergistic antinociceptive effects in humans and cats for reasons that remain poorly defined (Table 23-5). The administration of opioid agonist-antagonist drugs or antagonists with full μ-agonists has not been evaluated in horses or cattle and remains controversial.

OTHER POTENTIALLY EFFECTIVE METHODS
FOR PRODUCING ANALGESIA

Other potentially effective methods for providing long-term analgesia include electromagnetic and shockwave therapies and complementary therapies including acupuncture therapy, chiropractic manipulation, massage, and hydrotherapy.

REGIONAL ANALGESIA

Regional analgesia can be used as an alternative or adjunct to systemic analgesic therapy for long-term pain control with minimal side effects (Box 23-2). Many diagnostic and surgical procedures can be performed safely and humanely in the standing horse and cow using sedation, physical restraint, and regional analgesia. The ability to produce effective anesthesia of the spinal nerves requires a working knowledge of the local anatomy, an understanding of the pharmacology of the analgesic drugs used, and the technical proficiency to complete the appropriate injection technique. To desensitize spinal nerves, analgesic drugs must be deposited in the epidural or subarachnoid spaces.

EPIDURAL ANALGESIA

Epidural analgesia is produced by depositing local anesthetics outside of the dura mater. Epidural analgesia is generally easier to perform than subarachnoid anesthesia and has a reduced potential for nerve damage,

TABLE 23-5	Drug Antagonists
Drug	**Intravenous Dose (mg/kg)**
OPIOIDS	
Naloxone	0.01-0.02
Nalmefene	0.001-0.005
α_2-AGONISTS	
Atipamezole	0.1-0.2
Tolazoline	2.0
Yohimbine	0.075
BENZODIAZEPINE	
Flumazenil	0.01
ANALEPTIC (STIMULANT)	
Doxapram	0.5-1.0

BOX 23-2

Procedures Amenable to Regional Anesthetic Techniques

Standing surgery of the rectum, anus, perineum, tail, vulva, vagina, penis, and inguinal region:

- Rectal prolapses
- Perirectal abscesses
- Rectal tears
- Rectovaginal lacerations
- Ovariectomy
- Removal of urinary calculi

Flank approach to the abdomen:

- Abdominal exploratory
- Abomasal displacement (cattle)
- Cesarean section (cattle)
- Uterine torsion
- Loop colostomy
- Surgical embryo transfer
- Aid in the relief of postoperative straining
- Obstetric manipulations during dystocia
- Relief of inflammatory, traumatic, intraoperative and postoperative, or chronic pain

---

especially when the injection site is caudal (coccygeal-sacral) to the termination of the conus medullaris. Drugs administered epidurally have a longer duration of action but produce incomplete, inconsistent, or asymmetric analgesia because of the presence of a septum within the epidural space or the influence of fat accumulations.

TABLE 23-6	Drugs Used to Produce Regional Analgesia in Horses		
Drug	**Dosage (mg/kg)**	**Route**	**Duration of Analgesia**
LOCAL ANESTHETICS			
Mepivacaine HCl	0.20	S3-S4, S4-S5 (CE)	1-1½ hours
	0.14-0.25	S2-S3, S3-S4, S4-S5 (CE)	1½-2 hours
Mepivacaine HCl	0.06	S2-S3 (CSA)	20-80 minutes
	0.05-0.08	S2-S3 (CSA)	1-1½ hours
Lidocaine HCl	0.16-0.22	Co1-Co2 (CE)	30-60 minutes
	0.22-0.44		1-2½ hours
	0.45		2-3 hours
Lidocaine HCl	0.28-0.37	S3-S4, S4-S5 (CE)	1½-3 hours
α₂-AGONISTS			
Xylazine	0.03-0.35	Co1-Co2 (CE)	3-5 hours
Detomidine HCl	0.06	S4-S5 (CE)	2-3 hours
OPIOID			
Morphine	0.05-0.10	Co1-Co2 (CE)	8-16 hours
COMBINATIONS			
Lidocaine	0.22	Co1-Co2 (CE)	5½ hours
Xylazine	0.17		
Lidocaine	0.25	Co1-Co2 (CE)	2½ hours
Butorphanol	0.04		
Morphine	0.20	S1-L6 (CE)	>6 hours
Detomidine	0.03		

CE, Caudal epidural; *CSA*, caudal subarachnoid.

SUBARACHNOID ANALGESIA

Subarachnoid analgesia is produced by depositing local anesthetics within the dura mater. Subarachnoid analgesia by contrast produces a more consistent response because the roots of the spinal nerves within the subarachnoid space are not protected by the dura. Lower total drug doses and more predictable analgesic responses characterize subarachnoid anesthesia. The technique, however, is more difficult to perform and requires more sophisticated and expensive equipment.

REGIONAL ANALGESIC DRUGS

Historically, local anesthetics (e.g., lidocaine and mepivacaine) were the only drugs used to produce caudal regional anesthesia (Tables 23-6 and 23-7).

TABLE 23-7	Drugs Used to Produce Epidural Analgesia in Cattle		
Drug	**Dosage (mg/kg)**	**Onset of Action**	**Duration of Analgesia**
LOCAL ANESTHETICS			
Lidocaine HCl	0.2	5 minutes	10-115 minutes
α₂-AGONISTS			
Xylazine	0.05	20-40 minutes	2-3 hours
Clonidine	0.002-0.003	9-19 minutes	3-5 hours
Medetomidine	0.015	5 minutes	6½ hours
DISSOCIATIVES			
Ketamine	250 mg*	6½ minutes	17 minutes
Ketamine	500 mg*	5 minutes	34 minutes
Ketamine	1000 mg*	5 minutes	1 hour
COMBINATIONS			
Morphine	0.1	10 minutes	12 hours
Romifidine	0.05		
Lidocaine	80 mg*	10-15 minutes	Up to 8½ hours
Xylazine	20 mg*		

*Total dose.

LOCAL ANESTHETICS

Local anesthetics provide profound relief from pain by preventing the transmembrane flux of sodium ions, thereby inhibiting depolarization of the nerve membrane and the conduction of nerve impulses. Unmyelinated Aα and C (pain) fibers are preferentially blocked by local anesthetics because of their small size compared with the myelinated Aα and Aβ fibers, which are responsible for proprioception, touch and pressure sensation, and motor activity.

◆ Local anesthetic desensitization is dose dependent, nonspecific, and not always predictable. Full analgesic effect occurs within 10 to 20 minutes of drug administration for epidurally administered local anesthetics.

◆ Additional local anesthetic drug should not be administered during this period (10 to 20 minutes) to prevent overdosing, which can result in hypotension, and occasionally bradycardia, from sympathetic blockade.

◆ Complete sensory and inadvertent motor blockade results in significant ataxia and potentially recumbency.

α_2-AGONISTS

Although local anesthetics are effective analgesics for regional anesthesia, they can produce profound ataxia or recumbency as a result of their nonselective blockade of motor and sensory neurons. α_2-Adrenergic receptors are located throughout the CNS and are found in great numbers in the superficial laminae of the dorsal horn sensory fibers of the spinal cord and brainstem nuclei. α_2-Agonists (e.g., xylazine) produce effective, long-term analgesia with a reduced incidence of ataxia. Additionally, the notable sedative and cardiopulmonary effects of epidurally administered xylazine are diminished compared with the response after their intravenous or intramuscular administration. α_2-Receptors are colocalized with opioid receptors in the CNS; thus when α_2-agonists are coadministered with opioids, synergism frequently occurs.

◆ Epidural administration of xylazine (0.17 to 0.22 mg/kg of body weight; 1% solution) at the first coccygeal interspace produces surgical analgesia 30 to 45 minutes after administration, which lasts 3½ hours.

◆ Epidural administration of 0.06 mg/kg body weight detomidine hydrochloride (1% solution) via an epidural catheter advanced to the caudal sacral (S5 to S4) space produces variable analgesia extending from the coccyx to spinal cord segment S1 and from the coccyx to T16, respectively. Analgesia is achieved within 10 to 25 minutes after drug administration and lasts for more than 2 hours.

◆ Sedation after subarachnoid administration of xylazine or detomidine hydrochloride solution can be prominent.

OPIOIDS

Opioids have been successfully used in humans, dogs, and horses to produce effective caudal regional analgesia with a low incidence of systemic side effects. The use of opioids in horses and cattle, however, is relatively limited and for the most part has not provided clinically relevant analgesia. Epidural opioids produce analgesia without motor or sympathetic blockade by reducing the local release of presynaptic neurotransmitters and hyperpolarizing postsynaptic dorsal horn neuronal membranes.

◆ The onset of opioid drug effects is more rapid with the highly lipid-soluble opiates (e.g., fentanyl). Conversely, less lipid-soluble opiates such as morphine are retained within the cerebrospinal fluid for longer durations after single-dose administration, thereby producing prolonged analgesia (Table 23-6).

♦ Epidural opioid administration in horses has been limited primarily to morphine and butorphanol administered alone or in combination with lidocaine.

♦ Epidural opioid administration in cattle has been performed in combination with romifidine.

"BALANCED" EPIDURAL ANESTHESIA

The selective combination of drugs that produce analgesia by different mechanisms (e.g., α_2-agonists and opioids) with subanesthetic concentrations of local anesthetics has the advantage of (1) reducing the drug dose, (2) enhancing the degree of pain relief, and (3) reducing the adverse effects produced by larger doses of an individual drug. Functional interactions may result from simultaneous drug effects at different sites. For example, activation of presynaptic and postsynaptic mechanisms simultaneously, by a combination of drugs, may magnify the effects of one drug acting independently at one site.

♦ The combination of lidocaine with the α_2-adrenergic agonist xylazine produces a faster onset of analgesia than with xylazine alone and a longer duration than with lidocaine alone (Table 23-6).

♦ Butorphanol added to lidocaine increases the duration of visceral and cutaneous analgesia and extends the area of cutaneous analgesia.

♦ Morphine sulfate (0.2 mg/kg), in combination with the α_2-adrenergic agonist detomidine hydrochloride (30 µg/kg), produces profound hind limb analgesia in horses with experimentally induced tarsocrural joint synovitis. Long-term (14 days) administration of this combination is without apparent adverse systemic effects.

♦ Ketamine, a noncompetitive NMDA antagonist, may also be an effective regional analgesic when administered epidurally in combination with drugs that produce effects by different mechanisms. Epidural ketamine significantly decreases the amount of halothane required to maintain anesthesia during pelvic limb stimulation in ponies.

REGIONAL ANESTHETIC TECHNIQUES

Various regional nerve blocks have been developed to produce caudal analgesia in standing horses and cows, including caudal epidural analgesia, continuous caudal epidural analgesia, continuous caudal subarachnoid analgesia, segmental thoracolumbar subarachnoid analgesia, and segmental thoracolumbar epidural analgesia. These techniques can be used to perform standing surgery of the rectum, anus, perineum, tail, vulva, vagina, penis, and inguinal region; to allow a flank approach to

TABLE 23-8	Equipment for Regional Analgesic Techniques in Horses	
Technique	**Location of Needle Placement**	**Equipment Required**
Caudal epidural	Co1-Co2	18-gauge, 5- to 7.5-cm spinal needle
Continuous caudal epidural	Co1-Co2	18-gauge, 10.2-cm Tuohy needle
	S1-L6	20-gauge, 91.8-cm epidural catheter or 17-gauge, 19.5-cm Huber-point Tuohy needle 30-cm Formocath polyethylene catheter (0.095-cm OD) with spring guide (0.052-cm OD)
Continuous caudal subarachnoid	S1-L6	17-gauge, 19.5-cm Huber-point Tuohy needle 30-cm Formocath polyethylene catheter (0.095-cm OD) with spring guide (0.052-cm OD)
Segmental thoracolumbar subarachnoid	S1-L6	17-gauge, 17.5-cm Huber-point Tuohy needle 100-cm Formocath polyethylene catheter (0.095-cm OD) with spring guide (0.052-cm OD)
Segmental thoracolumbar epidural*	S1-L6	17-gauge, 17.5-cm Huber-point Tuohy needle 100 cm Formocath polyethylene catheter (0.095-cm OD) with spring guide (0.052-cm OD)

*Not recommended for clinical patient.

the abdomen; to aid in the relief of postoperative straining; to facilitate obstetric manipulations during dystocia; or to relieve inflammatory, traumatic, postoperative, or chronic pain.

GENERAL CONSIDERATIONS

Different injection sites and equipment are required for the various caudal regional anesthetic techniques (Table 23-8). The needle puncture site should be clipped and a surgical, aseptic preparation performed. The skin should be desensitized (superficial block) using a small-gauge needle (25 gauge, 1 inch), and 1 to 2 ml of local anesthetic should be

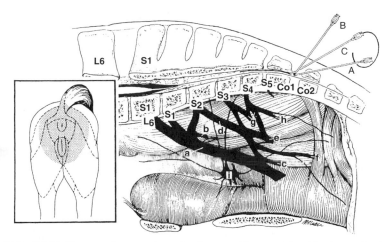

FIG. 23-7. Neuroanatomy and needle placement for caudal epidural anesthesia (**A** and **B**), and needle and catheter placement at Co1-Co2 for continuous caudal epidural anesthesia (**C**). Ventral nerve branches give rise to the following: *a,* sciatic nerve; *b,* caudal cutaneous femoral nerve; *c,* deep perineal nerve; *d,* pudendal nerve; *e,* distal cutaneous pudendal nerve; *f,* caudal rectal nerve; *g,* pelvic nerve; *h,* caudal rectal nerve; *i,* pelvic plexus. *Inset,* Stippled area delineates extent of subcutaneous desensitization after caudal blockade.

injected subcutaneously to reduce any local discomfort associated with the insertion of larger needles (18 to 16 gauge).

CAUDAL EPIDURAL ANESTHESIA

Correctly performed, anesthetic deposited epidurally produces regional anesthesia of the anus, rectum, vulva, vagina, perineum, urethra, and bladder (Fig. 23-7; Table 23-9). Caudal epidural anesthesia is produced by inserting a needle between the first and second coccygeal vertebrae (Co1 to Co2). The first coccygeal interspace is readily located in most horses and cows by palpating the first movable coccygeal articulation with the finger while raising and lowering the tail. In obese or well-muscled animals, the site may be difficult to palpate but can be located at the point where the angle of the tail is the steepest, about 5 cm cranial to the origin of the first tail hairs. The site may be ossified in older cows. After desensitizing the skin, an 18-gauge spinal needle with fitted stylet (5 to 7.5 cm) is inserted through the skin perpendicular to the contour of the croup (Fig. 23-7, *A*). Alternatively, the 18-gauge needle may be advanced at a 45-degree angle to the skin (Fig. 23-7, *B*). A distinct "pop" is generally noted as the needle passes through the dorsal interarcuate

TABLE 23-9	Regional Analgesic Techniques in Horses			
Technique	**Area Blocked**	**Site of Drug Deposition**	**Spinal Cord Segments Affected**	**Indications**
Caudal epidural	Caudal region*	Co1-Co2	S2-coccyx	Standing surgery to the anal and perianal regions; obstetric manipulations
Continuous caudal epidural	Caudal region*	S3-S5 S2-S3	S2-coccyx	Extend surgery time for standing procedures, relief of tenesmus, management of chronic pain
Continuous caudal sub-arachnoid	Caudal region*	S2-S3	S2-coccyx	Extend surgery time for standing procedures of anal and perianal regions
Segmental tho-racolumbar subarachnoid	Flank	T18-L1	T12-L3	Standing surgery for flank approach
Segmental tho-racolumbar epidural	Flank	T18-L1	T12-L3	Standing surgery for flank approach Not recommended for clinical patients

*Caudal region includes the anus, rectum, vulva, vagina, perineum, urethra, and bladder.

ligament, which indicates that the needle is properly placed. Proper needle placement is verified by applying (1) a drop or two of local anesthetic to the hub of the needle, which should be drawn into the epidural space by the negative pressure ("hanging drop technique"), or (2) by aspiration followed by resistance-free injection of 3 to 5 ml of air or local anesthetic. Aspiration of blood or cerebrospinal fluid suggests needle placement in the subarachnoid space. If this occurs, the needle should be withdrawn slightly and reaspirated.

◆ Caudal epidural anesthesia has the advantages of being relatively simple to perform, requiring no special equipment, thus limiting cost primarily to that of the drug itself.

◆ The potential for nerve damage is minimized because the spinal cord and its meninges end in the midsacral region, cranial to the injection site (Fig. 23-7).

◆ Disadvantages of the technique include inconsistent results, the limited duration of analgesic action, and the possibility for the development of rear limb ataxia or even lateral recumbency when increased drug doses

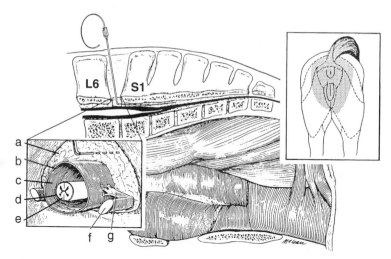

FIG. 23-8. Catheter introduction at the lumbosacral (L6-S1) intervertebral junction for continuous caudal epidural anesthesia. *Left inset,* Proper placement of needle and catheter within the epidural space: *a,* epidural space with fat and connective tissue; *b,* dura mater; *c,* subarachnoid space; *d,* pia mater; *e,* spinal chord. *Right inset,* Stippled area delineates extent of subcutaneous desensitization after caudal blockade.

are administered. This may induce an undesirable panic response in horses. Lateral recumbency also hinders the surgical team.

CONTINUOUS CAUDAL EPIDURAL ANESTHESIA

The limited duration of caudal epidural anesthesia can be overcome by placement of a catheter to provide continuous caudal epidural anesthesia (Table 23-9). The establishment of a route for repeated administration of small doses of anesthetic drug extends surgery time, reduces the risk of rear limb ataxia, and avoids the development of fibrosis of the epidural space that results from repeated needle trauma. The disadvantages of catheter placement include greater cost of equipment, complications associated from kinking and curling of the catheter, and lack of documentation for the optimal times and doses required for repeated spinal administration of anesthetics. In the horse a 10.2-cm, 18-gauge thin-walled Tuohy needle with stylet is inserted at the first coccygeal interspace, and a 20-gauge Teflon epidural catheter is advanced cranially toward the lumbosacral junction to the desired level (Fig. 23-7, *C*). Alternatively, in horses and in cattle, a 17.5- cm, 17-gauge Huber-point Tuohy directional needle can be used to place and pass a catheter to the caudal portion of the sacral (S3 to S5) epidural space from the lumbosacral intervertebral junction (Fig. 23-8).

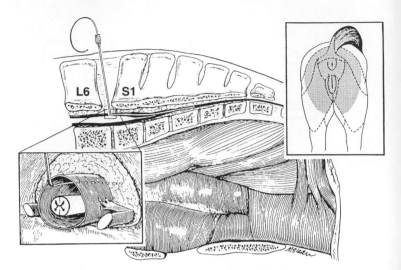

FIG. 23-9. Catheter introduction at the lumbosacral (L6-S1) intervertebral junction for continuous caudal subarachnoid anesthesia. *Left inset,* Proper placement within the subarachnoid space. *Right inset,* Stippled area delineates extent of subcutaneous desensitization after caudal blockade.

◆ Introduction of morphine and detomidine into an epidural catheter advanced to the lumbosacral region produces effective hind limb analgesia to the tarsocrural joint, lasting more than 6 hours in the horse.

◆ The caudal epidural injection of 60 to 100 mg of mepivacaine hydrochloride in aqueous solution into a catheter placed at the caudal portion of the sacral (S3 to S5) epidural space in the horse produces unilateral or bilateral analgesia extending from spinal cord segment S1 to the coccyx.

CONTINUOUS CAUDAL SUBARACHNOID ANESTHESIA

Continuous caudal subarachnoid anesthesia produces analgesia for prolonged periods in standing horses (Table 23-9). The technique is similar to that used to produce continuous caudal epidural anesthesia but provides the added advantage of producing a faster onset of action and shorter duration of effect with reduced drug doses. A 17.5-cm, 17-gauge Huber-point Tuohy needle with stylet is inserted into the subarachnoid space at the lumbosacral (L6 to S1) intervertebral space. Proper placement of the needle in the subarachnoid space is verified by the free flow of spinal fluid from the needle hub. The stylet is removed, and a 20-gauge Teflon catheter (0.036 cm outside diameter) or polyethylene tubing (0.095 cm outside diameter) reinforced with a stainless steel spring guide (0.052 cm outside diameter) is advanced to the midsacral (S2 to S3) subarachnoid space (Fig. 23-9).

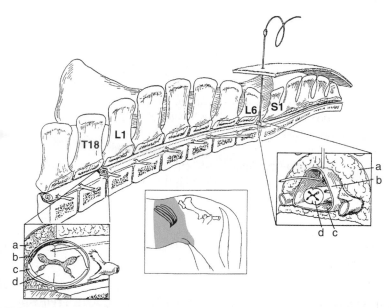

FIG. 23-10. Catheter introduction at the lumbosacral (L6-S1) intervertebral site and advancement to the thoracolumbar junction T18-L1 for segmental thoracolumbar subarachnoid anesthesia. *Left inset,* Proper placement of Tuohy needle and catheter within the subarachnoid space. *Middle inset,* Correctly positioned catheter and spring guide at T18-L1 intervertebral space. *Right inset,* Stippled area delineates extent of subcutaneous desensitization after blockade in the standing horse. *a,* Epidural space with fat and connective tissue; *b,* dura mater; *c,* subarachnoid space; *d,* spinal cord.

- Continuous caudal subarachnoid anesthesia requires approximately one third the amount of drug used to produce the same effect as epidural anesthesia.
- The onset of drug effect is faster, and the duration of effect is approximately half as long as that produced after epidural drug administration, conferring the advantage of increased control over the intensity of analgesia and associated side effects.
- Subarachnoid administration of drugs, however, carries the risk of trauma to the conus medullaris and associated nerve fibers and is much more difficult to perform than epidural anesthesia.

SEGMENTAL THORACOLUMBAR SUBARACHNOID ANESTHESIA

Segmental thoracolumbar subarachnoid anesthesia is used to produce anesthesia for standing flank surgery in the horse and cow (Table 23-9). Segmental thoracolumbar subarachnoid anesthesia requires adherence to strict aseptic technique. A 17.5-cm, 17-gauge Huber-point Tuohy needle with stylet is inserted into the subarachnoid space at the lumbosacral (L6 to S1) intervertebral space (Fig. 23-10). The L6 to S1 interspace is located 1 to 2 cm caudal to the cranial edges of the tuber sacral on the dorsal midline. A 100-cm–long catheter with a 0.095-cm outside diameter is passed through the needle and advanced approximately 60 cm to the midthoracic area. Desensitization of dorsal nerve roots T14 to L3 in the horse and T9 to L3 in the cow is produced within 5 to 10 minutes by injecting 1.5 to 2 ml of 2% mepivacaine hydrochloride and lasts for 30 to 60 minutes.

◆ Anesthesia can be prolonged by fractional bolus administration of half the initial drug dose at approximately 30-minute intervals.

◆ The advantages of this technique include a rapid onset, minimal drug dosage, and a selective analgesic effect.

◆ Disadvantages include the potential for traumatizing the conus medullaris, kinking and curling of the catheter, loss of motor control to the pelvic limbs, and meningitis if strict asepsis is not observed.

SEGMENTAL THORACOLUMBAR EPIDURAL ANESTHESIA

Segmental thoracolumbar epidural anesthesia is not commonly used in the horse compared with cattle because it is difficult to perform, provides variable results, and requires special equipment (Table 23-9). Furthermore, the T18 to L1 epidural space can be catheterized from the lumbosacral epidural space to desensitize spinal nerves T12 to L2. Segmental (T12 to L2) analgesia involving the flank and extending caudally to the area of the stifle is achieved in 10 to 20 minutes after the injection of 80 mg (4 ml at 2% solution) mepivacaine hydrochloride, with a duration of analgesia lasting approximately 1 to 1½ hours. A 10.2-cm, 18-gauge Tuohy needle is inserted into the epidural space in well-restrained cattle at the thoracolumbar or L1-L2 interspace. L1-L2 is located 1.5 to 2 cm caudal to an imaginary line between the cranial edges of the transverse processes of L2. T13-L1 can be identified between the last rib and the cranial edge of the transverse process of L1.

◆ Segmental thoracolumbar epidural anesthesia should not be routinely used in horses because, as stated previously, it is difficult to perform and requires a specially designed catheter and wire guide.

◆ Catheter placement carries the risk of catheter kinking or curling at the lumbosacral intervertebral space, causing the injectant to be deposited in the region of the femoral and ischial nerves and predisposing the horse to a loss of pelvic limb function and panic.

◆ Unilateral block may develop, and if the catheter tip passes into the paravertebral space, an absence of blockade will be observed.

PROXIMAL PARAVERTEBRAL THORACOLUMBAR ANESTHESIA (CATTLE)

An alternative to simple infiltration of the incision line with local anesthetic for standing laparotomy in cattle is proximal paravertebral thoracolumbar anesthesia. The dorsal and ventral branches of spinal nerves T13-L2 are blocked, along with L3-L4 if anesthesia of the caudal paralumbar fossa is required (e.g., cesarean section). The cranial aspect of the transverse process of L1 is palpated. A spinal needle (4.25 to 15 cm, 18 gauge) is passed ventrally and walked off the bone cranially after desensitizing the skin 2.5 to 5 cm from the dorsal midline. An initial 10 to 15 ml of 2% lidocaine is deposited ventral to the intertransverse fascia before withdrawing the needle 1 to 2.5 cm and injecting another 5 ml in order to anesthetize the ventral and dorsal branches of the spinal nerves. Blockade is accompanied by scoliosis toward the side of anesthesia.

♦ This technique provides a wide, uniform area of anesthesia.
♦ The time required to perform the block is less than for a line block.
♦ Although technically more difficult, landmarks are easily palpated except in fat cattle.
♦ Hind limb weakness may be seen with L3-L4 blockade.
♦ Scoliosis may make surgical orientation and closure of the incision more difficult.

SIDE EFFECTS

Caudal regional anesthesia carries the risks of nerve or spinal cord trauma, infection and ataxia, and recumbency resulting from motor blockade. Judicious use and application of regional anesthetic techniques, however, provides a low-cost, safe, efficacious means of producing analgesia for many standing surgical procedures and can be used as an adjunct to general anesthesia to reduce the amount of injectable and/or inhalant drug required to maintain surgical anesthesia.

CONCLUSION

The development of evaluation techniques, assessment tools, and treatment options for pain in horses and ruminants lags behind recent advances in small animal pain management. Current research into development of pain scoring systems and scales, evaluation of newer tools such as pressure algometry, evaluation of the pharmacodynamics and pharmacokinetics of new drugs and reevaluation of established ones, and critical assessment of the efficacy of complementary therapies should provide increased options for treatment of pain in horses and cattle in the future.

ACKNOWLEDGMENT

Some of the information in this chapter is reprinted from Grosenbaugh DA, Skarda RT, Muir WW: *Equine Veterinary Education* 11:98-105, 1999; Muir WW: *Equine Veterinary Education* 10:335-340, 1998. Where regional anesthesia technique differs for cattle, it is noted in the text.

SUGGESTED READINGS

Anderson DE, Muir WW: Pain management in cattle, *Vet Clin North Am Food Anim Pract* 21:623-635, 2005.

Ashley FH, Waterman-Pearson AE, Whay HR: Behavioral assessment of pain in horses and donkeys: application to clinical practice and future studies, *Equine Vet J* 37:565-575, 2005.

Broom DM: Animal welfare: concepts and measurement, *J Anim Sci* 69:4167-4175, 1991.

de Leon-Casasola OA, Lema MJ: Postoperative epidural opioid analgesia: what are the choices? *Anesth Analg* 83:867-875, 1966.

Dickenson AH: Mechanisms of the analgesic actions of opiates and opioids, *Br Med Bull* 47:690-702, 1991.

Doherty TJ, Geiser DR, Rohrbach BW: Effect of high-volume epidural morphine, ketamine, and butorphanol on halothane minimum alveolar concentration in ponies, *Equine Vet J* 29:370-373, 1997.

Eisenach JC, Kock MD, Klimscha W: α_2-Adrenergic agonists for regional anesthesia, *Anesthesiology* 85:655-674, 1996.

Fikes LW, Lin HC, Thurman JC: A preliminary comparison of lidocaine and xylazine as epidural analgesics in ponies, *Vet Surg* 18:85-86, 1989.

Gan TJ, Ginsgerg B, Glass PSA et al: Opioid-sparing effects of a low-dose infusion of naloxone in patient-administered morphine sulphate, *Anesthesiology* 87:1075-1081, 1997.

Gaynor JS, Hubbell JAE: Perineural and spinal anesthesia, *Vet Clin North Am Equine Pract* 7:501-519, 1991.

Green EM, Cooper RC: Continuous caudal epidural anesthesia in the horse, *J Am Vet Med Assoc* 184:971-974, 1984.

Grosenbaugh DA, Skarda RT, Muir WW: Caudal regional anesthesia in horses, *Equine Veterinary Education* 11:98-105, 1999.

Grubb TL, Riebold TW, Huber MJ: Comparison of lidocaine, xylazine for perineal analgesia in horses, *J Am Vet Med Assoc* 210:1187-1190, 1992.

Haussler KK, Erb HN: Pressure algometry: objective assessment of back pain and effects of chiropractic treatment, *Proceedings of the American Association of Equine Practitioners* 49:66-70, 2003.

Haussler KK, Erb HN: Mechanical nociceptive thresholds in the axial skeleton of horses, *Equine Vet J* 38:70-75, 2006.

Joyce J, Hendrickson DA: Comparison of intraoperative pain response following intratesticular or mesorchial injection of lidocaine in standing horses undergoing laparoscopic cryptorchidectomy, *J Am Vet Med Assoc* 229:1779-1783, 2006.

Kehlet H, Dahl JB: The value of "multimodal" or "balanced analgesia" in postoperative pain treatment, *Anesth Analg* 77:1048-1056, 1993.

Knobloch M, Portier CJ, Levionnois OL et al: Antinociceptive effects, metabolism and disposition of ketamine in ponies under target-controlled drug infusion, *Toxicol Appl Pharmacol* 216:373-386, 2006.

Lankveld DP, Driessen B, Soma LR et al: Pharmacodynamic effects and pharmacokinetic profile of a long-term continuous rate infusion of racemic ketamine in healthy conscious horses, *J Vet Pharmacol Ther* 29:477-488, 2006.

LeBlanc PH: Regional anesthesia, *Vet Clin North Am Equine Pract* 6:693-704, 1990.

LeBlanc PH, Caron JP: Clinical use of epidural xylazine in the horse, *Equine Vet J* 22:180-181, 1990.

LeBlanc PH, Caron SP, Patterson JS et al: Epidural injection of xylazine for perineal analgesia in horses, *J Am Vet Med Assoc* 193:1405-1408, 1988.

LeBlanc PH, Eberhart SW: Cardiopulmonary effects of epidurally administered xylazine in the horse, *Equine Vet J* 22:189-191, 1990.

Lee I, Yamada H: Epidural administration of fixed volumes of xylazine and lidocaine for anesthesia of dairy cattle undergoing flank surgery, *J Am Vet Med Assoc* 227:781-744, 2005.

Malone E, Ensick J, Turner T et al: Intravenous continuous infusion of lidocaine for treatment of equine ileus, *Vet Surg* 35:60-66, 2006.

Mills PC, Cross SE: Regional differences in transdermal penetration of fentanyl through equine skin, *Res Vet Sci* 82(2):252-256, 2007. Prepublished on Sep 29, 2006, as DOI 10.1016/j.rvsc.2006.07.015.

Muir WW: Anesthesia and pain management in horses, *Equine Veterinary Education* 10:335-340, 1998.

Muir WW, Skarda RT, Sheehan WC: Hemodynamic and respiratory effects of a xylazine-acetylpromazine drug combination in horses, *Am J Vet Res* 40:1518-1522, 1979.

Muir WW, Skarda RT, Sheehan WC: Hemodynamic and respiratory effects of a xylazine-morphine sulfate in horses, *Am J Vet Res* 40:1417-1420, 1979.

Natalini CC, Linardi RL: Analgesic effects of epidural administration of hydromorphone in horses, *Am J Vet Res* 67:11-15, 2006.

Orsini JA, Moate PJ, Kuersten K et al: Pharmacokinetics of fentanyl delivered transdermally in healthy adult horses: variability among horses and its clinical implications, *J Vet Pharmacol Ther* 29:539-546, 2006.

Price J, Catriona S, Welsh EM et al: Preliminary evaluation of a behavior-based system for assessment of post-operative pain in horses following arthroscopic surgery, *Vet Anaesth Analg* 30:124-137, 2003.

Robertson S: The importance of assessing pain in horses and donkeys, *Equine Vet J* 38:5-6, 2006.

Schelling CG, Klein LV: Comparison of carbonated lidocaine and lidocaine hydrochloride for caudal epidural anesthesia in horses, *Am J Vet Res* 46:1375-1377, 1985.

Skarda RT: Local and regional analgesic techniques: horses. In Thurman JC, Tranquilli WJ, Benson GJ, editors: *Lumb & Jones' veterinary anesthesia*, ed 3, Philadelphia, 1996, Williams & Wilkins.

Skarda RT, Muir WW: Segmental thoracolumbar spinal (subarachnoid) analgesia in conscious horses, *Am J Vet Res* 43:2121-2128, 1982.

Skarda RT, Muir WW: Segmental epidural and subarachnoid analgesia in conscious horses: a comparative study, *Am J Vet Res* 44:1870-1876, 1983.

Skarda RT, Muir WW: Continuous caudal epidural and subarachnoid anesthesia in mares: a comparative study, *Am J Vet Res* 44:2290-2298, 1993.

Skarda RT, Muir WW: Caudal analgesia induced by epidural or subarachnoid administration of detomidine hydrochloride solution in mares, *Am J Vet Res* 55:670-680, 1994.

Skarda RT, Muir WW: Analgesic, hemodynamic, and respiratory effects of caudal epidurally administered xylazine hydrochloride solution in mares, *Am J Vet Res* 57:193-200, 1996.

Skarda RT, Muir WW: Comparison of antinociceptive, cardiovascular, and respiratory effects, head ptosis and position of pelvic limbs in mares after caudal epidural administration of xylazine and detomidine hydrochloride solution, *Am J Vet Res* 57:1338-1345, 1996.

Skarda RT, Muir WW, Ibrahim AL: Plasma mepivacaine concentrations after caudal epidural and subarachnoid injection in the horse: a comparative study, *Am J Vet Res* 45:1967-1971, 1984.

Solomon RE, Gebhart GF: Synergistic antinociceptive interactions among drugs administered to the spinal cord, *Anesth Analg* 78:1164-1172, 1994.

Spadavecchia C, Arendt-Nielsen L, Anderson OK, et al: Effect of romifidine on the nociceptive withdrawal reflex and temporal summation in conscious horses, *Am J Vet Res* 66:1992-1998, 2005.

Sylvester SP, Stafford KJ, Mellor DJ, et al: Behavioural responses of calves to amputation dehorning with and without local anaesthesia, *Aust Vet J* 82:697-700, 2004.

Sysel AM, Pleasant RS, Jacobson JD et al: Efficacy of an epidural combination of morphine and detomidine in alleviating experimentally induced hindlimb lameness in horses, *Vet Surg* 25:511-518, 1996.

Sysel AM, Pleasant RS, Jacobson JD, et al: Systemic and local effects associated with long-term epidural catheterization and morphine-detomidine administration in horses, *Vet Surg* 26:141-149, 1997.

Taylor PM, Pascoe PJ, Mama KR: Diagnosing and treating pain in the horse: where are we today?, *Vet Clin North Am Equine Pract* 18:1-19, 2002.

Valverde A, Little CB, Dyson DH: Use of epidural morphine to relieve pain in a horse, *Can Vet J* 31:211-212, 1990.

Wolf L: The role of complementary techniques in managing musculoskeletal pain in performance horses, *Vet Clin North Am Equine Pract* 18:107-115, 2002.

24 PAIN MANAGEMENT FOR THE PET BIRD

JOANNE PAUL-MURPHY

RECOGNIZING PAIN BEHAVIOR IN PET BIRDS

All animals possess the neuroanatomic and neuropharmacologic components necessary for the transduction, transmission, and perception of noxious stimuli. It stands to reason, therefore, that all animals can experience pain even if they cannot give verbal expression to the emotional component of pain. Although humans are incapable of assessing emotion in birds, emotional behaviors may have been preserved in evolution so that there is no survival advantage to emotional display for some avian species, whereas for another there may be benefit. For the purposes of this chapter, it is accepted that birds perceive and respond to noxious stimuli and that birds feel pain.

Birds are often undertreated for pain. Poor understanding of avian behaviors makes it difficult to identify when birds are in pain and the severity of their pain (Box 24-1). The difficulty is compounded when birds are isolated in a hospital setting because social isolation can alter the bird's response to pain.[1] Additionally, lack of scientific information about appropriate therapies has hampered knowledge of avian pain management, having the effect of minimizing veterinary treatment of avian pain.

BOX 24-1
Birds are often undertreated for pain. Poor understanding of avian behaviors makes it difficult to identify when birds are in pain and the severity of the pain.

Assessment of pain must consider the species, gender, age, environment, and concurrent disease. When a bird is in pain, there is a change or absence of one or more normal behaviors (Table 24-1). Social interactions decrease in species of birds that have complex

TABLE 24-1	Effect of Chronic Pain on Pet Bird Behavior
Behavioral Changes	**Examples**
Decreased social interactions	Perching away from other birds
	Decreased grooming of self and/or conspecifics
	Decreased interactions with owner
Guarding behavior	Change in posture to protect a painful area
	Decreased activity
Increased aggression	Toward conspecifics
	Toward owner
Grooming behavior: at painful site or generalized	Feather destructive behaviors
	Self-mutilation

The effect of chronic pain on a bird's behavior can be subtle. When an owner reports changes in the bird's behavior such as listed above, consider the possibility of a painful condition.

social systems. This may be an obvious change, such as perching away from the flock, or might be more subtle, such as a reduction in social grooming. When birds are housed as single pets, their social interactions with the owner may be reduced. Birds in pain may display guarding behavior, which may be manifested as antisocial behaviors, to protect a painful area. Some forms of aggression have been linked to painful conditions in birds when these aggressive behaviors dissipate following treatment of the painful condition. A behavioral change in feather grooming is common to solitary and social birds with painful conditions. Decreased self-grooming is a withdrawal behavior that can occur when a bird's focus is on pain; however, increased self-grooming or grooming of cagemates has also been reported when birds are stressed or painful. Grooming and feather picking may increase over a specific area directly related to the region of discomfort. Studies using chickens with induced sodium urate arthritis demonstrated that shifting the bird's attention reduced the severity of pain and may potentially reduce peripheral inflammation.[2]

PHYSIOLOGY OF AVIAN PAIN

The physiology of pain in all animals involves detection of a noxious stimulus in the periphery (mechanical, thermal, or chemical) and transmission of the impulses to the spinal cord, where they are modulated and projected to the brain for central processing of the information, which determines the perception of the noxious stimulus. Taxonomic differences in central nervous system anatomy and complexity are apparent, but anatomic, physiological, and biochemical studies in nonmammalian vertebrates have found that pain perception is expected to be analogous to mammals.

Peripheral nociceptors have been studied in birds and include high-threshold mechanothermal, mechanochemical, mechanical, and thermal. Mechanothermal nociceptors are multifunctional and respond to mechanical stimulation and temperatures higher than 40° C. These nociceptors are similar to cutaneous free nerve endings in mammals with slow-conducting unmyelinated C-fiber components. Compared with mammals, the receptive fields of some of the polymodal fibers are greater in birds. As stimulus intensity increases, the number of responses increases. Some fibers have continuous response up to 56° C, whereas other fibers peak at lower temperatures, and increasing the thermal stimulus above this peak results in a reduction of impulses.

Thermal and mechanical nociceptors are polymodal and can be Aσ or C fibers with discharge patterns and receptor field size similar to mammals.[3] The avian counterpart may be less sensitive to low temperatures and have a greater threshold to high temperatures, perhaps related to the higher body temperatures of birds. Recent studies have demonstrated polymodal nociceptors (mechanochemical) in the nasal and oral mucosa of chickens similar to mammals, with chemical sensitivity to a range of compounds.[4] Birds have multiple ascending pathways in the dorsal horn laminae of the spinal cord transmitting pain signals to the midbrain and forebrain. The distribution of neurons in the nociceptive spinothalamic tract cells is similar between birds and mammals.[5]

Peripheral sensitization occurs when inflammation at the site of injury creates an increased response to a normally painful stimulus. Cell damage and leakage leads to a series of responses resulting in increased sensitivity of the peripheral receptors. Central sensitization is an increase in the excitability of spinal cord neurons and a recruitment of neurons not involved in pain perception under normal circumstances. When stimulation from the peripheral nociceptors to the spinal cord continues for an extended period, a wide range of spinal neurons becomes sensitized and hyperresponsive.[6] Although sensitization has not been experimentally demonstrated in birds, mammalian studies have demonstrated that when analgesics are given before a painful event rather than after the start of the stimulation, the spinal excitability can be dampened.[7,8] The earlier pain is treated, the less total drug is required to maintain analgesia during and after surgery (Box 24-2).

A study of pigeons undergoing orthopedic surgery demonstrated that pigeons receiving butorphanol before and after surgery returned to normal behaviors sooner than pigeons receiving butorphanol in the postoperative period only.[9]

BOX 24-2
Treat for pain before and during surgery so that less total drug will be required to maintain analgesia during and after the procedure.

TREATMENT OF PAIN

Diagnosing the cause of pain can be challenging in birds, and identification of the disease process or site of tissue damage affects the choice of analgesic drugs and supportive care. Therapy should be directed at resolving the injury or disease in addition to using analgesics to decrease peripheral pain signals and their effect on the central neural processing of the pain. Conversely, the patient's signs of pain may be recognized before a diagnosis is reached, and in these cases, treatment of the pain becomes a critical component of the symptomatic therapy (Box 24-3). Election of analgesic drugs may need to be conservative when the cause of pain is unknown.

BOX 24-3
The patient's signs of pain may be recognized before a diagnosis is reached. In these cases, treatment of the pain becomes a critical component of the symptomatic therapy.

Combining analgesics that act by different mechanisms can augment the pain relief. Administration of two or more analgesics frequently produces a synergistic effect. Surgical analgesia commonly includes a local anesthetic at the incision site, an opioid administered directly before and after surgery, and a nonsteroidal antiinflammatory drug (NSAID) given during surgery and for several days following the procedure (Box 24-4). This combination of drugs usually allows the dosage of each drug and the concentration of inhalation anesthetic to be reduced, thereby reducing the side effects of each drug. Adjunctive

---

BOX 24-4 | MULTIMODAL SURGICAL ANALGESIA
1. Local anesthetic (lidocaine) at incision site
2. Opioid (butorphanol) immediately before and after surgery
3. Nonsteroidal antiinflammatory drug (NSAID; meloxicam) given intramuscularly following induction
4. Oral NSAID administration for 3 to 5 days following the procedure

drugs, such as tranquilizers, used in conjunction with analgesic drugs can enhance the analgesia by reducing anxiety. The most common sedatives used in avian medicine are the benzodiazepines, which calm birds before handling for anesthesia.

Supportive care is important to the management of pain. This includes keeping the avian patient warm, dry, and clean. Hospital environment stressors such as barking dogs or strong smells of cats, ferrets, or other "predators" can be minimized by having a separate area for avian critical care. Gentle human contact and using a soothing voice are beneficial for the pet bird.

REGIONAL ANESTHESIA AND ANALGESIA

Local anesthetics such as lidocaine and bupivacaine block sodium channels in the nerve axon, which interferes with the conduction of action potentials along the nerve. When local anesthetics are used preoperatively, the number and frequency of impulses are reduced, thereby reducing nociceptor sensitization, which has the beneficial effect of minimizing central sensitization.

Regional infiltration using a local line or splash block is the most common method used. A 25- or 27-gauge needle is used to make several subcutaneous (SC) injections of small volumes of dilute solution into the operative area. The SC space in the bird is very thin. A line block follows the course of the intended incision by injecting a small bleb of dilute anesthetic SC, then withdrawing the needle and reinserting it at the edge of the bleb. Another bleb is made under the skin, and the process is repeated until the length of the incision is blocked.

Local anesthetic dosage recommendations for birds are lower than mammals because birds may be more sensitive to the effects of the drug (Box 24-5). Systemic uptake of the drug can be rapid in birds, and metabolism may be prolonged, increasing the potential for toxic reactions. Toxic side effects include fine tremors, ataxia, recumbency, seizures, stupor, cardiovascular effects, and death. Toxic effects can be acute if accidentally injected intravenously. Chickens given intraarticular injections of high doses of bupivacaine (2.7 to 3.3 mg/kg) showed immediate signs of toxicity such as drowsiness and

---

BOX 24-5

Local anesthetic dosage recommendations are lower for birds than mammals because birds may be more sensitive to the systemic effects of the drug.

recumbency.[10] The duration of action of local anesthetics depends on the molecular properties and lipid solubility of the drug. Neither the time to effect nor duration of action has been determined for these drugs in birds. In a study of bupivacaine using mallard ducks, the absorption rate was slower than the elimination rate.[11]

Dosage recommendations for lidocaine are 2 to 3 mg/kg; thus the commercial preparation of 20 mg/kg should be diluted 1:10 with sterile water. Using a 2-mg/kg concentration of lidocaine increases accuracy of dosing and provides the volume needed for blocking a surgical site (Box 24-6). The commercial preparation of bupivacaine is a 0.5% solution (5 mg/ml). No bupivacaine dosage has been established for birds, but 1 mg/kg total dose has been safely administered to large birds. Dilution of bupivacaine is also recommended to increase the volume for administration. Intraarticular administration of bupivacaine (3 mg in 0.3 ml saline) was studied for its analgesic effects in chickens with experimentally produced acute arthritis. Chickens given bupivacaine were able to feed, peck, and stand on the affected limb similar to birds without arthritis.[10] Topical benzocaine has been used for minor wound repair in small birds.[12] Topical bupivacaine/dimethyl sulfoxide mixture applied to the amputation site of beak-trimmed chickens provided 4 hours of analgesia.[13]

BOX 24-6
Dosage recommendations for lidocaine are 2 to 3 mg/kg. The commercial preparation of 20 mg/kg should be diluted 1:10 with sterile water. Using a 2-mg/kg concentration of lidocaine increases accuracy of dosing and provides the volume needed for blocking a surgical site.

Local anesthetics in the form of transdermal patches and transdermal creams have not been studied for use in birds. Additionally, epidural infusions, spinal blocks, intravenous blocks, and peripheral nerve blocks are difficult to perform in birds; therefore the use of local anesthesia through these applications has not been reported.

OPIOIDS

Opioids reversibly bind to specific receptors in the central and peripheral nervous system. Opioids vary in their receptor specificity and efficacy in mammals, which results in a wide variety of clinical effects in different species. Clinical effects are also influenced by the commercial preparation of opioid and the dose and route of administration to the species receiving the drug. It stands to reason that the type of opioid and the dose also have a wide range of clinical effects in different avian species. The distribution, number, and type of opioid receptors are conserved across vertebrate species in the brainstem and spinal cord but vary substantially in the forebrain. Autoradiography was used to identify μ, κ, and δ opioid receptors in the forebrain of rats, mice, and humans, and κ-receptors represented 9%, 13%, and 37% of the total opioid receptor population, respectively. In contrast, the pigeon forebrain has a relatively high proportion (76%) of κ-receptors.[14] κ-Receptors have multiple physiological functions in the bird, and the analgesic function of these receptors still needs further investigation.

Physiological and analgesic effects of butorphanol have been studied in parrots using the isoflurane-sparing technique. With this method, healthy birds are anesthetized with isoflurane with determination of the minimum anesthetic concentration (MAC) by using a noxious stimulus (toe pinch) and observing a withdrawal response with a cognitive movement. Each bird is then treated with butorphanol (1 mg/kg), and the MAC is redetermined. If the concentration of isoflurane can be lowered, then this "sparing effect" is considered to be due to the analgesic effects of butorphanol. Butorphanol (1 mg/kg) was administered to three species of parrots, and the isoflurane MAC could be significantly lowered in cockatoos and African grey parrots, but not Amazon parrots.[15,16] A higher dosage of butorphanol may be necessary to demonstrate an effect in Amazon parrots. When turkeys were given a low dose of butorphanol (0.1 mg/kg) in a similar gas anesthesia–sparing model, the halothane MAC was not changed. A similar type of study using chickens compared three dosages of morphine (0.1, 1.0, and 3.0 mg/kg) and an experimental κ-opioid. Both drugs had isoflurane-sparing effects in this study.[17]

The effect of different opioids on conscious parrots was evaluated by studying the change in withdrawal threshold from noxious electrical and thermal stimuli before and after receiving an opioid. When African grey parrots were given butorphanol 1 mg/kg intramuscularly (IM), 50% of the birds had significant analgesia; and when given 2 mg/kg, a greater percentage of birds experienced significant analgesia. Butorphanol dosages of 3 to 6 mg/kg had similar analgesic effects on Hispaniolan Amazon parrots. Doses of 3 mg/kg demonstrated significant analgesia, but increasing the dosage to 6 mg/kg did not increase the effect.[18,19] Buprenorphine at 0.1 mg/kg IM in African grey parrots did not show an analgesic effect when tested by analgesiometry, but pharmacokinetic analysis suggests that this dose may not achieve effective plasma levels.[20] Pigeons given 0.25 and 0.5 mg/kg buprenorphine showed an increased latency period for withdrawal from a noxious electrical stimulus of 2 and 5 hours, respectively.[21] Fentanyl 0.02 mg/kg was evaluated using cockatoos, and it did not affect the withdrawal threshold of the cockatoos. A tenfold increase in the dosage of fentanyl (0.2 mg/kg SC) did produce an analgesic response, but many birds were hyperactive for the first 15 to 30 minutes after receiving the high dose.[19] These three opioids had rapid absorption and rapid elimination in parrots, with mean residence times of less than 2 hours.

Butorphanol 1 to 3 mg/kg IM is the current recommendation for opioid analgesia in parrots, but it needs to be administered every 2 to 3 hours (Box 24-7).

BOX 24-7
Butorphanol 1 to 3 mg/kg intramuscularly is the current recommendation for opioid analgesia in parrots but needs to be administered every 2 to 3 hours to maintain effect.

NONSTEROIDAL ANTIINFLAMMATORY DRUGS

Cyclooxygenase (COX) enzymes initiate a cascade of reactions that result in polyunsaturated acids being converted to eicosanoids such as prostaglandins and thromboxane.[22] These eicosanoids are released at sites of tissue injury and cause inflammation and sensitization of nerve endings. NSAIDs inhibit COX enzymes, thereby disrupting eicosanoid synthesis and reducing inflammation at the site of injury. NSAIDs also decreases sensitization of nerve endings and have a modulating effect within the central nervous system. The relative expression of COX-1 and COX-2 enzymes varies between species. Both enzymes are important in avian peripheral inflammation and in spinal pain transmission, but more information is needed to differentiate their physiological effects in avian species.

NSAIDs are used to relieve visceral and musculoskeletal pain, acute pain associated with trauma, and chronic pain such as arthritis and to decrease inflammation and sensitization associated with surgery. The most common NSAIDs used in current avian medicine are meloxicam, carprofen, ketoprofen, piroxicam, and celecoxib (Table 24-2). Specific NSAIDs such as diclofenac and flunixin meglumine are not recommended for birds because of significant toxic effects reported in vultures and quail, respectively.[23,24] The inhibition of COX enzymes can have potential unwanted effects and should be monitored and evaluated in each patient. In birds, toxic effects include renal impairment and hepatic enzyme elevations; therefore, increased monitoring is indicated with high-risk patients—establishing a baseline of plasma uric acid, phosphorous, and hepatic enzyme concentrations—before NSAID administration and reevaluation of these parameters at fixed intervals.

Drug	Route	Dosage(mg/kg Unless Otherwise Stated)	Frequency	Comments
Acetylsalicylic acid	PO	0.5-1.0	Every 8-12 hours	Anecdotal clinical application. Wide species variation in pharmacokinetic studies.
	Per 250 ml drinking water	325 mg	Change water every 8 hours	Alters taste/smell of water and may not be well accepted
Carprofen	SC, PO	1.0-3.0	Every 8-12 hours	Raised pain threshold for 90 minutes
Celecoxib	PO	10	Every 24 hours	Anecdotal use for neuropathic gastric dilation symptoms
Flunixin meglumine	IM	1.0-5.0	Every 12-24 hours	May cause muscle necrosis at injection site; hydration is essential; use only for short duration; potential nephrotoxicity
Ibuprofen	PO	5-10	Every 12-24 hours	Anecdotal use in small birds; use pediatric suspension
Indomethacin	PO	2	Every 8-10 hours	Pharmacokinetic in chickens
	IM	0.4		Anecdotal clinical application
Ketoprofen	PO	2.0	Every 12-24 hours	Higher dose effective in ducks; effective period may be only 30-70 minutes. Mortality associated with male Eiders.
	IM	5.0		
	IV			
Meloxicam	PO	0.5-2.0	Every 8-12 hours	Anecdotal clinical application; prolonged therapy well tolerated. Wide species variation in pharmacokinetic studies.
	IM			
	SQ			
Phenylbutazone	PO	3.5-7.0	Every 8-12 hours	Anecdotal clinical application
Piroxicam	PO	0.5	Every 12 hours	Anecdotal application for chronic osteoarthritis; prolonged therapy well tolerated

NSAIDs should not be used if there is any indication of renal impairment, hepatic dysfunction, severe hypovolemia, or gastric ulceration. A fecal occult blood test can determine upper gastrointestinal bleeding in pet birds when they are not fed meat products. Use one NSAID at a time, and in cases of chronic pain, review the response to therapy frequently and change to a different formulation of NSAID if the response is diminishing. For treatment of mild to moderate chronic pain, NSAIDS can be given on an as-needed basis. Safety of meloxicam was studied in three vulture species at dosages as high as 2 mg/kg, and serum uric acid concentrations were not increased.[25]

Analgesic efficacy of NSAIDs related to dose and frequency of administration has not been well studied in any avian species. Pharmacokinetic trials in several species of birds have found NSAID serum concentrations to be highly variable between species, and information is lacking about any parrot species.

Three NSAIDs (sodium salicylate, flunixin, and meloxicam) were administered intravenously and found to have rapid elimination in five species of birds (chickens, ostriches, ducks, turkeys, and pigeons).[26] The half life of 0.5 mg/kg meloxicam was three times longer in chickens and pigeons than other avian species tested, 3.2 hours and 2.4 hours respectively, compared to 13.7 hours in humans.[26] Pharmacokinetics of ketoprofen 2 mg/kg given orally, IM, and intravenously to quail *(Coturnix japonica)* showed a very short half-life and low bioavailability orally (24%) and IM (54%) compared with humans and dogs.[27] An analgesia study using mallard ducks undergoing a skin incision found no detectable analgesia using ketoprofen at 0.5 to 2.0 mg/kg.[28] However, ketoprofen 5 mg/kg IM administered to wild mallard ducks anesthetized with isoflurane had an analgesic effect 30 to 70 minutes after administration.[29] A field anesthesia study using ketoprofen, propofol, and bupivacaine in Eider ducks, associated ketoprofen administration with mortality of males with histopathologic renal lesions.[30] A carprofen dose of 1 mg/kg SC given to chickens raised their threshold to pressure-induced pain for at least 90 minutes.[31] Another study using chickens concluded that 30 mg/kg IM carprofen was required to eliminate behaviors associated with experimental arthritis.[32] Carprofen (1 mg/kg) given to chickens with chronic lameness improved their ability to walk and navigate a maze with peak plasma levels occurring at 1 to 2 hours after SC administration.[33] Unfortunately, plasma concentrations do not have a direct correlation to physiological activity of the NSAID because NSAIDs tend to accumulate in areas of inflammation. In mallard ducks, 5 mg/kg flunixin and 5 mg/kg ketoprofen significantly suppressed thromboxane B_2 levels within 15 minutes of intramuscular administration and maintained this physiological effect for 4 hours.[34]

CHRONIC PAIN

Assessment of analgesia is challenging when the condition is progressive, such as chronic degenerative joint disease or neoplasia. Response to analgesia therapy is based on evaluation of a set of behaviors particular for each bird.

NSAIDS are the first course of therapy for chronic disorders because they have no sedative effect and have a longer duration of analgesic effect than opioids. Carprofen or meloxicam are the current drugs of choice because of the widespread use and low incidence of reported toxicities. Both can be orally administered once daily, but meloxicam has an advantage because it is available in an oral suspension and can be easily dosed for small birds. NSAIDs are initiated at the low-end dosage and monitored for response to treatment. If pain gradually increases over time, the dosage can be increased. Monitoring the complete blood count and renal (uric acid, phosphorous) and hepatic (aspartate aminotransferase and creatinine kinase) plasma values every 2 to 4 months is recommended, especially in the older bird. If pain recurs following several months of treatment, the next set of options includes changing to another NSAID such as piroxicam. Piroxicam may have synergistic action with anticancer drugs and is also an effective NSAID for degenerative joint disease in birds. Piroxicam is noted for renal toxicity and gastric ulceration in mammals. In a study using chickens with ascites syndrome, a high dose of piroxicam (0.6 mg/kg) caused gastrointestinal ulceration.[35] However, long-term use of low-dose piroxicam (0.1 mg/kg) has been administered and closely monitored for several consecutive months to captive cranes with chronic degenerative joint disease and has not caused clinical problems.[36] If pain persists or increases, especially with neoplasia, opioid therapy may be indicated. Butorphanol, although short acting, was shown to reduce painful behaviors associated with chronic arthritis in turkeys.[37] Unfortunately, parenteral forms of recommended opioids are only effective for a few hours. Experimental studies using long-acting liposome-encapsulated butorphanol in parrots with experimental arthritis showed effectiveness for 3 to 4 days and greater efficacy at reducing pain and lameness than NSAIDs.[38] No information is available regarding orally administered opioids in birds, but in mammals, much higher dosages are required for oral administration to reach effective plasma levels.

CONCLUSION

Avian analgesia is finally recognized as a critical component of avian medicine and surgery. The need to recognize pain and to provide pain relief is the first step, and many anecdotal therapeutic dosages extrapolated from other companion animals have developed. Several published research investigations, using several species of birds, have begun to provide avian analgesia therapeutics with empirical information for clinical application. The challenge is to continue pushing this research forward with appreciation that there are approximately 10,000 known species of birds, perhaps 200 species commonly kept as pets, and that each species has a range of behaviors as varied as their species-specific pharmacokinetics and pharmacodynamics to each analgesic drug.

REFERENCES

1. Jones RB, Harvey S: Behavioral and adrenocortical responses of domestic chicks to systematic reduction in group size and to sequential disturbances of companions by experimenter, *Behav Processes* 14:291-3030, 1987.
2. Gentle MJ, Tilston VL: Reduction in peripheral inflammation by changes in attention, *Physiol Behav* 66(2):289-292, 1999.
3. Gentle MJ, Hunter LN, Waddington D: The onset of pain-related behaviors following partial beak amputation in the chicken, *Neurosci Lett* 128:113-116, 1991.
4. McKeegan DEF: Mechano-chemical nociceptors in the avian trigeminal mucosa, *Brain Res Rev* 46:146-154, 2004.
5. Zhai XY, Atsumi S: Large dorsal horn neurons which receive inputs from numerous substance-P like immunoreactive axon terminals in the laminae I and II of the chicken spinal cord, *Neurosci Res* 28:147-154, 1997.
6. Roughan JV, Flecknell PA: Effects of surgery and analgesic administration on spontaneous behavior in singly housed rats, *Res Vet Sci* 69:283-288, 2000.
7. Woolf CJ: A new strategy for the treatment of inflammatory pain: prevention or elimination of central sensitization, *Drugs* 47(suppl 5):1-9, 1994; discussion, pp 46–47.
8. Woolf CJ, Chong MS: Preemptive analgesia: treating postoperative pain by preventing the establishment of central sensitization, *Anesth Analg* 77(2):362-379, 1993.
9. Paul-Murphy J: Unpublished data.
10. Hocking PM, Gentle MJ, Bernard R et al: Evaluation of a protocol for determining the effectiveness of pretreatment with local analgesics for reducing experimentally induced articular pain in domestic fowl, *Res Vet Sci* 63:263-267, 1997.
11. Machin KL, Livingston A: Plasma bupivacaine levels in mallard ducks *(Anas platyrhyncos)* following a single subcutaneous dose. Proceedings of the Joint Conference of the American Association of Zoo Veterinarians, American Association of Wildlife Veterinarians, Association of Reptilian and Amphibian Veterinarians, and National Association of Zoo and Wildlife Veterinarians, Orlando, Fla, pp 159–163, 2001.
12. Clubb SL: Round table discussion: pain management in clinical practice, *J Avian Med Surg* 12(4):276-278, 1998.
13. Glatz PC, Murphy LB, Preston AP: Analgesia therapy of beak-trimmed chickens, *Aust Vet J* 69(1):18, 1992.

14. Mansour A, Khachaturian H, Lewis ME et al: Anatomy of CNS opioid receptors, *Trends Neurosci* 11(7):308-314, 1988.

15. Curro TG, Brunson D, Paul-Murphy J: Determination of the ED50 of isoflurane and evaluation of the analgesic properties of butorphanol in cockatoos (*Cacatua* spp.), *Vet Surg* 23:429-433, 1994.

16. Curro TG: Evaluation of the isoflurane-sparing effects of butorphanol and flunixin in psittaciformes, *Proc Assoc Avian Vet pp* 17-19, 1993.

17. Concannon KT, Dodam JR, Hellyer PW: Influence of a mu and kappa opioid agonist on isoflurane minimal anesthetic concentration in chickens, *Am J Vet Res* 56:806-812, 1996.

18. Paul-Murphy JR, Brunson DB, Miletic V: Analgesic effects of butorphanol and buprenorphine in conscious African grey parrots (*Psittacus erithacus erithacus* and *Psittacus erithacus timneh*), *Am J Vet Res* 60(10):1218-1221, 1999.

19. Paul-Murphy J, Ludders J: Avian analgesia, *Vet Clin North Am Exot Anim Pract* 4(1):35-45, 2001.

20. Paul-Murphy J, Hess J, Fialkowski J: Pharmacokinetic properties of a single intramuscular dose of buprenorphine in African grey parrots (*Psittacus erithacus erithacus*), *J Avian Med Surg* 18(4):224-228, 2004.

21. Gaggermeier B, Henke J, Schatzmann U, et al: Investigations on analgesia in domestic pigeons (*C. livia*, Gmel., 1789, var. dom.) using buprenorphine and butorphanol, *Proc Eur Assoc Avian Vet* 70-73, 2003.

22. Vane JR, Bakhle YS: Blotting RM: Cyclooxygenases 1 and 2, *Annu Rev Pharmacol Toxicol* 38:97-120, 1998.

23. Oaks JL, Gilbert M, Virani MZ et al: Diclofenac residues as the cause of vulture population declines in Pakistan, *Nature* 427:630-633, 2004.

24. Klein PN, Charmatz K, Langenberg J: The effect of flunixin meglumine (Banamine) on the renal function in northern bobwhite (*Colinus virginianus*): an avian model. Proceedings of the Association of Reptilian and Amphibian Veterinarians and American Association of Zoo Veterinarians, Pittsburgh, pa, 1994, pp 128–131.

25. Swan G, Naidoo V, Cuthbert R et al: Removing the threat of diclofenac to critically endangered Asian vultures, *PLoS Biol* 4(3):66, 2006.

26. Baert K, De Backer P: Comparative pharmacokinetics of three non-steroidal anti-inflammatory drugs in five birds species, *Comp Biochem Physiol C* 134:25-33, 2003.

27. Graham JE, Kollias-Baker C, Craigmill AL et al: Pharmacokinetics of ketoprofen in Japanese quail (*Coturnix japonica*), *J Vet Pharmacol Ther* 28:399-402, 2005.

28. Machin KL: Assessment of pain in captive and free-ranging ducks after intraabdominal transmitter placement. Proceedings of the Joint Conference of the American Association of Zoo Veterinarians and American Association of Wildlife Veterinarians, Omaha, Neb, 1998, pp 470–473.

29. Machin KL, Livingston A: Assessment of the analgesic effects of ketoprofen in ducks anesthetized with isoflurane, *Am J Vet Res* 63(6):821-826, 2002.

30. Mulcahy DM, Tuomi P, and Larsen SR: Differential Mortality of Male Spectacled Eiders (*Somateria fischeri*) and King Eiders (*Somateria spectabilis*) Subsequent to Anesthesia With Propofol, Bupivacaine, and Ketoprofen, *J Avian Med Surg* 17:117-123, 2003.

31. Danbury TC, Weeks CA, Chambers JP et al: Self-selection of the analgesic drug carprofen by lame broiler chickens, *Vet Rec* 146(11):307-311, 2000.

32. Hocking YR: Effects of non-steroidal anti-inflammatory drugs on pain-related behaviour in a model of articular pain in the domestic fowl, *Res Vet Sci* 78(1):69-75, 2005.

33. McGeown D, Danbury TC, Waterman-Pearson AE et al: Effect of carprofen on lameness in broiler chickens, *Vet Rec* 144:668-671, 1999.

34. Machin KL, Tellier LA, Lair S, Livingston A: Pharmacodynamics of flunixin and ketoprofen in mallard ducks, *J Zoo Wildl Med* 32:22-29, 2001.

35. Valle K, Dian-Cruz A, Avila E et al: Antioxidant action of piroxicam on liver, heart and lung in broiler chicks, *J Vet Pharmacol Ther* 24(4):291-293, 2001.

36. Paul-Murphy J, Sladky K, Krugner-Higby L: Evaluation of butorphanol and carprofen for arthritic pain in parrots. Proceedings of the American Association of Zoo Veterinarians. Tampa, Fla, 2006, p 273.

37. Buchwalder T, Huber-Eicher B: Effect of the analgesic butorphanol on activity behaviour in turkeys *(Meleagris gallopavo)*, *Res Vet Sci* 79(3):239-244, 2005.

38. Sladky KK, Krugner-Higby L, Meek-Walker EB et al: Serum concentrations and analgesic efficacy of liposome-encapsulated and standard butorphanol tartrate in Hispaniolan parrots *(Amazona ventralis)*, *Am J Vet Res* 67(5):775-781, 2006.

25 CLINICAL APPROACHES TO ANALGESIA IN REPTILES

CRAIG MOSLEY

The analgesic management of reptiles can be challenging because of their unique physiological, anatomic, and behavioral adaptations. Although reptile pain and nociception have not been extensively studied, there is strong evidence that reptiles are capable of nociception. The neuroanatomic components necessary for nociception have been described.[1,2] In addition, endogenous antinociceptive mechanisms[2,3] and a demonstrable modulation of nociception with pharmacologic agents known to be analgesics in other species have been demonstrated.[4-8] In lizards *(Gekko gecko),* spinal projections originating in the brainstem region (nucleus raphes inferior) that project to the superficial layers of the dorsal horn have been identified, and these structures suggest the presence of tracts, similar to those found in mammals, that mediate descending inhibition of nociception.[7] Neurotransmitters that are important in nociceptive modulation in mammals have been identified in reptiles.[9] Although endogenous opioids and opioid receptors involved in reproduction and thermoregulation have been identified in reptiles, little is known about the role of opioids in nociception.[9-12] This information suggests that, at least at the physiological level, reptiles are capable of responding to noxious stimuli in a manner similar to mammals. The question of whether reptiles can "feel" pain or what significance pain or nociception has for physiological homeostasis is a far more complex question to answer. Until further evidence is available, it would seem most ethical to assume that reptiles are capable of feeling pain and to treat or manage pain when there is reasonable evidence that pain is present. Interestingly, in a recent survey of the membership of the Association of Reptile and Amphibian Veterinarians, 98% of the respondents indicated their belief that reptiles do feel pain. However, only 39% of respondents in this survey reported using analgesics in more than 50% of their patients.[13] The reasons for failure to use analgesics were not specifically addressed in this study. However, some possibilities include a failure to recognize painful patients, lack of efficacy data, concern of adverse effects, and little or no experimentally determined drug dose or pharmacokinetic information.

Reptiles are capable of nociception. Analgesic techniques to minimize the negative effects of nociception should be used in these animals.

The benefits of providing adequate analgesia are well recognized in mammals. The consequences of untreated pain are consistent with impaired patient homeostasis. These alterations can result in negative energy balance, lead to immune system compromise, inhibit healing, and interfere with normal behavioral process required for health (see Chapter 3).[14,15]

The benefits of preemptive analgesia have also been demonstrated and not only does it reduce postoperative pain by decreasing central sensitization but also may facilitate healing and prevent and/or limit the actions of detrimental neurohumoral responses to pain.[16,17] In addition, the use of analgesics as part of a balanced anesthetic protocol can reduce the doses of other anesthetics. This may help reduce the negative cardiopulmonary effects of general anesthesia. Overall, it has been demonstrated in humans and other mammals that appropriate analgesia is an important part of complete medical care in health and disease.

ASSESSING PAIN IN REPTILES

Assessing pain in nonverbal species, including human infants, is a challenging endeavor. Pain is defined as a sensory or emotional experience. Adult humans can express their individual level and significance of pain. In nonverbal humans and animals, behavioral assessment tends to be the best indicator of pain.[18-20] However, with more than 8000 different reptile species identified that exhibit a wide range of unique physiological and behavioral adaptations, it is exceedingly difficult to assess behavioral changes in these animals. This makes the identification of behavioral alterations that may be associated with pain particularly difficult. Recognition of abnormal behavior in reptiles requires careful, often time-consuming observation, and changes may be subtle. An approach similar to pain assessment in other veterinary species can be adapted for use in reptiles (Box 25-1). If possible, it is probably best to observe reptiles remotely (using a remote camera) because evidence indicates that reptiles may suppress some pain behaviors when an

---

BOX 25-1

An Approach to Pain Assessment in Reptiles

A. Behavior

Species Considerations

Requires proper species identification and familiarity with species-specific behaviors. Basic species differences affect behavioral patterns, and these are important when attempting to differentiate normal from abnormal behaviors.

- Predominant activity pattern (diurnal, nocturnal)
- Predated or predator species
- Habitat (arboreal, aquatic, terrestrial, fossorial)

Individual Patient Considerations

- Stage of ecdysis
  - Some may become more aggressive during this time.
- Hibernation status
  - Hibernating animals or those inclined to hibernate may be more docile and less responsive than normal.
- Socialization
  - Altered response to human interaction (normally docile animal to biting) occurs; poor response to caregiver occurs.
- Concurrent illness
  - Patient may be incapable of exhibiting behaviors associated with pain, or behaviors associated with disease may be mistaken for pain behaviors.
- Owner assessment
  - Owners are often more familiar with their animal's normal behavior; however, owners may also be biased based on their own understanding and belief regarding their animal's conditions.

Environmental Considerations

- Enclosure
  - Home enclosures often more "interesting" compared with hospital enclosures, providing animal with plenty of opportunity to exhibit normal behaviors.
- Preferred optimal body temperature
  - Ambient environmental temperature is one of the main determinants of metabolic rate in resting reptiles, and consequently normal behavior may influenced by alterations in metabolic rate.
- Observer
  - Good evidence that reptiles may suppress behaviors and activity that may be associated with pain in the presence of an observer (i.e., may not withdraw from painful stimulus)

Locomotor Activity

- Posture
  - Hunched, guarding of affected body area, not resting in normal posture
- Gait
  - Must differentiate neurologic and mechanical dysfunction from pain-induced lameness
- Other
  - Excessive scratching or flicking foot, tail, or affected area
  - Unwillingness to perform normal movements (look up, step up, thrash with tail)
  - Exaggerated flight response

— Continued

BOX 25-1

An Approach to Pain Assessment in Reptiles—*cont'd*

Miscellaneous
- Appetite
  - Reduced appetite may be related to underlying disease but may also be related to pain.
- Eyes
  - Eyelids may be held closed when animal is painful or ill.
- Color change
  - Species capable of color change may do so in response to stress and/or pain.
- Abnormal respiratory movements
  - Respirations may be associated with primary respiratory disease but also pain affecting the muscles and tissues involved in respiration.

B. Anticipated Level of Pain
The anticipated level of pain is commonly used to evaluate pain in reptiles and is based on the likelihood and severity of tissue trauma associated with a particular procedure or condition. This is a well-accepted approach in veterinary medicine, particularly when dealing with less familiar species.[41] However, in addition to significant species differences, significant individual differences in response to therapy and response to tissue trauma can be seen.

C. Physiological Data
Most physiological parameters have been shown to be poor indicators of pain in most species. Physiological parameters can be influenced by disease and excitement. In addition, the physiological parameters of reptiles may be influenced by a number of metabolic processes, such as activity level, temperature alterations, and feeding.

D. Response to Palpation
In some species a negative response to palpation can be a useful indicator of pain. However, in reptiles this may be less sensitive because most reptiles withdraw from touch regardless of whether the animal is experiencing pain.

---

observer is present.[21] This behavior may be a protective response similar to that seen in some reptiles subjected to brief physical restraint[4] and is likely a normal protective behavioral response to a perceived threat, similar to that found in many other vertebrate species.[22] In a survey of reptile veterinarians, it was found that the anticipated level of pain extrapolated from other species (76%), behavioral changes (66%), anticipated level of pain based on prior experience in reptiles (57%), and physiological changes (32%) were commonly used to evaluate pain in reptiles.[13]

Pain assessment in reptiles is challenging and requires a good understanding of normal reptile behavior, physiology, and unique species-specific adaptations. An approach similar to pain assessment in other veterinary species can be adapted for use in reptiles. Remote observation may be required to evaluate pain in reptiles accurately.

ANALGESIC THERAPY IN REPTILES

A carefully designed analgesic plan should include not only the specific analgesic drugs and route of drug administration but also steps to monitor patient response to therapy and address the provision of ongoing supportive patient care.

ROUTE OF DRUG ADMINISTRATION

It is probably important to consider the route of drug administration in reptiles for many reasons, including ease of drug administration, unique anatomic or physiological structures, and variability in drug bioavailability and uptake among various routes of drug administration. Intramuscular drug administration is commonly used in reptiles. Historically, hind limb and tail injection sites have been avoided because of concerns related to the first-pass effect associated with passage of any administered drug through the kidneys via the renal portal system. However, at least in some species, this may be more of a theoretical than practical concern because only a small amount of blood from the hind limbs and tail passes through the kidney,[23,24] whereas in other species a small amount from the hind limbs passes through the renal portal system but a substantial amount of blood from the tail passes through the renal portal system.[25] Regardless, it may be best to avoid hind limb and tail administration of potentially nephrotoxic drugs or those highly metabolized or excreted by the kidneys. Some recent evidence from the green iguana indicates that the bioavailability of intramuscularly administered ketoprofen may be reduced.[26] In addition, time to effect may vary depending on the absorption rate of the drug from the site of deposition. Absorption may be affected by the physiochemical properties of the drug, tissue blood flow, and cardiac output. Oral drug administration may be more desirable for patients who require chronic analgesic therapy, for most become intolerant of repeated intramuscular injections. Oral drug administration can be difficult in some patients, although the use of feeding tubes can greatly simplify and facilitate this process. A more important consideration when contemplating oral drug administration may be the considerable differences in gastrointestinal function among reptile species. Many are strict carnivores (snakes) and may fast for days to months between meals, whereas others are primarily herbivores (turtles, tortoises, and some lizards) and tend to feed more or less continuously. These differences presumably affect the bioavailability and pharmacokinetics of drugs given orally among the different reptile species. However, recently a study in green iguanas found that the bioavailability and pharmacokinetics of meloxicam given orally to be essentially the same as intravenous drug administration.[27] Although intravenous drug administration is not always feasible in reptiles, the combination of good technique, practice, appropriate patient selection, and skilled physical restraint can facilitate predictable venous access. Intravascular injection ensures complete bioavailability of a drug and may avoid the tissue irritation associated with some drugs when given intramuscularly.

Significant pharmacokinetic and pharmacodynamic differences exist between reptiles and mammals, making the extrapolation of drug dosing difficult. When available, species-specific analgesic drug studies in reptiles can provide valuable insight to help guide analgesic therapy. However, critical evaluation is required to interpret the results of these studies accurately.

DRUGS

The three primary classes of analgesic drugs used in reptiles are local anesthetics, nonsteroidal antiinflammatory drugs (NSAIDs), and opioids (Table 25-1).

CLASSES OF ANALGESIC DRUGS COMMONLY USED IN REPTILES ARE THE FOLLOWING:
- Opioids
- Local anesthetics
- Nonsteroidal antiinflammatory drugs

OPIOIDS

It is well documented that reptiles have opioid receptors in the central nervous system and that the proopiomelanocortin system (one of the three molecular systems from which all naturally occurring opioids are derived) is well preserved among vertebrates.[9-12,28,29] The importance of the different opioid receptors in modifying pain perception is far less clear. Opioids are the only class of analgesic drugs that have been assessed for clinical analgesic properties in reptiles. However, each study should be carefully evaluated for the quality of experimental design and strength of its conclusions. Based on recent studies, butorphanol (despite its frequent use) does not appear to produce significant analgesic effects in some reptiles.[8,21,30] However, other studies suggest that butorphanol, at least at some doses, may reduce the intensity of motor reactions in response to an electrical stimulus applied to the tails of green iguanas.[31]

In the same study, buprenorphine (0.02 and 0.04 mg/kg IM) did not significantly alter the motor reaction in response to an electrical stimuli compared with saline. Evidence indicates that morphine may be effective as an analgesic in at least some reptile species.[5,6,8,31] It should be noted that time for onset of action appears to be prolonged (2 to 8 hours) following morphine administration and that the duration of effect may vary considerably among species.[5,6,8] Delayed onset of action may be related to slow receptor binding kinetics or slow absorption from the intramuscular or subcutaneous injection site. Opioids appear to be safe for use in reptiles, producing no discernible alterations in heart rate and behavior (sedation or excitement), but they do cause significant respiratory depression in some species.[8]

LOCAL ANESTHETICS

Local anesthetics act by interrupting transmission of sensory and motor neurons. In reptiles, local anesthetics are commonly used to facilitate minor surgical interventions, but they can also be used as analgesics. Recently, a technique has been described to block the mandibular nerve in crocodilians.[32] The limited duration of analgesic effect and accompanying motor paralysis associated with local anesthetics limit their use primarily to the immediate perioperative period or when hospitalized. Local anesthetic toxicity can be avoided by careful attention to total dose of local anesthetic administered to a patient. It must be kept in mind that many reptile patients are very small, and large doses can be administered accidentally. In general, the toxic doses of local anesthetics in mammals (dogs) should not be exceeded: for example, lidocaine (toxic dose 10 to 22 mg/kg) and bupivacaine (toxic dose 5 mg/kg).[33] Additionally, excessive dilution of local anesthetics may decrease their efficacy. Dilution of commercially available concentrations of local anesthetics should probably not exceed 50% on a per volume basis. A 1% lidocaine solution is available commercially and may be preferred for use in patients at greater risk for local anesthetic toxicity (i.e., small patients).

NONSTEROIDAL ANTIINFLAMMATORY DRUGS

The role of cyclooxygenase in the pathophysiology of pain and inflammation of reptiles has not been studied. However, reported clinical experience strongly supports the efficacy of NSAIDs in reptiles, and they continue to be popular. Recent studies examining the pharmacokinetics of meloxicam in the green iguana showed

TABLE 25-1 Dosages of Drugs with Potential Analgesic Effects in Reptiles

Drug	Route	Dosage	Comments	References
Butorphanol*	IM	1-8 mg/kg	May not be effective as an analgesic in reptiles	8, 30, 31
Buprenorphine*	IM, IV, SC	0.4-1.0 mg/kg	May not be effective as an analgesic in reptiles	31
Morphine	IC, IM	0.05-4.0 mg/kg (crocodiles) 1.5-6.5 mg/kg (turtles) 1.0 mg/kg (green iguanas)	Ceiling effect seen at 0.3 mg/kg in Nile crocodiles (*Crocodylus niloticus africana*) Duration of action may persist for up to 24 hours in turtles	5, 6, 8, 31
Meperidine	IC	1-4 mg/kg	Ceiling effect seen at 2 mg/kg in Nile crocodiles (*C. niloticus africana*)	6
Ketamine	IM, IV, SC	10-100 mg/kg	High doses are associated with anesthesia Low doses <10 mg/kg likely associated with analgesia without sedation	34, 35
Xylazine*	IM	1-1.25 mg/kg		38
Medetomidine	IM, IV, IO	50-100 µg/kg (tortoises) 150-300 µg/kg (aquatic) 150 µg/kg (snakes and lizards)	Lower doses may be effective for analgesia	36, 37, 39, 41

Meloxicam	IM, IV, PO	0.1-0.2 mg/kg q24-48h†	Bioavailability and pharmacokinetics for oral and intravenous administration in green iguanas (Iguana iguana)	27, 42
Carprofen*	IM, IV, SC	2-4 mg/kg followed by 1-2 mg/kg q24-72h†		42
Ketoprofen	IM, SC	2 mg/kg q24-48h†		26, 42
Flunixin meglumine*	IM	0.1-0.5 mg/kg q24-48h†		42
Lidocaine (2%)*	Local infiltration	Toxic dose unknown; recommend <5 mg/kg	Dilute to 0.5% to increase volume	42
Bupivacaine (0.5%)*	Local infiltration	Toxic dose unknown; recommend <2 mg/kg	Dilute to 0.25% to increase volume	42

IC, Intracoelomic; *IO*, intraosseous.

*Doses not determined experimentally; extrapolated or anecdotal.

†Repeat dosing pharmacokinetics has not been studied and is based on extrapolation.

excellent bioavailability of this drug given orally.[27] There is also some evidence of enterohepatic or possibly urinary resorption of meloxicam. The results suggest that plasma levels associated with analgesia are maintained for 24 hours after a single dose. However, it should be noted that plasma levels of NSAIDs do not always correspond to their clinical effect, and thus it is difficult to recommend effective and safe dosing intervals. A pilot examination of the pharmacokinetics of ketoprofen administered intravenously and intramuscularly in green iguanas has also been completed and revealed that bioavailability (78%) was decreased when ketoprofen was administered intramuscularly and that terminal half-life was greater than that in comparable studies in dogs.[26] Again this may suggest that dosing intervals in reptiles should be greater compared with mammals. This recommendation is routinely followed for other drugs in reptiles, especially those associated with significant toxicity. Limited toxicity studies involving meloxicam were not associated with any clinically apparent abnormalities, nor were there any histopathologic lesions that could be associated with toxicity present at necropsy. However, mild biochemical and hematologic abnormalities were noted that could not be clearly explained.[27] Thus, until further studies in reptiles become available, it is probably still best to consider the possibility that side effects similar to those seen in mammals (gastrointestinal irritation, renal compromise, platelet inhibition) may occur in reptiles. Therefore, hydration status, concurrent medications (steroids), presence of coagulopathy, gastrointestinal disease, and renal disease should be addressed before administering these drugs.

OTHER DRUGS

Ketamine administered at subanesthetic doses is being used as an analgesic in many mammalian species, but its analgesic potential in reptiles has not been studied. Ketamine alone and used at anesthetic doses is associated with hypertension, tachycardia, bradypnea, and hypoventilation.[35-37] Ketamine may be a useful analgesic adjunct in select cases. The α_2-agonists produce analgesia, sedation, and muscle relaxation in mammals. The analgesic effects of α_2-agonists have not been evaluated in reptiles, but clinical impressions suggest that they may be capable of producing an analgesic effect. Medetomidine induces cardiopulmonary effects in reptiles similar to those seen in mammals: bradycardia, hypertension, and a reduction in arterial oxygen partial pressures.[36,37,39,40] Other analgesic drugs and adjuncts such as tramadol, gabapentin, amantadine, the tricyclic antidepressants, and various forms of nutraceutical and physical therapy have not been explored in reptiles but may have a role to play as our understanding of nociception, pain, and analgesic treatments in reptiles increases.

CONCLUSION

Reptiles are a unique and diverse class of animals that have developed distinctive mechanisms not found in most other animals for managing alterations in body temperature and metabolic rate. An approach to pain management based on current understanding of reptile physiology, nociception, pain, and analgesia represents a generalized approach to pain management in this class of animals. As our knowledge and understanding increase, it is likely that our approach to pain management in this class of animals will also be modified and refined to address reptile pain more specifically. New information should be evaluated objectively and without the influence of personal bias or beliefs. Reptiles are likely to have evolved unique mechanisms for managing pain and avoiding the negative consequences associated with pain that we do not yet completely understand.

REFERENCES

1. Liang YF, Terashima S: Physiological properties and morphological characteristics of cutaneous and mucosal mechanical nociceptive neurons with A-delta peripheral axons in the trigeminal ganglia of crotaline snakes, *J Comp Neurol* 328:88-102, 1993.
2. Stoskopf MK: Pain and analgesia in birds, reptiles, amphibians, and fish, *Invest Ophthalmol Vis Sci* 35:775-780, 1994.
3. Gans C, Gaunt AS: Muscle architecture and control demands, *Brain Behav Evol* 40:70-81, 1992.
4. Mauk MD, Olson RD, LaHoste GJ et al: Tonic immobility produces hyperalgesia and antagonizes morphine analgesia, *Science* 213:353-354, 1981.
5. Kanui TI, Hole K, Miaron JO: Nociception in crocodiles: capsaicin instillation, formalin and hot plate tests, *Zoological Science* 7:537-540, 1990.
6. Kanui TI, Hole K: Morphine and pethidine antinociception in the crocodile, *J Vet Pharmacol Ther* 15:101-103, 1992.
7. ten Donkelaar HJ, de Boer-van Huizen R: A possible pain control system in a non-mammalian vertebrate (a lizard, *Gekko gecko*), *Neurosci Lett* 83:65-70, 1987.
8. Sladky KK, Miletic V, Paul-Murphy J, et al: Analgesic efficacy and respiratory effects of butorphanol and morphine in turtles. *J Am Net Med Assoc* 230:1356-1362, 2007.
9. de la Iglesia JA, Martinez-Guijarro FI, Lopez-Garcia C: Neurons of the medial cortex outer plexiform layer of the lizard *Podarcis hispanica*: Golgi and immunocytochemical studies, *J Comp Neurol* 341:184-203, 1994.

10. Reiner A: The distribution of proenkephalin-derived peptides in the central nervous system of turtles, *J Comp Neurol* 259:65-91, 1987.

11. Lindberg I, White L: Reptilian enkephalins: implications for the evolution of proenkephalin, *Arch Biochem Biophys* 245:1-7, 1986.

12. Ng TB, Hon WK, Cheng CH et al: Evidence for the presence of adrenocorticotropic and opiate-like hormones in the brains of two sea snakes, *Hydrophis cyanocinctus* and *Lapemis hardwickii, Gen Comp Endocrinol* 63:31-37, 1986.

13. Read MR: Evaluation of the use of anesthesia and analgesia in reptiles, *J Am Vet Med Assoc* 224:547-552, 2004.

14. Kona-Boun JJ, Silim A, Troncy E: Immunologic aspects of veterinary anesthesia and analgesia, *J Am Vet Med Assoc* 226:355-363, 2005.

15. Muir WW: Pain and stress. In Gaynor J, Muir WW, editors: *Handbook of veterinary pain management*, St Louis, 2002, Mosby.

16. Lascelles BD, Waterman AE, Cripps PJ et al: Central sensitization as a result of surgical pain: investigation of the pre-emptive value of pethidine for ovariohysterectomy in the rat, *Pain* 62:201-212, 1995.

17. Woolf CJ, Chong MS: Preemptive analgesia: treating postoperative pain by preventing the establishment of central sensitization, *Anesth Analg* 77: 362-379, 1993.

18. Holton L, Reid J, Scott EM et al: Development of a behaviour-based scale to measure acute pain in dogs, *Vet Rec* 148:525-531, 2001.

19. Pritchett LC, Ulibarri C, Roberts MC et al: Identification of potential physiological and behavioural indicators of post-operative pain in horses after exploratory celiotomy for colic, *Applied Animal Behaviour Science* 80:31-43, 2003.

20. van Dijk M, de Boer JB, Koot HM et al: The association between physiological and behavioral pain measures in 0- to 3-year-old infants after major surgery, *J Pain Symptom Manage* 22:600-609, 2001.

21. Fleming GJ, Robertson S: Use of thermal threshold response to evaluate the antinociceptive effects of butorphanol in juvenile green iguanas *(Iguana iguana)*, Tampa, Fla, 2006, American Association of Zoo Veterinarians.

22. Porro CA, Carli G: Immobilization and restraint effects on pain reactions in animals, *Pain* 32:289-307, 1988.

23. Holz P, Barker IK, Burger JP et al: The effect of the renal portal system on pharmacokinetic parameters in the red-eared slider *(Trachemys scripta elegans)*, *J Zoo Wildl Med* 28:386-393, 1997.

24. Holz P, Barker IK, Crawshaw GJ et al: The anatomy and perfusion of the renal portal system in the red-eared slider *(Trachemys scripta elegans)*, *J Zoo Wildl Med* 28:378-385, 1997.

25. Benson KG, Forrest L: Characterization of the renal portal system of the common green iguana *(Iguana iguana)* by digital subtraction imaging, *J Zoo Wildl Med* 30:235-241, 1999.

26. Tuttle AD, Papich M, Lewbart GA et al: Pharmacokinetics of ketoprofen in the green iguana *(Iguana iguana)* following single intravenous and intramuscular injections, *J Zoo Wildl Med* 37:567-570, 2006.

27. Hernandez-Divers SJ, McBride M, Koch T, et al: Single-dose oral and intravenous pharmacokinetics of meloxicam in the green iguana *(Iguana iguana)*. Naples, Fla, 2004, Association of Reptilian and Amphibian Veterinarians.

28. Zagon IS, Sassani JW, Allison G et al: Conserved expression of the opioid growth factor, [Met5]enkephalin, and the zeta (zeta) opioid receptor in vertebrate cornea, *Brain Res* 671:105-111, 1995.

29. Polzonetti-Magni A, Facchinetti F, Carnevali O et al: Presence and steroidogenetic activity of beta-endorphin in the ovary of the lizard, *Podarcis s. sicula raf, Biol Reprod* 50:1059-1065, 1994.

30. Mosley CA, Dyson D, Smith DA: Minimum alveolar concentration of isoflurane in green iguanas and the effect of butorphanol on minimum alveolar concentration, *J Am Vet Med Assoc* 222:1559-1564, 2003.

31. Greenacre CB, Takle G, Schumacher JP et al: Comparative antinociception of morphine, butorphanol, and buprenorphine versus saline in the green iguana, *Iguana iguana*, using electrostimulation, *J Herp Med Surg* 16:88-92, 2006.

32. Wellehan FX, Gunkel CI, Kledzik D et al: Use of a nerve locator to facilitate administration of mandibular nerve blocks in crocodilians, *J Zoo Wildl Med* 37:405-408, 2006.

33. Liu PL, Feldman HS, Giasi R et al: Comparative CNS toxicity of lidocaine, etidocaine, bupivacaine, and tetracaine in awake dogs following rapid intravenous administration, *Anesth Analg* 62:375-379, 1983.

34. Custer RS, Bush M: Physiologic and acid-base measures of gopher snakes during ketamine or halothane-nitrous oxide anesthesia, *J Am Vet Med Assoc* 177:870-874, 1980.

35. Schumacher J, Lillywhite HB, Norman WM et al: Effects of ketamine HCl on cardiopulmonary function in snakes, *Copeia* pp 395-400, 1997.

36. Sleeman JM, Gaynor J: Sedative and cardiopulmonary effects of medetomidine and reversal with atipamezole in desert tortoises *(Gopherus agassizii)*, *J Zoo Wildl Med* 31:28-35, 2000.

37. Dennis PM, Heard DJ: Cardiopulmonary effects of a medetomidine-ketamine combination administered intravenously in gopher tortoises, *J Am Vet Med Assoc* 220:1516-1519, 2002.

38. Bennett RA: Reptile anesthesia, *Semin Avian Exotic Pet Med* 7:30-40, 1998.

39. Greer LL, Jenne KJ, Diggs HE: Medetomidine-ketamine anesthesia in red-eared slider turtles *(Trachemys scripta elegans)*, *Contemp Top Lab Anim Sci* 40:9-11, 2001.

40. Chittick EJ, Stamper MA, Beasley JF, et al: Medetomidine, ketamine, and sevoflurane for anesthesia of injured loggerhead sea turtles: 13 cases (1996-2000), *J Am Vet Med Assoc* 221:1019-1025, 2002.

41. Lock BA, Heard DJ, Dennis P: Preliminary evaluation of medetomidine/ketamine combinations for immobilization and reversal with atipamezole in three tortoise species, *Bull Assoc Reptil Amphib Vet* 8:6-9, 1998.

42. Funk R: Reptile formulary. In Mader D, editor: *Reptile medicine and surgery*, ed 2, St Louis, 2006, Saunders Elsevier.

26 CLINICAL APPROACH TO ANALGESIA IN FERRETS AND RABBITS

MATTHEW JOHNSTON

O ver the past 10 to 15 years, the standard of care for treatment of small and exotic mammals has been steadily increasing. During this same period, there has been a growing surge of interest and research in the field of veterinary pain management. Unfortunately, however, only a limited number of publications relate to analgesia in pet small mammals such as rabbits and ferrets. Most of the literature dealing with pain in rabbits and ferrets relates to these animals as laboratory specimens, and focus on pets has been mostly overlooked. No doubt, however, rabbit and ferret ownership continues to increase, and it follows that more and more often, veterinarians are being asked to provide these animals with the same quality of care given to more traditional pets.

Several excellent reviews have been written on analgesia in small mammals,[1-3] but none of these reviews focus especially on rabbits and ferrets, and none are written from the standpoint of these animals as pet species. The goal of this chapter is to focus on a practical, clinical approach to pain management in ferrets and rabbits. It should be understood that because of the shortage of published studies relating to analgesia in these two species, the author is drawing from his own clinical experience and extrapolating from what is known in other species. Whenever possible, reference is made to published information.

RECOGNITION OF PAIN

In some circumstances, it is not difficult to recognize when a rabbit or ferret is in pain. Stimuli that cause pain in other animals such as surgery or tissue trauma should be assumed also to cause pain in these species. Though

Adapted from Johnston MS: Clinical approaches to analgesia in ferrets and rabbits, *Seminars in Avian and Exotic Pet Medicine: Anesthesia and Analgesia,* 14(4): 299-335, 2005.

this concept seems simple, in a survey of British veterinarians published in 1999, only 22% of veterinarians administered some form of analgesia perioperatively to small mammals. Additionally in this survey, veterinary surgeons were more likely to administer analgesics to rabbits than to ferrets.[4] Though surgical pain should be easy to identify, some stimuli that cause pain in ferrets and rabbits are more difficult to recognize, and an understanding of these species' unique physiology and behaviors is important.

Stimuli that are known to cause pain in other species should be assumed to also cause pain in ferrets and rabbits.

Ferrets and rabbits could not be any more different from a physiological and behavioral standpoint. Ferrets are strict carnivores and predators that generally have a boisterous and gregarious demeanor, even when in an unfamiliar environment such as a veterinary hospital. Rabbits, however, are strictly herbivorous prey animals that are generally quiet and reserved and can be anxious when in unfamiliar territory. Observations of normal ferrets and rabbits help the practitioner gain insight into behaviors associated with pain. Some behaviors are not specific for pain but could be associated with an underlying disease process, so the patient's entire clinical picture should be taken into account when assessing pain.

Painful ferrets may prefer to stay curled into a ball and exhibit aggressive biting behavior or teeth-bearing when disturbed. Additionally, ferrets with visceral pain may have a decreased appetite and exhibit bruxism when presented with food. A hunched abdominal posture as seen in Fig. 26-1 is common in ferrets after laparotomy incisions when pain management is not adequate. Uncomfortable ferrets may shiver despite a normal body temperature. Other signs of pain in ferrets include a bristle tail, when the fur on the tail stands on end, resembling a pipe cleaner; eyelids that are held half-closed; focal muscle fasciculations; high-pitched vocalization or grunting when handled; lameness; and general disinterest in the surroundings.

Signs of pain in ferrets include the following:
- Immobility
- Bruxism
- Shivering
- "Bottle brush" tail

In rabbits, the most easily identifiable sign of pain is anorexia. Rabbits are normally grazing animals that eat continuously, and when painful, this grazing behavior ceases. Painful rabbits also grind their teeth, especially when visceral or dental pain is present. Though most painful rabbits choose to sit motionless in a far corner of a cage, some rabbits may have fits of rapid

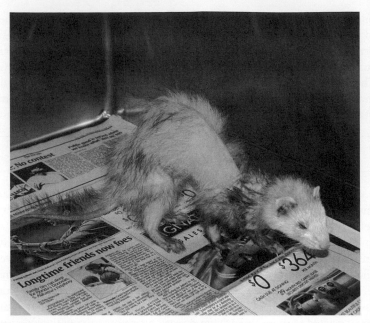

FIG. 26-1. Exhibition of abdominal pain in a ferret following laparotomy for a left adrenalectomy. Note the hunched posture and tucked abdomen characteristic of this species when experiencing moderate to severe abdominal pain.

and uncontrolled locomotion when handled. Painful rabbits may vocalize or exhibit a decreased respiratory rate characterized by a pronounced nasal flare and deep breathing pattern. Rabbits normally have a very rapid respiratory pattern characterized by short, shallow breaths. The painful rabbit may appear unkempt because of a lack of grooming behavior and may avoid rearing up on its hind legs to accept treat items. Epiphora and serous nasal discharge are sometimes present in rabbits that are in severe acute pain.

Signs of pain in rabbits include the following:
- Anorexia
- Bruxism
- Nasal flaring
- Immobility

ACUTE AND CHRONIC PAIN

As is true in most traditional pets, in general, it is easier to recognize the signs of acute pain in ferrets and rabbits. However, besides surgical and traumatic pain, there are several medical conditions that lead to acute pain that are often overlooked. Analgesic management should be part of the therapeutic plan for any medical condition that causes acute pain. For example, otitis interna is an acute infectious/inflammatory medical condition that is common in rabbits. This condition is likely painful based on the degree and extent of inflammation that is present within the ears, as well as the orthopedic postural abnormalities that result from the severe torticollis; furthermore, most rabbits with the condition are anorectic. However, many practitioners skip pain management in the treatment of this condition. At our hospital, we have found that rabbits with this condition benefit clinically from the administration of analgesic drugs, specifically nonsteroidal antiinflammatory drugs. In rabbits, ileus leads to gastric and cecal dilation, which activates nociceptive fibers associated with the stretch receptors in the gastrointestinal tract. A similar pain pathophysiology occurs in ferrets with gastrointestinal foreign bodies or trichobezoars. Both conditions lead to acute pain, but in many instances, analgesia is not part of the veterinarian's initial treatment regimen. Experimentally in rabbits, several opioids were shown to decrease painful behaviors following colorectal distention,[5] suggesting that this class of drugs may be useful for managing pain during these clinical presentations. Clinically, at our hospital, we have found that constant rate infusions of butorphanol (rabbits) or fentanyl (ferrets) can reduce the outward signs of pain associated with these gastrointestinal problems.

Conditions that lead to chronic pain are often harder to recognize in ferrets and rabbits. A thorough history from the caretaker that suggests changes in behavior may hint at chronically painful conditions. Neoplasia, arthritis, and dental problems are three common causes of chronic pain in ferrets and rabbits. Though some of these conditions cannot be cured, the quality of life of the pet can be greatly increased when analgesia is used to help manage these conditions. Often, simple corrections of husbandry can lead to alleviation of the pain, and pharmacologic intervention is not always necessary. For example, geriatric rabbits with stifle and coxofemoral arthritis may benefit from a heavily bedded cage, whereas ferrets with chronic periodontitis may be kept comfortable by feeding of a softened food.

PREVENTION OF PAIN

Several modalities may help prevent the cascade of factors that lead to pain. Gentle surgical technique leads to a reduction in inflammation and subsequent pain postoperatively. Crushing and pulling of tissues activates Aδ and C-nociceptive fibers, which are not immediately recognized by the central nervous system when the animal is anesthetized. However, these noxious stimuli lead to central nervous system changes that are exhibited as painful behaviors upon recovery from anesthesia.[6]

Known in humans and assumed to be true in animals is that memory of a painful stimulus correlates strongly with the maximal intensity of pain. Therefore, if therapy can intervene and prevent central stimulation, the intensity of pain should be reduced. This concept is the basis for preemptive analgesia, or administration of antinociceptive drugs before the noxious stimulus in order to improve postoperative analgesia.[6] Preemptive analgesia should be a part of the anesthetic regimen for all rabbits and ferrets undergoing procedures that may lead to pain postoperatively.

Preemptive analgesia such as opioid premedicants and preincisional line blocks with local anesthetics are simple and highly effective means of reducing or blocking the sensation of pain, making for a more comfortable recovery from surgical procedures in ferrets and rabbits.

ANALGESIC AGENTS AND THEIR APPLICATION IN FERRETS AND RABBITS

Table 26-1 gives dosage information on drugs discussed in the text.

OPIOIDS

The use of opioid drugs remains a mainstay of analgesic therapy, especially when facing situations of moderate to severe acute, postsurgical or traumatic pain. Opioids exert their effects via inhibition of pain transmission in the dorsal horn of the spinal cord, activation of inhibitory pathways from the brain, inhibition of supraspinal afferent nerves, and by causing a decrease in the release of neurotransmitters in the spinal cord.[7] Some examples of opioids commonly used in ferrets and rabbits are butorphanol, buprenorphine, morphine, hydromorphone, oxymorphone, and fentanyl.

The beneficial analgesic effects of opioids in ferrets and rabbits far outweigh the potential for side effects. Side effects can be minimized in certain situations by using opioids epidurally or as constant rate infusions.

Some practitioners have been wary of using this class of drugs because of its potential for adverse side effects such as sedation, respiratory depression, and ileus. However, the beneficial analgesic properties of

TABLE 26-1	Doses of Analgesic Drugs for Ferrets and Rabbits	
Drug	**Ferret**	**Rabbit**
Butorphanol	0.1-0.4 mg/kg q2-4h IV, IM, or SC 0.1-0.2 mg/kg per hour IV CRI*	0.5 mg/kg q2-4h IV or SC 0.1-0.3 mg/kg per hour IV CRI*
Buprenorphine	0.01-0.03 mg/kg q6-10h IV, SC, or transmucosally†	0.01-0.05 mg/kg q6-10h IV or SC
Morphine	0.2-2 mg/kg IM single dose preoperatively 0.1 mg/kg epidurally	0.5-5 mg/kg IM single dose preoperatively 0.1 mg/kg epidurally
Hydromorphone	0.1-0.2 mg/kg IV, IM, or SC q6-8h 0.005-0.015 mg/kg per hour IV CRI*	0.05-0.2 mg/kg IV, IM, or SC q6-8h
Oxymorphone	0.05-0.2 mg/kg IV, IM or SC q6-8h	0.05-0.2 mg/kg IV, IM or SC q6-8h
Fentanyl	20-30 μg/kg per hour IV CRI* during anesthesia to reduce volatile inhalant concentrations 1-4 μg/kg per hour IV CRI* for analgesia	20-30 μg/kg per hour IV CRI* during anesthesia to reduce volatile inhalant concentrations‡ 1-4 μg/kg per hour IV CRI* for analgesia‡ 25 μg/h transcutaneous patch‡
Meloxicam	0.1-0.2 mg/kg SC or PO q24h	0.1-0.5 mg/kg SC or PO q12-24h
Lidocaine	<2 mg/kg SC 4.4 mg/kg epidurally	<2 mg/kg SC
Bupivacaine	<1.5 mg/kg SC 1.1 mg/kg epidurally	<1.5 mg/kg SC
Ketamine (analgesic)	0.5 mg/kg IV before surgery 10 μ/kg per minute IV CRI* during surgery 2 μg/kg per minute IV CRI* for 24 hours postoperatively§	0.5 mg/kg IV before surgery 10 μg/kg per minute IV CRI* during surgery 2 μg/kg per minute IV CRI* for 24 hours postoperatively§
Tramadol	5 mg/kg PO q12h	5-10 mg/kg PO q12-24h

Note that many of these dosages are based on clinical experience and extrapolation from other species. The attending veterinarian is responsible to monitor for adverse effects associated with administration of these drugs.

*CRI, Constant rate infusion.

†Administer directly into space between molars and buccal mucosa.

‡May be associated with ileus; generally not recommended.

§Must be combined with an additional analgesic agent such as an opioid to provide adequate analgesia.

these drugs far outweigh the potential adverse effects in the majority of cases. Ferrets seem especially sensitive to the sedative and respiratory depressant effects of opioids, so lower dose ranges and careful monitoring should be used with this species. The ileus-inducing effects of opioids are a major concern for practitioners working on rabbits; however, pain-induced ileus is much more difficult to treat than that brought on by the administration of opioids, so this concern does not justify their exclusion from analgesia protocols. Usually the institution of forced feedings and adequate fluid therapy is enough to counteract the motility-slowing effects of opioids. In addition, because there are several different opioids available to practitioners, in most cases, a relatively safe drug can be found.

Opioids are classified as mixed agonist-antagonists, pure agonists, and pure antagonists. Pure antagonists are not discussed in this chapter because they are used primarily to reverse the effects of the other two classes and by themselves have no analgesic properties. Three different classes of opioid receptors are recognized: μ, κ, δ. The μ receptors are further broken down into μ-1, μ-2, and μ-3 subgroups. In mammals, μ-1 and κ receptors are the primary receptors responsible for analgesia.[7]

The most commonly used mixed agonist-antagonists are butorphanol and buprenorphine. Butorphanol has agonist effects mainly at κ-receptors, with minimal to no μ effects, hence its classification as a μ-antagonist.[7] Pharmacokinetic data are available for rabbits for this drug and suggest that a 0.5-mg/kg dose intravenously results in a half-life of elimination of just over 1½ hours. The same dose given subcutaneously resulted in an elimination half-life of just over 3 hours.[8] No pharmacologic studies are available for this drug in ferrets. Butorphanol is suitable for mild-moderate pain in rabbits because of its κ effects, but the frequency of administration makes it impractical for many situations. However, butorphanol can be given as an intravenous constant rate infusion (CRI) to counteract the need for frequent dosing. As mentioned before, this method of administration is especially good at addressing visceral pain associated with gastrointestinal disorders. In ferrets, butorphanol is mainly used for its sedative effects because the analgesic effects seem limited in this species.

Buprenorphine is classified as a partial μ-agonist and κ-antagonist. Buprenorphine binds strongly to the μ-receptors, and because of this, buprenorphine can be difficult to reverse.[7] Buprenorphine, like butorphanol, is suitable for management of mild to moderate pain. Unlike butorphanol, the analgesic effects of buprenorphine seem to last longer, though no pharmacologic data are available in ferrets or rabbits. Clinically, analgesic effects seem to persist for 6 to 10 hours in both species following subcutaneous administration. However, one study demonstrated that behavior attributed to pain in rabbits was not diminished after administration of buprenorphine.[9] In addition, buprenorphine has been shown to have transmucosal absorption in cats,[10] and this route is used with clinical success in ferrets. Because transmucosal absorption of buprenorphine depends on the pH of the saliva, it would make sense that animals with similar digestive physiology (cats and ferrets) should respond similarly, though no studies have been done to back up this assumption.

Morphine is considered the prototype opioid to which all other opioids are compared. Morphine has the added benefit of being inexpensive, hence its use as the primary opioid in most veterinary practices.[7] Because of its rather large array of side effects, especially respiratory depression in ferrets and induction of ileus in rabbits, repeated systemic dosing of morphine is rarely performed. Morphine is used commonly as a one-time premedication before noxious stimulus to provide preemptive analgesia. However, epidurally administered morphine can be an excellent analgesic technique for abdominal and hind limb procedures in both species. In ferrets and rabbits, epidural or spinal morphine administration is known to attenuate postoperative pain responses.[11,12] For more complete analgesia, a local anesthetic such as lidocaine or bupivacaine may be combined with the morphine and administered epidurally. The analgesic effects of epidurally administered morphine last approximately 12 to 24 hours, and the adverse effects noted before are virtually eliminated.

The procedure for lumbosacral epidural puncture in ferrets and rabbits is similar to that described for dogs and cats,[13] except that there is rarely a definitive "popping" feel when the epidural space is entered. Landmarks used for lumbosacral epidural puncture in both species are the wings of the ileum and the dorsal prominence of the first sacral vertebra. The three landmarks form a triangle, and the lumbosacral space is in the center of this triangle, directly on midline. Epidural puncture can be performed with the ferret or rabbit in ventral recumbency or in lateral recumbency. In both positions the coxofemoral and lumbosacral joints should be hyperflexed to help open up the space (Fig. 26-2). It should be noted that in rabbits, the spinal cord continues caudally into the sacral vertebrae, so the potential for accidental spinal puncture during lumbosacral epidural injection is higher.[14] If cerebrospinal fluid is seen in the hub of the needle during epidural puncture, half of the volume of drug should be administered because the drug will be confined to the subarachnoid space and may distribute further cranially.

Hydromorphone and oxymorphone are similar drugs and so are discussed together. Currently, hydromorphone is significantly less

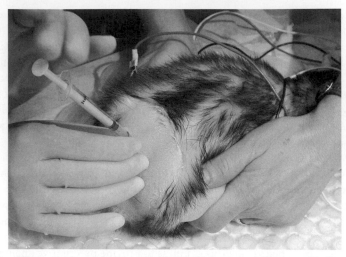

FIG. 26-2. Epidural injection in a ferret. Note the positioning with the hind legs flexed at the coxofemoral joint to allow maximal opening of the lumbosacral space, located by palpation of the wings of the ileum and the dorsal prominence of the first sacral vertebra.

expensive than oxymorphone and so is used more frequently in veterinary practice. The analgesic effects of both drugs are similar to morphine, but both have the advantage of decreased adverse side effects.[7] Both drugs have been used extensively by the author in ferrets and rabbits, with minimal adverse side effects. No data are available for either drug in either species short of anecdotal clinical reports. Hydromorphone and oxymorphone can be used as premedications to provide preemptive analgesia, postoperatively to manage moderate to severe pain, or as primary analgesics following trauma or painful medical conditions. In ferrets, both drugs cause profound sedation, making assessment of their analgesic properties difficult. In ferrets and rabbits, subcutaneous injection seems to provide approximately 6 hours of analgesia. In ferrets the sedative effects of the hydromorphone seem attenuated when it is used as an intravenous CRI along with ketamine.

Fentanyl is a very short-acting pure μ-agonist with analgesic effects similar to morphine. The effects of fentanyl last less than 30 minutes after a single intravenous injection.[7] Fentanyl is used commonly in ferrets intraoperatively as a CRI to decrease volatile inhalant anesthetic concentrations and as a CRI to provide analgesia for moderate to severe pain. A fentanyl CRI is the most commonly used analgesic modality for ferrets in the immediate postoperative period at our hospital. Fentanyl is also available as a transdermal patch, the use of which has been evaluated in rabbits. Though this study reported therapeutic blood concentration using a 25-µg/h patch in rabbits, it also reported a loss in body weight of the fentanyl-treated rabbits.[15] This observation correlates with the author's experience with fentanyl in rabbits, whether administered transcutaneously or intravenously. Rabbits administered fentanyl seem to have a severely decreased appetite, and management of ileus associated with fentanyl can be difficult. For this reason, fentanyl is used sparingly in rabbits at our hospital.

NONSTEROIDAL ANTIINFLAMMATORY DRUGS

Nonsteroidal antiinflammatory drugs (NSAIDs) as a class share common therapeutic actions, including antiinflammatory, analgesic, and antipyretic effects. This discussion focuses on the analgesic effects. NSAIDs are the most commonly used analgesic drugs in veterinary medicine, owing to the fact that they are effective for acute and chronic pain and have few side effects. NSAIDs exert their analgesic effects via inhibition of the cyclooxygenase enzyme, which thereby decreases tissue inflammation.[16] NSAIDs are contraindicated in ferrets or rabbits that are pregnant, have hepatic or renal dysfunction, are in shock or have other conditions limiting perfusion, or have known gastrointestinal ulceration.

Many NSAIDs have been used in rabbits and ferrets throughout the past 10 to 15 years, but by far the most commonly used NSAID today in these animals is meloxicam. The increased use of meloxicam in ferrets and rabbits is primarily because of its relative safety, ease of administration, and apparent effectiveness. Meloxicam is a cyclooxygenase-2–selective NSAID, which means that clinically its side effects are minimal, though usually gastrointestinal when seen. Meloxicam is available as a palatable liquid 1.5-mg/ml solution (Metacam, Boehringer Ingelheim, St. Joseph, Missouri) that is readily accepted by ferrets and rabbits. Though caution should be used with long-term administration of NSAIDs in ferrets, owing to their apparent sensitivity to certain NSAIDs,[17] it appears that meloxicam is safe to use for short-term administration. Any ferret or rabbit receiving a long-term NSAID regimen should have plasma liver enzymes, blood urea nitrogen, and creatinine monitored periodically to ensure that toxicosis is not occurring. Rabbits seem to tolerate meloxicam especially and NSAIDs generally very well, with minimal adverse effects. Meloxicam has been used in numerous rabbits with chronic painful conditions (dental root overgrowth, arthritis, neoplasia) for long periods at doses higher than that for dogs with apparent clinical efficacy and no changes in plasma biochemistry values or gastrointestinal signs. It is always prudent to use the lowest possible clinically effective dose, however, until further studies on safety and efficacy are performed. One clinical study involving meloxicam in rabbits was performed to assess the isoflurane-sparing effects of meloxicam in rabbits, and the results of this study showed that when used alone, meloxicam was not successful in reducing the minimum alveolar concentration of isoflurane. However, a meloxicam-butorphanol combination had greater isoflurane-sparing effects than butorphanol alone, suggesting that meloxicam indeed has analgesic effects in rabbits.[18] A second study looked at single dose and repeated-dose pharmacokinetics of oral meloxicam administration in rabbits. This study concluded that a dose of greater than 0.3 mg/kg given once daily was necessary to achieve optimal plasma levels over a 24-hour period.[19] This latter study supports the higher dose regimen recommended in Table 26-1.

Meloxicam is a commonly used nonsteroidal antiinflammatory drug (NSAID) in ferrets and rabbits. Rabbits seem particularly resistant to any of the side effects of NSAIDs. Monitoring of gastrointestinal health and for renal and hepatic parameters should be performed on any ferret or rabbit receiving NSAID therapy long term.

LOCAL ANESTHETICS

Local anesthetics such as lidocaine and bupivacaine are also commonly used in veterinary practice. Local anesthetics work to provide regional anesthesia by reversibly blocking the transmission of nociceptive stimulation from nerve endings or fibers. Local anesthetics can be used topically, via direct infiltration into soft tissue containing nerve endings, intraarticularly (not practical in ferrets or rabbits), intravenously, or epidurally.[20] Care must be taken when using these drugs in small patients such as rabbits or ferrets to avoid reaching toxic drug concentrations. When injecting subcutaneously, always aspirate back on the syringe to ensure that the drug is not being accidentally administered intravenously. Practically, for bupivacaine and lidocaine, use less than 1.5 and 2 mg/kg, respectively, of drug to avoid accidental toxicosis. When used epidurally, bupivacaine may lead to motor weakness in the hind limbs for up to 12 hours after injection. This motor weakness can be agitating to rabbits and may lead to increased morbidity postoperatively. For this reason, our hospital uses bupivacaine epidurally in ferrets only. One of the best uses of local anesthetics is as a line block before surgical incisions. For abdominal procedures, a 2½-inch spinal needle with the trocar removed is used to infiltrate the subcutaneous tissue with lidocaine before incision. Care should be taken not to puncture the abdominal wall and viscera accidentally when performing this technique.

KETAMINE

Ketamine is known primarily for its sedative properties. Ketamine is used frequently in ferrets and rabbits as a premedication and has recently been used to augment analgesia by administration of a microdose CRI intraoperatively and postoperatively. Recently, ketamine has been shown to act as preemptive analgesic by inhibiting the N-methyl-D-aspartate (NMDA) receptor in the central nervous system. NMDA stimulation has been shown to increase central nervous system sensitization. Therefore, blockade of this receptor aids in prevention of pain perception.[21] It should be noted that no studies confirm this effect in rabbits or ferrets and that ketamine alone is not an acceptable analgesic in most instances. However, a ketamine CRI may allow a lower dosage of an opioid or other analgesic to be administered.

TRAMADOL

Tramadol has recently become popular in veterinary medicine as an analgesic agent for treatment of mild to severe chronic pain. The popularity of tramadol stems from the fact that it is efficacious in certain circumstances, is not controlled, and is cost-effective. The mechanisms of action of tramadol are not completely understood, but it appears to have opioid-like properties and serotonin and norepinephrine reuptake inhibition.[21] Though evidence of the use of tramadol is limited in clinical applicability for rabbits[22] and is nonexistent for ferrets, tramadol has been used with variable clinical efficacy in both of these species. Doses have been extrapolated for other mammals and applied to rabbits and ferrets. One important consideration when administering tramadol to ferrets and rabbits is its palatability. Tramadol is intensely bitter, and because rabbits and ferrets generally require medications to be compounded into a liquid formulation, a strong flavoring agent is necessary to mask this bitter taste.

REFERENCES

1. Flecknell PA: Analgesia of small mammals, *Vet Clin North Am Exot Anim Pract* 4:47-56, 2001.
2. Flecknell PA: Analgesia in small mammals, *Seminars in Avian and Exotic Pet Medicine* 7:41-47, 1998.
3. Flecknell PA: Pain relief in laboratory animals, *Lab Anim* 18:147, 1984.
4. Lascelles BDX, Capner CA, Waterman-Pearson AE: Current British veterinary attitudes to perioperative analgesia for cats and small mammals, *Vet Rec* 145:601-604, 1999.
5. Borgbjerg FM, Frigast C, Madsen JB et al: The effect of intrathecal opioid-receptor agonists on visceral noxious stimulation in rabbits, *Gastroenterology* 110:139-146, 1996.

6. Muir WW: Physiology and pathophysiology of pain. In Gaynor JS, Muir WW, editors: *Handbook of veterinary pain management*, St Louis, 2002, Mosby.

7. Wagner AE: Opioids. In Gaynor JS, Muir WW, editors: *Handbook of veterinary pain management*, St Louis, 2002, Mosby.

8. Portnoy LG, Hustead DR: Pharmacokinetics of butorphanol tartrate in rabbits, *Am J Vet Res* 53:541-543, 1992.

9. Robinson AJ, Muller WJ, Braid AL et al: The effect of buprenorphine on the course of disease in laboratory rabbits infected with myxoma virus, *Lab Anim* 33:252-257, 1999.

10. Robertson SA, Taylor PM, Sear JW: Systemic uptake of buprenorphine by cats after oral mucosal administration, *Vet Rec* 152:675-678, 2003.

11. Sladky KK, Horne WA, Goodrowe KL et al: Evaluation of epidural morphine for postoperative analgesia in ferrets *(Mustela putorius furo)*, *Contemp Top Lab Anim Sci* 39:33-38, 2000.

12. Kero P, Thomasson B, Soppi AM: Spinal anaesthesia in the rabbit, *Lab Anim* 15:347, 1981.

13. Gaynor JS, Mama KR: Local and regional anesthetic techniques for alleviation of perioperative pain. In Gaynor JS, Muir WW, editors: *Handbook of veterinary pain management*, St Louis, 2002, Mosby.

14. Greenaway JB, Partlow GD, Gonsholt NL et al: Anatomy of the lumbosacral spinal cord of rabbits, *J Am Anim Hosp Assoc* 37:27-34, 2001.

15. Foley PL, Henderson AL, Bissonette EA et al: Evaluation of fentanyl transdermal patches in rabbits: blood concentrations and physiologic response, *Comp Med* 51:239-244, 2001.

16. Budsberg S: Nonsteroidal antiinflammatory drugs. In Gaynor JS, Muir WW, editors: *Handbook of veterinary pain management*, St Louis, 2002, Mosby.

17. Richardson JA, Balabuzsko RA: Ibuprofen ingestion in ferrets: 43 cases, *Journal of Veterinary Emergency and Critical Care* 11:53-39, 2001.

18. Turner PV, Kerr CL, Healy AJ et al: Effect of meloxicam and butorphanol on minimum alveolar concentration of isoflurane in rabbits, *Am J Vet Res* 67:770-774, 2006.

19. Turner PV, Chen HC, Taylor WM: Pharmacokinetics of meloxicam in rabbits after single and repeat oral dosing, *Comp Med* 56:63-67, 2006.

20. Mama KR: Local anesthetics. In Gaynor JS, Muir WW, editors: *Handbook of veterinary pain management*, St Louis, 2002, Mosby.

21. Gaynor JS: Other drugs used to treat pain. In Gaynor JS, Muir WW, editors: *Handbook of veterinary pain management*, St Louis, 2002, Mosby.

22. Küçük A, Kadioglu Y, Celebi F: Investigation of the pharmacokinetics and determination of tramadol in rabbit plasma by a high-performance liquid chromatography-diode array detector method using liquid-liquid extraction, *J Chromatogr B Analyt Technol Biomed Life Sci* 816:203-208, 2005.

27

PHYSICAL THERAPY AND REHABILITATION IN DOGS

DARRYL L. MILLIS

The use of physical modalities in the treatment of acute and chronic pain has received little attention. The focus of pain management has largely relied on the pharmacologic management of pain, with application of these agents in a number of ways. However, there are other modalities that appear to be efficacious in treating pain, alone or in combination with pharmaceuticals. Commonly used physical agents include cryotherapy, thermotherapy, physical rehabilitation and therapeutic exercises, transcutaneous electrical nerve stimulation, low-level laser, massage, pulsed electromagnetic field therapy, static magnet therapy, and extracorporeal shock wave treatment. Although most of these have their greatest application in the management of chronic pain, such as osteoarthritis, some modalities are also useful as adjunctive management of acute pain. This chapter reviews the use of these modalities, evidence for efficacy, indications, contraindications, and application.

In humans, there is limited but positive evidence that some physical modalities are effective in managing chronic pain associated with specific conditions, with the most support for the modality of therapeutic exercise. Different physical modalities have similar magnitudes of effects on chronic pain. The effect on pain by various modalities is generally strongest in the short-term immediately after the intervention, but effects can last as long as 1 year after treatment. Veterinarians applying physical modalities should obtain training that includes the risks and precautions for these modalities. If practitioners lack training in the use of physical modalities, it is important to consult with other health care professionals who have specialized training.

CRYOTHERAPY

Cryotherapy is used to reduce inflammation, pain, and edema, which facilitates improved mobility. Cryotherapy decreases tissue blood flow by causing vasoconstriction and reduces tissue metabolism, oxygen use, and muscle

---

Cryotherapy

Cold aids pain relief. Cryotherapy has effects locally and at the level of the spinal cord via neurologic and vascular mechanisms.

- Cold temporarily numbs the affected area by constricting the blood vessels.
- Cold raises the activation threshold of tissue nociceptors.
- Nerve cooling also increases the duration of the refractory period, the time when a nerve cannot be stimulated by a second impulse.
- Cold reduces the nerve conduction velocity of pain nerves. This effect is thought to be linear until 10° C, when neural transmission is blocked.
- Cold receptors may be overstimulated by cryotherapy, resulting in pain control at the spinal level by preventing pain transmission to higher centers via the spinal gate control theory of pain transmission.
- The result is a local anesthetic effect called cold-induced neuropraxia.
- Cryotherapy may reduce painful reflex muscle spasms.

---

spasm. Treatment with ice provides short-term analgesia and minimizes hematoma formation. Cryotherapy following contusion reduces the number of leukocytes adhering to endothelial cells and should therefore reduce edema.

INDICATIONS FOR CRYOTHERAPY

Cryotherapy is best applied during the acute inflammatory phase of tissue healing and after exercise to minimize any inflammatory response. Cryotherapy is effective in reducing pain, particularly acute postoperative pain. In addition, cryotherapy is effective in reducing edema when combined with compression and elevation. Cold also decreases the metabolic rate of reactions involved in tissue injury and healing. At joint temperatures of 30° C (86° F) or lower, the activity of cartilage-degrading enzymes—including collagenase, elastase, hyaluronidase, and protease—is inhibited.

Precautions and Contraindications for Cryotherapy

- If there is a history of frostbite to the area, further cold application is contraindicated. Observe for signs of frostbite during and after cryotherapy application.
- Caution should be exercised when applying cryotherapy around superficial peripheral nerves because cases of cold-induced nerve palsy of the ulnar and superficial peroneal nerves have been reported in humans.
- Cold should also not be used in patients with generalized or localized vascular compromise or who possess an impaired thermoregulatory capacity.
- Use caution in applying cold over open wounds, areas of poor sensation, or in very young or old dogs.

APPLICATION OF CRYOTHERAPY

Topical cold treatment decreases the temperature of the skin and underlying tissues to a depth of 2 to 4 cm. Techniques for cryotherapy include the application of cold or ice packs, ice bath immersion, and massage with ice over painful areas or acupoints. Cryokinetics combines cryotherapy with motion (passive, active-assisted, or active) to facilitate normal, pain-free movement and to reduce edema through muscle pump action to return lymphatic fluid to the vascular system. The primary benefit of cryokinetics is to facilitate the patient's ability to perform pain-free exercise as long as the level of exercise remains below levels that cause further injury.

To prevent frostbite or cold-induced injuries, it is critical to observe the skin for response to cold. Near the end of a 20-minute treatment, the skin may normally be erythematous, but pale or white skin is an indication that cold-induced tissue damage may be occurring. The range of expected sensations during cryotherapy include an initial sensation of cold, followed by burn, sting, and ache, and finally a numb sensation. Because animal patients cannot describe these sensations, careful observation of the animal's behavioral responses and skin condition every few minutes during the treatment session is critical.

Ice Packs

The simplest method of ice application is to wrap a freezer bag containing crushed ice in a thin damp cloth (such as a pillow case) and apply it directly over the affected area. Another ice pack may be made by combining one-third part isopropyl alcohol and two-thirds part water and placing it in a resealable plastic bag and then in a freezer. The resulting slush more easily conforms to irregular dog extremities (Fig. 27-1). A compression wrap to secure the bag to the body results in more effective tissue cooling. Cold compression units are commercially available and combine compression with cryotherapy. Cold water circulates in a fabricated sleeve that is applied to provide compression to the area. If crushed ice is not available, cold packs may be prepared by mixing three parts water to one part rubbing alcohol and double bagging with sealed bags and placing in a freezer. The resulting slush may then be molded around irregular body parts. To prevent skin damage, apply a towel or cloth to prevent direct contact of the ice pack with the animal's skin. Apply the cryotherapy treatment for 15 to 25 minutes at a time, inspecting the tissue for its response after the first 5 to 10 minutes. Monitor closely for signs of frostbite.

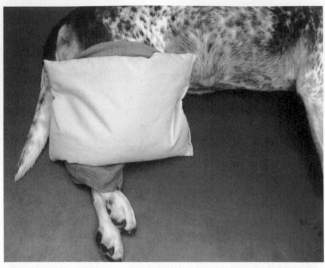

FIG. 27-1. An ice pack may be wrapped in a thin towel before placing it on a dog's limb.

Cold Immersion Baths

Cold immersion results in the greatest decrease in tissue temperature because it exposes the greatest body surface area to cold. The body part is immersed in an ice "slush" bath as part of the immediate first aid following injury. The analgesia from the immersion allows the animal to perform cryokinetics with relative ease.

Ice Massage

Ice massage is a quick and effective method of applying cryotherapy to the affected area with the muscle in a position of gentle stretch. Placing tongue depressors in paper cups filled with water and freezing them is a low-cost method to perform ice massage. Ice massage is applied parallel to the muscle fibers. The pressure from the ice massage stimulates mechanoreceptors more than other forms of cryotherapy. This technique is particularly useful for small, irregular areas. Treatment time is generally 5 to 10 minutes or until the affected area is erythematous and numb.

TREATMENT DURATION AND FREQUENCY

The duration and frequency of cryotherapy depend on the severity of the injury, the area of injury, and the desired outcome. Treatment times may be cycled to 20 to 45 minutes on, followed by an equal amount of

---

Thermotherapy

Heat therapy may reduce pain.
- Heat causes vasodilation, which increases blood flow. This effect may reduce tissue ischemia by supplying oxygen and nutrients while simultaneously removing metabolites that accumulate during tissue damage or exercise.
- Thermoreceptor afferent input may act via the gate control theory of pain control by acting on the dorsal horn of the spinal cord to block transmission of pain to higher pain centers.
- Heat causes general relaxation of painful muscle spasms.
- Heat may also act on muscle spindles and sensory nerve conduction. A decrease in neuronal activity of secondary nerve endings and an increase in activity of primary nerve endings and Golgi tendon organs have been measured following heat application to nerve endings and muscle spindles. This results in a net inhibition of motor neurons, which helps to break the pain-spasm-pain cycle.

---

time off. Practically, cryotherapy is typically administered two to six times daily. Cryotherapy may be applied following an exercise session to minimize reactive swelling and pain.

THERMOTHERAPY

Heat therapy, which can be superficial or deep, is like cryotherapy in that it provides analgesia and decreased muscle tonicity. Unlike cryotherapy, thermotherapy increases tissue temperature, blood flow, metabolism, and connective tissue extensibility; aids muscle relaxation; and reduces stiffness. Because heat increases circulation to the affected area, there is some concern that this may worsen inflammation and edema.

INDICATIONS

Heat therapy is indicated for patients with chronic pain, especially pain due to muscle spasm. Heat is also beneficial for patients where stretching is indicated to help enhance collagen extensibility.

APPLICATION OF HEAT THERAPY

Superficial thermal therapy may be applied using commercially available packs containing cornhusks, gel material that can be used for hot or cold application, or packs containing iron filings (activation of such packs produced heat for several hours following a chemical reaction resulting in oxidation; Fig. 27-2). Commercially available wraps may also be used for heat application by placing heat packs inside the wraps.

Contraindications and Precautions for Superficial Heat Applications

- Superficial heat is contraindicated during acute inflammation because it may exacerbate the inflammatory process, over an area of subcutaneous or cutaneous hemorrhage, if thrombophlebitis is present, or over malignant tissue.
- Superficial heat should be used with caution in patients with poor thermoregulatory capacity, edema, impaired circulation, or over open wounds.
- Dogs should be monitored closely because they cannot verbalize their intolerance.
- A tissue burn may result if the patient is not able to dissipate the heat load via vasodilation or if too much heat (too hot or too long) is applied. Burns can be avoided by using materials that cool as the treatment progresses, increasing the insulation layer between the patient and the hot pack, or limiting the initial temperature increase.
- Caution should be used with products generating high-intensity heat (greater than 45° C), such as with Hydrocollator packs or electric heating pads.
- Monitor the skin condition before, during, and after treatment for any adverse effects.

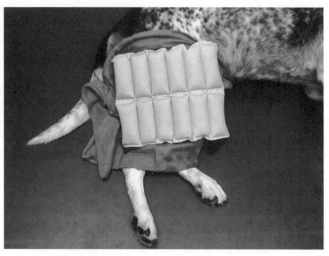

FIG. 27-2. A hot pack applied to a dog.

TREATMENT DURATION AND FREQUENCY

The duration and frequency of thermal treatment depend on the severity of the injury, the stage of tissue healing, the area of the injured part, and the desired outcome. Treatment times may be cycled to 30 to 45 minutes on, followed by an equal amount of time off. Thermal modalities should be applied to support the goal of pain-free function to obtain the best results in the shortest time.

CONTRAST THERMOTHERAPY

Contrast thermotherapy, in which the affected body part is immersed in cold water followed by immersion in hot water, is commonly used in rheumatic conditions and regional pain in humans. Contrast baths induce cyclic vasodilation and vasoconstriction to facilitate flushing debris and inflammatory mediators from the injured area. However, some authors do not agree with this proposed mechanism.

Few research studies have been performed regarding the efficacy of contrast thermotherapy for management of pain, but it is commonly used for sports injuries. Two well-controlled studies have shown that contrast thermotherapy has no effect on muscle tissue temperature.

INDICATIONS AND CONTRAINDICATIONS FOR CONTRAST THERMOTHERAPY

Contrast baths are most appropriate during the early phase of tissue healing, or in cases of chronic edema. Clinically, it may be appropriate to use contrast baths during the transition from acute to subacute injury management. Contrast baths are not indicated in the immediate acute inflammatory phase.

APPLICATION OF CONTRAST BATHS

The body part is immersed in alternating cold and hot baths, in a ratio anywhere from 4 minutes cold, 1 minute hot near the end of the acute phase of inflammation to 2 minutes hot, 2 minutes cold in the chronic phase of injury. This cycle is repeated three to five times for a total of 15 to 30 minutes. If the injury is relatively acute, the final cycle should be in the cold bath to help reduce edema formation and the cold-to-hot ratio should be weighted toward longer times in cold. If contrast baths are used before exercise in subacute or chronic conditions, then the final cycle should be in the hot bath.

PHYSICAL REHABILITATION AND THERAPEUTIC EXERCISES

Active and passive exercise programs have been recommended for treatment of chronic pain, particularly OA. Reduced activity and deconditioning lead to decreased muscle mass and strength, loss of endurance, increased joint stiffness, and loss of cardiovascular fitness.

Exercise treatment in OA is useful to reduce pain and disability. This is achieved through improvement of muscle strength, stability of joints,

ROM, and aerobic fitness. These functions are often impaired in patients with OA, presumably contributing to pain and disability. Improving these functions is assumed to reduce pain and disability.

APPLICATION OF PHYSICAL REHABILITATION

A specific exercise program must be developed for each patient that addresses the patient's impairments and functional needs. Therapeutic exercise should include stretching and ROM, aerobic conditioning, muscle strength and endurance training, and correction of gait abnormalities if possible. Baseline values should be established for exercise time and intensity. Exercise duration and intensity may then be increased in a stepwise fashion until aerobic activity is maintained for 25 to 30 minutes per session. Goals should also be set for any strengthening activities. Although the program should be monitored by the veterinary team, owners are encouraged to participate in a home exercise program with their pet. A log of the home exercise program should be maintained by the owner and reviewed by the veterinary team at regular intervals.

JOINT MOBILITY

The normal ROM should be established as much as possible. Joint mobility, muscle tightness, and muscle weakness must be addressed to establish more normal ROM. OA often results in joint stiffness, and muscles secondarily become stiff and shortened. If this process continues, there is a cycle of continued weakness, tightness, abnormal movement, and pain. Treatment consists of ROM and stretching exercises.

PASSIVE RANGE OF MOTION

- ◆ Treatment should be administered in a quiet and comfortable area, away from distractions, such as loud noises, other pets, and other persons that are not helping with the treatment.
- ◆ A muzzle should be applied for initial treatments or if the dog is painful, resistant to treatment, or overly anxious.
- ◆ The patient is placed in lateral recumbency with the affected limb up. Help may be required to restrain the animal and to help keep it quiet and relaxed. In all forms of ROM activities, the therapist should be comfortable and use proper body mechanics to avoid injury to himself or herself.
- ◆ Place one hand on the limb above the joint. Place the other hand on the limb below the affected joint. Be certain that the entire limb is supported to avoid any undue stress to the involved joint (Fig. 27-3).

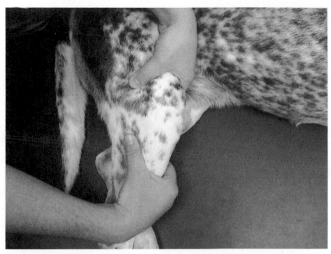

FIG. 27-3. Placement of hands for passive range of motion to a dog's stifle.

- Begin by slowly and gently flexing the joint. The other joints of the limb should be allowed to remain in a neutral position (a position as if the animal were standing). Try not to move the other joints while working on the affected joint because some joints may be restricted by the position of the joints above or below the target joint. Slowly continue to flex the joint until the patient shows initial signs of discomfort, such as tensing the limb, moving, vocalizing, turning the head toward the therapist, or trying to pull away, but do not cause undue discomfort.
- With the hands maintained in the same positions, slowly extend the joint. Again, try to keep the other joints in a neutral position and minimize any movement of the other joints. Slowly continue to extend the joint until the patient shows initial signs of discomfort.
- Alternatively, a number of joints may be simultaneously placed through a ROM, a technique sometimes referred to as ROM functional patterns. This form of ROM exercise may be appropriate as an animal nears active use of a limb. Flexing and extending all of the joints of a limb in a pattern that mimics a normal gait pattern may also be beneficial for neuromuscular reeducation.
- For most routine conditions, 15 to 20 repetitions, performed 2 to 4 times per day, are adequate. As the ROM returns to normal, the frequency may be reduced.
- Also important is to maintain normal ROM in the other joints of the affected limb.

STRETCHING

Stretching is often combined with ROM exercises to increase flexibility of tissues. Performance of some low-intensity active exercise is beneficial before stretching if possible. Application of superficial heat or therapeutic ultrasound before stretching may improve tissue extensibility. If the tissues are warmed first, less damage to the tissues may occur. The combination of muscles, tendons, skin, and joint capsule should be considered, and their relative contributions to restricted motion should be assessed. For example, the target tissue for lengthening a muscle that is contracted is the muscle belly, not the tendon.

- The patient should be in a comfortable position, which is generally in lateral recumbency, and should be on a padded surface. The patient should be as relaxed as possible, and in some cases, mild sedation or tranquilization may be beneficial.
- One hand should stabilize the bone proximal to the joint, and the other should stabilize the bone distal to the joint. The distal bone should be moved relative to the proximal bone.
- The affected joint should be slowly placed through one end of a ROM (usually beginning in flexion) until a restriction to motion is felt. Very gentle traction may be applied to the joint while slowly stretching to the point of initial restriction.
- The patient may indicate that it feels mild discomfort, such as turning the head or mildly tensing the muscles in the affected limb. Under no circumstances should more severe pain be inflicted, which might be indicated by vocalizing, trying to move away, or attempting to bite.
- The stretch should be prolonged, ideally for at least 15 seconds. During the stretch, a conscious effort should be made to try to increase the joint excursion without increasing the level of discomfort. There should be no bouncing motions during the stretch.
- Following the stretch at one end of the motion range, the pressure is slowly released and the opposite end of the ROM should be stretched.
- Each muscle group should be stretched three to five times in a session before other activities begin.
- The therapist should be patient and not try to achieve full ROM in one or two sessions. The ideal daily frequency of stretching is unknown for dogs. In general, two to four sessions per day may initially be required, with the frequency decreased as normal ROM and tissue extensibility improve. The process must be applied consistently and regularly to obtain good results, and it may take 2 to 3 weeks to see noticeable improvement.

ACTIVE RANGE OF MOTION

More active ROM exercises may be initiated to encourage voluntary joint motion through a wider range than is typically achieved with only walking or trotting. Joint ROM is limited during normal walking and trotting, so the joints do not go through a complete normal ROM. If joint restriction is present, patients may benefit by performing activities that encourage a more complete ROM.

- Swimming or walking in water results in greater flexion of joints and greater ROM. Decreased joint extension may occur with swimming, but walking in water maintains relatively normal active joint extension while increasing joint flexion, resulting in greater overall joint ROM.
- Other activities that may be performed include walking in snow, sand, or tall grass, and crawling through a play tunnel.
- Climbing stairs may increase joint excursion while also increasing strength.
- Walking over cavaletti rails is an excellent method of achieving normal limb extension for walking while increasing joint flexion and overall ROM of the elbow, stifle, and tarsal joints as the dog negotiates the rails. In addition, the rails may be raised or lowered to encourage increased or decreased joint flexion, based on the needs of the individual patient.

THERAPEUTIC EXERCISES

Strength and endurance improve if the level of exercise provides stress to tissues so that adaptation occurs while avoiding excessive loading that may exacerbate structural weaknesses. In general, endurance, cardiovascular fitness, and obesity are initially addressed through endurance activities. It is critical to be certain that joints are stable before initiating an exercise program. For example, performing weight-bearing exercises on a limb with a cranial cruciate ligament rupture hastens the development of OA.

- The level of activities is modified by *first increasing the frequency* of the activity, with adequate rest periods between sessions.
- Owners should be warned that patients may initially experience increased soreness, discomfort, and fatigue for the first week or two as a result of muscle soreness, but care should be taken to be certain that joint inflammation is not exacerbated.
- After appropriate adaptation and conditioning have occurred at this level of activity, the *length of the activities* may be increased to provide further challenges.

◆ Finally, additional strength and conditioning may be achieved by *increasing the speed* of activities and *adding strengthening exercises.*

Daily exercise is preferable to exercise only once or twice a week. Caution should be used early in the exercise period to avoid overuse injuries and pain after exercise. In general, patients should initiate a conservative exercise program. Depending on the level of the disability and deconditioning, two exercise periods per day may be enough. If lameness and pain are not exacerbated at this level, exercise may be increased to three periods per day the next week, and four periods per day the following week, being certain that lameness and pain do not increase.

Chronic pain is not a static condition, and exercise periods must adapt to occasional "bad days." The level of activity should be decreased on days of worsened pain or lameness because forced exercise may exacerbate the inflammatory process in arthritic joints. When the degree of pain and lameness return to previous levels, the activity may be increased more gradually. The next step should be to increase the length of the walks.

A reasonable rule of thumb is to increase the length of activity by 10% to 15% per week, being vigilant for any exacerbation of pain or lameness; if pain or lameness is noted, the level of activity is decreased by 50% until the patient returns to baseline, and then the level of activity is increased more gradually.

Controlled leash walking, walking on a treadmill, jogging, swimming, and going up and down stairs or ramp inclines are excellent low-impact exercises. The length of the exercise should be titrated so there is no increased pain after activity. Also, it is better in the early phases of training to provide three 10-minute sessions rather than one 30-minute session. Avoiding sudden bursts of activity helps avoid acute inflammation of arthritic joints.

Slow Walks

◆ Slow leash walks are perhaps the most important therapeutic exercise for patients with debilitating chronic diseases. These walks are also frequently performed incorrectly.
◆ Leash walks must be performed very slowly to allow the dog to bear weight without undue stress on painful joints.
◆ Leash walks must be performed for the speed of the dog, not the handler.
◆ Leash walks are performed for only 5 minutes, two or three times daily to begin. If the lameness or limb use is not worse after the first couple of days, the length and time of the walks may be gradually increased by 1 to 3 minutes per session every few days.
◆ Dogs may be walked up and down inclines, hills, or ramps to add more challenges and to encourage muscular and cardiovascular fitness.

Treadmill Walking

◆ Treadmill walking reduces stress and pain of limb movement in some conditions, such as the pain of hip extension in dogs with hip dysplasia or the pain of stifle extension following repair of a cranial cruciate ligament.

◆ Most dogs trained to leash readily take to treadmill walking.

◆ Many treadmills are available, and some models for humans may be adapted for canine use.

◆ A harness to provide support and prevent falls, side walls to prevent stepping off the treadmill, variable speed of the treadmill, a timer, and the ability to change the incline angle are useful features for canine treadmills.

◆ Do not face the treadmill toward a wall; have it face down a hallway or toward the middle of a room.

◆ One person may be in front of the dog to encourage it or provide treats.

◆ One person may stand over the dog to help keep it moving straight.

◆ A sling may be used to help support especially weak dogs.

◆ The treadmill may be angled up or down to reduce or increase stress on the forelimbs or rear limbs.

◆ Joint motion is similar between walking on a treadmill and normal walking over ground, but the treadmill provides some active assistance for movement of painful joints. In addition, the stance time of weight bearing is greater on a treadmill.

Ramp Walking and Stair Climbing

◆ Ramp walking and stair climbing are useful to improve power in rear limb extensors.

◆ The dog may begin ramp walking or stair climbing if the dog is consistently using the limb at a walk with decreasing lameness over time.

◆ Exercises must begin slowly to encourage proper use of rear limbs. The dog should step up with each limb rather than skipping up steps or jumping up steps by using both rear limbs ("bunny hopping"; Fig. 27-4)

◆ This therapy is best started with ramp walking, then low, gradually rising steps, and progressing to increasingly steeper steps.

◆ Begin with ramp walking for 5 minutes, then five to seven steps, and increase to two to four flights once to three times daily.

Jogging

◆ Jogging may be initiated in many cases in dogs that are walking on the limb with minimal lameness and pain.

◆ Begin jogging slowly to improve muscle strength and cardiovascular fitness 2 to 3 minutes two or three times daily, and increase up to 20 minutes two to four times daily.

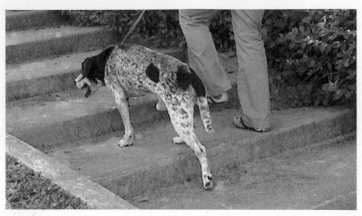

FIG. 27-4. Dogs may begin slowly walking up low-rise stairs in the early phases of rehabilitation if the surgical repair (if surgery has been performed) is stable and the dog is increasingly less lame with lower-level rehabilitation activities such as leash walking.

- Be certain that lameness is not worse after jogging. If so, the dog should rest for several days and receive antiinflammatory medication; and when jogging is reinitiated, it should be at slower speeds and for less time.
- The dog may jog up hills for greater effect if there are no problems jogging on flat surfaces.

Sit-to-Stand Exercises

- Sit-to-stand exercises help to strengthen hip and stifle extensors without causing extension of the hip, stifle, and hock more than is achieved with walking. The exercises may be beneficial for dogs with hip dysplasia, in which full extension of the hips is painful.
- Sit-to-stand exercises should be combined with training, occasionally using a low-calorie treat.
- It may be easier to back the dog into a corner, with the affected leg against a wall. This encourages the dog to push up evenly with both rear limbs when rising, and not pushing up with a good leg while pushing the affected leg out away from the body (Fig. 27-5).
- The handler should concentrate on having the dog sit and stand correctly, with both rear limbs flexing equally while sitting, and pushing off evenly with both rear limbs to stand.
- Start with 5 to 10 repetitions once or twice daily and work up to 15 repetitions 3 to 4 times daily.

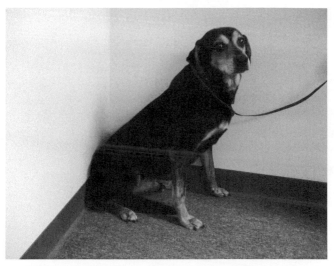

FIG. 27-5. Proper positioning for sit-to-stand exercises.

Wheelbarrowing

◆ Wheelbarrowing exercises are designed to improve use of the forelimbs and strengthening of the weight-bearing muscles.

◆ The rear limbs are lifted off of the ground, and the dog is moved forward. Dogs with normal proprioception will move the forelimbs so that they do not fall.

◆ Some dogs with weakness of the forelimbs may require support to prevent them from collapsing.

◆ As dogs become stronger and endurance improves, dogs may be wheelbarrowed up and down inclines for greater effect.

Dancing Exercises

◆ Dancing exercises are designed to improve use and strength of the rear limbs.

◆ Because it may be difficult to encourage some dogs to exercise on an affected limb, it is recommended to apply a muzzle to the dog.

◆ The forelimbs are lifted off the ground, and the dog is moved forward or backward. Dogs with normal proprioception will move the limbs so that they do not fall.

◆ Most dogs dance forward, but others may stretch until they are nearly on the ground. In these situations, the handler should get behind the dog and place the arms under axillary region of the dog to support it and walk forward.

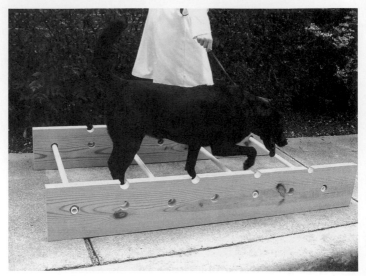

FIG. 27-6. Walking over cavaletti rails increases active flexion of the elbow, stifle, and tarsal joints.

Forward dancing results in less extension of the hip joint and may be beneficial for dogs with painful hips. Backward dancing results in a more vertical position of the dog, and hip joint extension is much greater compared with forward dancing.

◆ As dogs become stronger and endurance improves, dogs may dance up and down inclines for greater effect.

Cavaletti Rails

◆ Cavaletti rails are raised rails or poles that are spaced apart on the ground. In some cases a ladder that is laying on the ground may act as cavaletti rails (Fig. 27-6).
◆ Cavaletti rails are useful to help with increasing stride length, limb use, and active ROM of joints.
◆ The height of the rails may be raised to encourage greater active flexion and extension of the elbow, stifle, and tarsal joints, but care should be taken to prevent jumping over the rails.
◆ The rails are spaced equally or with varying widths. Initially, it is a good idea to space the rails equally, somewhat less than the normal stride length of the patient. As the animal improves, the rails may be spaced at varying distances to provide challenges to proprioception, or they may be spaced wider apart to encourage a longer stride length.

Pole Weaving

- Weaving back and forth between vertical poles is an exercise that is useful for encouraging lateral flexion of the spinal column, proprioceptive training, and weight shifting during gait to encourage use of limbs and strengthening of muscles in preparation for more challenging exercises, such as turning sharply while running.
- A series of vertical poles is placed in a straight line.
- The distance between the poles should be less than the length of the dog to encourage lateral bending of the spinal column and weight shifting.

MUSCLE STRENGTHENING ACTIVITIES

Exercises that concentrate on strengthening muscles are designed to improve power and speed. These exercises include pulling or carrying weights, working against elastic bands, playing ball, and running for short distances at high speed.

Pulling or Carrying Weights

- Pulling or carrying weight is a method of increasing the force that muscles must use and encourages muscle strengthening. These exercises are similar to weight lifting in humans.
- Many harnesses are available to pull sleds or carts. The harnesses should be well-designed and padded and should fit the patient very well to avoid problems with pressure sores. Dogs may pull various weights, depending on the stage of recovery and the dog's strength.
- The position of the dog's head and neck is important when pulling weight. If strengthening of the forelimb muscles is desired, the dog's head should be lower than the back to encourage transfer of weight to forelimbs to allow pulling; if strengthening of the rear limb muscles is desired, the dog's head should be higher than the back to encourage transfer of weight to the rear limbs to allow the animal to drive off of the rear limbs for pulling weight.
- Backpacks are also available, and various weights may be placed in the backpack to allow strengthening of multiple muscle groups.
- Strap-on leg weights may be used to help strengthen flexor muscles during gait. Initially, the weights should be placed relatively proximal on the limb to reduce the muscle force and stress on joints during the early rehabilitation period. As strength and stamina improve, the weights may be moved further distally to provide more challenges. In general, 0.25-kg, 0.5-kg, 1-kg, and 2-kg weights may be used for small, medium, large, and very large dogs, respectively.

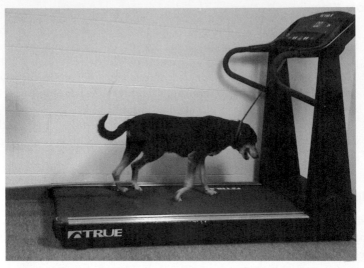

FIG. 27-7. Elastic bands may be placed on a dog's limb while walking on a treadmill to provide resistance while walking.

Elastic Bands

◆ Various stiffnesses of elastic bands are available that may be fastened to a dog's limb to provide resistance while walking.

◆ It is important that the resistance not be so great that the normal gait is hindered; rather, the therapist should provide mild resistance to allow the dog to walk or jog normally.

◆ The band should be held parallel and close to the ground to allow normal joint flexion and extension.

◆ Elastic bands may also be used with treadmill walking (Fig. 27-7).

Controlled Ball Playing

◆ Controlled ball playing is a fun activity for dogs and their owners and is an excellent method to establish strength and speed. However, control and gradual introduction of ball playing are essential to avoid reinjury.

◆ Begin ball playing on a relatively short leash or in an enclosed kennel or room to avoid overly explosive activity in the early postoperative period.

◆ Progress to ball playing in an enclosed area, such as a small dog run or room.

◆ As the animal nears full return to function, activity on a long leash is instituted, and if there are no problems, off-leash activity is introduced in a safe environment.

Swimming and walking in water are some of the best activities for dogs with chronic OA (Fig. 27-8). The buoyancy of water is significant

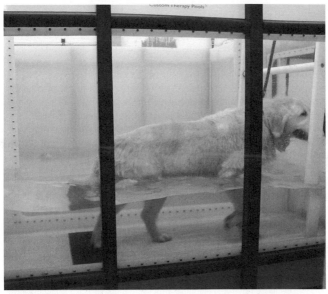

FIG. 27-8. Walking on an underwater treadmill provides buoyancy for painful joints and results in increased active joint movement compared with walking over ground.

and limits the impact on the joint while promoting muscle strength and tone and joint motion. Training in an underwater treadmill may increase peak weight bearing forces by 5% to 15%, which is comparable to achievements obtained using medication in many patients.

Following exercise, a 10-minute warm-down period allows muscles to cool down. A slower-paced walk may be initiated for 5 minutes, followed by ROM and stretching exercises. A cooldown massage may help decrease pain, swelling, and muscle spasms. Finally, cryotherapy may be applied to painful areas for 15 to 20 minutes to control postexercise inflammation.

TRANSCUTANEOUS ELECTRICAL NERVE STIMULATION

Transcutaneous electrical nerve stimulation (TENS) is an inexpensive, safe, noninvasive modality with few side effects that can be used to treat a variety of painful conditions. The clinical application of TENS involves the delivery of an electrical current, usually from a small battery-operated device, to the skin by surface electrodes. A variety of stimulators are available with a wide range of stimulation parameters to choose from, including frequency, intensity, pulse duration, and electrode placement sites.

Transcutaneous Electrical Nerve Stimulation

- Transcutaneous electrical nerve stimulation (TENS) provides analgesia by several potential mechanisms of action.
- Conventional TENS provides peripheral stimulation with electrical impulses that activate nonnoxious large myelinated afferent Aβ nerve fibers in the skin and inhibit small unmyelinated "C" fibers within the dorsal horn of the spinal cord.
- This "gate theory" is based on the principle that there is a gateway in the dorsal horn of the spinal cord that regulates the flow of pain signals that are ascending by small-diameter afferent nerve fibers and descending from higher levels of the brain for central processing, thus reducing the perception of pain.
- Most devices have a stimulation of approximately 100 Hz, which is thought to be comfortable to most persons. Individuals describe a "pins-and-needles" sensation under the electrodes, resulting in paresthesia.
- Some TENS units produce a more noxious high-intensity stimulus at 2 Hz. This stimulates small-diameter afferent fibers and results in the release of endogenous opiates and pain relief by stimulating the descending pain-inhibiting pathway.
- Different frequencies of TENS may act through different neurotransmitter systems.
- Low-frequency TENS analgesia may be mediated by activation of serotonin and μ-opioid receptors, whereas conventional TENS activates δ-opioid receptors. However, conclusive evidence regarding the more effective method of TENS is lacking. Five studies comparing conventional TENS and low-frequency TENS found no differences in pain-reducing effect.
- Pulse duration and stimulus intensity are also factors in providing analgesia. Greater analgesia has been achieved by increasing the stimulus intensity or pulse duration.
- Electrode placement may also influence the effectiveness of TENS. In general, electrodes are placed over the painful region.

Three important factors that determine the quality of TENS application include (1) the type of device (e.g., stimulators, electrode type, and design); (2) the wave form of the device, which is modified by adjusting the amplitude, rate, and width controls; and (3) the proper location of electrodes. Although four types of TENS device settings are currently used in human clinical practice, high-frequency (40- to 150-Hz, 50- to 100-microsecond pulse width, low to moderate intensity) or conventional TENS stimulators are most commonly used in animals because they are more comfortable and create less anxiety in small animal patients.

INDICATIONS FOR TENS

TENS is a form of neuromuscular electrical stimulation (NMES). TENS is used for pain control, primarily in chronic conditions, but there may also be use for acute conditions. Other forms of NMES are commonly used in the rehabilitation of patients that have had orthopedic or neurologic injury, such as fracture repair, cruciate ligament reconstruction, and meniscal

Precautions and Contraindications for Transcutaneous Electrical Nerve Stimulation

- Contraindications include high-intensity stimulation directly over the heart, animals with pacemakers, animals with seizure disorders, over infected areas or neoplasms, over the carotid sinus, or over the trunk during pregnancy.
- Precautions include application over areas with impaired sensation; over abdominal, lumbar, and pelvic regions during pregnancy; over areas of skin irritation or damage, or possible interference with electronic sensing devices such as electrocardiographic monitors.

débridement or repair. Patients that have neurologic conditions, such as cerebrovascular accidents, closed head injuries, spinal cord injuries, or other neurologic disease involving paralysis or paresis may also benefit from NMES. NMES has been used to increase joint mobility, decrease joint contracture, decrease edema, enhance circulation, minimize disuse atrophy, improve muscle strength, retard loss of volitional control, improve sensory awareness, decrease spasticity, diminish pain, and correct gait abnormalities.

APPLICATION OF TENS

In determining whether to use TENS in a patient, the use of other concurrent methods of pain control should be assessed. Some patients cannot tolerate medications, and in these cases, TENS may provide an acceptable alternative. In other patients, the use of TENS may provide additional pain control.

The hair over the area to which electrical stimulation will be applied must be clipped to lower impedance. The skin may be cleaned with alcohol before treatment. Carbon electrodes may be placed over the region to receive TENS. In general, up to four electrodes may be placed over the affected area. If four electrodes are used, they are typically placed in a crossed fashion. Water-soluble electrode gel may be applied as a coupling agent, and the electrodes may be further secured with nonadhesive bandage material or Velcro straps.

For TENS application, premodulated electrical stimulation (70 Hz) is applied to the affected area. In some situations, interferential current may be applied with four electrodes.

Amperage (intensity) may be increased to the tolerance level of the animal and should be reduced if gross movement of the area is noted or if the animal displays any signs of distress or discomfort including turning its head in recognition of the stimulus or becoming agitated. Amperage may be reduced to a level just below that which produces these signs. Although the optimum time of treatment and the frequency of treatment are unknown, most clinicians believe that TENS should be applied to the desired area(s) for 30 minutes, three to seven times per week.

Precautions should be taken to avoid injury to the handler and animal. A muzzle should be applied, and the animal should be placed in lateral recumbency during the initial treatment. In some cases, tranquilization may be necessary if the animal is anxious. It is recommended that treatment only be given under the supervision of trained personnel.

LOW-LEVEL LASER THERAPY

Low-level laser therapy (LLLT) is a light source that consists of pure light of a single wavelength and has been recommended for managing chronic pain, especially in those with chronic OA. The effect is not thermal but is related to photochemical reactions in the cells.

Until recently, LLLT devices were not widely used in the United States, but several have been approved by the Food and Drug Administration (FDA) in recent years. The effectiveness of laser therapy is still unclear, and the interpretation of studies regarding the efficacy of LLLT is hindered by specifics regarding the wavelengths and dosages of laser.

The results of studies regarding pain management with the use of laser have been controversial. However, studies performed have resulted in FDA approval of 635-nm low-level lasers for the management of chronic, minor pain such as OA and muscle spasms.

Low-Level Laser Therapy

- Although the mechanisms of action of low-level laser therapy on pain are unclear, several mechanisms of action have been postulated.
- Laser therapy may have some analgesic effects by blocking pain transmission to the brain. Some studies have shown changes in the conduction of the radial and median nerve after low-level laser therapy, but others have shown no effect.
- Laser treatment may also increase the release of endorphins and enkephalins, which may further provide analgesic benefits.
- Laser therapy has been used to stimulate muscle trigger points and acupuncture points, which may provide pain relief.
- Nociceptive stimulation may be affected. The effects of diode laser irradiation (830 nm, 40 mW, 3 minutes, continuous wave) on peripheral nerves was examined by monitoring neuronal discharges elicited by application of various stimuli to the hind limb skin of rats. Laser treatment of the saphenous nerve inhibited neuronal discharges elicited by pinch, cold, and heat stimulation. Injection of a chemical irritant into the hind paw skin elicited neuronal discharges in the ipsilateral dorsal root, and these discharges were significantly inhibited or abolished by laser irradiation. These results suggest that laser irradiation may selectively inhibit nociceptive neuronal activities.

Precautions and Contraindications for Low-Level Laser Therapy

- Protective eye gear should be worn to prevent damage to the retina if the laser shines into the area.
- Pregnant women should avoid laser treatment.
- Laser should not be applied to open fontanels.
- Laser should not be applied over malignancies.
- Do not apply laser directly into the cornea.
- Avoid laser application over tattoos because of the high absorption of laser light by pigmented areas.
- Do not apply laser over growth plates of immature animals.
- Do not apply laser over photosensitive areas of the skin.

APPLICATION OF LOW-LEVER LASER THERAPY

The area should be clipped because 50% to 99% of the laser light may be absorbed by hair. Little is known about the transmission of laser light to deeper tissues in darker dogs, but HeNe laser energy is likely to be absorbed because of the pigment. Any iodine or povidone-iodine should be washed off the area to allow greater transmission of light. Drugs, such as cortisone, that reduce inflammation may have a negative effect on healing. The therapist should wear protective eye wear because damage may occur to the retina if the laser shines into the eyes.

The three variables for lasers used for LLLT are (1) the wavelength, (2) the number of watts or milliwatts, and (3) the number of seconds to deliver joules of energy. With these factors known, the length of time needed to hold the laser on a point to deliver the appropriate joules of energy must be calculated. For example, if a 904-nm laser with a maximum output power of 250 mW is used, it will take 4 seconds to deliver 1 J. Unfortunately, the optimal wavelengths, intensities, and dosages have not been adequately studied in animals, and information in humans is difficult to interpret because of different conditions and treatment regimens.

Wavelengths of low-power lasers commonly used are 632.8 nm (HeNe, gas) in the visible light range, 810 nm (Ga/Al/As, diode), and 904 nm (Ga/As, diode) in the infrared region of the light spectrum. Other wavelengths are used in surgical settings. The wavelength is the prime determinant of tissue penetration. Lasers that do not penetrate as deeply (630 to 740 nm) are suitable for acupuncture point stimulation and wound healing but have not proved their clinical efficacy with deep-seated musculoskeletal conditions. Infrared lasers (750 to 1500 nm) penetrate more deeply and are used to treat trigger points, ligaments, joint capsules, and intraarticular structures.

Power is measured in watts and is often expressed as milliwatts. One watt is equivalent to 1 J/s. Power density is the power delivered under the area of the probe. Energy density is the amount of energy, or dose, per square centimeter of tissue. The greater the power density and higher the wavelength, the deeper the penetration through tissues. More laser dosage is not better, however, and overdosing may retard the desired effect.

The following example illustrates how to calculate the number of seconds to apply the laser to a particular area to deliver a given dose of laser energy for a laser delivering 250 mW/s, for a total dose of 1 J:

0.250 W = 1 J/X seconds

(0.250 W)(X seconds) = 1 J

X seconds = 1 J/0.250 W

X = 4 seconds

With this particular laser, it is necessary to hold the laser on one point for 4 seconds to deliver 1 J of energy. The following doses have been suggested for treating pain:

Analgesic effect:

Muscle pain: 2 to 4 J/cm^2

Joint pain: 4 to 8 J/cm^2

Antiinflammatory effect:

Acute and subacute: 1 to 6 J/cm^2

Chronic: 4 to 8 J/cm^2

LLLT is generally administered with a handheld probe, with a small beam area that is useful to treat small surfaces. Laser energy may be applied with the laser probe in contact with the skin, which eliminates reflection for the skin and minimizes beam divergence, or with the probe not held in contact (Fig. 27-9). With the noncontact method, it is necessary to hold the probe perpendicular to the treatment area to minimize wave reflection and beam divergence. The appropriate dosage may be applied to larger areas by administering the calculated dose to each site in a grid fashion, or by slowly moving the probe over the entire surface, being certain to distribute the energy evenly to each site. In any case, the probe should be held perpendicular to the skin. A coupling medium is not necessary, as in ultrasound, because the laser beam is not attenuated by air.

MASSAGE

Massage has been reported to relieve pain, aid relaxation, and promote a feeling of well-being in humans. In addition to helping to improve lymphatic drainage, circulation, and tissue movement, soft tissue massage is also thought to provide symptomatic relief of pain.

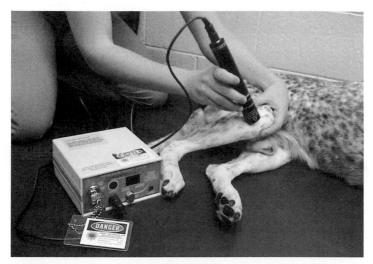

FIG. 27-9. Application of a low-level laser.

Massage and Pain Relief

Suggested mechanisms of pain relief include the following:
- Relaxation
- Increasing the pain threshold through the release of endorphins and the gate control theory of pain
- Increase in pain threshold

Massage causes traction at tissue interfaces. Horizontal plexuses lie at interfaces in the tissues, and gentle pulling on these vessels may stimulate the accompanying sympathetic nerves, which supply the mechanoreceptors. These receptors may be distorted by the massage, possibly lowering mechanoreceptor sensitivity and reducing pain and tenderness.

The flushing effect of massage on tissue fluids and removal of inflammatory mediators may increase the speed at which the inflammation resolves in humans with delayed-onset muscle pain following exercise.

INDICATIONS FOR MASSAGE

Massage may be indicated for dogs having surgery to maintain mobility and ease pain, after exercise to reduce muscle soreness, in patients with edema, and in patients with chronic OA to help ease muscle tension.

Precautions and Contraindications for Massage

- Massage is contraindicated in patients with open wounds, unstable fractures, severe pain, coagulation disorders, infections, or neoplasia.

APPLICATION OF MASSAGE

- ◆ Select a quiet area that is free of interruptions.
- ◆ Provide a soft, padded surface for the patient.
- ◆ Work in a systematic way.
- ◆ The therapist should relax and maintain proper body posture.
- ◆ Use larger muscles such as the shoulder muscles instead of the hands to minimize fatigue.
- ◆ Massage may be performed to isolated areas or to the entire limb and body. If the dog has a specific condition, local massage may be appropriate on a regular basis. General massage helps with treatment of compensatory conditions and biomechanical changes.

MASSAGE TECHNIQUE
Stroking

- ◆ Use good technique to start the treatment.
- ◆ Run hands over the dog from neck to tail and down the limbs with medium pressure.
- ◆ This aids relaxation of the dog and allows assessment of tissues; note muscle tone, any swelling, masses, or temperature differences between body areas.

Effleurage

- ◆ Beginning at a distal area, such as the foot, the hands move proximally, using medium pressure.
- ◆ This helps to move fluids to the lymph nodes and aids drainage.

Petrissage

- ◆ Petrissage promotes muscle relaxation, decreases muscle stiffness, increases blood flow.
- ◆ One rolls or kneads the soft tissues (Fig. 27-10).
- ◆ Muscle bellies may be lifted and rolled.

Trigger Point Therapy

- ◆ Trigger point therapy is used for small areas of spasm felt within a muscle belly.
- ◆ Nodules are located, and ischemic compression is applied using one or two fingers.
- ◆ Compression is held for approximately 20 seconds and released for 10 seconds before reapplying compression.
- ◆ Generally, three or four repetitions may be required.

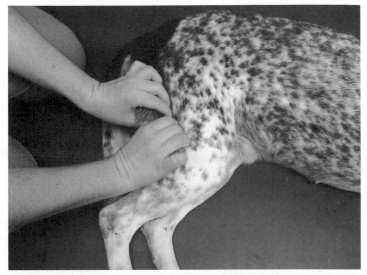

FIG. 27-10. Applying petrissage massage technique to the caudal thigh muscles of a dog.

STATIC MAGNETIC FIELD THERAPY

The use of static magnets for medical purposes is relatively common in humans and is becoming more popular in animals. Owners can purchase magnets that are embedded in wraps, collars, or pet beds. Static magnets provide a continuous magnetic field that is thought to alter physiological processes, including an increase in local blood flow.

Static Magnetic Field Therapy

Proposed mechanisms for pain relief include the following:
- Possible release of endorphins
- Antiinflammatory effects

INDICATIONS FOR THE USE OF STATIC MAGNETS

Static magnets may be used as a complementary modality to other forms of OA treatment.

Precautions and Contraindication to the Use of Static Magnets

- No specific contraindications or precautions exists for use of static magnets, with the exception that they should not be used in patients with pacemakers.

USE OF STATIC MAGNETS

Static magnets are cheap and are easy to apply. The strength of static magnets is measured in gauss. Therapeutic magnets are in the range of 2500 to 6000 gauss, whereas the earth's magnetic field is 0.5 gauss. Magnetic resonance imaging units produce magnetic fields that are 2 to 4 times greater than therapeutic magnetic pads. In contrast, common refrigerator magnets are about 50 to 200 gauss. In general, the amount of gauss delivered to the skin is less than that directly in contact with the magnet because the magnetic field decreases rapidly with distance. In fact, the amount delivered to the skin may be only about one third of the amount of the magnet.

Static magnets may be combined with other treatments. The magnets must be placed directly over affected joints because of the rapid decrease in magnetic field over short distances. However, it may be difficult to maintain them over the affected area(s). Static magnets should be considered as a complement to OA treatment, not as a sole or alternative treatment. The biggest potential danger of static magnets is that they may delay conventional treatment and result in progression of disease or result in undue discomfort.

EXTRACORPOREAL SHOCK WAVE TREATMENT

Extracorporeal shock wave treatment (ESWT) involves the application of high-energy, high-amplitude acoustic pressure waves to tissues. Shock waves are characterized by an extremely short build-up time of approximately 5 to 10 nanoseconds with an exponential decay to baseline. Shock waves behave like sound waves in tissue, in that the waves travel through soft tissue and fluid and release their energy into the tissues when a change in tissue density is encountered, such as the interface between bone and ligament. This energy release is thought to stimulate healing. Two primary methods are used to deliver the energy. Focused shock waves have the ability to focus the energy to different tissue depths. The shock waves are focused by means of a parabola to deliver an intense shock to a small area with a focused depth, up to 110 mm. Radial shock waves are delivered to the surface of the body. From there, the shock waves rapidly disperse through the tissues, releasing their energy rapidly to a wide area. Because of the energy dissipation, it is difficult to deliver energy to deeper tissues.

Orthopedic applications of ESWT in humans include delayed or nonunion fractures, plantar fasciitis, lateral epicondylitis, Achilles and patella tendinitis, and with limited experience, OA. Focal ESWT is currently FDA approved in the United States for use in chronic heel pain (plantar fasciitis) and tennis elbow (lateral epicondylitis). Other potential applications include the use of ESWT to provide analgesia for humans with avascular necrosis of the femoral head, to treat calcified tendinitis of the shoulder, and to stabilize loose press-fit total hip replacements. Patients with humeral epicondylitis or plantar fasciitis tend to respond better to ESWT if the condition is chronic (>35 months) rather than more acute (3 to 12 months).

In veterinary medicine, ESWT has been used in horses for the treatment of suspensory ligament desmitis, tendinopathies, navicular disease, back pain, OA, and stress fractures. Although the treatment of dogs with shock wave therapy is new, tendinitis, desmitis, spondylosis, nonunion fractures, and OA have been treated.

Extracorporeal Shock Wave Treatment

Pain may be modulated in patients receiving extracorporeal shock wave treatment, but the mechanisms of action are unclear. The following effects have been described that may contribute to analgesia:

- Reduced inflammation and swelling
- Short-term analgesia
- Production and release of growth factors
- Stimulation of nociceptors that may inhibit afferent pain signals

---

INDICATIONS FOR ESWT

ESWT may be beneficial to patients with chronic OA of the major joints, especially if they cannot tolerate NSAIDs or other forms of treatment. In addition, ESWT may be useful as a nonpharmacologic form of adjunctive treatment along with medical management to obtain additional improvement. In addition, patients with OA of the vertebral column may benefit from ESWT, as well as patients with chronic nonunion fractures.

APPLICATION OF ESWT

Heavy sedation or anesthesia is required for focused ESWT. Because many patients requiring treatment are geriatric, adequate health screening should be performed before treatment, including a complete physical examination and appropriate ancillary tests such as radiographs, complete blood count, serum chemistry profile, and urinalysis.

A complete understanding of the anatomy of the treatment area and the spatial relationships of various anatomic landmarks is critical because ESWT is a localized treatment. Because shock waves may cause petechiation and bruising, aspirin and other non–cyclooxygenase-selective drugs should be discontinued before treatment because these drugs inhibit platelet function and may worsen the bruising.

Precautions and Contraindications for Extracorporeal Shock Wave Treatment

- Dogs with immune-mediated joint disease or neurologic deficits should not be treated with extracorporeal shock wave treatment (ESWT) because this treatment has no known effects on these conditions.
- Neoplastic joint disease, infectious arthritis, and diskospondylitis should not be treated with ESWT because of the risk of spreading the disease process with treatment.
- Acute unstable fractures and patients with unstable hardware are also not candidates for ESWT, even though this treatment has shown efficacy in treating nonunion fractures, because some stability of the fracture must be present to allow bone healing.
- Shock waves can have adverse effects if they are applied at excessively high energy levels, if a large number of shocks are used, or if they are focused on structures sensitive to their effects. Excessive and violent cavitation can lead to the production of free radicals, which can cause chemical or thermal damage to cells and tissues.
- Concurrent use of nonsteroidal antiinflammatory drugs that affect platelet function is not recommended before ESWT because of the risk of petechiation and bruising.
- Shock waves should not be delivered over the lung field, brain, heart, major blood vessels, nerves, neoplasms, or a gravid uterus.

The treatment area should be clipped, and the skin should be cleaned with alcohol if it is excessively oily. Ultrasound gel is liberally applied to the area (Fig. 27-11). Do not use other lotions or creams because these contain too much air, and this attenuates the sound waves.

At this time, the optimal energy level or number of shocks for various conditions are not known. Based on the manufacturer's directions and the area(s) to be treated, the energy level and number of shocks to be delivered are selected. In general, treatments should not be repeated more frequently than every 2 weeks. Most conditions are treated two or three times.

When treating joints, it is important to direct the probe at the insertion sites of the joint capsule, not the articular cartilage. If treating the supraspinatus or biceps tendons, direct probe over these areas from proximal to distal. Do not direct the probe over the thorax or lungs if treating conditions of the forelimbs. Patients may be a bit sedate for the rest of the day after treatment and may develop some bruising, petechiation, or a hematoma over the treatment site. Some patients may be sore for several days after treatment and then have relative relief from pain. During this time, consider use of NSAIDs or other medications to provide analgesia. Continued improvement may be seen for up to several weeks after treatment. Some conditions seem to be more responsive to shock wave treatment than others. For example, the hips and back may respond well, whereas stifles may not respond to the same extent. Anecdotally, initial response rates of up to 80% may be seen, and the effects may last as long as 1 year.

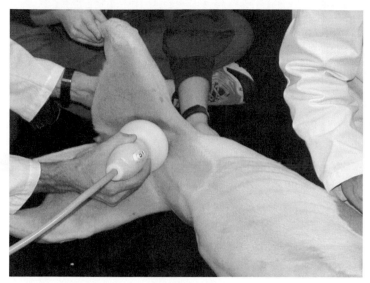

FIG. 27-11. Application of extracorporeal shock wave treatment.

SUGGESTED READINGS

Beckerman H, de Bie RA, Bouter LM et al: The efficacy of laser therapy for musculoskeletal and skin disorders: a criteria-based meta-analysis of randomized clinical trials, *Phys Ther* 72:483-491, 1992.

Carreck A: The effect of massage on pain perception threshold, *Manipulative Physiotherapist* 26(2):10-16, 1994.

Collacott EA, Zimmerman JT, White PT, Rindone JP: Bipolar permanent magnets for the treatment of chronic low back pain, *JAMA* 283:1322-1325, 2000.

Harlow T, Greaves C, White A et al: Randomised controlled trial of magnetic bracelets for relieving pain in osteoarthritis of the hip and knee, *BMJ* 329:1450-1454, 2004.

Meeusen R, Lievens P: The use of cryotherapy in sports injuries, *Sports Med* 3:398-414, 1986.

Nadler SF, Weingand K, Kruse RJ: The physiologic basis and clinical applications of cryotherapy and thermotherapy for the pain practitioner, *Pain Physician* 7:395-399, 2004.

Sluka KA, Walsh D: Transcutaneous electrical nerve stimulation: basic science mechanisms and clinical effectiveness, *J Pain* 4:109-121, 2003.

Sutton A: Massage. In Millis DL, Levine D, Taylor RA, editors: *Canine physical therapy and rehabilitation*, Philadelphia, 2004, Saunders.

Wittink H, Cohen LJ, Michel TH: Pain rehabilitation: physical therapy treatment. In Wittink H, Michel TH, editors: *Chronic pain management for physical therapists*, ed 2, Boston, 2002, Butterworth and Heinemann.

Yurtkuran M, Kocagil T: TENS, electroacupuncture and ice massage: comparison of treatment for osteoarthritis of the knee, *Am J Acupunct* 27:133-140, 1999.

28 REHABILITATION METHODS AND MODALITIES FOR THE CAT

SANDRA HUDSON

- ◆ The field of feline rehabilitation has been slow to take hold because of the perceived idea that the cat will not cooperate with the modalities or perform exercises.
- ◆ Physical rehabilitation is effective in providing pain management in cats, provided that feline behavior and personality are taken into account.
- ◆ Cat owners have begun to enjoy increased expectations for the health and recovery of their pet by incorporating principles and applications from human physical therapy to enhance recovery from injuries, to reduce pain, and to improve the daily life of their cat.

PRINCIPLES OF REHABILITATION

- ◆ Physical therapy is the application of techniques that help restore function, improve mobility, relieve pain, and prevent or limit permanent physical disabilities of patients suffering from injuries or disease.
- ◆ Identical modalities and similar exercises used in the human field can be applied to the animal.
- ◆ Rehabilitation for the cat provides controlled activities and therapeutic modalities that enhance the recovery of the cat.
- ◆ Feline rehabilitation is designed to provide the most complete return to function possible while reducing the risk of additional injury.
- ◆ Feline rehabilitation can be used to promote advanced conditioning, gait training, management of chronic pain, and conservative management for certain conditions or as an alternative to some surgeries (Table 28-1).

TABLE 28 1	Primary Areas of Rehabilitation		
Phase	**Primary Goals**	**Type**	**Example**
Immediate postoperative (cat may still be recovering from anesthesia)	Reduce pain, swelling, and edema Maintain range of motion and muscle mass	Passive	Cryotherapy
Early postoperative/ early weight bearing (Non–weight bearing to toe touching)	Improve strength, increase range of motion, improve proprioception	Passive and active	Passive range of motion Balance board exercises
Progressive weight bearing	Increase muscle strength and endurance, joint range of motion, and proprioception	Passive and active	Therapeutic ultrasound Underwater treadmill
Gait training	Return to normal stride length and gait pattern	Active	Cavaletti rails, inclines or declines
Conditioning	Improve body composition	Active	Underwater treadmill

---

BOX 28-1

Factors That Facilitate Productive and Safe Rehabilitation Session for the Cat

- Quiet environment free of other animals
- Owner presence
- Patience
- Confident application of modality or introduction of exercise
- Sedation

If the second attempt at an exercise is more difficult than the first, it is best to wait until another session.

SPECIAL CONSIDERATIONS FOR THE CAT

◆ Effective rehabilitation of the cat requires special attention and consideration of the individual animal's personality (Box 28-1).
◆ It is recommended to have several alternative ways to reach rehabilitation goals.

OBJECTIVES OF REHABILITATION

◆ The goal of rehabilitation is the restoration of the quality of life and function for the cat through improvement of the bones, joints, and muscles.
◆ The five primary objectives of rehabilitation are as follows:
  • Pain management
  • Strength
  • Endurance
  • Range of motion
  • Proprioception

PAIN MANAGEMENT

◆ Pain management techniques assist in reducing the suffering experienced by the cat with acute or chronic pain. Physical therapy is a critical element in the pursuit to regain the function that has been lost.
◆ Pain can cause a cat to stop moving because it may fear that increased movement will increase the pain.
◆ In many cases the way to reduce the pain and increase function is to start moving in a relaxed and low-stressed manner.

STRENGTH

◆ Atrophy can occur because of disease, injury, lack of use, or lack of nerve impulse.
◆ Strength activities increase the size of muscle fibers. Increasing strength can improve the stability of an injured joint.

ENDURANCE

◆ Prolonged contraction of a muscle leads to muscle fatigue because of the inability of the metabolic process of the fibers to supply nutrients at the level required for the workout.

◆ Endurance exercises increase the oxidative capacity of the muscle, making it more resistant to fatigue.
◆ Improving endurance facilitates the cat's return to its normal level of activity.

RANGE OF MOTION

◆ Range of motion is the capability of a joint to go through its complete spectrum of movements.
◆ Range of motion of a joint can be passive or active.
◆ Passive range of motion can be defined as the range of motion that is achieved when an outside force (such as a therapist) causes movement of a joint and is usually the maximum range of motion that a joint can move.
◆ Active range of motion is the range of motion that can be achieved when opposing muscles contract and relax, resulting in joint movement. For example, the active range of motion to allow the elbow to bend requires the biceps to contract while the triceps muscle relaxes. Active range of motion is usually less than passive range of motion.
◆ Range of motion therapy is beneficial in healing and in recovery from soft tissue and joint lesions, maintaining existing joint and soft tissue mobility, minimizing the effects of contracture formation, assisting neuromuscular reeducation, and enhancing synovial movement.
◆ Observation of the cat's gait can help determine gross deficits in range of motion. However, the evaluation of the quality of the resistance of the joint as the end point of a passive movement of the joint provides information about the complete range of motion for that joint (Table 28-2).

PROPRIOCEPTION

◆ Proprioception and kinesthesia, the sensation of joint motion and acceleration, are the sensory feedback mechanisms for motor control and posture.
◆ These mechanisms along with the vestibular system help the body remain oriented and balanced.

REHABILITATION PROGRAM

◆ The rehabilitation program begins with the evaluation of the cat.
◆ The owner is the key factor in providing information for the optimal outcome for the cat because the cat rarely behaves or moves as it does in its own environment.

TABLE 28-2	Joint End Feels		
End Feel	**Description**	**Example (Normal)**	**Example (Abnormal)**
Bone on bone	Abrupt halt to movement when two hard surfaces meet	Carpal extension Cervical extension	Shoulder flexion
Capsular	Elastic arrest of movement with some give	Hip flexion Shoulder flexion Hip extension Shoulder extension	
Empty	Unable to reach end range because of painful reaction of cat; no tissue tension felt		All joints
Spasm	Muscle spasm actively occurs when attempting range of motion		All joints
Springy block	Rebound of both extreme ends of range of motion because of intraarticular displacement		Common with meniscal injury
Tissue approximation	Range of motion stopped because of secondary engagement against a muscle	Stifle flexion	

OWNER-PROVIDED HISTORY

◆ Age, breed, and the general appearance and disposition of the cat help determine how cooperative the cat will be.
◆ Details about the onset of the problem or injury identify how long the animal has been favoring a leg, and any pertinent medical history may indicate that an exercise or modality should or should not be used.

- The presence of other pets is also a consideration because in the early to middle phase of rehabilitation it is often necessary to restrict unsupervised activity with other animals to reduce the risk of injury.
- The cat's baseline activity level helps determine the cat's condition and the owner's expectation of what the cat should be able to do after rehabilitation.
- Identification of medication and supplements the cat is currently receiving and how the owner believes they are or are not working can be helpful in assessing benefits from rehabilitation.
- Questions should be asked to help determine whether the cat's normal activities have changed.

CLINICAL FINDINGS

- Lameness evaluation
- Evaluation of the cat in standing and sitting positions
- Ability to rise
- Evaluation of the appearance of the scar and any discoloration, swelling, edema, or warmth of the affected tissue before range of motion of the affected and unaffected joints is measured to determine any loss of movement
- Evaluation of passive and active range of motion

REHABILITATION GOALS

- It is important to set reasonable goals at the beginning of the rehabilitation program.
- Thorough evaluation and assessment of the cat's current condition, the expectations of the cat's owner, and the commitment of the owner to the rehabilitation program provide necessary information to develop the proper program for each cat.
- Expectations vary greatly. Owners should be given the information and time to determine their personal rehabilitation goals for their cat.
  - Goals can be set for each phase of the rehabilitation.
- Phase I (within 1 week): Strengthen pelvic limbs so that cat is able to bear weight for a minimum of 20 seconds without outside support.
- Phase II: Strengthen pelvic limb so that cat is able to walk.

OUTCOME MEASUREMENTS

◆ Ensure that rehabilitation goals are being met.
◆ Determine how the animal is progressing as objectively as possible.
◆ Provide the information needed to improve or change the rehabilitation protocol to ensure the most benefit for each cat.
◆ Provide progress information to owner, therapist, and veterinarian.

PASSIVE RANGE OF MOTION

◆ Passive range of motion is measured with a goniometer. A goniometer is a protractor-like instrument with two blades that are attached to a 360-degree marked hinge that pivots to measure the angle formed by two bones across a joint. The two bones are moved to extreme flexion and extension, and a measurement is taken at each extreme. Limited range can be at flexion only, extension only, or both. Measurements taken in the conscious cat can indicate pain-free range of motion. Measurements made in the sedated cat can indicate the maximal range of motion because the cat cannot respond to pain in joint manipulation when sedated.
◆ Initial goniometry measurements can provide information needed to decide the rehabilitation exercises and modalities to be used and to measure the effectiveness of the interventions. Affected and nonaffected joints are measured. Range of motion can be limited by pain or a mechanical problem such as contracted muscle (Fig. 28-1).

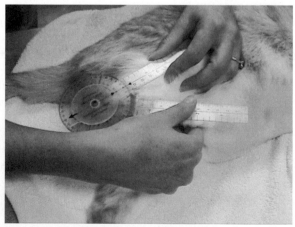

FIG. 28-1. Measuring flexion of hock of cat with goniometer.

ACTIVE RANGE OF MOTION

◆ Active range of motion is evaluated by encouraging or allowing the cat to sit, rise, and lie down.
◆ The cat can be asked to climb stairs or walk over poles for additional data.

MUSCLE MASS

◆ Measurement of thigh or arm circumference helps assess changes in muscle mass throughout the rehabilitation program.
◆ Measurement of the circumference is taken with a special measuring tape called an oliometer.
◆ The special gauge at the end of the tape ensures that the same amount of stress is placed on the tape to ensure repeatability of measurement and to help give accurate results (Fig. 28-2).

BODY COMPOSITION

◆ Body composition is a term used to describe the percentage ratio of body fat to lean muscle.

GAIT ANALYSIS

◆ Motion is a result of a combination of nerves stimulating muscle to move bone.
◆ Abnormal motion occurs when this chain of events is disrupted.

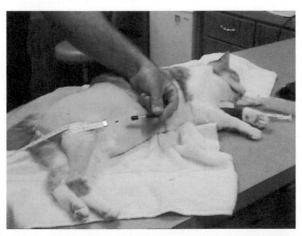

FIG. 28-2. Measurement of thigh circumference using the oliometer.

- Locomotion of the cat is described as its gait.
- Chronic pain or traumatic injury can cause a cat to alter its movement. Alteration in gait may cause pain or injury to unaffected limbs.
- Gait-training techniques and exercise focus on returning the cat to as near normal movement as possible.
- Therapists and owners must identify the specific limitations of the individual cat. In some cases, improvements can be made, but the cat may never return to normal movement. Gait analysis can also be used to assess any subclinical factors that might affect performance.

LAMENESS EVALUATION

- Lameness is defined as a difference from normal gait.
- The walk and trot are the easiest gaits to evaluate for lameness because of the symmetric movement of the trot and walk.
- Evaluation of the gait is called gait analysis.
- Subjective gait analysis is the most common diagnostic tool to assess lameness. Analysis is best done before ever touching the cat. Analysis starts by observing the animal while it is still. The analyst looks for conformation abnormalities such as turned out toes or abnormalities in stance such as the cat holding one leg up or putting most of its body weight on a particular leg. After these observations are noted, the animal is analyzed while moving.
- Gait analysis of the cat should be done in a closed room. The evaluation of normal movement of a cat may only be possible through a videotape of the cat in its home environment.

TYPES OF REHABILITATION MODALITIES

Rehabilitation can be divided into two specific categories:
- Passive rehabilitation modalities, which require no participation from the cat
- Active rehabilitation, which requires the cat to participate in the therapy

PASSIVE REHABILITATION MODALITIES
Thermal Agents

- The application of heat or cold is used to increase or decrease the temperature of the tissue around a joint and can be used throughout a rehabilitation program.
- The use of heat versus cold is determined by the stage of recovery of the tissue.

♦ Heat and cold treatments can reduce the stiffness and pain, especially for joint problems such as arthritis.

The application of cold is used to do the following:

♦ Reduce bleeding
♦ Reduce inflammation
♦ Decrease pain

Specific indications for the use of cold include the following:

♦ Musculoskeletal injury
♦ Following orthopedic surgery
♦ Treatment of muscular pain
♦ Postexercise soreness

Application of Cold Therapy

- Place a thin layer of material between the cold pack and the cat's skin to increase the comfort level.
- Place a towel over the cold pack to avoid loss of cold to the environment.
- Cold therapy is usually applied for 20 minutes, 1 to 4 times a day.
- Even one application of cold during the first 24 hours of trauma has been shown to be beneficial in reducing swelling and pain in the human patient.
- Immediately postoperative, while the cat is still under anesthesia, application of cold may be the only application tolerated by the cat (Fig. 28-3).
- Subsequent applications are best performed with cat resting in the lap of therapist with a blanket wrapped around the cat.

Contraindications. Cold should not be applied if the cat has the following:

- Cold hypersensitivity
- Decreased or absent sensation

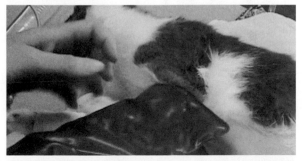

FIG. 28-3. Application of cold pack to limb following orthopedic surgery while cat still recovering from anesthesia.

- Compromised circulation (Do not place cold directly over these areas.)

Application of Heat Therapy.   Superficial heat therapy is used to do the following:

- Increase metabolism
- Increase soft tissue extensibility
- Decrease pain

Heat should be used only after signs of inflammation are gone. Specific uses for heat include the following:

- Subacute and chronic traumatic and inflammatory conditions
- Muscle spasm
- Tissue tightness
- Adhesions
- Pain

In the management of osteoarthritis, heat may be used to help loosen tight muscles around a joint to improve flexibility.

- Superficial heat can be applied using heat packs (Fig. 28-4).
- Application time is 20 minutes 2 to 4 times per day. Inspect the skin at least every 5 minutes.
- Remove the heat source if the cat shows any signs of discomfort.

Contraindications.

- Heat therapy should not be used if any signs of inflammation are present, such as redness or swelling.
- Heat should not be used on animals with decreased or absent sensation, over malignancies, or over an active infection.

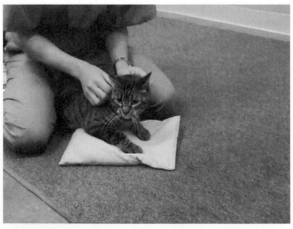

FIG. 28-4. Most cats tolerate application of heat well.

Electrical Stimulation

Electrical stimulation recruits muscle fibers to reverse volitional contractions. Electrical stimulation recruits the fast-twitch fibers first.

♦ Electrical stimulation can be used to do the following:
- Increase muscle strength
- Attenuate atrophy
- Reduce pain
- Reduce edema

Contraindications
- Cats with pacemakers or seizure disorders
- Over the trunk of pregnant females
- In patients that cannot give feedback
- Over infected areas
- Over areas of thrombosis
- Any time active motion is contraindicated

Animal reaction to electrical stimulation should be carefully monitored. Two types of current are generally recommended for use on felines:
- Continuous alternating current for pain and edema
- Pulsed current for strengthening and edema

The area to be stimulated must be clipped and cleaned before the electrodes can be properly applied.

Electrical Stimulation for Pain Management.   Two wave forms
are generally used for the management of pain caused by posttraumatic, postoperative, or chronic pain:
- Interferential waveform consists of two channels, each with a sinusoidal waveform, one fixed and one of variable frequency. The electrodes are positioned so that the two channels cross each other to stimulate large-impulse fibers. These frequencies interfere with the transmission of pain messages at the spinal cord. Interferential stimulation allows for a deep penetration of the tissue with more comfort and therefore more compliance than a transcutaneous electrical nerve stimulation application.
- A premodulated waveform is an amplitude-modulated sine wave that is similar to the beat frequency created by the interferential current. This waveform is often used when four electrodes cannot be placed.
- The electrode placement should cover the entire area suspected of pain. Specific frequency and phase duration of the stimulation varies with each patient and condition. Many electrical stimulation units are available with a variety of variables and recommended parameters.

Electrical Stimulation for Attenuation of Muscle Atrophy

- Two waves that can be used for muscle contraction are high volt and Russian.
- Locate the area where the motor nerve enters the muscle. This location allows for optimum muscle contraction with as low a current as possible to increase the comfort level of the treatment.
- Apply the gel to the skin of the cat, and place the electrode over the expected area of the motor point.
- Turn the unit on and move the electrode until the desired contraction is observed.
- Once identified, the motor points can be marked on the cat with a indelible marker for subsequent treatments.
- Optimum time and frequency of treatment are unknown.
- Common clinical use has been 15 to 20 minutes, 3 to 7 times per week.
- Generally accepted frequency is 25 to 50 Hz.

Therapeutic Ultrasound

◆ Ultrasound is produced by applying an electric current to a crystal (Fig. 28-5). The current causes the crystal to vibrate at a resonant frequency, emitting pressure waves that are absorbed by the tissue.

◆ Therapeutic ultrasound generates ultrasonic energy in continuous or pulsed form to produce thermal, mechanical, and chemical effects in tissues.

◆ Ultrasound is capable of separating collagen fibers and changing the tensile strength of tendons to permit a greater amount of stretching.

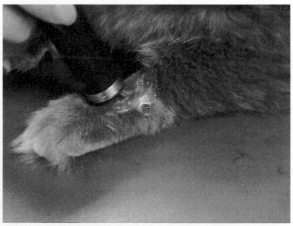

FIG. 28-5. Application of therapeutic ultrasound to the carpal joint of the cat.

- Exercise caution when using ultrasound over plastic or metal plate implants because the reflection may cause more intense heating, leading to burns or discomfort.
- Choose a sound head that provides absolute continuous contact with the skin.

  Therapeutic ultrasound can be used to do the following:
- Increase collagen extensibility (stretch)
- Increase blood flow and increase range of motion
- Decrease pain and muscle spasm
- Accelerate wound healing

  The treatment protocol is as follows:

1. Determine the depth of tissue to be treated.
   - If tissue to be treated is from skin to 3 cm deep, select 3.3-MHz frequency.
   - If tissue to be treated is 2 to 5 cm deep, select 1.0-MHz frequency.
2. Determine the amount of soft tissue in the area to select the rate at which the energy is delivered into the area.
   - Choose 1 to 2 W/cm^2 for areas with large amount of soft tissue such as the caudal thigh muscle.
   - Choose 1 to 1.5 W/cm^2 for areas with less soft tissue, and 0.5 to 1.0 W/cm^2 for areas with little soft tissue, such as the carpus.
   - Choose the mode pulsed or continuous depending on type of thermal effects desired. Both modes give thermal and nonthermal effects, but the pulsed ultrasound has a lower average energy so that the thermal effects are minimal. Pulsed ultrasound is available in 20% pulse and 50% pulse. Pulsed ultrasound is selected when healing effects are desired with as little heating as possible.
   - Treatment time can be calculated by determining the number of transducer heads that fit into the treatment area and multiplying that number by 2.5.
   - The transducer head is moved at a rate of 4 cm/s in overlapping circles in the treatment area.
   - Keep the beam at less than 15 degrees to the surface of the skin.
   - Select a treatment area that requires no more than 20 minutes of treatment time.
   - If a large treatment area is desired, select a larger transducer head or divide the area into different treatment session areas.
   - Sessions are usually repeated 2 to 3 times per week.

Massage

- Therapeutic massage is the manipulation of soft tissue that includes holding, causing movement, and applying pressure to the body.

- Massage therapy may improve functioning of the circulatory, lymphatic, muscular, skeletal, and nervous system and may improve the rate at which the body recovers from injury or illness.
- Massage can be used to relax and reduce anxiety of the cat in the postoperative stage of recovery.

  Two basic massage techniques are as follows:

- Effleurage massage is a gliding stroke using the whole hand. The stroke is applied along the lines of the muscle and affects the superficial tissues. Effleurage is mostly used to assist with circulation, so the strokes are always performed toward the heart.
- Petrissage uses a kneading compression stroke with skin rolling. Petrissage is used for muscle tension, knots, and spasms.

Passive Range of Motion

- Passive range of motion is the manipulation of a joint through its complete possible flexion and extension.
- Passive range of motion provides controlled movement along the normal lines of stress, which can result in stronger scar and connective tissue.
- The motion of the joint affects muscles, joint surfaces, capsules, ligaments, fasciae, vessels, and nerves. Reduction in the normal range of motion can be caused by orthopedic or neurologic surgery, trauma, immobilization, or inactivity.

  Range of motion therapy is beneficial in the following:

- Healing and in recovery from soft tissue and joint lesions
- Maintaining existing joint and soft tissue mobility
- Minimizing the effects of contracture formation
- Assisting neuromuscular reeducation and enhancing synovial movement

  Passive range of motion will not do the following:

- Prevent muscle atrophy
- Improve strength and endurance

  Passive range of motion may be the most important exercise for a cat recovering from a fracture because of the restrictive nature of the movement allowed by splinting or casting.

  General Instruction.   Allow the cat to be in a comfortable position. This may be sitting, standing, or lying. Isolate the range of motion of the joint as much as possible so that pain or stiffness does not influence the range of the focus joint.

  Carpus. Support the leg with one hand. With the leg in a neutral position begin the extension. Continue to extend the carpus to the end feel. Then, to get maximum extension, extend the digits to end feel. Press on the pads of the foot. This simulates the normal position of the leg during stance phase of movement, giving the cat proprioceptive feedback and making it more aware of the leg. Hold for 10 seconds, and then begin flexion of the carpal joint. Continue flexing the joint until the end feel, and then for maximum flexion, flex or fold the digits to the back of the leg. Hold for 10 seconds. Repeat 5 to 10 times.

Elbow. The carpal joint must be flexed and extended to flex and extend the elbow. Begin with the carpal joint supported by one hand and the other hand behind the elbow. Gently push the elbow into extension end feel. The carpal joint will extend at the same time. Push gently on the carpal joint to get maximum extension of the carpal joint and elbow. Hold for 10 seconds. Begin the flexion by flexing the carpal joint, and then, supporting the elbow joint to keep in same location, flex to end feel. Hold for 10 seconds. Repeat 5 to 10 times (Fig. 28-6).

Sholder. Begin with one hand supporting the leg in a neutral position. Hold one hand on the top of the shoulder. Begin extending the elbow, which will also extend the carpus. Bring the elbow to end range and continue to push gently on the elbow until the end feel of shoulder is reached. Usually the leg will reach just above the eye if the head is in normal position. Hold for 10 seconds. Begin the flexion. Fold the elbow and gently push up against the supporting hand to end feel. Hold for ten seconds. Repeat 5 to 10 times.

Stifle. Combine passive range of motion for these two joints to get maximum extension and flexion. Supporting the tarsus in a neutral position, begin to push gently on the stifle until end feel is reached. Gently push on the tarsus to reach maximum extension. Digits can be extended and the pads of the foot pressed as if the cat were standing. Hold for 10 seconds; begin flexion by folding the tarsus to maximum flexion and then folding the knee to maximum flexion. Hold for 10 seconds; repeat 5 to 10 times.

Hip. Support the limb and begin to push the stifle gently into extension. Keeping the knee in extension and one hand on the ischial tuberosity to prevent movement, gently bring the leg back until end feel of the hip is reached. Hold for 10 seconds. Begin flexion by folding the stifle and tarsus and bringing the knee up to hip joint end feel. Hold for 10 seconds. Repeat 5 to 10 times.

Phototherapy (Cold Laser)

♦ Phototherapy is application of low-power light to areas of the body in order to stimulate healing.
♦ Phototherapy can accelerate wound and tissue repair by as much as 30% to 40%.

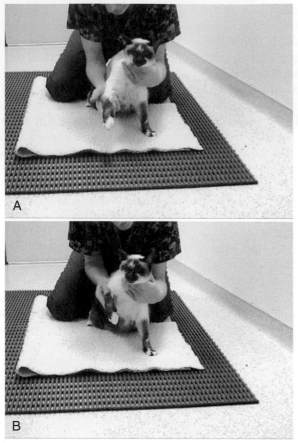

FIG. 28-6. A, Passive range of motion of elbow joint—extension. **B,** Passive range of motion of elbow joint—flexion.

- Cell proliferation and wound healing can be enhanced by 150% to 200%.
  Phototherapy works as follows:
- Photons, electromagnetic energy, are emitted from the low-power laser and enter the tissue.
- The energy is absorbed by the mitochondria of the cell.
- The energy is converted to chemical energy within the cell.
- The permeability of the cell membrane changes, which affects a variety of cell types including macrophages, fibroblasts, endothelial cells, and mast cells.

Phototherapy can be used for the following:

- Soft tissue injuries such as sprains, strains, and tendinitis
- Osteoarthritis
- Chronic pain
- Wound management of ulcers, pressure sores, and burns
- Skin infections
- Healing of incision sites

Cover wound or phototherapy device with clear protective barrier if the skin is broken. Apply the laser with gentle contact for duration of treatment (Fig. 28-7).

ACTIVE REHABILITATION

Aquatic Therapy

Aquatic therapy is the use of the therapeutic properties of water to provide exceptional exercise for the following while reducing the risk of injury:

- Strength
- Range of motion
- Endurance

Aquatic therapy allows for active muscle contraction while limiting peak vertical force.

Aquatic therapy is beneficial for the following:

- Soft tissue injuries
- Osteoarthritis
- Postoperative fracture care
- Muscle weakness

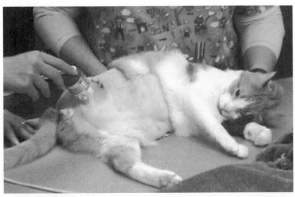

FIG. 28-7. Application of phototherapy to incision site of amputation.

◆ Neurologic impairment
◆ Geriatric care
◆ Postoperative amputee care

  Contraindications
  • Cardiac dysfunction
  • Respiratory dysfunction
  • Surface infection
  • Danger of bleeding or hemorrhage
  • Severe peripheral vascular disease
  • Diarrhea

The therapeutic properties of water include the following:

  • Thermal—Transfer of heat to the submerged tissue
  • Buoyancy—The upward thrust of water on immersed body
  • Hydrostatic pressure—Pressure exerted by water on immersed body
  • Cohesion—The tendency for water molecules to adhere to each other
  • Turbulence—The whirlpools in water caused by movement

The therapeutic thermal effects of water are the same as for superficial heat, only more systemic.

  • Passive range of motion can be performed in warm water to increase stretch and range of motion because of the increase in tissue extensibility.
  • The soothing effects of warm water reduce pain and may increase the cat's ability to exert more effort.
  • Increasing the water temperature can stimulate metabolism, relax tight muscles, help reduce pain, and increase soft tissue extensibility.

The buoyancy property of water is used to increase or decrease the amount of weight bearing on joints and bones.

  • The actual effect of buoyancy can be dramatic.
  • Reducing the body weight of the cat can reduce the amount of stress on a weak joint to allow the cat to exercise in more natural gait pattern and move more comfortably.

The effect of hydrostatic pressure increases with water depth.

  • This effect encourages upward flow of edema.
  • Exercising the cat in deeper water enhances the effect of hydrostatic pressure.

Cohesion and turbulence contribute to the resistance the cat has while moving through the water.

  • The cohesion property of water is used to increase the specific flexion of the joint at water level.

The unique effects of the underwater treadmill include the following:
- Ability to vary the water depth to increase or decrease the amount of weight bearing the cat has while exercising
- Vary the speed of exercise
- Control the water temperature closely because of the small body of water

Introduction
- Special attention is required for safe and productive introduction of the cat to aquatic therapy.
- The therapist must be relaxed and confident in the process to ensure the cooperation of the cat.
- Instructions of how to hand over and then to retrieve the cat after the exercise should be carefully explained to the owner or handler.

Recommendations
- Prepare a towel and place to put the cat at the immediate end of the exercise session. This can be in the towel-wrapped arms of the owner or another technician.
- Water temperature should be 90° to 92° F.
- While standing in the exercise chamber of the underwater treadmill, the therapist should raise the water level to the desired level.
- Turn the treadmill on the desired speed.
- Normal walking speed for the cat in treadmill is 0.8 to 1.3 mph.
- Have the owner hand the cat to the therapist in the chamber with a smooth confident motion with the cat facing the direction it will walk (Fig. 28-8).
- Place the cat in the water, and guide the cat with hands supporting trunk of the cat if needed (Fig. 28-9).

When the session is complete, do the following:
- Do not turn off the treadmill.
- Lift and remove the cat from the water, and place it on the prepared towel and wrap the cat (Fig. 28-10).
- Hand the cat to the owner or assistant, and then turn off and drain the treadmill (Fig. 28-11).
- Gently towel dry the cat (Fig. 28-12).

Feline Exercise Therapy

- ◆ Feline exercise therapy is an active rehabilitation technique using the cat's natural ability to complete activities.
- ◆ This form of therapy is designed to return the cat to normal function sooner and to lessen the risk of future injuries. The level of each exercise varies with the condition or postoperative stage of the cat.

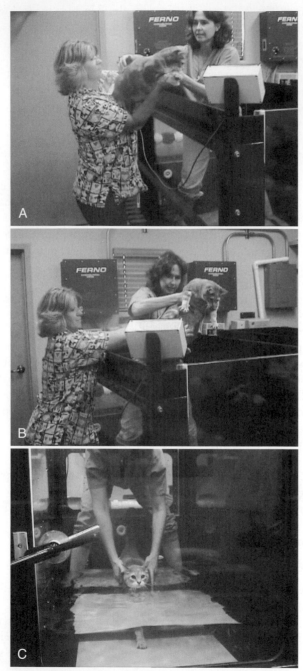

FIG. 28-8. A, The client passes the cat to the therapist. **B,** The therapist confidently takes the cat and in one smooth movement moves the cat toward the water. **C,** The therapist gently releases the cat so that it can begin walking on the treadmill.

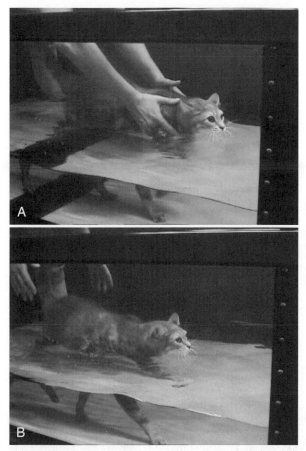

FIG. 28-9. A, The therapist supports the cat for the first several strides. **B,** The therapist remains near to guide the cat but allows the cat as much independence as possible in the treadmill.

- An exercise therapy program begins with short-duration, low-impact activities and progresses to longer periods with more strenuous activities. Modification of the program to accommodate the cat's comfort level is important.
- The exercise therapy program is divided into three stages: warm-up, the exercise activities themselves, and the postexercise therapy.
  The warm-up portion of the program is as follows:
- Assess the cat's physical and mental condition, and prepare the cat for the exercise session. Assessment of the cat is important in order to evaluate the impact of previous sessions and to make changes necessary to keep progressing toward therapy goals.

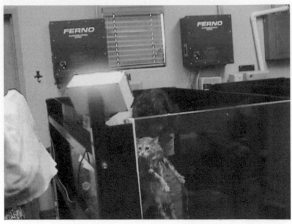

FIG. 28-10. The therapist lifts the cat from the water without turning off the treadmill.

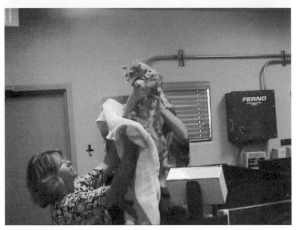

FIG 28-11. The therapist smoothly prepares to hand the cat to the client waiting with a towel.

◆ The cat is prepared for the exercise session by warming the affected area with a warm pack, passive range of motion, massage, or stretch. A combination of superficial heat and stretch is an excellent way to prepare the cat to get the most from the exercise session.

Gait Training

◆ Chronic pain or traumatic injury can cause a cat to alter its movement.
◆ This alteration in gait may cause pain or injury to even unaffected areas.

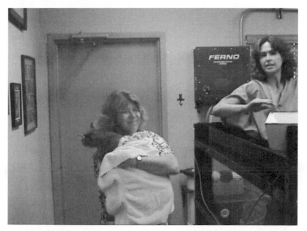

FIG. 28-12. The client begins gently to towel dry the cat.

♦ Gait-training techniques and exercise focus on returning the cat to as near normal movement as possible.

Early Proprioception Exercises

Physioroll

- Choose the appropriate size of ball for the cat and for the type of exercise.
- The ball should be at the wither height of the cat when it is standing.
- Air can be added or removed to help make the ball the right size.

Although many cats may resist being placed on the ball initially, most cats relax after rhythmic movement or bouncing begins. The relaxation can help prevent muscle guarding and subsequent stiffness following surgery or trauma (Fig. 28-13).

- Place the cat on the ball so that the trunk is supported.
- Gently roll the ball until the front legs come in contact with the ground.
- Hold and bounce gently for 10 to 20 seconds.
- Then gently roll the ball so the front feet come off the ground and the back feet touch the ground.
- Gently bounce for 10 to 20 seconds.
- The weight is gradually shifted from front to hind limbs and then back again.
- The amount of weight can be increased or decreased depending on the amount of roll and pressure on the ball.
- The cat will use trunk muscles to stabilize itself.

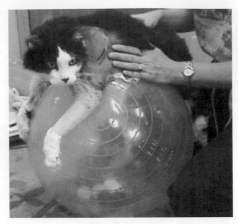

FIG. 28-13. Cat relaxing on ball following surgery to repair dog bite wound.

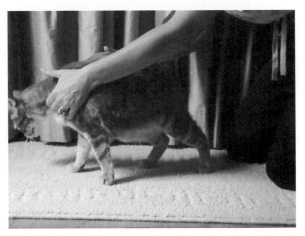

FIG. 28-14. Standing resistance exercise: The cat resists and pushes against the gentle resistance.

Standing Resistance

- Once the cat can stand, gently press on the shoulder, slowly increasing pressure (Fig. 28-14).
- The cat will push back to remain standing.
- If the push is too hard, the cat will be knocked off balance.
- Release the pressure slowly or the cat may fall.
- Try to keep the cat in the same spot.
- Shoulder, hip, and trunk on both sides of the cat are good locations for resistance exercises.

Balance Board

- The balance board is usually 20 inches with a 14-degree angle.
- Homemade versions may vary from these specifications and are still suitable.
- Balance board exercise can assist in the restoration of stability and proprioception of cats following back, rear limb, or front limb surgery.
- Balance board exercise can also be used as an early weight-bearing exercise following knee or hip surgery, elbow or shoulder surgery, or fracture repair (Fig. 28-15).

Benefits of balance board exercise include the following:
- Improved balance and coordination
- Better proprioceptive awareness for injury prevention
- Greater trunk and pelvic girdle stability
- Increased leg and ankle range of motion

Perform the balance board exercise as follows:
- Position the cat centrally over the board with feet shoulder width apart.
- Begin by slowly moving the board front to back for 20 repetitions.
- Support the cat as needed. Be sure to keep the rocking motion under control.
- Then lift the cat and rotate the board 90 degrees and rock side to side for 20 repetitions.
- The cat will contract its muscles and shift its weight to stay on the balance board.

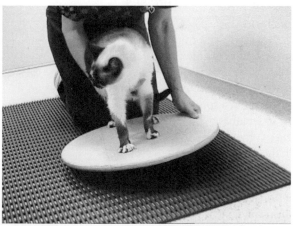

FIG. 28-15. The therapist supports the cat while slowly rocking the board.

Early Weight-Bearing Exercises

These exercises encourage static weight bearing.

One Leg Standing (Fig. 28-16)

- Lift the contralateral leg. Hold for 10 to 15 seconds.
- Repeat 2 to 3 times.
- Increase time and repetitions as cat's strength increases.

Cross Leg Standing (Fig. 28-17)

- Lift the contralateral leg.
- Once the cat is balanced, lift the diagonal rear leg.
- Hold for 10 to 15 seconds. Repeat 2 to 3 times.
- Increase time and repetitions as cat's strength increases.

Dancing

- Support the cat under front legs and lift to encourage increased weight bearing on rear legs.
- Hold for 10 to 15 seconds.
- Repeat 2 to 3 times. Increase time and repetitions as cat's strength increases.
- When the cat's strength increases to the point that it is no longer difficult to support its weight in the stationary position, begin with 2 to 3 steps and increase until the cat is able to move forward 10 steps.

Carts and Slings (Fig. 28-18)

- Carts and slings can be used to support the animal during the early stages of recovery from most neurologic conditions.
- Carts and slings provide the needed support for the dog to assist the therapist during range of motion and floor exercises.

Examples of Rear Limb Exercises

Sit to Stand (Fig. 28-19)

- Place the cat in a sit position.
- Allow or encourage the cat to stand.
- Repeat several times.

Down to Stand (Fig. 28-20)

- Place the cat in a sphinx down position.
- Allow or encourage the cat to rise.

Incline

- Walk the cat up incline.
- Gradually increase the grade.

Gait-Training Exercises

Cavaletti Exercises. Cavaletti poles can be used for the following (Fig. 28-21):

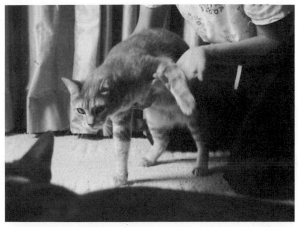

FIG. 28-16. One leg standing encourages low-impact early weight bearing. While supporting the cat, lift the noninjured limb and hold for 10 to 15 seconds.

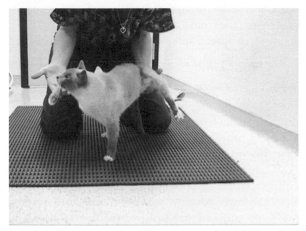

FIG. 28-17. Cross leg stand encourages increased weight bearing during the early weight-bearing phase. Gently lift a noninjured front leg and then a noninjured diagonal rear leg to allow the cat to stand with 50% of its weight on an injured leg in a standing or still position.

- Increase range of motion
- Increase stride length

Perform Cavaletti exercises as follows:
- Start with poles approximately the same distance apart as the height of the cat's elbow.
- Encourage cat to go through the poles.

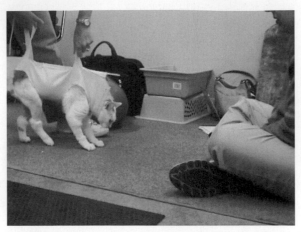

FIG. 28-18. Supported walking with a cat in sling.

- This can be done by luring the cat with food, calling, or allowing the cat to go over poles into a closet or carrier.
- Raise, lower, or spread apart the poles to reach desired gait.

Examples of Front Limb Exercises

Wheelbarrow (Fig. 28-22)
- Lift both rear legs.
- Hold for 10 to 15 seconds.
- Repeat 2 to 3 times.
- Increase time and repetitions as cat's strength increases.

When the cat's strength is increased to the point that it no longer has difficulty supporting its weight in the stationary position, begin to walk the cat slowly forward while holding both rear legs. Begin with 2 to 3 steps and increase until cat is able to move forward 10 steps.

Down to Sit
- Start with the cat in the down position.
- Lure the cat to the sitting position by raising your hand above its head with food in your hand.

Physioroll or Physioball (Fig. 28-23)
- Fold and hold the contralateral limb to the injured limb, and roll the cat forward.
- The cat will reach for the ground with the injured limb.
- Gently bounce the cat with the limb on the ground.

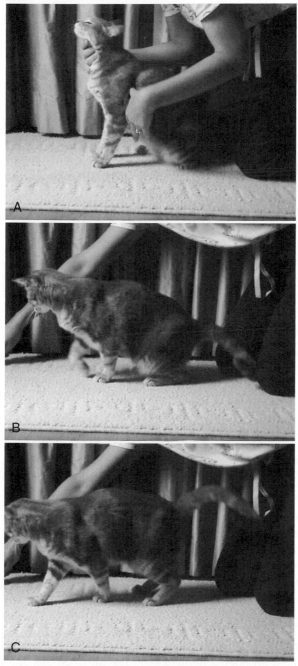

FIG. 28-19. A, Place the cat in a sitting position. **B,** Point to something on the floor in front of the cat while releasing the cat. **C,** Allow the cat to rise into the stand.

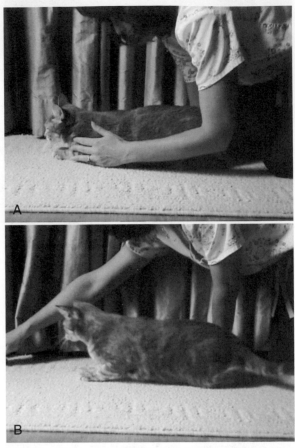

FIG. 28-20. A, Place and support the cat in a down position. **B,** Point to something in front of the cat while releasing the cat.

Trail of Treats (Fig. 28-24)
- Place treats on the floor about 1 foot apart.
- Allow the cat to walk slowly, sniffing the ground.
- This keeps the cat's weight over its feet and encourages weight bearing on both front feet.

Decline (Fig. 28-25)
- Walk the cat down hills or ramps to encourage front limb weight bearing.

Tunnel (Fig. 28-26)
- Walking through a tunnel causes the cat to crouch and increases weight bearing on front limbs.

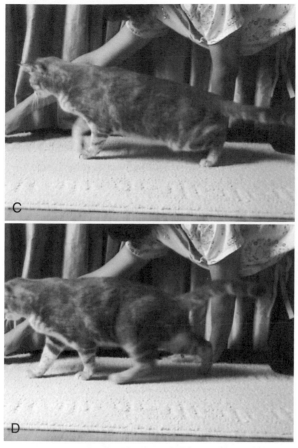

FIG. 28-20—Cont'd. C, Allow the cat to rise without taking a step. **D,** Allow the cat to take one to two steps to be sure of a complete stand.

Rear Limb Rehabilitation Program

Hip

- Problem: Loss of extension (range of motion)
  - Exercises
    - Passive range of motion
    - Active range of motion
      - Cavaletti exercises
      - Walking in 6 inches of high grass
      - Walking in 6 inches of water

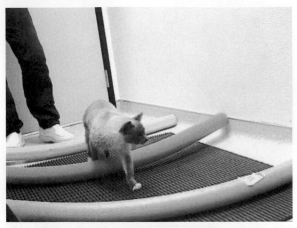

FIG. 28-21. Cat walking over Cavaletti rails.

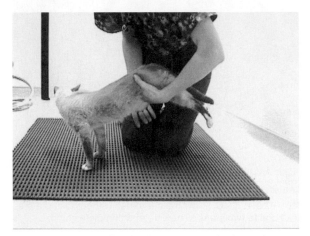

FIG. 28-22. Wheelbarrow: Gently lift and support both rear legs to encourage early weight bearing on front limbs.

- Problem: Loss of pelvic muscle mass
  - Exercises
    - Stationary weight-bearing exercises
    - One leg standing
    - Cross leg standing
    - Sit to stand
    - Down to stand
  - Moving weight-bearing exercises
    - Slow walking
    - Incline

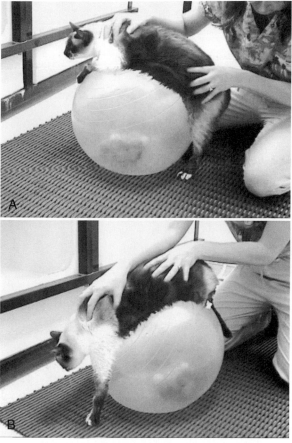

FIG. 28-23. A, Place cat on ball. **B,** Gently roll the cat forward to encourage active range of motion and weight bearing on a front limb.

- Underwater treadmill
- Serpentine walking
- Problem: Muscle guarding
  - Exercises
    - Physioball
    - Active stretching
    - Balance board
  - Modalities
    - Massage therapy
    - Therapeutic ultrasound
    - Electrical stimulation for pain control

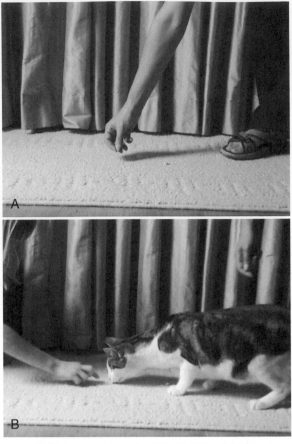

FIG. 28-24. A, Place small pieces of food about 6 inches apart on floor. **B,** Point at food and allow cat to sniff and eat trail of treats to encourage weight bearing on front limbs.

Knee

- Problem: Loss of range of motion
  - Exercises
    - Passive range of motion
    - Active range of motion
      - Cavaletti exercises
      - Walking in 6 inches of high grass
      - Walking in 6 inches of water

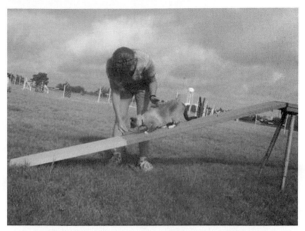

FIG. 28-25. Decline: Allow the cat to walk down the incline slowly. Food may be used to encourage the descent.

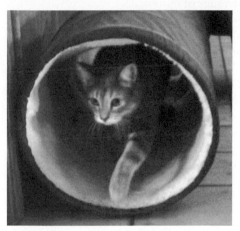

FIG. 28-26. Cat walking through tunnel to encourage flexion of front limbs.

- Problem: Loss of forelimb muscle
  - Exercises
    - Stationary weight-bearing exercises
      - One leg standing
      - Cross leg standing
      - Down to sit
    - Moving weight-bearing exercises
      - Slow walking
      - Decline

- Underwater treadmill
- Trail of treats
- Serpentine walking
- Problem: Muscle guarding
  - Exercises
    - Physioball
    - Active stretching
    - Balance board
  - Modalities
    - Massage therapy
    - Therapeutic ultrasound
    - Electrical stimulation for pain control

Hock

- Problem: Loss of extension (range of motion)
  - Exercises
    - Passive range of motion
    - Active range of motion
      - Cavaletti exercises
      - Walking in 6 inches of high grass
      - Walking in 6 inches of water
      - Exercise in underwater treadmill
- Problem: Muscle guarding
  - Exercises
    - Physioball
    - Active stretching
    - Balance board
  - Modalities
    - Massage therapy
    - Therapeutic ultrasound
    - Electrical stimulation for pain control

Front Limb Rehabilitation Program

Shoulder

- Problem: Loss of extension (range of motion)
  - Exercises
    - Passive range of motion
    - Active range of motion
      - Cavaletti exercises
      - Walking in 6 inches of high grass
      - Walking in 6 inches of water

- Problem: Loss of shoulder cuff muscle
  - Exercises
    - Stationary weight-bearing exercises
      - One leg standing
      - Cross leg standing
      - Down to sit
    - Moving weight-bearing exercises
      - Slow walking
      - Decline
      - Underwater treadmill
      - Tunnel
      - Trail of treats
- Problem: Muscle guarding
  - Exercises
    - Physioball
    - Active stretching
    - Balance board
  - Modalities
    - Massage therapy
    - Therapeutic ultrasound
    - Electrical stimulation for pain control

Elbow

- Problem: Loss of range of motion
  - Exercises
    - Passive range of motion
    - Active range of motion
      - Cavaletti exercises
      - Walking in 6 inches of high grass
      - Walking in 6 inches of water
- Problem: Loss of arm muscle
  - Exercises
    - Stationary weight-bearing exercises
      - One leg standing
      - Cross leg standing
      - Down to sit
      - Wheelbarrow
      - Physioball
    - Moving weight-bearing exercises
      - Slow walking
      - Decline
      - Underwater treadmill
      - Wheelbarrow

- Problem: Muscle guarding
  - Exercises
    - Physioball
      - Active stretching
      - Balance board
    - Modalities
      - Massage therapy
      - Therapeutic ultrasound
      - Electrical stimulation for pain control

Carpal

- Problem: Loss of range of motion
  - Exercises
    - Passive range of motion
    - Active range of motion
      - Cavaletti exercises
      - Walking in 6 inches of high grass
      - Walking in 6 inches of water
      - Exercise in underwater treadmill
- Problem: Hyperextension
  - Exercises
    - Underwater treadmill

Back

- Problem: Rear limb atrophy
  - Exercises
    - Underwater treadmill
    - Serpentine walking
- Problem: Muscle spasm
  - Exercises
    - Physioball
    - Active stretching
    - Balance board
  - Modalities
    - Massage therapy
    - Electrical stimulation for pain control

Obesity

- Problem: Exercise intolerant
  - Exercises
    - Underwater treadmill
    - Slow walking
- Problem: Joint pain
  - Exercises
    - Physioball

- Active stretching
- Balance board
- Underwater treadmill
- Modalities
  - Massage therapy
  - Electrical stimulation for pain control
  - Therapeutic ultrasound

29 QUALITY OF LIFE ISSUES

M. LESLEY WISEMAN-ORR, JACQUELINE REID,
ANDREA M. NOLAN, AND E. MARIAN SCOTT

MEASURING THE IMPACT OF CHRONIC PAIN UPON HEALTH-RELATED QUALITY OF LIFE

Acute pain is associated with tissue damage or the threat of it and serves the vital purpose of rapidly altering behavior in order to avoid damage or minimize further damage and to optimize the conditions in which healing can take place, stopping when healing is complete. In contrast, chronic pain persists beyond the expected course of an acute disease process and tends to have a significant impact on the psychology of the sufferer. Human chronic pain is often associated with fear, anger, anxiety, or depression, all of which may be caused by a patient's pain and in their turn may exacerbate it. Chronic pain therefore can have a widespread impact on patients' social, psychological, and physical well-being, thereby affecting their quality of life (QOL).

QOL is a general term used in a variety of disciplines in which it is accepted that QOL is, like pain, a multidimensional construct that is subjectively experienced by and is uniquely personal to the individual. Health-related quality of life (HRQL) is concerned with those aspects of QOL that change as a result of ill health and medical interventions. HRQL has not previously been defined for animals, and no widely accepted definition for QOL in animals exists. We propose the following simple definition, intended to be relevant in any circumstances (including those of ill health): QOL is the subjective and dynamic evaluation by the individual of its circumstances and the extent to which these meet its expectations, which results in an affective (emotional) response to those circumstances. Consequently, HRQL is the subjective evaluation of circumstances that include an altered health state and related interventions.

Recognition of the effects of chronic pain on HRQL in humans has led to the development of instruments to measure chronic pain through such impacts, and many of the instruments now used in people are concerned primarily with the way in which the chronic condition disrupts activities of daily living and alters HRQL. Indeed, HRQL measures may be more responsive to clinical changes in patients with a chronic condition than are pain measures themselves.

The application of the term *quality of life* to animals is less common, at least in formal veterinary or scientific contexts in which the focus has been on "welfare" and welfare measurement. Some use these terms interchangeably, but the authors believe that there is a distinction between the two as follows. Welfare (and similarly well-being) is a complex construct that combines subjective and objective aspects of the conditions of life for animals, for example, as described in the "five freedoms" of the Farm Animal Welfare Council. Although the importance to its welfare of how the animal feels is now widely recognized, practical welfare measurement is still most usually concerned with ensuring that minimum standards of care are provided. Consequently, the focus is on ensuring that animals do not feel too bad, rather than on helping to make them feel good or very good. If we adopt for animals a conceptualization and definition of QOL that is similar to that for people, then consideration of QOL in veterinary and animal science offers the opportunity to make explicit the importance of the individual's perspective and to shift the focus in animal welfare significantly from the avoidance of poor QOL to the attainment of good and even excellent QOL (Box 29-1).

Although the subjective nature of the pain experience renders impossible any scientific certainty about its perception (even about how it is perceived by another person), most scientists now consider that, unless proved otherwise, the morally correct stance is to assume that many nonhuman animal species may suffer pain in a similar way to humans. Accordingly, we should assume that chronic pain may have a negative effect on an animal's HRQL as it does on our own, and anecdotal evidence and recent studies have provided some evidence for this.

IMPORTANCE OF MEASURING CHRONIC PAIN AND HRQL IN ANIMALS

The incidence of chronic pain in companion animals is increasing. In the past two decades small animal practitioners have seen a considerable change in the demographics of the pet population with an increase in the geriatric population of dogs and cats, resulting in more frequent

---

BOX 29-1

QOL and HRQL of People and Animals in Pain

- Quality of life (QOL), like pain, is a multidimensional construct that is subjectively experienced by and is uniquely personal to the individual.
- Until relatively recently, the term *welfare* rather than *quality of life* has been applied to animals. However, whereas welfare measurement ensures that minimum standards of care are provided so animals do not feel too bad, QOL measurement, by focusing on the animal's perspective, attempts to ensure that the animal feels good or very good.
- When ill health or medical intervention leads to changes in QOL, the term *health-related quality of life* (HRQL) is used.
- In humans, chronic pain can adversely affect a person's social, psychological, and physical well-being, thereby affecting HRQL, and we believe that this also applies to animals.
- In humans, chronic pain is measured by its impact on HRQL, and recent evidence supports the use of similar methodology in animals.

---

presentations of painful, chronic conditions such as osteoarthritis and painful tumors.

The current trend in managing chronic osteoarthritis in dogs is toward using combinations of therapeutic agents accompanied by lifestyle and dietary management, and in oncology, clinicians must choose from a range of therapeutic options. To assess clinical change, gauge treatment efficacy, and guide treatment decisions, including decisions regarding the appropriateness of euthanasia, many clinicians and their clients would find it helpful to have access to valid, reliable, and responsive measures of pain and HRQL as they attempt to identify the best course of action for the treatment of a patient that cannot speak for itself. With greater choice of treatment options and increased affordability has come increasingly demanding ethical decision making in general veterinary practice and in specialist veterinary practice. This is particularly true in the field of oncology, in which increased survival is often achieved by the aggressive use of potentially aversive treatment protocols that may adversely affect HRQL during and after treatment. In palliative care, too, treatments can have negative and positive impacts on QOL that must be weighed against each other and against *quantity* of life valuations. An instrument that could be used with confidence to measure QOL and to monitor clinical change in an individual, as well as to provide data that would facilitate the development and selection of treatments with known effectiveness and impact, should reliably inform such decision making and so lessen the moral distress often suffered by those involved in such decisions, whether veterinary practitioner or client. Until now, there have been no such instruments, and measurement of an animal's pain and QOL has used indirect clinical measures and subjective judgment by veterinarian and/or client: an assessment approach of questionable validity, reliability, and sensitivity and one that is at risk of positive and negative bias.

The current emphasis on evidence-based veterinary medicine, in which decisions on adopting, modifying, or abandoning treatment methodologies are made according to peer-reviewed evidence, requires that robust measures of clinical impact be developed. Furthermore, a recent international workshop of experts in animal and human pain concluded that the creation of valid and acceptable instruments to measure animal pain is one of the most important tasks requiring immediate action. The unpleasant feelings associated with pain—the emotional component of pain—cause an animal to suffer. Measuring that emotional component of an animal's pain or HRQL represents a huge challenge. In the past two decades the medical profession has recognized the importance, however difficult, of the valid and reliable measurement of how people are feeling, and we have much to learn from the methods established by our medical colleagues in pursuit of that aim.

QUICK ASSESSMENT QUALITY OF LIFE QUESTIONNAIRE

The Quick Assessment Quality of Life Questionnaire is for use by pet owners and is designed to assess the QOL of pets (species unspecified), regardless of disease condition; that is, it is a generic instrument (Box 29-2). However, it is not clear on what basis the items in the questionnaire were generated, leading to the assumption that it was ad hoc and that the questionnaire was not validated before publication. Furthermore, no guidance is given as to how the questionnaire should be used by the pet owner; it appears that the answers to questions 1 to 5 inform a global impression of the pet's QOL, recorded by the owner on a 1-to-10 numeric rating scale.

QUESTIONNAIRE FOR EVALUATING HEALTH-RELATED QUALITY OF LIFE IN DOGS WITH SIGNS OF PAIN SECONDARY TO CANCER

The 12 items in the Questionnaire for Evaluating Health-Related Quality of Life in Dogs with Signs of Pain Secondary to Cancer were based on those used in a questionnaire to assess HRQL in people with cancer and cover three domains, namely, physical, psychological, and social functioning (Box 29-3). Responses are scored from 0 to 3 and are summed to give an overall score (0 to 36), with lower scores indicating lower HRQL.

BOX 29-2

Quick Assessment Quality of Life Questionnaire

1. How many pleasures does your pet currently have in his life? _____ How many pleasures did your pet have in his life when he was feeling his best, physically and emotionally? _____

2. How many things does your pet currently have or do in his life that could be called fun? _____ How many things did your pet have or do in his life that could be called fun when he was feeling his best, physically and emotionally? _____

3. On a scale of 1 to 10, 1 being unaffected and 10 being severely distressed (suffering), how much discomfort is your pet currently experiencing from unpleasant feelings (such as nausea, ill feelings, difficulty breathing, pain, itchiness, constipation, loneliness, fear, anxiety, depression)? _____

4. All things considered, what do you consider to be your pet's current enjoyment of life overall, on a scale of 1 to 10 (1 means no enjoyment, and 10 is the highest possible level of enjoyment)? _____

5. On a scale of 1 to 10, 1 being very unwilling and 10 being very willing, how willing would you be to take on the life your pet is now living? _____

6. Based on the answers given to the above five questions, rate your pet's current quality of life using a scale of 1 to 10, 1 being the lowest and 10 being the highest possible quality of life an animal could have. _____

From McMillan FD: *J Am Anim Hosp Assoc* 39:227-235, 2003.

The questionnaire was shown to be acceptable to respondents, easy to use, and quick to complete. Scores demonstrated a difference between healthy dogs, those with skin disease (pruritus, not pain), and dogs with cancer, but whether the instrument is sensitive enough to detect differences in dogs with different degrees of pain related to cancer requires further investigation.

KARNOFSKY'S SCORE MODIFIED FOR CATS

Karnofsky's score was developed to determine the ability of a human patient to carry on normal activities in life by using a scale of 0% to 100%. This scale was modified for use in cats, based on eating, playing, sleeping, and social behaviors, as well as general health.

The Karnofsky's score for cats is calculated by adding the score from an owner questionnaire (Box 29-4) to a general condition score generated by the attending clinician (Box 29-5). The owner compares the actual behavior of the cat to its behavior when well and has to judge the difference, choosing between five scores (0 = behavior not present any more; 1 = behavior shown only rarely; 2 = behavior is shown half as often as before; 3 = behavior is shown almost as often as before; 4 = behavior is shown as often as before). Thereafter each item

BOX 29-3

Questionnaire for Evaluating Health-Related Quality of Life in Dogs with Signs of Pain Secondary to Cancer

How much do you think that the disease is disturbing your dog's quality of life?
  Very much (0)
  Much (1)
  Alittle (2)
  Not at all (3)
Does your dog still do what it likes (e.g., play or go for a walk)?
  Nu (0)
  Rarely (1)
  Frequently (2)
  In a normal way (3)
How is your dog's mood?
  Totally altered (0)
  Some episodes of alteration (1)
  Changed a little bit (2)
  Normal (3)
Does your dog keep its hygienic habits (i.e., does your dog clean itself)?
  No (0)
  Rarely (I)
  Less than beforc (2)
  Yes (3)
How often do you think that your dog feels pain?
  All the tlme (0)
  Frequently (I)
  Rarely 12)
  Never (3)
Does your dog have an appetite?
  No (0)
  Only eats when forced; will eat more of what it likes (1)
  Little (2)
  Normal (3)
Does your dog get tired easily?
  Yes, always (0)
  Frequently (1)
  Rarely (2)
  No (3)
How is your dog sleeping?
  Very badly; not sleeping at all (0)
  Badly (1)
  Almost normally (2)
  Normally (3)
How often does your dog vomit?
  Always (0)
  Frequently (1)
  Rarely (2)
  Never (3)

—Continued

BOX 29-3

Questionnaire for Evaluating Health-Related Quality of Life in Dogs with Signs of Pain Secondary to Cancer—*Cont'd*

How are the intestines of your dog functioning?
  Very badly (0)
  Badly (1)
  Almost normally (2)
  Normally (3)
Is your dog able to position itself to defecate and urinate?
  Never positions itself to urinate or defecate (0)
  Rarely positions itself to urinate or defecate (1)
  Sometimes positions itself to urinate or defecate (2)
  Urinates and defecates normally (3)
How much attention is your dog giving to the family?
  Indifferent (0)
  Little attention (1)
  Increased attention; the dog is needy (2)
  Has not changed (3)
  Scores (values in parentheses) for all 12 questions are summed to determine the health-related quality of life score. Possible scores range from 0 to 36.

From Yazbeck KVB, Fantoni DT: *J Am Vet Med Assoc* 226:1354-1358, 2005.

score (0 to 4) is multiplied by a weighting factor attributed to that particular item (as in Box 29-4). Summing the weighted scores gives the questionnaire score out of 50. The clinician determines the general condition of the patient by choosing one of six scores (5 = completely normal general condition; 4 = minor changes; 3 = medium changes; 2 = major changes in general condition; 1 = severely diseased; 0 = dead). The score chosen is multiplied by 10 to give a maximum of 50.

Thus the score is calculated as follows:

$$\text{General condition score (0 to 50)} + \text{Questionnaire}$$
$$\text{score (0 to 50)} = \text{Karnofsky's score (0 to 100)}$$

The usefulness of the Karnofsky's score was demonstrated in a study of naturally feline immunodeficiency virus–infected cats undergoing treatment in which treated cats showed improved HRQL compared with untreated controls, but to the authors' knowledge, further validation has not been carried out. Additionally, no information as to how the weights for the items in the owner's questionnaire were derived is available, leading to the assumption that it was ad hoc.

BOX 29-4

Karnofsky's Score Modified for Cats (Owner Questionnaire)

Questionnaire is to be answered by the cat owners. The owner has to compare the actual behavior of the cat to the behavior before he noticed any signs of disease and has to judge the difference. He can choose between five scores (0 = behavior is not present any more; 1 = behavior is only shown rarely; 2 = behavior is shown about half as often as in earlier times; 3 = behavior is shown almost as often as in earlier times; 4 = behavior is shown as often as in earlier times). The points are multiplied with the factor individually for every question. The maximum (max.) points are listed at the right side.

Questions About the Cat's Behavior (Factor/Max. points)

Eating Behavior (Max. points = 10)
Your cat is eating the whole amount of what you feed:	1.5/6
Your cat is eating with appetite every time you feed:	0.25/1
Your cat is eating immediately after receiving its food:	0.25/1
Your cat is eating everything that is offered:	0.25/1
Your cat is eating something it did not like in earlier times:	0.125/0.5
Your cat is catching mice:	0.125/0.5

Excretion Behavior (Max. points = 5)
Your cat is always house-trained:	1/4
Your cat is burying its excretions in a proper way:	0.25/1

Sleeping Behavior (Max. points = 10)
The duration of its nonsleeping periods is normal:	1.5/6
Your cat is very energetic:	1/4

Comfort Behavior (Max. points = 10)
Your cat is cleaning and grooming itself often and carefully:	1/4
Your cat is very self-content:	0.5/2
Your cat sunbathes regularly:	0.5/2
Your cat visits its favorite places regularly:	0.5/2

Playing Behavior (Max. points = 8)
Your cat plays frequently:	0.25/1
Your cat is interested in new toys:	0.25/1
Your cat is coming regularly to you for the routine contact:	1/4
Your cat shows a curious behavior toward other people:	0.5/2

Social Behavior (Max. points = 7)
Your cat is often leaving the house for a walk:	0.5/2
The duration of time spent outside is normal:	0.5/2
Your cat behaves interestedly in other animals:	0.5/2
Your cat is fighting or having sexual activities as often as usual:	0.25/1

From Hartmann K, Kuffer M: *Eur J Med Res* 3:95-98, 1998.

In conclusion, there are remarkably few measurement instruments available to the veterinary surgeon who wishes to measure companion animal QOL or HRQL. Increasingly, such measurement is becoming more and more necessary in clinical practice as medical advances facilitate the keeping of animals with painful chronic disease for a longer time, and evidence-based medicine requires that robust measures of clinical impact be developed. The development of valid, reliable, and

---

BOX 29-5

Karnofsky's Score Modified for Cats (Clinician Questionnaire)

100%—Normal behavior, no complaints, no evidence of disease
90%—Minor signs of disease, still normal eating, resting, and social behavior
80%—Some signs of disease, eating behavior not influenced, social behavior slightly reduced, normal activities like playing and grooming only with effort, increased sleeping time
70%—Playing, comfort, and social behavior reduced, more lethargy than normal, less appetite
60%—Requiring assistance sometimes in cleaning and special feeding care
50%—Requiring assistance all the time in cleaning and feeding, and sometimes medical care
40%—Requiring assistance for everything and depending on medical care; wild, roaming cats without human help in acute danger to life
30%—Severely disabled, taking no food, appropriate medical care difficult at home, hospitalization indicated
20%—Very sick, life not possible without hospitalization, active supportive treatment necessary for staying alive
10%—Danger to life, fatal process progressing rapidly
0%—Dead

---

sensitive measurement instruments for QOL and HRQL in animals is time-consuming, challenging, and costly, but in the authors' view, the resourcing and carrying out of such research are mandatory if we are to maintain rigorous scientific standards in modern veterinary medicine.

Suggested Readings

Association of Veterinary Teachers and Research Workers: Guidelines for the recognition and assessment of pain in animals, *Vet Rec* 118:334-338, 1986.

Brearly JC, Brearly MJ: Chronic pain in animals. In Flecknell PA, Waterman-Pearson A, editors: *Pain management in animals*, London, 2000, WB Saunders.

Cambridge AJ, Tobias KM, Newberry RC, Sarkar DK: Subjective and objective measurements of postoperative pain in cats, *J Am Vet Med Assoc* 217(5):685-690, 2000.

Conzemius MG, Hill CM, Sammarco JL, Perkowski SZ: Correlation between subjective and objective measures used to determine severity of postoperative pain in dogs, *J Am Vet Med Assoc* 201(11):1619-1622, 1997.

Holton L, Scott EM, Nolan AM, et al: The development of a composite measure scale to assess pain in dogs, *J Vet Pharmacol Ther* 20(suppl 1):167-168, 1997.

McMillan FD: Maximising quality of life in ill animals, *J Am Anim Hosp Assoc* 39:227-235, 2003.

Paul-Murphy J, Ludders JW, Robertson SA, et al: The need for a cross-species approach to the study of pain in animals, *JAMA* 224(5):692-697, 2004.

Wiseman-Orr ML, Nolan AM, Reid J, Scott EM: Development of a questionnaire to measure the effects of chronic pain on health-related quality of life in dogs, *Am J Vet Res* 65:1077-1084, 2004.

Wiseman-Orr ML, Scott EM, Reid J, Nolan AM: Validation of a structured questionnaire as an instrument to measure chronic pain in dogs on the basis of effects on health-related quality of life, *Am J Vet Res* 67:1826-1836, 2006.

Wojciechowska JI, Hewson CJ: Quality-of-life assessment in pet dogs, *J Am Vet Med Assoc* 226(5):722-728, 2005.

30 HOSPICE AND PALLIATIVE CARE

TAMI SHEARER

Not surprisingly, as the human population ages and has more personal exposure to palliative and hospice care, pet owners are aware that there are benefits to having those services available for pets too. Consequently, a growing number of pet owners are requesting palliative and hospice care services for their pets. Ultimately, the goal of palliative and hospice care in veterinary medicine is to relieve suffering while enhancing the quality of life for the pet and family.

Often the trend in veterinary medicine is to shadow advances in human care. However, when it comes to palliative and hospice care, the profession is adopting a philosophy rather than a diagnostic test. Little information is available to guide the veterinary practitioner through this philosophy and process of palliative and hospice care, until now.

The availability of euthanasia for pets has created a delay in embracing palliative care and hospice care in the veterinary profession. Because of advances in veterinary medicine, the profession is now able to recognize and treat symptoms better than before, and veterinarians are less dependent on the option of euthanasia to alleviate suffering. The result is an overall qualitative improvement and extension of life for pets.

The American Veterinary Medical Association recognizes hospice care as an important part of a pet's care and has guidelines that support the practice of good veterinary medicine. A copy of the guidelines can be obtained from the association.

The term *hospice* comes from the Latin word *hospitium*, which means to host. Hospice is defined as a facility or program designed to provide a caring environment for supplying the physical and emotional needs of the terminally ill. The term *palliate* comes from the Latin word *palliare*, which means to cloak or conceal. Palliative care is focused on the relief of suffering to achieve the best quality of life regardless of the disease outcome. Palliative care is not hospice care, but the services may overlap during the approach of death.

A human study of 122 caretakers showed that a lack of preparedness when a person was dying resulted in a prolonged grieving period of more than 9 months, with major depression. Because of the strong bond between some people and their pets, it is reasonable to assume that similar data may apply to the loss of a pet, thus highlighting the need for palliative and hospice care for pet owners.

The following information should help any veterinarian use the philosophy of palliative and hospice care immediately. This care can provide aid in many situations (Box 30-1).

BOX 30-1

Qualifications/Circumstances That Warrant Palliative or Hospice Care

1. A decision not to pursue curative treatments
2. Diagnosis of a terminal illness
3. Diagnosis of a chronic illness
4. Symptoms of a chronic illness that are interfering with the routine of the pet
5. Disease process in which curative treatment was possible but failed
6. Problems that require long-term intensive care
7. Illnesses that are progressive
8. Diseases or traumas that have health complications associated with them

---

Veterinarians should keep in mind that palliative or hospice care should always be relationship centered. Palliative and hospice care should be family oriented with the focus on the pet's quality of life. Any veterinarian interested in providing palliative care and hospice services should be a good listener, patient, and empathic and should have good time management skills.

If possible, a palliative or hospice care program should begin as soon as a qualifying diagnosis is made, even before the onset of symptoms. All curative treatments need to be discussed with pet owners before entering into palliative or hospice care. With every new case, careful review of diagnostic tests and response to treatment may prevent the mistake of developing a hospice plan for a pet with a treatable illness. Accurate diagnostic and prognostic information should help to transition from curative treatment to supportive care, and then from palliative to hospice care.

Patient evaluation should consist of the following:
- Physical examination findings
- List of all problems
- Assessment of quality of life

The location where hospice care is carried out is less important than the philosophy behind the care. Having a quiet designated area in a veterinary hospital to see patients for palliative or hospice consultations is preferable, but not necessary. The care can be carried out in standard examination rooms or at the pet owner's house. To offer the service is better than not to offer it because of lack of a specialized area. The pet should be comfortable in the chosen surrounding.

PALLIATIVE AND HOSPICE CARE PROTOCOL

It makes sense to follow an established protocol to ensure that all details of care are provided. Every pet's condition and family relationship is different; the protocol serves as the template for the veterinarian and the pet's family to share information. A Five-Step Strategy for Comprehensive Care developed by the nonprofit Pet Hospice and Education Center provides such a protocol (Box 30-2).

BOX 30-2

Five-Step Strategy for Comprehensive Care

1. Evaluation of the pet owner's needs, beliefs, and goals for the pet
2. Education about the disease process
3. Development of a personalized plan for the pet and pet owner
4. Application of hospice or palliative care techniques
5. Emotional support during the care process and after the death of the pet

---

EVALUATION OF THE PET OWNER'S NEEDS, BELIEFS, AND GOALS FOR THE PET

For the program to be successful, the care delivered by the veterinary professional must be consistent with the beliefs of the pet owner. Investigation of these psychosocial concerns allows for proper development of a personalized program. Communication is a major part of the foundation upon which palliative and hospice care is built. For example, if a family does not believe in euthanasia, then the course of action and recommendations need to be tailored to meet this belief. If the goal is to keep the pet out of the hospital, then this should be understood, and alternatives to hospitalization should be discussed. Keep in mind that it is not unusual for pet owners to abandon their original palliative or hospice care plan and pursue additional treatment in the hope of a cure.

To ask the proper questions so as to prepare for the medical plan adequately is important, especially as the end of life nears. Whether the pet owner has had any past experiences (good or bad) with health care is helpful to know because this can play a role in understanding the decision-making process. A pet owner's goals of care may vary. The owner may strive for a cure despite the prognosis or instead may choose just to keep the pet comfortable. The owner's attitude regarding nutritional support is important because there are support options ranging from free feeding to esophagostomy and percutaneous endoscopic gastrostomy tubes. The veterinarian should explain the risks and benefits of the various support options. Forced feeding by placing food in the mouth of a dying pet that is not hungry should be discouraged.

When designing a plan for an ill pet, it is important to consider whether the pet owner has desires for diagnostic testing to track the disease trajectory or to make treatment adjustments. The owner may also have a preference regarding where a pet spends its time. For example, some pet owners choose not to consider hospitalization but opt for outpatient or home care for their pet.

Financial concerns on the pet owner's part should be taken into consideration but should not alter the sharing of information about all treatment options. There may be benefit in using alternative/complementary care if the pet owner is open to these options. An example of complementary therapy is the use of milk thistle (silymarin) to aid in the treatment of liver disease.

Early on, the veterinarian should discuss final event details with the pet owner. Specifically, the veterinarian should determine where a pet owner wants the pet to die and whether the owner wants to be with the pet at that time. The veterinarian shou ld inform the owner regarding the pet's body if the pet dies at home. Several choices may be available for handling the pet's remains, and there is benefit in asking about this ahead of time.

Veterinarians should be prepared to go where the clients need them to go to improve a pet's quality of life (Box 30-3).

EDUCATION ABOUT THE DISEASE PROCESS

The veterinarian should become familiar with the disease process to be able to share factual information with the pet owner about life expectancy, symptoms of the disease, and common side effects. This shared knowledge allows the pet owner to be able to make better choices on the pet's behalf. An accurate diagnosis is important before initiating

> **BOX 30-3**
>
> **Psychosocial Concerns Assessment**
>
> Medical experiences
> Belief regarding death and euthanasia
> Preferences for testing to track illness trajectory
> Preferences regarding hospitalization versus outpatient versus home care
> Role of financial concerns on health care choices
> Preferences regarding alternative/complementary care
> Preferences on where a pet dies and whether owner wants to be present
> Discussion of what to do with the body if the pet dies at home
> Choice of how to handle the remains

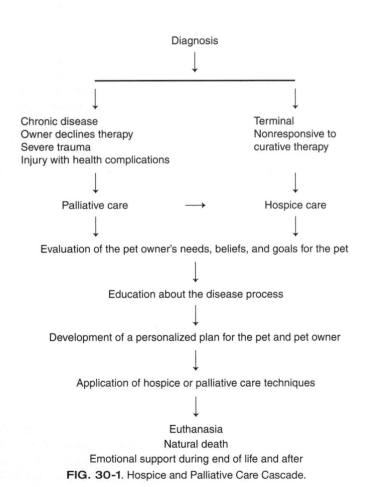

Diagnosis

↓

Chronic disease
Owner declines therapy
Severe trauma
Injury with health complications

Terminal
Nonresponsive to
curative therapy

↓   ↓

Palliative care ⟶ Hospice care

↓   ↓

Evaluation of the pet owner's needs, beliefs, and goals for the pet

↓

Education about the disease process

↓

Development of a personalized plan for the pet and pet owner

↓

Application of hospice or palliative care techniques

↓

Euthanasia
Natural death
Emotional support during end of life and after

FIG. 30-1. Hospice and Palliative Care Cascade.

a hospice plan. Careful review of diagnostic tests and response to treatment may prevent the embarrassment of developing a hospice plan for a pet with a treatable illness.

Taking into account all the side effects associated with the disease and letting the pet owner know that these complications may respond to symptomatic treatment is important. For example, constipation is a common side effect of many illnesses and can often be prevented by educating the pet owner to look for the symptoms of small, hard stools, and/or decreased frequency of bowel movements and then providing early therapy for the condition before obstipation develops. Pet owners need to know that a decrease in appetite should be treated early with antacids, antiemetics, and appetite stimulants to maintain a better nutritional state longer. This may be of importance to delay cancer cachexia.

DEVELOPMENT OF A PERSONALIZED PLAN FOR THE PET AND PET OWNER

Development of a personalized plan for the pet and pet owner should take into consideration the previous discussion about the family's beliefs and desires for the pet. In addition to managing the symptoms of disease, the plan should take into account the willingness of the pet to take medications and how the pet reacts to the stress of hospital visits. In designing a palliative and hospice care plan, the program should be coordinated to extend across the different locations of the pet's care. For example, the coordinator may work with the family and internal medicine specialist to make sure that all the communication is being well directed and that all of the physical, emotional, and psychosocial needs are being met.

As a pet's condition begins to deteriorate, it is important to transition into hospice care. For this to happen, the family must acknowledge that the pet is actually dying and is showing no improvement or worsening with medical help. Even after an end of life plan has been developed, it is not uncommon for a pet owner suddenly to want to investigate curative options even after a disease has become unresponsive to curative attempts. If this happens, the veterinarian should review the disease process, indications, and contraindications of such options with the pet owner to promote the making of informed decisions.

While designing the end of life plan, veterinarians may come across dilemmas regarding treatment choices because of side effects of some medications. Veterinarians should take into account the principle of double effect in which interventions may have a positive and a negative consequence. The concept is used in human medicine to help ethically justify the treatment choices. For example, a medication used to alleviate pain may also risk death because of respiratory depression, but the importance of controlling pain may be overriding.

For pets that are difficult to medicate, oral medicines can be compounded into a more palatable medication. Also, many medicines can be given as a subcutaneous injection that the pet owner can be taught to administer. Not all dermal preparations are efficacious.

Part of the plan should address the nutrition of the pet. Pets that have a good appetite may be fed a prescription diet formulated for the specific disease process, but if a pet is not interested in food, a variety of creative options can be considered. Supplementing or relying on feeding tubes, such as esophagostomy and percutaneous endoscopic gastrostomy tubes, may be considered for certain disease processes. These options should be reviewed with the pet owner before plan development. Force feeding should not be recommended in a palliative or hospice care plan.

Treatment of all processes that interfere with quality of life is important. Appropriate drug therapy must take into consideration side effects and drug interactions. For example, veterinarians should treat a painful otitis even in a dying pet to prevent additional discomfort from the infection or inflammation.

People that are in respiratory distress report that opioids alleviate the feeling of distress better than oxygen therapy does. Placement of a fan directed at a dyspneic patient may also decrease anxiety from not being able to breathe easily.[2] Pets may be prescribed these therapies for breathing comfort if oxygen therapy is not a treatment option. An antianxiety drug may also be prescribed to minimize the anxiety of oxygen deprivation.

When treating wounds, distinction should be made between the actual pain of the wound itself versus the pain associated with tending to the wound. It may be helpful to give pain medication 1 to 2 hours before wound treatment.

Because pets that are in palliative or hospice care programs may have multiple symptoms, special care must be taken to lessen the side effects of polypharmacy therapy. The veterinarian must obtain a complete list of medications that a pet has been prescribed to avoid drug interactions such as serotonin syndrome or reactions between nonsteroidal antiinflammatory drugs and corticosteroids. Serotonin syndrome presents as mental status changes, autonomic hyperactivity, and neuromuscular abnormalities. Serotonin syndrome can be avoided by not combining an opioid with a serotonin reuptake inhibitor. If serotonin syndrome does occur, it can be controlled by removal of the offending drug combination and supportive therapy. Potential problems can also occur in chronic renal failure; be watchful of reactions with gabapentin and tricyclic antidepressants. Metoclopramide should not be prescribed for nausea and vomiting if there is a possibility of a digestive tract obstruction. In humans, opioid-induced urinary retention is treated with an opioid antagonist.

Distinguishing between dysphoria and pain is a necessary challenge. Some drugs may elicit whining and restlessness in pets. Choices to alleviate these symptoms include providing good pain relief, discontinuing the offending drug, providing an opioid blocker, and offering sedation. Even though care is taken when prescribing drugs, the pet owner should be advised to make the following observations (Box 30-4).

BOX 30-4

Medication Side Effect List for Clients

1. A rapid decline in condition especially after starting a new medication
2. Restlessness, excitability, salivation, licking of lips, or trembling after administration of a medication
3. Lack of appetite or vomiting after giving medication
4. Change in bowel movement consistency, frequency, or color
5. Development of skin irritation or itching
6. Development of depression or disorientation after administration of a medication

---

APPLICATION OF PALLIATIVE OR HOSPICE CARE TECHNIQUES

The pet owner should be taught how to carry out the techniques to provide comfort. The pet owner should be shown and then made to demonstrate understanding of the technique. For example, a client should demonstrate administration of subcutaneous fluids on the pet. A technical support team member for the pet owner should be available to contact when problems develop in carrying out the technique (Box 30-5).

BOX 30-5

Hospice Technique Tips

1. Provide technique demonstration
2. Provide written information describing the technique
3. Have the client repeat the technique in front of staff
4. If needed, provide compounded medications for ease of administration
5. Provide a list of medication side effects

EMOTIONAL SUPPORT DURING THE CARE PROCESS AND AFTER DEATH

End of life is defined as the period when death is imminent. Before and during this time, the pet owner needs a means of interpreting quality of life. Veterinarians should have a system to evaluate quality of life that takes into account not only the physical comfort of the pet but also the emotional well-being to aid the pet owner in the decision process. Dr. Alice Villalobos has designed a scale that defines the areas that make up quality of life called "HHHHMM." The scale takes into account how the pet is coping with hurt, hunger, hygiene, happiness, mobility, and more. The scale is an excellent resource for veterinarians to share with pet owners.

A description of the dying process, whether by natural causes or by euthanasia, should be shared with the pet owner based on the specific disease trajectory before the death of the pet.

If time permits, an emotional support system for the owner should be implemented before the end of life of the pet. This emotional support system might call on the services of other professionals including human hospice medical advisors, ethicists, clergy, psychologists, social workers, and volunteers who have advanced training in human palliative and hospice care. A team approach helps ensure that every psychosocial component of care for the pet and the family is covered.

Bereavement counseling should last as long as necessary. The veterinarian plays an important role in the emotional support regarding loss of a pet. The veterinary staff should be able to recommend more services to help pet owners grieve the loss of a pet, especially if the pet owner is depressed or has special needs. Many larger communities have pet loss support groups.

ROLE OF PHYSICAL REHABILITATION TECHNIQUES IN PALLIATIVE AND HOSPICE CARE*

The role of physical rehabilitation techniques in the management of caring for an ill pet can be valuable because it can add great benefit without the side effects associated with drug therapy. As with all treatment choices, it is best to have an understanding of the indications and contraindications for each modality.

Veterinarians should integrate rehabilitation techniques in the palliative and hospice care plans when possible (Table 30-1). Massage

---

*Details about physical rehabilitation can be found in Chapters 27 and 28.

may help decrease pain and improve circulation. Simple techniques such as assisted standing by the use of slings or a towel help to slow muscle atrophy. Weight shifting may help a pet stay mobile with less loss of balance. Use of exercise balls make supporting a pet's weight easier and may promote range of motion or stretching at the same time. Range of motion exercises may decrease pain while improving mobility and strength (Boxes 30-6 and 30-7).

Adjusting the position of the pet may prevent decubitus ulcers and pressure sores, as well as atelectasis and lung congestion. Respiratory secretions may be managed with manual therapy of percussion, vibration, postural drainage, and initiating a cough by palpating the trachea. This should not be attempted if there has been thoracic trauma, a low platelet count, subcutaneous emphysema, or a heart condition.

TABLE 30-1	Rehabilitation Techniques in Palliative and Hospice Care	
Therapies	**Indications**	**Contraindications**
Massage	Decrease pain	Shock
	Improve circulation	Fever
	Increase lymphatic flow	Over areas of acute inflammation and dermatitis
	Release endorphins	
Assisted standing	Maintain strength	Induces pain
	Slow muscle atrophy	
Weight shifting	Maintain mobility	Induces pain
	Improve balance	
	Build strength	
Range of motion/ stretching	Improve mobility	Induces pain
	Improve strength	
	Decrease pain	
Positioning	Prevent pressure sores	Induces pain or difficult breathing
	Prevent atelectasis	
	Prevent lung congestion	
Cryotherapy	Decrease inflammation	Decreased sensation
	Decrease pain	Unable to give feedback
	Decrease swelling	Hypertension
		Peripheral vascular disease

Continued

TABLE 30-1	Rehabilitation Techniques in Palliative and Hospice Care—*Cont'd*	
Therapies	**Indications**	**Contraindications**
Heat	Decrease pain Decrease muscle spasm Improve circulation Increase flexibility/tissue extensibility	Decreased sensation Unable to give feedback Obesity Peripheral vascular disease Over malignant neoplasia, dermatitis, infection, pregnancy
Electrical stimulation	Regain strength Reeducate muscles Decrease pain Reduce edema	Seizure disorders Peripheral vascular disease Over heart, dermal neoplasia, thrombophlebitis, pacemakers, uterus during pregnancy
Aquatic therapy	Decrease pain Build strength Improve balance Improve range of motion	Heart conditions Respiratory disorders Vascular disease Dermal infections Diarrhea
Therapeutic ultrasound	Improve wound healing Improve muscle circulation Decrease muscle spasm Decrease pain Increase extensibility of collagen	Over spinal cord after laminectomy, dermatitis, dermal neoplasia, thromboembolism, pacemakers, heart, growth plates, implants, carotid sinus
Low-level laser	Decrease muscle spasm Decrease pain Increase muscle circulation Improve wound healing	Induces pain Over uterus during pregnancy

---

BOX 30-6

Tips to Improve Comfort

Provide comfort with good pain management.

Tend to all secondary disease symptoms, such as nausea and vomiting.

Provide clean, soft bedding located in a thermally comfortable area with access to social interaction with family.

Provide nonslip flooring.

Provide thermal comfort by providing warmth or keeping the pet cool.

Prevent dry, sore mouth by use of a mouth moisturizer.

Prevent dry, sore eyes by the use of an eye lubricant or artificial tears.

Allow good access to palatable foods and fresh water.

Provide opportunities to urinate and defecate frequently, using assisted standing devices if needed.

Provide attention to satisfy the pet's emotional needs.

Avoid environmental dangers such as fly strike, heatstroke, and freezing.

Never restrict water availability, and keep food and water within reach.

When restraint is necessary, use conservative restraint to minimize breathing problems and pain from arthritis.

Keep pet clean around the genitals, rectum, feet, eyes, and mouth by using baby wipes or mild soap with lukewarm water.

Provide hygiene aids including disposable pads, diapers, and hygiene panties.

Block off stairs to prevent falls, and move furniture so that the pet does not get wedged between pieces.

Provide mobility aids, such as specially designed slings and carts.

BOX 30-7

Most Common Side Effects of the Disease Processes

Pain

Dyspnea

Nausea/vomiting

Constipation

Reflux

Anorexia

Pruritus

Bone marrow failure

Urine retention

Fatigue

Neurologic symptoms

From Engelberg R, Downey L, Curtis R: *J Palliat Care* 5:1086-1098.

CONCLUSION

Any veterinarian should be able to use the philosophy of palliative and hospice care. Veterinarians should keep in mind that this type of care should always be relationship centered. Ultimately, the goal of palliative and hospice care in veterinary medicine is to relieve suffering while enhancing the quality of life for the pet and family.

SUGGESTED READINGS

Millis DL, Levin D, Taylor R: *Canine rehabilitation and physical therapy*, Philadelphia, 2004, Elsevier.

Shearer TS: *The essential book for dogs over five*, Columbus, Ohio, 2002, Ohio Distinctive Publishing.

Villalobos A: *Canine and feline geriatric oncology: honoring the human-animal bond*, Ames, Iowa, 2006, Blackwell Publishing.

Drugs Used for the Treatment of Pain, Pain-Related Anxiety, and Anesthesia-Related Side Effects as Described in This Handbook

Drug	Trade Name	Dog Dose (mg/kg)	Cat Dose (mg/kg)	Equine Dose (mg/kg)	Cattle Dose (mg/kg)	Other Species Doses (mg/kg)
Acepromazine		0.025-0.1 max. 3 mg IV, SC, IM 0.5-2 PO	0.05-0.1 max. 1 mg IV 0.1-2.25 PO	0.02-0.05 IV	0.05-0.2 PO, 0.03-0.1 IM, 0.01-0.02 IV	Swine: 0.1-0.2 (adult) IM q12h
Acetaminophen	Tylenol	10-15 PO q8-12h Use with caution	Not recommended			Not recommended for birds
Alendronate	Fosamax	10-20 PO	3-5 PO			
Amantadine	Symmetrel	3-5 PO q24h	3-5 PO q24h			
Amitriptyline	Elavil	1-2 PO q12-24h	5-10 PO q24h			
Aspirin		10-25 PO q8-12h	10-25 PO q48h	25-50 PO q12h	100 PO q12h (ruminants)	Av: 1.0-5.0 PO q12h Swine: 10 PO q6-8h
Atenolol	Tenormin	0.25-1.0 PO q12-24h	2-3 PO q24h			
Atipamezole	Antisedan	50-100 µg/kg IM	50-100 µg/kg IM	50-100 µg/kg IV	0.1-0.2 IV, IM	Av: 0.02-0.04 SC, IM
Atropine		0.02-0.04 IV, SC, IM prn	0.02-0.04 IV, SC, IM prn			Toxic dose unknown recommend <2
Bupivacaine	Marcaine	1-2 SC, interpleural 1-1.5 epidural	1-2 SC, interpleural 1-1.5 epidural			F: <1.5 SC epidurally Ra: <1.5 SC Av: <1.0 SC Ck: Toxic at 2.7 intraarticularly

Buprenorphine	Buprenex, Carpuject	0.005–0.02 SC, IM, IV q4–8h	0.005–0.02 SC, IM, IV q4–8h 0.01–0.02 buccal q6–12h	0.01–0.04 IV		Re: 0.4–1.0 IM, SC, IV F: 0.01–0.03 q6–10h IV, SC Ra: 0.01–0.05 q6–10h IV, SC
Butorphanol	Torbugesic	0.2–1.2 SC, IM q2–6h 0.1–0.8 IV q0.5–2h 0.5–2 PO q6–8h	0.1–0.4 SC, IM q2–6h 0.1 IV q1–2h 0.5–2 PO q6–8h	0.02–0.1 IV q3–4h 0.04–0.2 IM	0.05–0.2 IV, IM (ruminants)	Re: 1 IM F: 0.1–0.4 q2–4h IV, IM, SC 0.1–0.2 mg/kg per hour IV CRI Ra: 0.5 q2–4h IV, SC 0.1–0.3 mg/kg per hour IV CRI *Parrot: 1–3 IM Camelids: 0.05–0.2 IV, IM
Carprofen	Rimadyl, Zenecarp	4.4 SC single dose 2.2 PO q12h 4.4 PO q24h	1–4 SC single dose Not recommended for oral use	0.5–1.1 IV		Re: 2–4 followed by 1–2 q24–72h IM, IV, SC Av: 1.0–2.0 q12–24h; oral doses may need to be higher
Chlorpromazine	Thorazine	0.05–0.50 SC, IM, IV q6–24h 0.8–4.4 PO q24h	0.5 IM, IV q6–8h 2–4 PO q24h		0.22 V once, 1.1 IM once Sheep, goats: 0.55 IV once, 2.2 IM once	Swine: 0.5 IM once

Continued

Drug	Trade Name	Dog Dose (mg/kg)	Cat Dose (mg/kg)	Equine Dose (mg/kg)	Cattle Dose (mg/kg)	Other Species Doses (mg/kg)
Clomipramine	Clomicalm	1-3 PO q12-24h	1-5 PO q12-24h			
Clonidine	Catapres	0.01 IV 0.1/15-20 kg transdermal patch	0.01 IV			
Codeine		0.5-1 PO q4-6h	0.5 PO q6h			
Deracoxib	Deramaxx	1-2 PO q24h 3-4 PO q24h 7-day limit				
Detomidine	Dormosedan			0.01-0.04 IV, IM	0.002-0.1 IV 0.005-0.04 IM	
Dexamethasone		0.10-0.15 SC, PO, IV	0.10-0.15 SC, PO, IV	0.01-0.15 IV, IM	0.01-0.15 IV, IM	
Dexmedetomi-dine	Dexdomitor Precedex	0.0005 mg/kg per hour IV (preanesthetic) 0.005-0.01 IV bolus (short-term sedation/analgesia) 0.0005-0.001 mg/kg per hour IV (extended sedation/analgesia—CRI)				
Dextrometho-rphan	Benylin	0.5-2 PO, SC, IV q6-8h	0.5-2.0 PO q6-8h			
Diazepam	Valium	0.1-0.5 IV, IM 0.5-2.2 PO	0.05-0.4 IV, IM 0.5-2.2 PO	0.05-0.1	0.02-0.08 IV	Av: 0.5-1.0 mg/kg IM, IV
Diltiazem	Cardizem, Dilacor	0.5-1.5 PO 0.125-0.035 IV	1.75-2.5 PO 0.125-0.0.35 IV	0.125 IV		
Dipyrone	Metamizole	25-100 IM, IV, SC, PO q8h	25 IM, IV, PO q12-24h	5-22 IV		
Doxapram	Dopram	1-5 IV	1-5 IV	0.5-1.0 IV	0.5-1.0 IV	

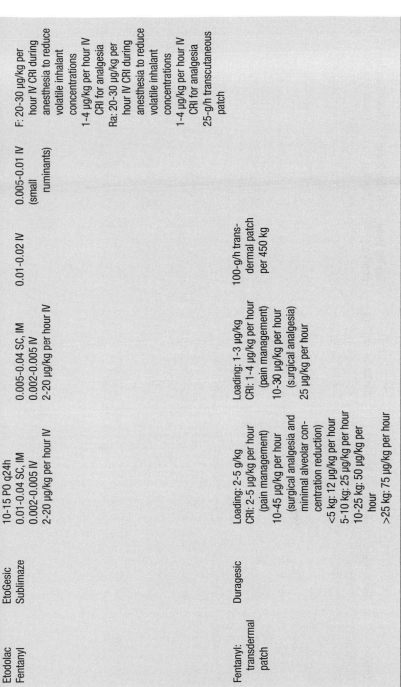

Drug	Trade name	Dog	Cat	Other
Etodolac	EtoGesic	10-15 PO q24h		
Fentanyl	Sublimaze	0.01-0.04 SC, IM 0.002-0.005 IV 2-20 μg/kg per hour IV	0.005-0.04 SC, IM 0.002-0.005 IV 2-20 μg/kg per hour IV	0.01-0.02 IV	0.005-0.01 IV (small ruminants)	F: 20-30 μg/kg per hour IV CRI during anesthesia to reduce volatile inhalant concentrations 1-4 μg/kg per hour IV CRI for analgesia Ra: 20-30 μg/kg per hour IV CRI during anesthesia to reduce volatile inhalant concentrations 1-4 μg/kg per hour IV CRI for analgesia 25-g/h transcutaneous patch
Fentanyl: transdermal patch	Duragesic	Loading: 2-5 g/kg CRI: 2-5 μg/kg per hour (pain management) 10-45 μg/kg per hour (surgical analgesia and minimal alveolar concentration reduction) <5 kg: 12 μg/kg per hour 5-10 kg: 25 μg/kg per hour 10-25 kg: 50 μg/kg per hour >25 kg: 75 μg/kg per hour	Loading: 1-3 μg/kg CRI: 1-4 μg/kg per hour (pain management) 10-30 μg/kg per hour (surgical analgesia) 25 μg/kg per hour	100-g/h transdermal patch per 450 kg	

Continued

Drug	Trade Name	Dog Dose (mg/kg)	Cat Dose (mg/kg)	Equine Dose (mg/kg)	Cattle Dose (mg/kg)	Other Species Doses (mg/kg)
Firocoxib	Previcox	5 PO q24h				
Flumazenil	Romazicon	0.2 mg/dog IV prn	0.2 mg/cat IV prn	0.02 IV	0.02 IV Sheep: 0.02 IV	Swine: 0.02 IV
Flunixin meglumine	Banamine	1.0 PO single dose 0.5-2.2 IV 1 IV, IM, SC once	1.0 PO single dose 0.5-2.2 IV 1 IV, IM, SC once	0.2-1.1 IV, IM q24h	1.1-2.2 IV q24h	0.1-0.5 q24-48h IM
Gabapentin	Neurontin	5-40 mg/kg PO q12h	5-20 mg/kg PO q12h			
Glycopyrrolate	Robinul-V	5-10 µg/kg IV, IM, SC	5-10 µg/kg IV, IM, SC	3.3-6.6 µg/kg IV	5-10 µg/kg IM, SC 2.5-5 µg/kg IV	Swine: 3.3 µg/kg
Hydrocortisone	Cortef	2.5-5 PO q12h	2.5-5 PO q12h	1-4 IV		
Hydromorphone	Dilaudid Hydrostat	0.05-0.2 SC, IM 0.05-0.1 IV q2-6h 0.05-0.1 mg/kg per hour	0.05-0.1 SC, IM q2-6h 0.03-0.05 IV q1h 0.01-0.05 mg/kg per hour			F: 0.1-0.2 IV, IM, SC q6-8h 0.005-0.015 mg/kg per hour IV CRI Ra: 0.05-0.2 IV, IM, SC q6-8h
Imipramine	Tofranil	0.5-1.0 PO q8h	2.5-5.0 PO q12h			

Ketamine (as N-methyl-D-aspartate receptor antagonist, not anesthetic)	Numerous: Ketalar, Vetalar, Ketaset, KetaFlo	0.5 IV, followed by 10 µg/kg per minute during surgery, followed by 2 µg/kg per minute for next 24 hours	0.5 IV, followed by 10 µg/kg per minute during surgery, followed by 2 µg/kg per minute for next 24 hours	Re: 10-100 IM, IV, SC F: 0.5 IV before surgery 10 g/kg per minute IV CRI for 24 hours postoperatively Ra: 0.5 IV before surgery 10 g/kg per minute IV CRI for 24 hours postoperatively
Ketoprofen	Ketofen, Anafen	1-2 IV, IM, SC initial dose 1 PO q24h up to 5 days	0.5-2 IV, IM, SC initial dose 0.5-1 PO q24h up to 5 days	1.1-3.3 IV, IM q24h 2.0 V, IM q24h Re: 2 q24-48h IM, SC Av: 1-5 IM, IV q24h
Ketorolac	Toradol	0.3-0.6 PO, IV, IM q8-12h	0.25 IM q12h	
Lidocaine		2-4 IV bolus then 25-75 µg/kg IV infusion 4.4 of 2% epidural	0.25-1.0 IV bolus, then 10-40 µg/kg IV infusion 4.4 of 2% epidural	0.16-0.45 sub-arachnoid/epidural Re: toxic dose unknown; recommend <5 F: <2 SC 4.4 epidurally Ra: <2 SC Av: 1-3; toxic at 4
Magnesium salts		5-15 IV 0.75-1 mEq Mg^{2+}/kg IV	5-15 IV 0.75-1 mEq Mg^{2+}/kg IV	

Continued

Drug	Trade Name	Dog Dose (mg/kg)	Cat Dose (mg/kg)	Equine Dose (mg/kg)	Cattle Dose (mg/kg)	Other Species Doses (mg/kg)
Medetomidine	Domitor	0.01-0.02 IM 0.005-0.01 IV (sedation/analgesia) 0.005-0.01 IM 0.003-0.005 IV (preanesthetic) 0.001-0.003 mg/kg per hour IV (supplemental CRI during inhalant anesthesia) 0.001-0.003 IV bolus (short-term sedation/analgesia) 0.001-0.002 mg/kg per hour IV (extended sedation/analgesia CRI)	0.015-0.03 IM 0.01-0.015 IV (sedation/analgesia) IM 0.005-0.01 IV (preanesthetic) 0.003-0.005 IV bolus (short-term sedation/analgesia)	0.01-0.02 IV		Camelids: 10-20 μg/kg Re: 50-100 μg/kg (tortoises) 150-300 μg/kg (aquatic) 150 μg/kg (snakes and lizards)
Meloxicam	Metacam	0.2 IV, SC 0.2 initial loading dose, then 0.1 PO q24h	0.3 SC 0.1 mg/kg loading dose, then 0.05 mg/kg PO q24h			Re: 0.1-0.2 IM, IV, PO q24-48h F: 0.1-0.2 SC, PO q24h Ra: 0.1-0.5 SC, PO q12-24h *Parakeets: 0.5-1.0 PO q12h
Meperidine	Demerol	3-10 IV, IM q2-3h or prn 2.5-6.5 IM (preanesthetic)	1-5 IV, IM prn 2.2-4.4 IM (preanesthetic)	0.2-1.0 IV		Re: 1-4 IC

Mepivacaine	Carbocaine-V	0.5 ml of 2% solution, q30sec, epidurally, until reflexes are absent	0.5 ml of 2% solution, q30sec, epidurally, until reflexes are absent	0.05-0.25 sub-arachnoid/ epidural	
Methadone	Dolophine	0.1-0.5 IV 0.5-1.0 IV, IM, SC q2-4h	0.1-0.5 IV, IM, SC q2-4h	0.05-0.1 IV	Swine: 0.1-0.2 IV
Methylpred-nisolone	Medrol, Depo-Me-drol, Solu-Medrol	0.5-1 PO q12h 0.22-0.44 PO q12-24h 30 IV followed by 5.4 mg/kg per hour for 24 to 48 hours	0.5-1 PO q12h 0.22-0.44 PO q12-24h 30 IV followed by 5.4 mg/kg per hour for 24 to 48 hours 20-40 mg IA	200 mg single total dose IM 40-240 mg total dose IA 0.1-0.5 IV	
Mexiletine	Mexitil	4-10 PO			
Midazolam	Versed	0.1-0.25 IV, IM	0.05-0.5 IV, IM		Av: 0.5-1.0 IV, IM Swine: up to 0.5 IM
Misoprostol	Cytotec	0.002-0.005 PO q8h	0.002-0.005 PO q8h		
Morphine		0.25-1.0 SQ, IM q4-6h 0.05-0.1 IV q1-2h 0.05-0.1 mg/kg per hour 0.1 epidurally q12-24h	0.05-0.1 IM, SC q4-6h	01-0.5 IV	Re: 0.05-4.0 (crocodiles) 1.5-6.5 (turtles) F: 0.2-2 IM single dose preoperatively epidurally Ra: 0.5-5 IM single dose preoperatively 0.1 epidurally

Continued

Drug	Trade Name	Dog Dose (mg/kg)	Cat Dose (mg/kg)	Equine Dose (mg/kg)	Cattle Dose (mg/kg)	Other Species Doses (mg/kg)
Morphine sulfate: sustained release	MS Contin	2-5 q12h	Not recommended			
Morphine sulfate tablets and oral liquid		1.0 PO q4-6h	Not recommended			
Nalbuphine	Nubain	0.5-1 SC, IM q1-4h 0.03-0.5 IV	0.2-0.4 IV, SC, IM q1-44h	0.02-0.08 IV		
Nalmefene	Revex	1-4 SC		0.001-0.005 IV	0.001-0.005 IV	
Naloxone	Narcan	0.002-0.04 IV, SC, IM as needed to reverse opiate	0.002-0.04 IV, SC, IM as needed to reverse opiate	0.01-0.02 IV	0.01-0.02 IV	
Naltrexone	Trexan	0.05-0.1 SC 2.2 PO q12h (behavioral problems)	0.05-0.1 SC	0.05-0.1 SC 0.04 IV, SC		
Oxymorphone	Numorphan	0.025-0.2 IV, IM, SC	0.02-0.2 IV, IM, SC	0.001-002 IV		F: 0.05-0.2 IV, IM, SC q6-8h Ra: 0.05-0.2 IV, IM, SC q6-8h
Pamidronate	Aredia	1-2 mg/kg diluted over 2-4 hours IV, SC	1-1.5 mg/kg diluted over 2-4 hours			
Pentazocine	Talwin-W	1.65-3.3 IM, IV, SC q4h	2.2-3.3 IM, IV, SC q4h	200-400 mg/ horse IV		

Generic	Brand					Swine: 4 IV q24h
Phenylbutazone	Butazolidin	10-22 PO, IV q8-12h (max. 800 mg/dog)	6-8 IV, PO q12h One time	2-4 IV q24h 4.4-8.8 PO q24h	17-25 loading dose, then 2.5-5 q24h or 10-14 q48h PO, IV	Swine: 4 IV q24h
Phenytoin	Dilantin	2-4 (max. 10) IV in increments 20-35 PO	2-3 PO			
Prednisone	Deltasone Meticorten	0.5-1 PO, IV, IM q12-24h initially, then taper to q48h	1-2 PO, IV, IM q12-24h initially, then taper to q48h	0.5-1 PO q12-24h		
Prednisolone	Cortisat-20 Delta-Cortef	0.5-1 PO, IV, IM q12-24h initially, then taper to q48h	1-2 PO, IV, IM q12-24h initially, then taper to q48h	100-200 mg/horse total IM		
Pregabalin	Lyrica	0.3-4 PO q8-12h				
Propranolol	Inderal	0.02-0.06 IV over 5-10 minutes 0.2-1 PO q8h (titrate dose to effect) 0.125-1.10 PO	0.4-1.2 (2.5-5 mg/cat) PO q8h 0.4-1.2 PO	Up to 0.1 IV slowly Repeat in 6-8 hours if necessary		
Omeprazole	Prilosec	20 mg/dog PO q24h	0.7 PO q24h			
Oxycodone	Percocet (with acetaminophen) OxyContin (sustained release)	0.1-0.3 PO q8-12h	Not recommended			

Continued

Drug	Trade Name	Dog Dose (mg/kg)	Cat Dose (mg/kg)	Equine Dose (mg/kg)	Cattle Dose (mg/kg)	Other Species Doses (mg/kg)
Oxymorphone	Numorphan Opana (sustained release)	0.05-0.2 IM, SC q2-4h 0.03-0.05 IV	0.05-0.2 IM, SC q3-4h 0.02 IM	0.01-0.02 IV		
Piroxicam	Feldene	0.3 PO q24h for 3 days, then every other day	0.01-0.03 IV 0.3 PO q48h 1 mg/cat PO q24h max. 7 days			Av: 0.1-0.5 PO q12h
Prazosin	Minipress	1 mg/15 kg (0.5-2 mg/dog) PO q8-12h	1 mg/15 kg (0.5-2 mg/cat) PO q8-12h			
Remifentanil	Ultiva	Loading: 4-10 μg/kg CRI: 4-10 μg/kg per hour (pain management) 20-60 μg/kg per hour (surgical analgesia)	Loading: 4-10 μg/kg CRI: 4-10 μg/kg per hour (pain management) 20-60 μg/kg per hour (surgical analgesia)			
Romifidine	Sedivet	0.02-0.04 IM, IV 0.01-0.02 IV (sedation/analgesia) IM 0.005-0.01 IV (preanesthetic)	0.09-0.18 IM, IV 0.03-0.06 IM 0.015-0.03 IV (sedation/analgesia) 0.02-0.03 IM 0.01-0.02 IV (preanesthetic)	0.008-0.12 IV, IM		
Ropivacaine	Naropin	1 ml of 0.2% or 0.5% per site intracostal nerve block 1-2 ml of 0.2%/kg intra-pleural regional block 0.5 epidural	1 ml of 0.2% or 0.5% per site intracostal nerve block 1-2 ml of 0.2%/kg intra-pleural regional block Total dose 1 SC for declaw 0.5 epidural			

Sufentanil	Sufenta	Loading: 5 g/kg 0.1 g/kg per minute			
Tolazoline		0.5-5 slow IV	0.5-5 slow IV	0.5-5 slow IV	2.0 IV
Tramadol	Ultram	5-10 IV (experimental dosage)	5-10 IV (experimental dosage)		F: 5 PO q12h Ra: 5-10 PO q12-24h
Triamcinolone	Vetalog Triamtabs Aristocort	0.5-1 PO q12-24h, then taper dose to 0.5-1 q48h 0.11-0.22 PO, IM, SC 1-3 IA	0.5-1 PO q12-24h, then taper dose to 0.5-1 q48h 0.11-0.22 PO, IM, SC	0.5-1 PO q12-24h 0.11-0.22 PO, IM, SC	
Xylazine	Rompun, TranquiVed	1.1 IV 1.1-2.2 IM, SC 0.05-0.1 IV prn 0.2 SC, IM q1-2h	1.1 IM, SC 0.05-0.1 IV prn 0.2-0.4 SC, IM q1-2h	0.5-1.0 IV 1-2 IM	0.03-0.1 IV 0.1-0.2 IM	Swine: 0.5-3 IM Sheep: 0.05-0.1 IV 0.1-0.3 IM Goats: 0.01-0.5 IV 0.05-0.5 IM Re: 1-1.25 IM
Yohimbine	Yobine	0.1-0.3 IV 0.25-0.5 SC, IM	0.1-0.3 IV 0.25-0.5 SC, IM	0.1-0.3 IV 0.3-0.5 IM 0.075 IV	0.125-0.2 IV 0.075 IV

Specific use of each drug and dose is described in greater detail in the appropriate chapter.

IA, Intraarticular; *Re*, reptile; *F*, ferret; *Ra*, rabbit; *Av*, avian; *Ck*, chicken; *CRI*, constant rate infusion; *IC*, intracardiac.

*, pharmacodynamics available. All other avian dosages are anecdotal from clinical use.

INDEX

Page numbers followed by a b, indicate boxes; f, figures; t, tables.

614